Markell and Voge's
Medical
Parasitology

Markell and Voge's
Medical Parasitology

DAVID T. JOHN, MSPH, PhD

Professor of Microbiology/Parasitology
Associate Dean for Basic Sciences and Graduate Studies
Oklahoma State University
Center for Health Sciences
College of Osteopathic Medicine
Tulsa, Oklahoma

WILLIAM A. PETRI, Jr., MD, PhD

Wade Hampton Frost Professor of Epidemiology
Professor of Medicine, Microbiology and Pathology
Chief of the Division of Infectious Diseases and International Health
Department of Internal Medicine
University of Virginia School of Medicine
Charlottesville, Virginia

NINTH EDITION

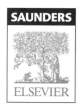
SAUNDERS

ELSEVIER

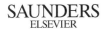

SAUNDERS
ELSEVIER

11830 Westline Industrial Drive
St. Louis, Missouri 63146

MARKELL AND VOGE'S MEDICAL PARASITOLOGY   ISBN-13: 978-0-721-64793-7
Copyright © 2006, Elsevier Inc.   ISBN-10: 0-7216-4793-6

Previous editions copyrighted 1958, 1965, 1971, 1976, 1981, 1986, 1992, 1999

ISBN-13: 978-0-721-64793-7
ISBN-10: 0-7216-4793-6

Executive Editor: Loren Wilson
Managing Editor: Mindy Hutchinson
Developmental Editor: Ellen Wurm
Publishing Services Manager: Melissa Lastarria
Project Manager: Rich Barber
Design Manager: Teresa McBryan

Working together to grow
libraries in developing countries
www.elsevier.com | www.bookaid.org | www.sabre.org
ELSEVIER   BOOK AID International   Sabre Foundation

Printed in the United States

Last digit is the print number: 9 8 7 6 5 4 3 2

Dedication

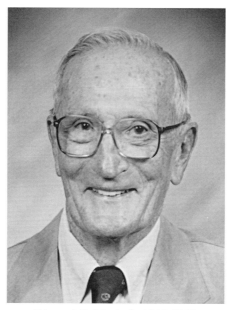

Edward K. Markell, 1918-1998

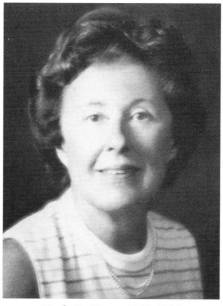

Marietta Voge, 1918-1984

Preface

The first edition of *Markell and Voge's Medical Parasitology* was published 48 years ago in 1958 under the title of *Diagnostic Medical Parasitology*. The name was abbreviated to *Medical Parasitology* with the second edition and remained as such until the eighth edition, at which time the current title was adopted. Marietta Voge passed away in 1984 at the age of 66 and Edward Markell in 1998 at the age of 80. The present edition is the first revision that one or both of them have not been involved with.

By way of historical note, Dr. Markell received his PhD in zoology from the University of California, Berkeley in 1942 and his MD from Stanford University in 1951. Dr. Voge received her PhD also from the University of California, Berkeley in 1950. They were both assistant professors at the University of California, Los Angeles, School of Medicine when they published the first edition of *Medical Parasitology*.

I became co-author with the sixth edition and Al Krotoski with the eighth edition. Dr. Krotoski and I both received our introduction to the field of parasitology through the first edition of *Medical Parasitology*. Dr. Krotoski retired from active professional work in 1995 and has decided not to participate in further editions of the book. My collaboration with Al Krotoski has been most enjoyable and productive and it was with regret that I accepted his decision to withdraw from authorship.

With the ninth edition, I am indeed fortunate to have William Petri become co-author. Dr. Petri earned his MD and PhD degrees from the University of Virginia, Charlottesville, where currently he is Professor and Chief of the Division of Infectious Diseases and International Health. Dr. Petri is a past president of the *American Society of Tropical Medicine and Hygiene* and his research has been with *Entamoeba histolytica* and amebiasis. His research has taken him around the world as an invited lecturer to Australia, Japan, Thailand, Bangladesh, India, Turkey, Israel, France, Germany, Argentina, Mexico, Canada, and throughout the United States.

Ed Markell was born in Brooklyn, New York, but he had a knack for recruiting "non-natives" to work with him on the book. Marietta Voge was born in Yugoslavia, Al Krotoski in Latvia, and I was born in Nigeria. Bill Petri was born in Washington, DC, so we have come full circle. A good sign, I believe.

This book is intended primarily for the medical student and the physician, but it is equally useful to the medical technologist and others who are concerned with the laboratory identification of the parasites of humans. All the chapters have been thoroughly updated and give current information on the life cycles of the human parasites and on the epidemiology, immunology, diagnosis, and treatment of the diseases they cause.

David T. John, MSPH, PhD

Acknowledgments

We are indebted to the people who contributed in various ways to this edition. Our special thanks to Terry Drenner, Joni Finfrock, Sheila Pete, and Marianna Wilson. We are grateful to our wives, Rebecca John and Mary Ann Petri, for their understanding, encouragement, and assistance during the months while the book was undergoing revision. The staff of Saunders, an imprint of Elsevier, as usual, has been most considerate and helpful. Our special appreciation to Ellen Wurm, Developmental Editor, and Mindy Hutchinson, Managing Editor, and the other members of their team, Missy Boyle, Heather Fogt, Alaina Webster, and Rich Barber.

Contents

Introduction

With the nearly simultaneous development of antibiotic drugs, synthetic pesticides, and various new antiparasitic agents, it was for a time widely believed that the infectious diseases would for all practical purposes disappear from the clinical scene. That this has not happened is obvious. Bacterial resistance appeared early; modifications of host resistance have resulted in the appearance of numbers of organisms in unfamiliar pathogenic roles. DDT and other insecticides not only have failed to eliminate the vectors of malaria, filariasis, and other parasitic diseases but have themselves brought on problems too well known to require mention here. The development of resistance to the synthetic antimalarials has been an ominous occurrence. The increased mobility of large segments of the population, and popularity of the tropics and subtropics as vacation areas, exposes them to a largely undiminished threat of parasitic infection, and the speed of transportation ensures that many will return to their native shores before their infections become patent. Refugees from war-torn areas have brought with them infections seldom encountered by physicians in North America and Europe. For these reasons it remains necessary that all physicians have some familiarity with the parasitic diseases, no matter how "exotic."

Modifications of the environment, as typified by construction of the Aswan Dam and the Transamazon Highway in Brazil, have brought about major increases in parasitic disease. Flooding of vast areas with the creation of Lake Nasser has resulted in new habitats for the snail hosts of schistosomiasis and in a tremendous upsurge in incidence of that disease, brought in by infected construction workers. Building the Transamazon Highway necessitated the importation into the area of large numbers of susceptible laborers, causing them to be exposed to the local enzootic diseases, notably leishmaniasis. It behooves us to consider the impact of such projects on the ecology before rather than after the damage is done.

Global warming is suggested as a possible reason for the eventual spread of diseases now seen primarily in the tropics to more temperature climes. In a provocative article, Killick-Kendrick (1996) suggests that visceral leishmaniasis may become endemic in southern England, based on a prediction that by the year 2025 that area will have a climate like that presently seen in the south of France. Carriers of the disease (both human and canine) are certainly present in Britain, but at the present time the sandfly vector has been seen only as close to England as the Channel Islands (it occurs in France), and while its larvae can overwinter in areas as cold as Britain, it requires a warmer summer for propagation.

An important development has been the appearance of the human immunodeficiency virus (HIV) and its sequeal, the acquired immunodeficiency syndrome (AIDS), which results in greatly increased prevalence and severity of a number of parasitic, viral, and bacterial diseases. As immunosuppression becomes more widespread, not simply because of AIDS, but also as necessitated by organ transplantation, the result of cancer chemotherapy, or the indiscriminate release of toxic chemicals and carcinogens into the environment, heretofore unknown or extremely rare infections are being reported from humans. A number of these infections are covered in Chapter 11, Parasitic Infections in Immunocompromised Hosts.

With the ever-increasing pressure of a crowded medical curriculum, the time allocated to the study of protozoan, helminthic, and arthropod parasites has been severely curtailed in many institutions. The same demands of an expanded technology have depleted the ranks of laboratory technologists with good training in parasitology. The primary purpose of this book is to serve as a guide both to the clinical diagnosis and treatment and to the laboratory diagnosis of the protozoan and helminthic diseases of medical importance, and to a lesser extent to the arthropods in relation to disease.

While it is intended primarily for medical students and physicians, it is hoped that this book will prove equally useful to medical technologists and all others concerned with laboratory identification of the animal parasites of humans. The success of the cooperative diagnostic efforts of the physician and laboratory technologist depends on a mutual appreciation of their several problems. In the chapters dealing with technical methods, the problems of technologists are discussed; physicians will be better able to utilize laboratory services if they understand them. The manner in which parasitic organisms are acquired and how they produce disease in humans are perhaps of no direct importance to technologists. Yet a basic understanding of these matters should not only make technologists' work more interesting but enable them to do it better and more efficiently.

Over the years, we have had requests to include more case histories. These are interesting reading and tend to make the subject come alive, but properly presented they take up more space than we can afford, and without adequate presentation they do not do justice to the subject. The "Case Records of the Massachusetts General Hospital," published in the *New England Journal of Medicine*, are excellent and include many that deal with parasitic diseases. References to those cases discussed in recent years are given at the end of this chapter.

A word of explanation is in order concerning the illustrations. They are largely original and have been planned to emphasize points of diagnostic importance. The drawings that accompany the chapter on intestinal protozoa are all made at the same magnification, to facilitate a comparison of size ranges between different organisms and within a single species. Structures not important from the standpoint of identification have been omitted from the majority of drawings, with the purpose of emphasizing the features to which special attention should be paid. Nuclear structure is of great importance in the identification of many species of intestinal protozoa, but the variation that may be encountered is often a source of confusion. Drawings of nuclei alone, illustrative of the range of nuclear variation in the different species, have been included. These are not drawn to scale, but are all shown at the same size.

With reference to therapy for parasitic infections, it must always be borne in mind that most drugs intended to disembarrass the host of parasites do so on the basis of differential toxicity. That is, the antiparasitic agent is, one hopes, more toxic to the parasite than to the host. However, in some cases the margin is slim, and individual variation in host resistance may render it even slimmer. Frequently, toxic side effects are to be expected as the price of therapeutic effectiveness. It is to be hoped that, before treatment, the clinician will always consider whether the parasite is causing, or has a reasonable potential of causing, more trouble than may be anticipated from the treatment to be used. Treatment of certain parasitic diseases is changing almost as rapidly as that of the bacterial infections, and it is essential for the physician to keep abreast of the advances in this field. Review articles on this subject appear every other year in *The Medical Letter on Drugs and Therapeutics* and in many journals on a less regular basis. The *Tropical Diseases Bulletin*, a monthly abstracting journal published in England, lists the worldwide literature in tropical medicine, and occasional comprehensive clinical reviews. Another source is *Drug Information for the Health Care Professional*, vol. I, published yearly, originally by the U. S. Pharmacopeia but, since January 2004, now maintained by Thomson Healthcare, Inc., in which the USP-approved drugs are listed by disease.

In this edition we have included references to papers on diagnosis (both clinical and laboratory) and to treatment throughout the text, but we have in large measure attempted to eliminate other references in which most readers will have marginal or no interest. Where several studies are quoted and one paper refers to all, only that paper is usually referenced.

A list of some of the more important texts and monographs written in English is given at the end of this chapter. English-language journals devoted to parasitology and tropical medicine are also listed.

Texts and Monographs

Abdalla SH, Pasvol G (eds.). *Malaria: A hematological perspective*, 448 pp, London, 2004, Imperial College Press.

Aden Abdi Y, Gustafsson LL, Ericsson O, Hellgren U. *Handbook of drugs for tropical parasitic infections*, eBook, Boca Raton, FL, 2003, CRC Press.

Ash LR, Orihel TC. *Atlas of Human Parasitology*, ed. 4, 410 pp, Chicago, 1997, ASCP Press.

Binford CH, Connor DH (eds.). *Color atlas of tropical and extraordinary diseases*, vols. I and II, Washington, DC, 1976, Armed Forces Institute of Pathology.

Cook GC, Zumla AI (eds.). *Manson's tropical diseases*, ed. 21, 1864 pp, Philadelphia, 2002, WB Saunders.

Dalton JP (ed.). *Fasciolosis*, 544 pp, Wallingford, Oxon, UK, 1999, CABI.

Despommier DD, Gwadz RW, Hotez PJ, Knirsch CA. *Parasitic diseases*, ed. 4, 346 pp, New York, 1999, Apple Trees Productions.

Eddleston M, Pierini S. *Oxford handbook of tropical medicine*, 646 pp, New York, 1999, Oxford University Press.

Eldridge BF, Edman JD (eds.). *Medical entomology: A textbook on public health and veterinary problems caused by arthropods*, 672 pp, Berlin, 2000, Kluwer Academic.

Fayer R (ed.). *Cryptosporidium and cryptosporidiosis*, 272 pp, Boca Raton, FL, 1997, CRC Press.

Garcia LS. *Diagnostic medical parsitology*, ed. 4, 1112 pp, Herndon, VA, 2001, ASM Press.

Guerrant RL, Walker DH, Weller PF. *Essentials of tropical infectious diseases*, New York, 2001, Churchill Livingstone.

Guerrant RL, Walker DH, Weller PF (eds.). *Tropical infectious diseases: Principles, pathogens, and practice*, ed. 2, 1760 pp, Philadelphia, 2005, Elsevier.

Gilles HM (ed.). *Protozoal diseases*, New York, 2000, Oxford University Press.

Gilles HM, Warrell DA (eds.). *Bruce-Chwatt's essential malariology*, New York, 1999, Oxford University Press.

Gillespie SH, Pearson RD (eds.). *Principles and practice of clinical parasitology*, Hoboken, NJ, 2002, John Wiley & Sons.

Goddard J. *Physician's guide to arthropods of medical importance*, ed. 4, Boca Raton, FL, 2002, CRC Press.

Gutierrez Y. *Diagnostic pathology of parasitic infections with clinical correlations*, New York, 1999, Oxford University Press.

Jong EC, McMullen R. *The travel and tropical medicine manual*, ed. 3, 644 pp, Philadelphia, 2002, WB Saunders.

Joynson DHM, Wreghitt TG (eds.). *Toxoplasmosis: A comprehensive clinical guide*, 395 pp, Cambridge, UK, 2001, Cambridge University Press.

Killick-Kendrick R. Leishmaniasis—an English disease of the future? *Bull Trop Med Int Health* 4:5, 1996.

Mahmoud AAF (ed.). *Schistosomiasis*, 524 pp, London, 2001, Imperial College Press.

Marr JJ, Nilsen TW, Komuniecki RW (eds.). *Molecular medical parasitology*, 496 pp, New York, 2002, Academic Press.

Muller R. *Worms and human disease*, ed. 2, 320 pp, Wallingford, Oxon, UK, 2001, CABI.

Nutman TB (ed.). *Lymphatic filariasis*, 292 pp, London, 2000, Imperial College Press.

Olson BE, Olson ME (eds.). *Giardia: The cosmopolitan parasite*, 352 pp, Wallingford, Oxon, UK, 2002, CABI.

Orihel TC, Ash LR. *Parasites in human tissues*, 386 pp, Chicago, 1995, ASCP Press.

Peters W, Pasvol G. *Tropical medicine and parasitology*, ed. 5, 334 pp, Philadelphia, 2002, Elsevier Mosby.

Ravdin JI. *Amebiasis*, 196 pp, London, 2000, Imperial College Press.

Service MW (ed.). *The encyclopedia of arthropod-transmitted infections*, 608 pp, Wallingford, Oxon, UK, 2001, CABI.

Singh G, Prabhakar S (eds.). *Taenia solium cysticercosis: From basic to clinical science*, 480 pp, Wallingford, Oxon, UK, 2002, CABI.

Strickland GT (ed.). *Hunter's tropical medicine and emerging infectious diseases*, ed. 8, 1192 pp, Philadelphia, 2000, WB Saunders.

Thompson RCA, Lymbery AJ (eds.). *Echinococcus and hydatid disease*, 447 pp, Wallingford, Oxon, UK, 1995, CABI.

Warren KS. *Immunology & molecular biology of parasitic infections*, ed. 3, 610 pp, Oxford, UK, 1993, Blackwell Scientific.

Zuckerman JN (ed.). *Principles and practice of travel medicine*, 503 pp, Hoboken, NJ, 2001, John Wiley & Sons.

Some Journals Devoted Wholly or in Part to Medical Parasitology and Tropical Medicine

Acta Tropica
American Journal of Tropical Medicine and Hygiene
Annals of Tropical Medicine and Parasitology
Annals of Tropical Paediatrics
Current Therapy
Experimental Parasitology
Folia Parasitologica
International Journal of Parasitology
Journal of Parasitology
Journal of Parasitology and Parasitic Diseases
Journal of Tropical Medicine and Hygiene
Journal of Tropical Pediatrics
Malaria Journal
Molecular and Biochemical Parasitology
Parasite Immunology
Parasitology
Parasitology International
Parasitology Today
The Medical Letter
Transactions of the Royal Society of Tropical Medicine and Hygiene
Travel Medicine and Infectious Disease
Travel Medicine International
Tropical and Geographical Medicine
Tropical Diseases Bulletin
Tropical Doctor
Tropical Medicine and International Health
Tropical Medicine and Parasitology

Some "Case Records of the Massachusetts General Hospital" Dealing with Parasitic Diseases

References are to the *New England Journal of Medicine*, year indicated by case number.

Acanthamebiasis:
   Baum J, Albert D. Case No. 10–1985. *312*:634–641.

Amebiasis:
   Maynard EP, Nash, G. Case No. 37–1974. *291*: 617–623.
   Maynard EP, Vickery AL. Case No. 32–1977. *297*:322–330.
   Braasch JW, Compton CC. Case No. 7–1990. *322*:454–460.
   Fawaz KA, Compton CC. Case No. 18–1990. *322*:1298–1305.

Babesiosis:
Marcus LC, Mattia AR. Case No. 28–1993. *329*:194–199.
Gutman JD, Kotton CN, Kratz A. Case No. 29–2003. *349*:1168–1175.

Clonorchiasis:
Nishioka NS, Donnelly SS. Case No. 33–1990. *323*:467–475.

Cryptosporidiosis:
Blacklow NR, Wolfson JS. Case No. 39–1985. *313*:805–815.

Cysticercosis, Cerebral:
Schnur JA, Richardson EP. Case No. 40–1977. *297*:773–780.
Parker SW, Richardson EP. Case No. 48–1984. *311*:1425–1432.
Tarlov EC, Richardson EP. Case No. 11–1986. *314*:767–774.
Schmahmann JD, Vonsattel J-P. Case No. 20–1990. *322*:1446–1458.
Maguire JH, Tierney MR. Case No. 8–1993. *328*:566–573.
Bromfield EB, Vonsattel, J-P. Case No. 24–2000. *343*:420–427.

Cysticercosis, Noncerebral:
Kazanjian PH, Mark EJ. Case No. 26–1994. *330*:1887–1893.

Dirofilariasis, Pulmonary:
Kazemi H, Mark EJ. Case No. 13–1979. *300*:723–729.

Echinococcosis:
Maynard EP, Gordon RD. Case No. 25–1979. *300*:1429–1434.
Donaldson GA, Prat J. Case No. 31–1980. *303*:325–331.
Weller PF, Moskowitz G. Case No. 45–1987. *317*:1209–1218.
Baden LR, Ryan ET. Case No. 4–2003. *348*:447–455.

Fascioliasis:
MacLean JD, Graeme-Cook FM, Ryan ET. Case No. 12–2002. *346*:1232–1239.

Filariasis, Brugian (highly atypical case):
Jacoby GA, Goodman ML. Case No. 26–1974. *291*:35–42.

Leishmaniasis:
Lerner EA, von Lichtenberg FC. Case No. 7–1991. *324*:476–485.

Loiasis:
Nutman TB, Kradin RL, Ryan ET. Case No. 1–2002. *346*:115–122.

Malaria:
Diamond JR, Colvin RB. Case No. 35–1989. *321*:597–605.
Wyler DJ, Mattia AR. Case No. 11–1994. *330*:775–781.
Daily JP, Waldron MA. Case No. 22–2003. *349*:282–295.

Microsporidiosis:
Wanke CA, Mattia AR. Case No. 51–1993. *329*:1946–1954.

Schistosomiasis:
Locke S, Richardson EP. Case No. 21–1985. *312*:1376–1384.
Kaplan MM, Compton CC. Case No. 27–1988. *319*:37–44.
O'Leary MP, Mattia AR. Case No. 1–1994. *330*:51–57.
Liu LX, Compton CC. Case No. 4–1996. *334*:382–389.
Recht LD, Louis DN. Case No. 39–1996. *335*:1906–1914.
Blute Jr RD, Oliva E. Case No. 31–2000. *343*:1105–1111.
Ropper AH, Stemmer-Rachamimov A. Case No. 21–2001. *345*:126–131.

Schistosomal Dermatitis:
Maguire JH, Hooper DC. Case No. 27–1985. *313*:36–41.

Strongyloidiasis:
Weller PF, Gang DL. Case No. 13–1986. *314*:903–913.
May RJ, Compton CC. Case No. 47–1987. *317*:1332–1342.

Toxoplasmosis:
Kamitsuka PF, Southern JF. Case No. 36–1992. *327*:790–799.

Trypanosomiasis, African:
Moore AC, Ryan ET, Waldron MA. Case No. 20–2002. *346*:2069–2076.

Trypanosomiasis, American:
Acquatella H, Mattia AR. Case No. 32–1993. *329*:488–496.

Parasites, Parasitism, and Host Relations

In view of the tremendous numbers and diversity of living things and the varied circumstances of their existence, it is not surprising that they obtain their nourishment in many different ways. These various methods have basic similarities, so that frequently it is difficult to draw a firm line between one method of feeding and another. Many terms have been devised to describe the relationships that exist between different kinds of plants and animals at the fundamental food-seeking or food-supplying level. As these terms are not always used by everyone to denote the same thing, the result may be confusion rather than clarity. We need not concern ourselves here with many terms that have been created to designate slight differences in relationship and shall adopt somewhat rigid definitions of those that we do consider; however, it must be emphasized that any one organism may at different times exhibit different nutritional habits or at a given time obtain its nutriment in more than one way. *If a definition is helpful in the understanding of a biological process, it is worthwhile, but it should never be allowed to channel or limit one's ideas.*

In a consideration of the major nutritional relationships between different species, we shall limit ourselves to those involving different kinds of animals, with the understanding that much, but not all, of what is said may be extended to cover animal–plant interrelationships as well. Fundamentally, there are two ways in which an animal may obtain food at the expense of other animals. It may attack another living animal, consuming part or all of its body for nourishment, in the process frequently but not necessarily killing it. This process is known as *predation*; the attacker is the predator, and the victim the prey. Or an animal may derive its nutrition from already dead animals, either devouring those dead of natural causes or taking the leavings of a predator. Animals that subsist in this manner are known as *scavengers*. Some animals are pure predators, others pure scavengers, but many predators are not averse to an occasional bit of scavenging. Some animals always seek their food by their own efforts or in association with others of their own species. This is the most conspicuous and perhaps the most common way in which animals go about obtaining food; it is this large group to which we commonly refer when we speak of scavengers and predators.

Other animals, still in essence predators or scavengers, have become so modified that they are unable to obtain food except in close association, either continuous or at intervals, with members of another species. This association of two species, perhaps primarily for food getting on the part of one or both members of the group, is known as *symbiosis*.★ Literally, symbiosis means "living together," and it may also involve protection or other advantages to one or both partners. Different forms of symbiosis may be distinguished on the basis of whether or not the association is detrimental to one of the two partners. *Commensalism*, from

---

★The definitions given here for symbiosis, commensalism, and mutualism differ from those used by many authors. However, they conform to the recommendations of the Committee on Terminology of the American Society of Parasitologists.

the Latin for "eating at the same table," denotes an association that is beneficial to one partner and at least not disadvantageous to the other. A specialized type of commensalism known as *mutualism* occurs when such associations are beneficial to both organisms. *Parasitism*, on the contrary, is a symbiotic relationship in which one animal, the parasite, lives at the expense of the other animal, the host. Parasitism, like other forms of symbiosis, necessarily involves an intimate relationship between the two species, and it is this close and prolonged contact that differentiates parasitism from the predatory activities of many nonparasites.

Parasitism as a way of life may be the only possibility for a given organism, or it may be but one alternative. An organism that cannot survive in any other manner is called an *obligate parasite*. A *facultative parasite* is an organism that may exist in a free-living state or as a commensal and that, if opportunity presents itself, may become parasitic. It is implicit in this term that the organism does not of necessity have to be a parasite at any stage of its existence. Some animals are obligatory parasites at one or more stages of their life cycles but free living at others. The term "temporary parasite" is sometimes applied to such animals. Parasites living within the host may be described as *endoparasites*, whereas those that are found on the surface of the body are called *ectoparasites*.

Small organisms, such as mosquitoes, which must periodically seek out other and larger forms on which to nourish themselves, have occasionally been called intermittent parasites. This unhappy use of the term "parasite" comes from the assumption that a predator must be larger and stronger than its prey, whereas a parasite is small and weak. This generalization is certainly true of most predators and parasites, or at least of the most obvious ones. However, the essence of the parasitic relationship, which separates it from predation, is the protracted and intimate association between parasite and host. The association between the mosquito and its victim is neither prolonged nor intimate. Those blood-sucking arthropods, which lead an independent existence except for occasional nutritional forays, may be referred to as micropredators.

Many organisms customarily considered to be parasites are actually commensals. *Entamoeba coli* lives in the lumen of the intestine, subsists there on the bacterial flora of the gut, and does its host no appreciable harm. This is a symbiotic relationship in which no advantage or disadvantage accrues to the host, whereas the ameba is supplied with food and protected from harm. Other cases are less definite.

Adaptations to Parasitism

The parasitic relationship probably evolved early in the history of living organisms. We know little about how such relationships arose, but we may hypothesize that we can see in the facultative parasite one possible initial step along the road to obligate parasitism. The possibility of the adaptation of a parasitic mode of existence may depend on what is known as preadaptation, or evolutionary changes that make possible existence in an environment that otherwise would be unsuitable. Such preadaptive changes might be in the nature of increased resistance to the enzymatic activities of the host. Further physiologic adaptations to parasitism might involve the loss of enzymes or enzyme systems, which are then supplied by the host. Such losses may be expected to make a parasitic, or at least a symbiotic relationship, obligatory.

Certain groups of parasites exhibit profound morphologic adaptations to their way of life. As might be expected, these modifications are more striking in those groups that are wholly parasitic than in those that contain both free-living and parasitic species. Organs not necessary to a parasitic existence are frequently lost. The only groups of protozoans that contain nothing but parasitic forms are the phyla Apicomplexa and Microsporidia. Members of these phyla have no locomotor organelles, although the structures are present in one form or another in all other phyla of protozoa, even in their parasitic representatives. Most of the free-living turbellarian flatworms are provided with a ciliated epidermis in the adult stage.

Cilia are not found on the parasitic members of this group or on the related but strictly parasitic trematodes and cestodes. A digestive tract, moderately complex in the turbellarians, is generally reduced in the trematodes and is absent in the cestodes. The reproductive system is highly developed in the two latter groups; this seems a reflection of the difficulties inherent in transfer of these organisms to new hosts. Specialized attachment organs in the form of suckers and hooks have been developed by the parasitic flatworms. Body size may be greatly affected by the parasitic state. Although we think of parasites as small organisms, many of them are much larger than their free-living relatives. The majority of free-living turbellarians are less than a half centimeter in length, and while some land planarians may reach a half meter, none approaches the length of 10 m or more seen in some tapeworms. Most free-living nematodes barely attain naked-eye visibility as adults, but *Ascaris* can reach 35 cm and *Dracunculus* as much as 1 m.

On a more basic level, the parasitic mode of existence may result in profound biochemical changes. One of the most significant adaptations involves the loss of certain metabolic pathways common to free-living organisms, a process aptly referred to as "streamlining." The parasite, no longer able to synthesize certain necessary cellular components, obtains them instead from its host. Profound differences between metabolic pathways in parasite and host characterize the Kinetoplastida (*Leishmania* and *Trypanosoma* species in humans), *Entamoeba histolytica, Giardia lamblia,* and *Trichomonas vaginalis,* as well as most, if not all, of the helminth parasites. These metabolic differences between parasite and host may afford opportunity for strategic chemotherapeutic efforts, as will be seen later.

Specialized mechanisms for effecting entrance into the body or tissues are seen in some parasites. *E. histolytica* elaborates a proteolytic enzyme that aids its penetration of the intestinal mucosa. No such enzyme has been found in the commensal *E. coli.* The cercarial stage in the life cycle of the blood fluke is able to penetrate through the skin of humans to produce infection. It does this with the aid of penetration glands, which produce an enzyme capable of digesting the skin. The embryo of *Hymenolepis nana,* before developing into a cysticercoid larva, penetrates an intestinal villus with the help of the six hooklets it bears.

Once within the host's body, the parasite is subject to those defense mechanisms mobilized in the immune response. Continuation of a parasitic relationship depends on how successfully the immune response of the host is overcome. Many different defense mechanisms have evolved, and many of these will be discussed in consideration of the individual parasites. Immune evasion may involve such factors as location of the parasite in relatively protected sites, changes in the parasite surface antigenic structure brought about in a variety of ways, and active modification of the host immune response by products of parasite metabolism.

Increased reproductive capacity has already been mentioned as characterizing two parasitic groups in contrast with their free-living relatives. Most metazoan parasites exhibit such an increase, which in some cases involves larval stages as well as adults. The chances that a particular egg will successfully infect a new host are usually very small, and if more than one host species is involved, the chance of successful completion of the cycle becomes still smaller. If a parasite is successful in infecting an intermediate host, it is obviously advantageous if the larval stage that develops there can multiply to produce many additional organisms capable of infecting the definitive or a second intermediate host. Such a modification is seen in the trematodes and many of the cestodes, where in the intermediate host a single egg develops into a larva, which in turn produces many larvae of a more advanced kind.

Effects of the Parasite on the Host

A parasite, by definition, is an organism that lives at the expense of its host; however, we have already found that many organisms that are loosely termed parasites are in reality commensals. Some may be truly parasitic at times and at other times commensal in their relationship to the host. In many instances it cannot be said with certainty whether an organism injures the host. Even if we can be fairly sure that some injury is produced, we may not be able to detect it. Thus, a distinction is made between hookworm disease and hookworm infection on the basis of the presence or absence of clinical symptoms. Overt symptoms of infection with this parasite may depend on the number of worms present, the nutritional status of the host, or both.

Injury to the host may be brought about in many ways. Some of these mechanisms are common to all parasites, even if this term is used in its broad sense to include bacteria, viruses, and fungi. The most widespread type of injury is that brought about by interference with the vital processes of the host through the action of secretions, excretions, or other products of the parasite. Such interference is probably largely or exclusively on the level of the host enzyme systems. Parasites producing such effects may be in the tissues or organs of the host, in the bloodstream, or within the gastrointestinal tract, or they may even be ectoparasitic. Invasion and destruction of host tissue may be distinguished from injury that does not involve gross physical damage, although both types of injury reflect biochemical changes brought about in the host tissue by the parasites. When the giant intestinal fluke, *Fasciolopsis buski*, is present in large numbers, toxic symptoms are seen, but the precise cause is unknown. *E. histolytica* erodes the intestinal wall, destroying the tissues locally by means of a proteolytic enzyme. Malarial parasites invade and multiply in red blood cells, which are destroyed in the process and may also attach to the walls of smaller blood vessels in the brain, occluding them to produce localized ischemia. The helminth parasites, by virtue of their size, may damage the host in other ways impossible for the smaller parasites. In addition to its toxic effects, *F. buski* may produce severe local damage to the intestinal wall by means of its powerful suckers. *Ascaris* may perforate the bowel wall, cause intestinal obstruction if present in large numbers, and invade the appendix, bile duct, or other organs. Some parasites exert their effects by depriving the host of essential substances. Thus, hookworms suck blood and by so doing may deprive the host of more iron than is replaced by diet and so bring about an anemia. The broad fish tapeworm *Diphyllobothrium latum* selectively removes vitamin B_{12} from the alimentary tract, producing a megaloblastic anemia in some infected persons.

Effects of the Host on the Parasite

The effects of the parasite on the host are more obvious than those that operate in the opposite direction, but the latter are nonetheless important. The genetic constitution of the host may profoundly influence the host-parasite relationship. There are racial variations in resistance to *Plasmodium vivax*, which are related to the presence or absence of the Duffy blood group. There is also considerable evidence that possession of the sickle cell trait, an inherited characteristic, is also associated with increased resistance to infection with the malarial parasite *Plasmodium falciparum*.

The diet or nutritional status of the host may be of major importance in determining the outcome of a parasitic infection. A high-protein diet has been found to be unfavorable for the development of many intestinal protozoa, while a diet low in protein has been shown to favor the appearance of symptoms of amebiasis and the complications of this disease. It has been shown that a carbohydrate-rich diet favors the development of certain tapeworms, and the presence of carbohydrate in the diet is known to be essential for some of these worms. The general nutritional status of the host may be of considerable importance both in determining whether a particular infection will be accompanied by symptoms and in influencing their severity if present. Major nutritional disturbances may influence resistance through their effects on the immune mechanisms of the host.

While the fundamental immune processes are generally considered to be the same as in bacterial, viral, and mycotic infections, the details are much better known for bacteria and viruses than for protozoa and helminths. Every species of animal is naturally resistant to infection by many organisms that parasitize different species. As we have seen in the case of certain strains of malaria, resistance may also be a racial phenomenon. In some cases it has been possible to adapt parasites to hosts that they normally infect poorly or not at all. This does not necessarily involve changes in the host's natural resistance but rather changes in the parasite. Acquired immunity can be demonstrated in many parasitic diseases, and it is generally found to be at a lower level than that produced by bacteria and viruses. Absolute immunity to reinfection, as is generally seen following infection with smallpox, measles, whooping cough, and a number of other viral and bacterial diseases, occurs rarely following protozoal infections and probably never with helminth infections of humans. As yet, no useful vaccines have been developed against protozoal or helminthic infections. Although malaria is a likely candidate for a vaccine, recent field trials of potential malaria vaccines have failed to meet expectations. Primary infection with *Leishmania* seems to confer a degree of immunity to reinfection. While many protozoal and helminthic infections confer no long-lasting immunity to reinfection, they do seem to stimulate resistance while the parasites are still in the body. This resistance to hyperinfection, known as *premunition*, may be of great importance in endemic areas in limiting the extent of infection with plasmodia, hookworms, and other parasites.

Acquired immunity may be very important in modifying the severity of disease in endemic areas, particularly diseases such as malaria, schistosomiasis, and filariasis. Infants born in such areas to a semi-immune parent are at birth, and for some time thereafter, partially protected by maternal antibodies acquired transplacentally. If infection with one such parasite takes place during the first few months of life, it is likely not to be as severe as it would otherwise have been, and repeated infections over the years keep the acquired immunity at a high level and symptoms correspondingly mild. If, on the other hand, such a person leaves the endemic area for a protracted period, the acquired immunity wanes, and on returning to the endemic area that person may fare no better than someone becoming infected after entering the endemic area for the first time.

Exciting new areas of research have dealt with the role of eosinophils in killing young schistosomes and microfilariae, the ability of older schistosomes to induce immunosuppression in the host, the discovery of hostlike antigens on the surface of some parasites, and the phenomenon of antigenic variation in trypanosomes.

The role of cytokines, and particularly of tumor necrosis factor (TNF) or cachectin, has been the subject of much research activity. Cachectin, a major secretory product of activated macrophages, in low doses is protective against experimental malaria in mice, stimulates the killing of schistosomules by eosinophils in vitro, but paradoxically is thought to bring about the state of cachexia seen in trypanosomiasis. Side effects of administration of TNF to cancer patients are almost identical to the various signs and symptoms seen in severe falciparum malaria.

There is also increasing evidence of the importance of the "secretions and excretions" of protozoa and helminths as antigenic substances stimulating host resistance. In *Trypanosoma lewisi* infections in rats, the metabolic products of the parasites are more effective in producing immunity than are the dead trypanosomes themselves. Various immunologic tests have been devised based on the ability of the serum of an infected host to precipitate the secretions or excretions of eggs, larvae, or adults of a number of different helminths. Some of these are discussed in Chapter 16.

Parasites and the Compromised Host

This subject is covered in some detail in Chapter 11. We have already alluded to the compromised host in reference to the relationship between nutritional status and the outcome of a parasitic infection. Surgery, transfusion, intubation, and prolonged hospitalization are other ways in which the natural defenses of a patient may be compromised. The therapeutic armamentarium of the modern physician is also capable of compromising these defenses. Benefits to be derived from the use of corticosteroids and other immunosuppressive agents, and of the antimetabolites, must always be weighed against their effects on the defenses of the patient. Aggressive treatment of leukemia and other malignancies may pave the way for fatal *Toxoplasma* infection, and acute amebic colitis may follow the use of corticosteroids for presumed ulcerative colitis.

Parasitic infection of tissues compromised by malignant involvement is typified by the report of primary gastric amebiasis in a case of reticulum cell sarcoma in which the resistant normal gastric mucosa was largely supplanted by tumor cells. There is also good evidence to suggest that certain helminthic infections, notably strongyloidiasis and trichinosis, may flourish in immunologically compromised hosts.

Another type of immune compromise, the acquired immunodeficiency syndrome (AIDS), renders patients particularly susceptible to toxoplasmosis, cyclosporiasis, cryptosporidiosis, isosporiasis, and the disseminated form of strongyloidiasis, as well as a number of viral, fungal, and bacterial diseases and malignancies such as Kaposi's sarcoma.

Life Cycles of Protozoa and Helminths

Many parasitic organisms have but a single host, being transferred from one individual to another of the same species either through direct physical contact or by means of resistant or semiresistant forms that are able to survive a period outside or away from the host. *Entamoeba gingivalis*, a commensal organism that inhabits the mouth, has no cyst stage or other means of survival outside of the host, and it probably is transferred by direct contact. *Trichomonas hominis* likewise is unable to form cysts, but it probably can survive for short periods outside the body so that direct contact is not necessary. Many protozoa and helminths have cyst stages or eggs that survive for some time away from the host and by means of which new hosts become infected.

Parasitic infections may be carried from one host to another by arthropod *vectors*. A vector may also be a host if development of the parasite takes place within its body. If the arthropod is simply an instrument of passive transfer, we refer to it as *mechanical vector*. If a fly, feeding on fecal matter containing cysts of *E. histolytica*, becomes contaminated with some of these cysts, which it then transfers to food, it is acting as a mechanical vector of the ameba. When an anopheline mosquito sucks blood from a malaria patient, the parasites must develop in the mosquito before she is able to transmit the infection. In this instance the mosquito is both host and *biologic vector*.

Some protozoa and many helminths have complex life cycles, with not one but two, and sometimes more, hosts. When more than one host species is necessary to the development of the parasite, that host in which sexual reproduction occurs is called the *definitive host*. The species in which larval (or asexual if both sexual and asexual forms occur) stages of the parasites develop are called *intermediate hosts*; they are usually designated first and second intermediate hosts if there is more than one. Disconcerting as it may be to those with a strictly anthropocentric point of view, humans are but the intermediate host of the malarial parasite *Plasmodium*, which undergoes sexual reproduction in mosquitoes of the genus *Anopheles*. Many protozoa are asexual; if an arthropod host is required in the life cycle of an asexual parasite, one may refer to its vertebrate and invertebrate hosts.

Important Groups of Animal Parasites

The animal parasites of humans and most vertebrates are contained in five or more major subdivisions or phyla. The single-celled Protozoa, long considered to be one phylum, have recently been divided into a number of groups assigned phylum rank. Those containing organisms that can parasitize man include the Sarcomastigophora, Ciliophora, Apicomplexa, and Microsporidia. Other phyla containing parasitic species include the Platyhelminthes or flatworms; the Nematoda, or roundworms; the Acanthocephala, or thorny-headed worms; and the Arthropoda, which includes the insects, spiders, mites, ticks, and so forth. With the exception of the Apicomplexa, Microsporidia, and Acanthocephala, all these phyla contain both parasitic and free-living forms. Within each phylum only those groups that include species of medical importance are discussed here. Animal phyla may be subdivided into classes and the latter into orders. Each order may again be divided into families containing one or more genera and species. Assignment to these categories is made largely on the basis of morphologic characters; identification of any animal parasite requires some knowledge of its structure.

PHYLUM SARCOMASTIGOPHORA

This phylum is divided into two subphyla: the Mastigophora or flagellates, and the Sarcodina or amebae. The ameboflagellates partake of the characters of both groups.

The Mastigophora move by means of specialized structures known as flagella. A flagellum is a long, threadlike extension of cytoplasm that functions as a means of propelling the organism. Flagella always arise from small intracytoplasmic granules known as blepharoplasts. The number and position of flagella vary a great deal in different species. In addition to the flagella, and often associated with them, one may observe a variety of structures that serve supportive and other functions and give a characteristic appearance to each species. A number of flagellates are blood parasites or inhabit the tissues, whereas others are found in the alimentary canal. Most of the latter forms are commensals, but two species, *Giardia lamblia* and *Dientamoeba fragilis*, are pathogenic.

Sarcodina contains those forms that move by means of cytoplasmic protrusions called pseudopodia. This group includes all free-living amebae, as well as those that are symbiotic in the intestinal tract and elsewhere in the body. Most of the amebae of humans are commensals; one species, *Entamoeba histolytica*, is an important pathogen.

PHYLUM APICOMPLEXA

Members of this phylum, previously referred to as Sporozoa, are tissue parasites. While reproduction in the Mastigophora and Sarcodina is usually asexual, Apicomplexa have a complex life cycle with alternating sexual and asexual generations. Four species of *Plasmodium* are found primarily as blood parasites and cause malaria; species of *Isospora, Cyclospora, Cryptosporidium*, and *Sarcocystis* are parasitic in the mucosa of the intestinal tract, and *Toxoplasma* and *Sarcocystis* are found in various organs and tissues.

PHYLUM MICROSPORIDIA

Formerly classified with the Sporozoa, members of the Microsporidia are minute intracellular parasites of many kinds of vertebrates and invertebrates, and they differ significantly in structure from the Apicomplexa. Microsporidia rarely cause disease in immunocompetent persons, but may do so with greater frequency in immunosuppressed persons. A growing body of evidence suggests that the microsporidia may be fungi-related organisms (Metenier and Vivares, 2004).

PHYLUM CILIOPHORA

The ciliates include a variety of free-living and symbiotic species. Locomotion is accomplished by means of cilia, relatively short threads of cytoplasm arising from small basal granules.

Cilia are structurally similar to flagella but are usually shorter and more numerous. Some ciliates are multinucleate, while others contain but two nuclei, a large macronucleus and a small micronucleus. The only ciliate parasite of humans is *Balantidium coli*, found in the intestinal tract. Although rare, it is important, as it may produce severe intestinal symptoms.

PHYLUM PLATYHELMINTHES

The Platyhelminthes, or flatworms, are multicellular animals characterized by a flat, bilaterally symmetric body. Most flatworms are hermaphroditic, having both male and female reproductive organs in the same individual. The sexes are separate in the schistosomes. Adults may be less than 1 mm long or they may reach a length of many meters. Most members of the phylum are symbionts, living on or in the body of their hosts. Free-living species belong to the class Turbellaria, which also contains forms that are parasitic in lower animals. The classes Trematoda and Cestoda contain parasitic forms only.

The Trematoda, or flukes, are leaf-shaped or elongate, slender organisms that possess attachment organs in the form of hooks or cup-shaped muscular depressions called suckers. A simple digestive tract is present. Of the three orders of the Trematoda, the order Digenea contains all the species that are parasitic in humans. Members of this order have complex life histories, with at least one intermediate molluscan host. Included in the digenetic trematodes of humans are forms that parasitize the intestinal tract, the liver, the blood vessels, and the lungs.

Members of the class Cestoda typically have an elongate, ribbonlike, segmented body that bears a specialized attachment organ, the scolex, anteriorly. A digestive tract is absent. Adult cestodes or tapeworms inhabit the small intestine. With the exception of *Hymenolepis nana*, cestode larvae require an intermediate host for development. Humans may be host to either adult or larval stages, depending on the species of cestode.

PHYLUM NEMATODA

The nematodes, or roundworms, are elongate, cylindrical worms, frequently attenuated at both ends. They possess a stiff cuticle, which may be smooth or may be extended to form a variety of structures, particularly at the anterior and posterior ends. The sexes are separate, the male frequently being considerably smaller than the female. A well-developed digestive tract is present. While most nematodes are free living, a large number of species parasitize humans, animals, and plants. Intermediate hosts are necessary for the larval development of some forms. Parasites of humans include intestinal and tissue-inhabiting species.

PHYLUM ACANTHOCEPHALA

The thorny-headed worms are all endoparasitic organisms, the anterior end of which is modified into a hook-bearing, retractable proboscis that serves in attachment. A digestive tract is absent. Sexes are separate, and males are usually smaller than females. The life cycle requires an intermediate host. While thorny-headed worms are widely distributed among wild and domestic animals, only three genera have been reported in human beings.

PHYLUM ARTHROPODA

Arthropods are segmented and bilaterally symmetrical animals with a body enclosed in a stiff, chitinous covering or exoskeleton and bearing paired, jointed appendages. The digestive system is well developed. Sexes are separate. The phylum is subdivided into a number of classes, many of which are of medical importance.

The class Crustacea contains primarily aquatic forms, which breathe by means of gills. Included here are crabs, shrimps, crayfish, and copepods. Certain of these serve as intermediate hosts of human parasites.

The class Chilopoda contains the centipedes, which are characterized by the possession of one pair of legs on each body segment. The first pair of appendages is modified as poison claws.

The Arachnida, or spiderlike animals, possess a body divided into two parts, the cephalothorax and the abdomen. Adults have four pairs of legs. Included in this class are the scorpions, the spiders, and the ticks and mites. Scorpions and spiders produce venom, which in some species may be extremely toxic. Certain ticks and mites may transmit disease.

From a medical or economic point of view, the class Insecta includes by far the most important of the arthropods. Insects have three pairs of legs and a body divided into three distinct parts: head, thorax, and abdomen. Several orders of insects are worthy of special mention. The Anoplura, or sucking lice, are wingless, dorsoventrally compressed insects, among which are included human lice. The order Hemiptera, or true bugs, includes the wingless bedbugs as well as the more characteristic forms with wings. Two pairs of wings are seen in this group, and the first pair has thickened membranous bases. The cone-nosed bugs, or reduviids, are important as vectors of American trypanosomiasis. The coleoptera, or beetles, also have two pairs of wings, but the anterior pair is thickened throughout. Certain grain beetles are intermediate hosts of tapeworms. The Hymenoptera include ants, bees, wasps, and so forth. Bees, wasps, and fire ants are medically important because of the venom of their stings; other ants may serve as intermediate hosts for one of the human trematode parasites. The Siphonaptera, or fleas, are wingless and laterally compressed; in addition to their irritating bites, some fleas act as intermediate hosts of a species of tapeworm. The Diptera are insects with only one pair of true wings. This order includes several groups of medical importance, notably mosquitoes, flies, and gnats. Some larval flies are parasitic in humans and animals, while mosquitoes and gnats transmit many different diseases.

PHYLUM PENTASTOMIDA

Pentastomids are all endoparasitic forms, known as tongue worms, or linguatulids. The name is derived from their body shape, which is elongate and in some species tonguelike. Other species have a ringed or annulated body. Linguatulids lack external appendages and possess two pairs of hooks near the mouth. Adults live in the respiratory tract of vertebrates. Encysted larval stages may occur in the lungs and other internal organs of humans, and they are found principally in tropical areas.

Prevalence of Parasitic Infections

Estimates of the prevalence of parasitic diseases are at best extremely rough, as reporting of morbidity is essentially nonexistent in many of the areas in which these diseases occur. The following estimates are based on those of the World Health Organization (WHO) through 2002, the Centers for Disease Control and Prevention (CDC) through 2004, and others:

Amebiasis: approximately 1% of world population infected; annual deaths, to 100,000

Giardiasis: approximately 2.5 million annually

Malaria: population currently infected, more than 500 million; annual deaths, 2.5 million

Leishmaniasis: population currently infected, 2 million; annual deaths, 59,000

African trypanosomiasis: new cases per year, 100,000; annual deaths, 50,000

American trypanosomiasis: population currently infected, 16 million to 18 million; annual deaths, 50,000

Schistosomiasis: approximately 200 million infected (includes combined cases): *Schistosoma haematobium*, approximately 100 million infected; *Schistosoma mansoni*, approximately 80 million infected; *Schistosoma japonicum*, approximately 1.5 million infected; annual deaths, 500,000 to 1 million

Clonorchiasis and opisthorchiasis: 13.5 million infected

Paragonimiasis: 20 million infected
Fasciolopsiasis: 10 million infected
Lymphatic filariasis: 128 million infected
Onchocerciasis: 17.7 million infected with approximately 270,000 blind
Dracunculiasis: <75,000 infected in sub-Saharan Africa
Ascariasis: 1.3 billion infected: annual deaths, approximately 60,000
Hookworm: at least 1 billion infected
Trichuriasis: 900 million infected
Strongyloidiasis: 35 million infected
Trichostrongyliasis: 5.5 million infected
Cestodiases: 65 million infected

World Distribution of Parasitic Diseases

Figures 2-1 through 2-12 show in rough outline the world distribution of many of the important parasitic diseases. Those with a restricted distribution are omitted, as are those that occur essentially worldwide.

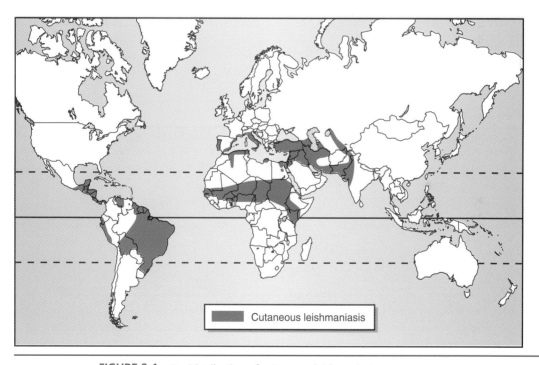

Cutaneous leishmaniasis

FIGURE 2-1 ▨ Distribution of cutaneous leishmaniasis.

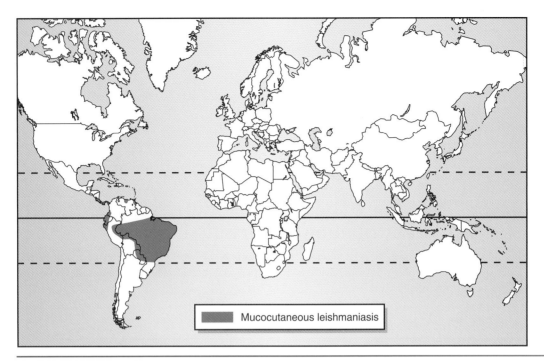

FIGURE 2-2   ▨   Distribution of mucocutaneous leishmaniasis.

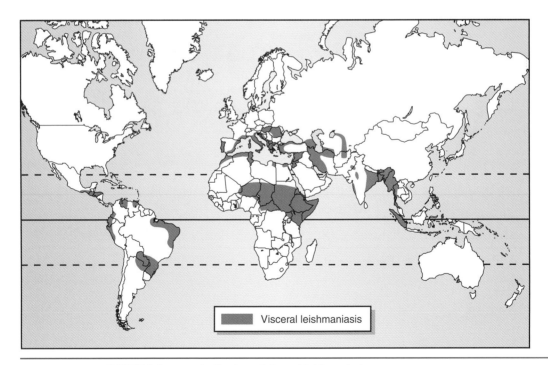

FIGURE 2-3   ▨   Distribution of visceral leishmaniasis.

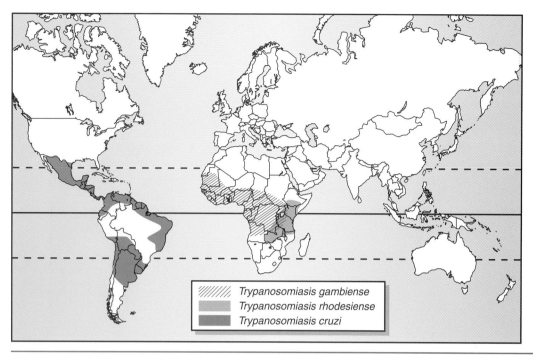

FIGURE 2-4 ■ Distribution of trypanosomiasis.

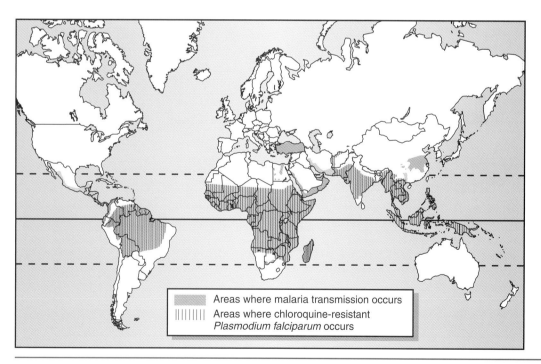

FIGURE 2-5 ■ Distribution of malaria; distribution of chloroquine resistance (2004).

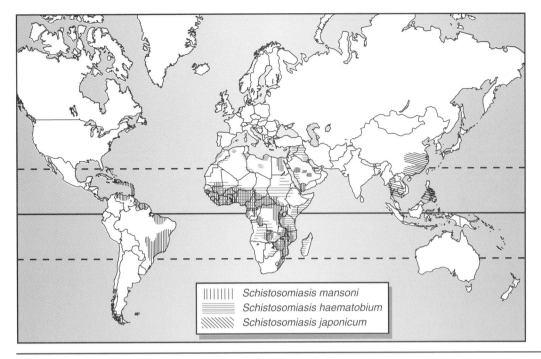

FIGURE 2-6 ▩ Distribution of schistosomiasis.

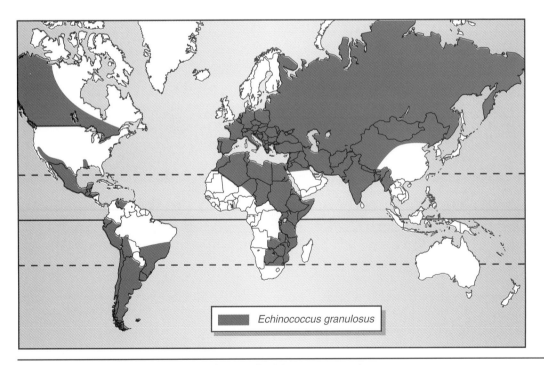

FIGURE 2-7 ▩ Distribution of *Echinococcus granulosus*.

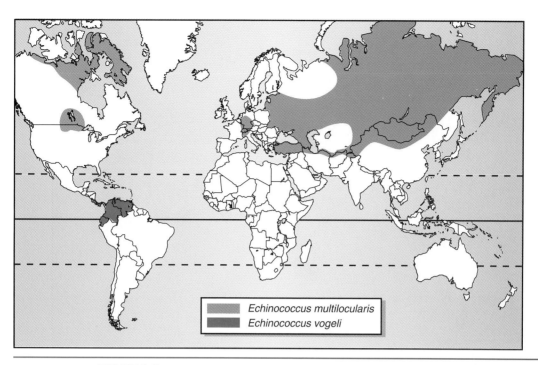

FIGURE 2-8 ▨ Distribution of *Echinococcus multilocularis* and *Echinococcus vogeli*.

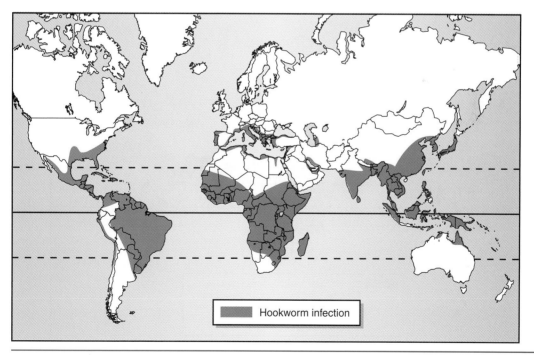

FIGURE 2-9 ▨ Distribution of hookworm infection.

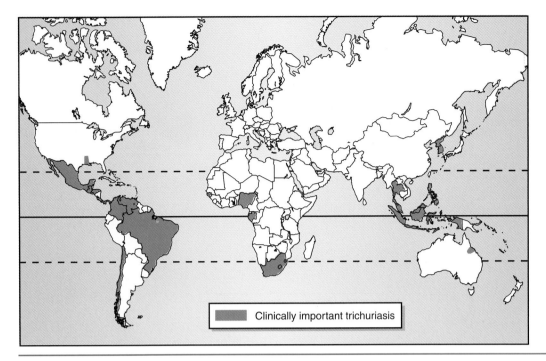

FIGURE 2-10 ▦ Distribution of clinically important whipworm disease.

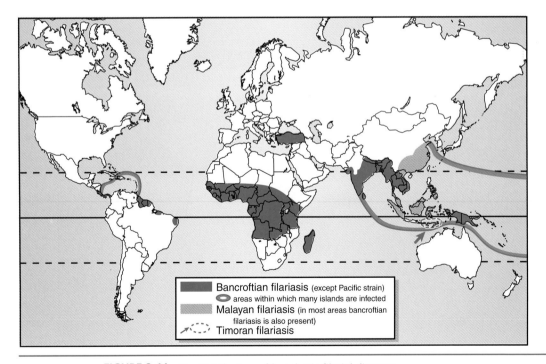

FIGURE 2-11 ▦ Distribution of lymphatic filarial diseases.

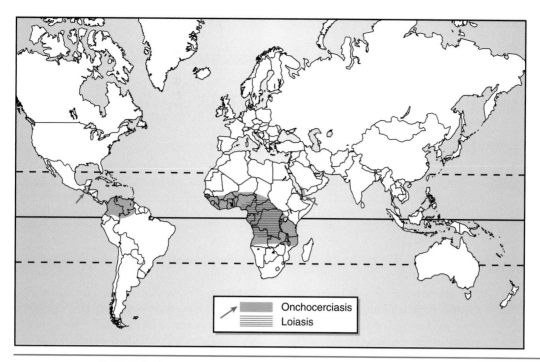

FIGURE 2-12 ■ Distribution of onchocerciasis and loiasis.

Reference

Metenier G, Vivares CP. Genomics of microbial parasites: The microsporidial paradigm, pp 207–236, 2004. In Hirt RP, Homer DS (eds.). *Organelles, genomes and eukaryote phylogeny: An evolutionary synthesis in the age of genomics.* Boca Raton, FL, 2004, CRC Press.

CHAPTER
3

Lumen-Dwelling
Protozoa

We have chosen to consider together not only the intestinal protozoa of humans but also protozoa found in the mouth, the upper respiratory passages, and the urogenital tract. The list includes the parasites *Entamoeba histolytica, Dientamoeba fragilis, Balantidium coli, Giardia lamblia, Trichomonas vaginalis, Isospora belli, Cryptosporidium parvum,* and *Cyclospora cayetanensis.* It also contains a number of commensals and some species of questionable pathogenicity. These organisms are generally of worldwide distribution; prevalence of the intestinal protozoa in the population correlates roughly with the level of sanitation. Color Plates I to IV illustrate some of the intestinal protozoa as they appear when stained with trichrome stain.

The Amebae

Six species of the genus *Entamoeba,* including the commensals *Entamoeba gingivalis, Entamoeba coli, Entamoeba hartmanni, Entamoeba dispar, Entamoeba moshkovskii,* and the pathogen *E. histolytica,* occur in humans. *Entamoeba polecki,* an intestinal ameba of pigs and monkeys, is seen occasionally in humans and may cause diarrhea. Other commensals are *Endolimax nana* and *Iodamoeba bütschlii.*

THE GENUS ENTAMOEBA

Amebae of this genus, widely distributed in both vertebrate and invertebrate animals, are characterized by possession of a vesicular nucleus with a comparatively small karyosome located at or near its center and with varying numbers of peripheral chromatin granules attached to the nuclear membrane. Morphologic differences distinguish all species except *E. histolytica, E. dispar, E. moshkovskii,* and *E. hartmanni. E. histolytica, E. moshkovskii,* and *E. dispar* are morphologically identical, and of the same size range, but can be differentiated by isoenzyme analysis, restriction fragment length polymorphism, and typing with monoclonal antibodies. *E. hartmanni,* formerly known as the "small race" of *E. histolytica,* is separated from the other two primarily on the basis of size.

Entamoeba histolytica

Until recently, the species-complex referred to as *E. histolytica* was considered to infect perhaps 10% of the world's population. With what is now common acceptance of the genetic distinctions between the pathogenic *E. histolytica* and commensal *E. moshkovskii* and *E. dispar,* and the finding that *E. dispar* is much more frequently encountered, the true prevalence of *E. histolytica* is perhaps closer to 1% to 5% worldwide. *E. histolytica* was first described in 1875, in a young Russian peasant in the port of Arkhangelsk, a scant 100 miles from the Arctic circle. Prevalence rates are highest in areas of crowding and poor sanitation, notably in the tropics.

E. histolytica principally inhabits the large intestine, where the trophozoites, or active forms, live in the intestinal lumen and on occasion may invade the mucosal crypts, where they feed on red blood cells and form ulcers. Ulceration of the intestinal wall may give rise to amebic dysentery. The invading amebae at times find their way into capillaries to be transported via the bloodstream to the liver or other organs, where abscess formation may occur. Amebae that remain in or reenter the lumen of the gut may, if intestinal motility is rapid, be passed out in liquid or semiformed stools as trophozoites, but if motility is normal they will "round up" and differentiate into the four nucleated resistant cyst stages. The life cycle of E. histolytica is illustrated in Figure 3-1.

Morphology. Living trophozoites of E. histolytica vary in size from about 12 to 60 μm in diameter (average slightly more than 20 μm). In preparations made from freshly passed stool, trophozoites are usually actively motile. They move by means of pseudopodia, cytoplasmic protrusions that may be formed at any point on the surface of the organism. The pseudopodium is quickly thrust out and may vary in form from short, blunt, and broad, to long and fingerlike. The clear glasslike ectoplasm, which forms the outer layer of the body of the ameba, flows out to form the pseudopodium, which in this species is characteristically hyaline when first formed. The more granular endoplasm flows slowly into the

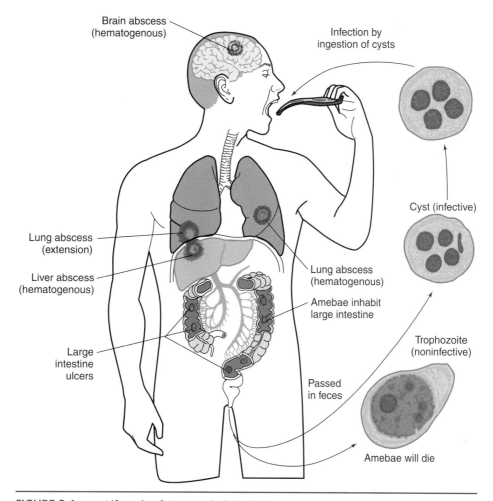

FIGURE 3-1 ■ Life cycle of *Entamoeba histolytica*.

pseudopodium as the ameba moves in the direction in which it was extruded. Motility is usually progressive and directional, rather than apparently aimless as in other amebae. The characteristic motility is seen only in freshly passed specimens. It may be enhanced by warming the slide by means of a thermostatically controlled "warm stage." A reasonably good substitute, and less expensive, is a copper coin, heated in the flame of a Bunsen burner and placed on the glass slide. It must be stressed that neither this expedient nor a warm stage will "revive" amebae that have been kept too long at room temperature.

Using scanning electron microscopy, researchers have described phagocytic stomata or endocytic food cups on trophozoites of *E. histolytica*. Present on the surface of amebae, phagocytic stomata are used in engulfment. Small endocytic stomata are used in pinocytosis, the engulfment of liquids, whereas larger stomata are involved in phagocytosis of bacteria and epithelial cells.

Red blood cells may be ingested but do not often appear in chronic infections. The freshly ingested erythrocytes appear as pale greenish, refractile bodies lying in the cytoplasm of the unstained ameba. Although ingestion of red blood cells has been reported to occur in rare instances in other amebae, for all practical purposes it may be considered to be confined to *E. histolytica*. The nucleus of the unstained trophozoite usually is not visible. Bacteria may at times be ingested by this ameba. They may also be seen in the cytoplasm if the ameba is degenerating. Death or degeneration of the parasites leads quickly to the formation of vacuoles in the cytoplasm—a "Swiss cheese" appearance—and such degenerate forms can never be identified with any accuracy. Similarly, even without such gross degenerative changes, if the amebae are kept too long at room temperature before being fixed, the finer structures of the nucleus undergo change. These structures are of great importance in specific identification of the amebae.

When seen properly fixed and stained with hematoxylin or trichrome stain, details of nuclear structure may be observed. The nuclear membrane appears as a delicate but distinct line, on the inner surface of which is seen the peripheral chromatin, a layer of granules, characteristically uniform and small. In the center of the nucleus is a small mass of chromatin, the karyosome; between the karyosome and the peripheral chromatin the faintly stained fibrils of the linin network sometimes are seen. Typical nuclear structure, as previously described, is depicted in most of the organisms in Figure 3-5. Some of the variations in morphology that may be encountered are shown in Figure 3-6. *It must be emphasized that, strictly speaking, there is no "characteristic" nuclear morphology for any species of Entamoeba.* While most conform to type, some may present a nuclear structure more like that usually associated with a different species.

Ingested red blood cells stain according to the degree to which they have been digested by the ameba. When stained with hematoxylin (Fig. 3-2), the cytoplasm of the ameba is grayish, nuclear structures are an intense bluish black, and freshly ingested erythrocytes stain similarly; the red blood cells become progressively paler as they are digested. In a trichrome stain (Fig. 3-3; Plate I, 1, 2), the cytoplasm is typically green, nuclear structures are dark red, and freshly ingested erythrocytes may be cherry-red or green; the cytoplasm of trichrome-stained amebae is occasionally a light pink, and sometimes green- and pink-staining forms alternate in the same preparation.

In preparation for formation of the resistant cyst stage, trophozoites extrude all ingested material and assume a rounded form. This stage, referred to as the precyst, may be distinguished by its single rounded nucleus, absence of ingested material, and lack of a cyst wall; however, nuclear morphology is often confusing at this stage, and it is best to rely on either trophozoites or cysts for specific identification.

Cysts (see Figs. 3-4, 3-5, 3-17; Plate I, 3, 4) may recognized by the presence of a hyaline cyst wall. They are usually spherical but may be ovoid or irregular in shape, and they vary from about 10 to 20 μm in diameter. In unstained preparations, the cyst wall is highly refractile. Cysts contain from one to four (or, rarely, more) nuclei. At times the nuclei may appear as small, refractile spheres within the cytoplasm of the unstained cyst, but more often

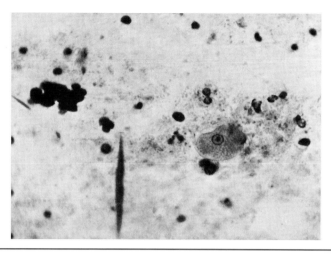

FIGURE 3-2   ■   Trophozoite of *Entamoeba histolytica* stained with iron hematoxylin. Note Charcot-Leyden crystals and clumped red blood cells. (From Hunter GW et al. *Tropical medicine,* ed. 5, Philadelphia, 1976, WB Saunders.)

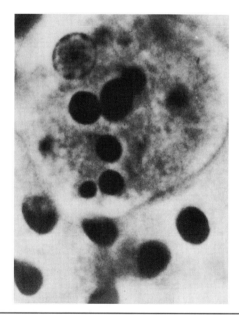

FIGURE 3-3   ■   *Entamoeba histolytica* trophozoite. Note ingested red blood cells (trichrome stain).

they are not visible. Chromatoidal bars, so named because they stain with hematoxylin like the chromatin of the nucleus, are composed of crystalline ribonucleic acid (RNA). If present, these are seen as rod-shaped, clear areas in the cytoplasm. When stained with iodine (see Fig. 3-35), the cytoplasm of the cyst is a light yellowish green to yellow-brown; the nuclear membrane and karyosome are distinct and light brown. Chromatoidal bars do not stain and appear as clear spaces in the cytoplasm. If the glycogen is present in vacuoles in the cytoplasm, it stains dark yellow-brown.

When cysts are stained with hematoxylin or trichrome, nuclear structure is similar to that seen in the trophozoites (see Figs. 3-5, 3-6, 3-17). The peripheral chromatin ring may appear to be thicker and less uniform in size. Some strains of *E. histolytica* consistently have eccentric karyosomes, and in some the peripheral chromatin, instead of appearing as a layer

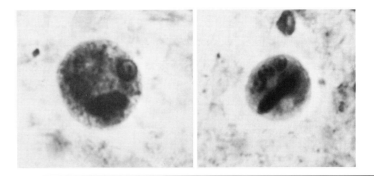

FIGURE 3-4 ■ *Entamoeba histolytica* cysts, showing nuclei and chromatoidal bodies. (Photomicrographs by Zane Price.)

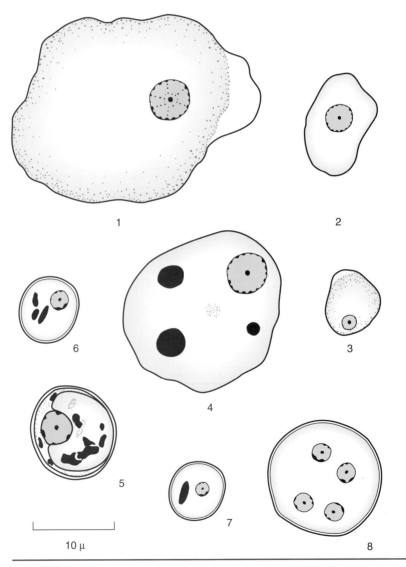

10 μ

FIGURE 3-5 ■ *Entamoeba histolytica*: *1*, trophozoite with hyaline pseudopodium; *4*, trophozoite containing red blood cells; *5*, early cyst containing glycogen mass and chromatoidals; *8*, mature quadrinucleate cyst without chromatoidals. *Entamoeba hartmanni*: *2, 3*, trophozoites; *6, 7*, mononucleate cysts (*2, 4, 6, 7*, and *8* show diagnostic features only).

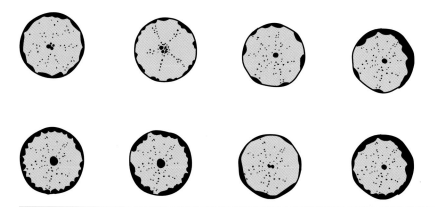

FIGURE 3-6 ■ *Entamoeba histolytica*. Variations in nuclear structure (some original, others adapted from various sources).

of spherical granules, forms thin plaques on the nuclear membrane. A third variant of nuclear structure is peripheral chromatin massed in crescent fashion at one side of the nuclear membrane. One or more chromatoidal bars may be found in the cytoplasm; they may be only slightly shorter than the diameter of the cyst or may be considerably shorter. Occasionally, especially in very young and usually mononucleate cysts, large numbers of very small chromatoidal bars are seen, usually surrounding a glycogen vacuole. The chromatoidals generally appear in the form of elongate bars with rounded or squared ends but may occasionally be ovoid or cigar shaped. Chromatoidal bars of this characteristic morphology are seen in *E. histolytica*, *E. dispar*, and *E. hartmanni* but may occur also in *E. polecki* (see Fig. 3-17). Chromatoidals are more frequently encountered in the mono- and binucleate cysts, and a large proportion of mature quadrinucleate cysts do not possess them. With hematoxylin, the chromatoidals take the same bluish black stain as the chromatin material of the nucleus, and with trichrome they stain bright red.

The following characteristics are valuable in the identification of the *E. histolytica/ E. dispar/E. moshkovskii* species complex:

I. *Trophozoites, unstained*	Suggestive: progressive motility; hyaline pseudopodia; no ingested bacteria; nuclei not visible
	Diagnostic: ingestion of red blood cells
II. *Trophozoites, stained*	Suggestive: clear differentiation of ectoplasm and endoplasm; no ingested bacteria
	Diagnostic: fine, uniform granules of peripheral chromatin and small central karyosome in nucleus; ingested red blood cells; average size over 12 μm
III. *Cysts, unstained*	Suggestive: four nuclei; rodlike chromatoidals
IV. *Cysts, stained*	Suggestive: maximum of four nuclei having both karyosome and peripheral chromatin; diameter over 10 μm
	Diagnostic: typical nuclear structure; chromatoidal bars with rounded or squared ends; diameter over 10 μm

Differentiation of *E. histolytica* from the commensals *E. dispar* and *E. moshkovskii* is not possible by morphology but requires the use of species-specific monoclonal antibodies or PCR techniques (Tanyuksel and Petri, 2003).

Symptoms and Pathogenesis. The following clinical classification is adapted from the World Health Organization (WHO) Report on Amebiasis (1969).

I. Asymptomatic infections

II. Symptomatic infections

A. Intestinal amebiasis
  1. Dysenteric
  2. Nondysenteric colitis
B. Extraintestinal amebiasis
  1. Hepatic
    a. Acute nonsuppurative
    b. Liver abscess
  2. Pulmonary
  3. Other extraintestinal foci (very rare)

The symptoms of amebiasis are far from clear cut and depend in large measure on the extent of tissue invasion and on whether the infection is confined to the intestinal tract or has spread to involve other organs. Intestinal amebiasis is the most common form of infection and may be asymptomatic. Certain patients with intestinal amebiasis have vague and nonspecific abdominal symptoms. Although these symptoms may improve or disappear after antiamebic therapy, they cannot specifically be related to the infection. Another group of patients have more definite symptoms, such as diarrhea or dysentery, abdominal pain and cramping, flatulence, anorexia, weight loss, and chronic fatigue. Frequently, all patients with symptomatic intestinal amebiasis are spoken of as having amebic dysentery. This term should be reserved for those who actually have dysentery, or blood and mucus in the stools. Amebic colitis is a term that can be used to denote any symptomatic intestinal infection.

It seems probable that strain differences in virulence—and, from time to time, differences in susceptibility of the host—both play a part in determining whether or not tissue invasion takes place. A parallel may be drawn between immunologic surveillance, thought to destroy and prevent the spread of malignant cells in normal persons, and an immunologic barrier created by the intestine; a breakdown of this immunologic barrier may occur in persons in whom tissue invasion takes place. Corticosteroid administration may provoke severe (and sometimes fatal) amebic colitis. Additionally, fatal necrotizing amebic enterocolitis in a severely burned patient has been described, in which the rapid worsening of the previously asymptomatic amebic infection was due in part to alteration of the immune response. The susceptibility of humans to *E. histolytica* infection is associated with specific alleles of the HLA complex. A statistically significant increase in mortality from amebic infection has been noted to occur in pregnancy and the puerperium, and a relationship of maternal stress to the severity of infection has been suggested. In addition, specific genotypes of *E. histolytica* are associated with amebic liver abscess formation and others with asymptomatic colonization. When *E. histolytica* succeeds in entering the intestinal mucosa, this penetration is generally not accompanied by inflammatory response. Because the local response is minimal, the constitutional response of the host is likewise. The amebae, secreting proteolytic enzymes, produce necrosis of the surrounding tissues (Fig. 3-7). Most frequently, the cecal area is involved, but the ascending colon and rectosigmoid—and indeed any part of the colon—may also be sites of primary invasion.

While the initial intestinal invasion may be accompanied by little local reaction and often no recognizable symptoms, diffuse inflammation, indistinguishable from the nonspecific inflammatory lesion of other types of colitis, may be seen in sections of biopsy specimens taken from patients with acute amebic colitis. The diarrhea thus provoked may be mild, with only a few loose stools daily, perhaps alternating with periods of constipation. Even in patients with mild diarrhea, or with normal stools, careful examination of the feces may reveal flecks of blood-tinged mucus, often containing numbers of motile *E. histolytica*. Patients with more acute illness may have a dozen or more explosive liquid stools daily, containing much blood and mucus and perhaps accompanied by abdominal cramps. Tenesmus, painful spasms of the anal sphincter, is a sign of rectal ulceration.

Despite extensive research, the molecular bases underlying pathogenicity and virulence of *E. histolytica* remain poorly understood. Proposed mechanisms for *E. histolytica* virulence include the production of enzymes or other cytotoxic substances, contact-dependent cell

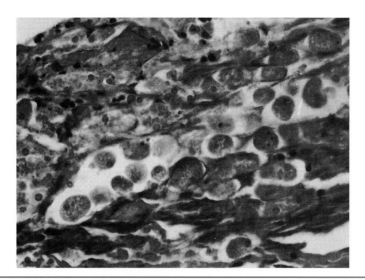

FIGURE 3-7 ■ Trophozoites of *Entamoeba histolytica* in ulcer of colon. (Photomicrograph by Zane Price.)

killing, and cytophagocytosis. At present, the steps believed to be involved in amebic killing of target cultivated mammalian cells are (1) receptor-mediated adherence of amebae to target cells, (2) amebic cytolysis of target cells, and (3) amebic phagocytosis of killed (or viable) target cells.

The attachment of *E. histolytica* trophozoites to the colonic mucosa is mediated by an amebal galactose-inhibitable adherence lectin. The addition of millimolar concentrations of galactose or *N*-acetyl-D-galactosamine inhibits attachment of *E. histolytica* trophozoites to cultivated mammalian cells. After attachment the parasite kills the host cell in an extracellular process that involves activation of host cell Caspase-3, leading to apoptotic death and engulfment of the host cell.

Little is known of the host-protective mechanisms in amebiasis. Intestinal secretory IgA against the parasite Gal/GalNAc lectin is associated with immunity to reinfection. Serum antibodies can be demonstrated in human infection by a variety of commonly used serologic techniques. It is generally assumed that serum antibodies are elicited after tissue invasion and that, although they are useful in serologic diagnosis of infection, antibodies do not seem to be involved in protection. To illustrate, the highest antibody titers are found in symptomatic infections. Nonetheless, serologic evidence must not preclude the possible existence of protective antibodies or antibody-dependent cellular mechanisms.

Trophozoites of *E. histolytica* have been shown to activate complement via the classical and alternative complement pathways. Although complement is amebicidal, pathogenic strains of *E. histolytica* may be resistant to complement-mediated lysis via inhibition of membrane attack complex formation.

Experimental hepatic amebiasis in immunodepressed mice suggests a protective role for cell-mediated immunity. Conversely, TH-2 phenotype immune response appear to exacerbate amebic colitis in the murine model. Additional experimental animal studies have demonstrated that host resistance is dependent on macrophages but not on T cell-mediated defense mechanisms. In fact, during acute invasive amebiasis, the host's T-lymphocyte responses to *E. histolytica* antigens appear to be specifically depressed by a parasite-induced serum factor. Trophozoites of a virulent strain of *E. histolytica* are able to kill normal human polymorphonuclear neutrophils, monocytes, and macrophages in vitro; however, activated macrophages are able to kill the same virulent amebae through a contact-dependent, antibody-independent mechanism.

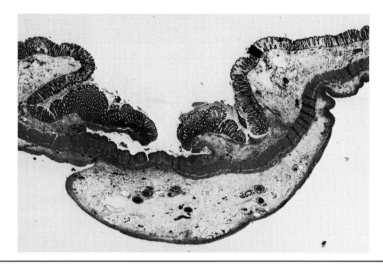

FIGURE 3-8 ■ Amebic ulcer of colon, showing characteristic undermining. (From Binford CH, Connor DH. *Pathology of tropical and extraordinary diseases*, Armed Forces Institute of Pathology, #74-2981.)

Amebae may penetrate the muscularis mucosae into the submucosa (Fig. 3–7), where they spread out into classic flask–shaped ulcers (Fig. 3–8) and erode blood vessels to give rise to the intraluminal bleeding characteristic of acute infections. If large numbers of ulcers are produced, they may coalesce by means of intercommunicating submucosal sinus passages. The undermined mucosa may remain fairly normal in appearance, or, if the undermining is extensive and there is secondary bacterial infection, there may be necrosis and sloughing of large portions of the intestinal wall. Rarely, intestinal casts may appear in the stools.

Sigmoidoscopic examination may demonstrate an almost normal mucosal pattern or one that is indistinguishable from those seen in ulcerative or granulomatous colitis. There may be scattered ulcerations up to a few millimeters in diameter, characterized by an erythematous border and yellowish center. In more advanced cases greater numbers of ulcers may be seen, ranging in diameter up to 10 or 12 mm, often with raised edges but with normal-looking mucosa elsewhere. Presence of a grossly normal mucosa between the ulcers serves to differentiate amebic from bacillary dysentery on sigmoidoscopic examination, the entire mucosa being involved in bacillary dysentery. As the amebic infection progresses, coalescence of the ulcers may produce irregularly wandering ulcer trenches, sometimes with hair-like remnants of the more resistant supportive structures projecting from their bases ("buffalo skin" or "Dyak hair" ulcers).

Abdominal palpation may reveal tenderness of the cecum, transverse colon, or sigmoid. Some hepatic enlargement and tenderness may be evident, but this does not necessarily indicate amebic invasion of that organ. Fever is not characteristic of uncomplicated amebic colitis. Mild leukocytosis may be seen, which is probably a response to the secondary bacterial infection so frequently present. The white blood cell count seldom rises above 12,000 per microliter; in bacillary dysentery the average may be not much higher, but counts may reach 16,000 to 20,000 per microliter. Even in moderately severe attacks of diarrhea or dysentery, spontaneous subsidence or alteration with periods of constipation is common.

Perforation of an amebic ulcer is generally a dramatic event, accompanied by the usual signs of peritoneal irritation or infection; however, slow leakage to the abdominal cavity through a severely diseased colonic wall may be more common. It is marked by distention, ileus, and gas in the peritoneal cavity, but not by the boardlike abdomen that marks acute perforation. Surgical intervention may be feasible in cases of acute perforation but not in the chronic type or in amebic appendicitis, as the infected gut is quite friable.

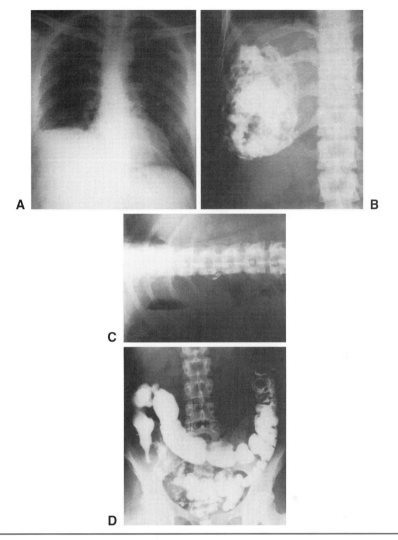

FIGURE 3-9 ▓ **A,** Elevation of right diaphragm and blunting of right costophrenic angle in amebic cyst of liver. **B,** Large amebic cyst of liver outlined by injection of contrast material. **C,** Amebic cyst of liver; note air in cyst cavity and fluid level after partial aspiration of contents. **D,** Amebiasis of the cecum; note funnel-shaped deformity seen on barium enema. (**A, B,** and **C** courtesy of Dr. Jerrold Turner, Harbor General Hospital, Torrance, CA.)

A chronic granulomatous lesion, known as an ameboma, develops most frequently in the cecal or rectosigmoid region. It may produce a so-called napkin-ring constriction of the bowel wall indistinguishable on x-ray examination from an annular carcinoma, or it may give rise to a characteristic (though nonspecific) conical configuration of the cecum (Fig. 3-9, *D*). In general, radiologic findings are similar to those seen in inflammatory bowel disease, although seldom with involvement of the terminal ileum.

Hepatomegaly and tenderness may occur in amebic colitis without any evidence of hepatic infection. The hepatic enlargement is thought to be a toxic response to intestinal infection, unrelated to the local presence of amebae. A condition known as amebic hepatitis has been postulated, but if defined as a diffuse early stage of liver infection, without abscess formation, it remains hypothetical. At any rate, it is clear that spread of the infection to the liver may occur in cases in which intestinal complaints never develop.

Hepatic infection is characterized by liver tenderness and enlargement, fever, weight loss, and sometimes a cough with evidence of pneumonitis involving the right lower lung field.

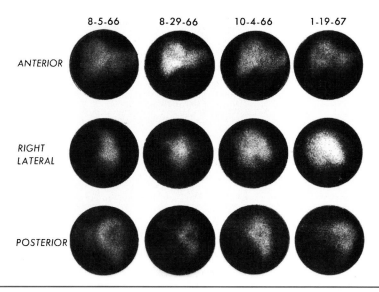

FIGURE 3-10 ▩ Hepatoscan of amebic abscess under treatment. (Courtesy of Dr. Paul Weber, Department of Clinical Pathology, San Francisco General Hospital, San Francisco, CA.)

The right leaf of the diaphragm may be elevated and fixed on position (Fig. 3-9, *A*). Multiplication of amebae in the liver may lead to the development of single or multiple abscesses, although the majority of amebae that reach the liver are probably destroyed there and do not produce abscesses. Single large abscesses (Fig. 3-9, *B, C*) may arise from the coalescence of multiple smaller ones. With abscess formation, hepatic pain becomes more severe and continuous; pain may also be referred to the right or left shoulder, depending on the position of the abscess. There is leukocytosis of 15,000 to 35,000 per microliter without a characteristic differential, and also fever and night sweats. The fever tends to occur daily in the afternoon, reaching a peak of about 102°F, and it is accompanied or followed by profuse sweating. Liver scans (Fig. 3-10) reveal areas of nonvisualization, most frequently single and in the right lobe, less often multiple or in other locations. Sonography, magnetic resonance imaging, and computed tomography (CT; Fig. 3-11) offer convenient means for evaluating the development and resolution when refined imaging techniques lead to early diagnosis and treatment. Liver function tests are of little value in the differential diagnosis of amebic abscess. Aspiration of an amebic abscess usually yields a thick, reddish brown fluid, which rarely contains amebae. Organisms are confined to the hepatic tissue of the abscess walls (Fig. 3-12). Under these circumstances, diagnosis by response to therapy is frequently the only practical approach, although modern techniques such as real-time PCR are highly sensitive for detecting *E. histolytica* DNA in the abscess. Results of serologic tests are usually positive in such cases.

Erosion of a hepatic abscess through the diaphragm into the lung may lead to pulmonary amebiasis. Pleurisy, with or without effusion or pleural rub, or right lower lobe pneumonitis may signal a subdiaphragmatic abscess without actual rupture into the pleural space. With rupture into the pleural cavity, a characteristic x-ray picture may result, with evidence of an effusion ascending the greater fissure, sometimes followed by rupture into the pleural space. If the abscess is localized in the left lobe of the liver, it may, of course, involve the left lung. If hepatic spread of the infection extends to involve a bronchus, amebae may be found in the sputum. Primary pulmonary amebiasis, blood-borne from an intestinal focus rather than arising from a hepatic abscess, has been reported. Amebic abscesses of other organs, such as the brain, pericardium, and spleen, are uncommon and when they occur are most often accompanied by amebic liver abscess. Signs of such infection are

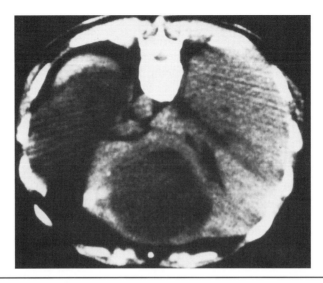

FIGURE 3-11 ▩ CT scan shows amebic abscess of liver. Space-occupying lesion in liver is clearly visible. (Courtesy of Dr. Herman Zaiman.)

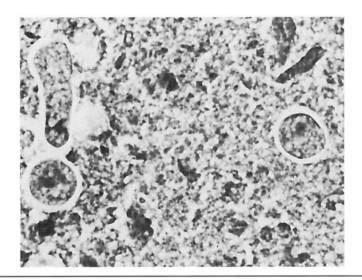

FIGURE 3-12 ▩ *Entamoeba histolytica* trophozoites in necrotic margin of amebic liver abscess (hematoxylin and eosin stain). (Photomicrograph by Zane Price.)

related to the organs involved. Amebic infection of the skin is rare but may produce extensive gangrenous ulcerations of the perineal tissues or affect the skin surrounding a colostomy or draining hepatic abscess. A case of cutaneous amebiasis of the face resulting in loss of vision in one eye, but without involvement of the mucocutaneous surfaces, has been described. Vaginal, urethral, and clitoral infections have been reported. Amebiasis of the penis is seen following intercourse with a partner who has vaginal amebiasis and also as a consequence of anal intercourse. In all of the conditions, trophic amebae may be recovered from the affected tissues.

The standard methods of stool examination are outlined in Chapter 14. The best way to diagnose *E. histolytica* infection is by a combination of stool antigen detection and serology. The traditional stool ova and parasite exam is both insensitive and notoriously nonspecific.

Amebae may often be found in specimens obtained by sigmoidoscopy. Material may be expressed from the ulcers by means of gentle pressure from a long-handled curette or loop and suspended in saline for microscopic examination. *E. histolytica* may be cultivated axenically in TYI-S-33 medium.★ Serologic techniques (see Chapter 16) have been employed for many years in the diagnosis of amebiasis. Indirect hemagglutination (IHA) and enzyme-linked immunosorbent assay (ELISA) tests are available. The IHA test is perhaps slightly more sensitive and may remain positive for many years. Enzyme immunoassays (EIA) are available to detect *Entamoeba*-specific antigen in fecal specimens. A monoclonal ELISA kit detects *E. histolytica* Gal/GalNAc lectin in stool and distinguishes it from *E. dispar* (see Chapter 16). A DNA hybridization probe will identify *E. histolytica* in stool samples. The polymerase chain reaction (PCR) technique has been used experimentally to differentiate *E. histolytica* from *E. dispar*.

Epidemiology. The prevalence of amebic infection, as of most enteric diseases, varies with the level of sanitation and is generally higher in the tropics and subtropics than in temperate climates. The severity of the disease and the incidence of complications may likewise be greater in the tropics, reflecting the higher incidence of infection. While various factors may play a role in determining the severity of the infection, severe disease is associated with malnutrition. In the United States, amebiasis is more common in immigrants and travelers from developing countries. In any region, it is more prevalent under crowded conditions, and may reach epidemic proportions in orphanages, prisons, and asylums. Outside such settings, in the United States, Canada, and Europe, the relatively few epidemic outbreaks can usually be traced to sewage-contaminated drinking water. *E. histolytica* and *E. dispar* infection is observed in men who have sex with men. A "pseudo-outbreak" of intestinal amebiasis was reported from Los Angeles County, California. Of 38 patients originally diagnosed as having intestinal amebiasis, upon reexamination only 2 (5.3%) actually were shown to have infection with *E. histolytica*. This is a reminder that identification of *E. histolytica* can be difficult.

Of 7914 autopsies performed in a general hospital in Mexico in the 1960s, amebiasis was found to be the fourth leading cause of death. In another report, amebiasis was identified as the third most prevalent infectious disease in Mexico and currently approximately 10% of the population has serologic evidence of prior amebiasis. Rates as high as 50% to 80% have been reported from some tropical areas, again not differentiating *E. dispar* from *E. histolytica*. It is, however, generally believed that the pathogenic *E. histolytica* is more prevalent in tropical areas. A study using modern diagnostic techniques demonstrated *E. histolytica* dysentery in 2% of children per year in Dhaka, Bangladesh.

From an epidemiologic standpoint, asymptomatic patients are of utmost importance in the transmission of the disease. Cysts are relatively resistant but are killed by drying, by temperatures over 55°C, and by superchlorination or the addition of iodine to drinking water. While contaminated water is a prime source of infection in many areas, food handlers may also play a role. The use of human feces (night soil) for fertilizer and the contamination of foodstuffs by flies, and possibly cockroaches, may be of epidemiologic importance in some areas.

A number of strains of amebae resembling *E. histolytica* are able to survive and multiply at room temperature (unlike *E. histolytica* itself) and have been isolated from human feces. The first such eurythermic ameba to be isolated and grown in culture is known as the Laredo strain, now classified as *E. moshkovskii*. It has an optimum growth temperature of 25° to 30°C and can survive at temperatures from 0° to 41°C, whereas the classic *E. histolytica* has an optimal temperature of 37°C and can survive a range of temperatures from 20° to 43°C.

★Available as a freeze-dried preparation (ATCC Medium PARA-215) from the American Type Culture Collection (ATCC), P.O. Box 1549, Manassas, VA 20108; (703) 365-2700; www.atcc.org.

TABLE 3-1 ■ Suggested Drug Regimens for Amebiasis*

Infection	Drug and Dosage
Asymptomatic intestinal amebiasis	Paromomycin 25-35 mg/Kg/D in 3 divided doses for 7 days *or* Diloxanide furoate (Furamide), 500 mg 3 times daily × 10 days *or* Metronidazole (Flagyl), 750 mg 3 times daily × 10 days
Amebic dysentery and liver abscess, ameboma	Metronidazole, as above × 10 days (total dose not to exceed 1.0 g) followed by luminal agent

*Acute symptoms of amebic dysentery will usually be brought under control within 3 to 5 days; there is seldom any marked toxicity with such curtailed use of these drugs.

E. moshkovskii is of limited pathogenicity to experimental animals and probably not pathogenic to humans. *Entamoeba moshkovskii* has been isolated from sewage plants in many parts of the world and in one study was shown to infect a substantial minority of children in Bangladesh.

Early studies involving the zymodemes (patterns of electrophoretic mobility of certain parasite isoenzymes) of various isolates of what was originally thought to be all one species (*E. histolytica*) demonstrated a difference between invasive and noninvasive strains. A seroepidemiologic survey of antibody responses to the zymodemes of *E. histolytica* showed that 94% to 100% of persons infected with amebae having pathogenic zymodemes were seropositive, even though some had no symptoms, whereas only 2% to 4% of persons infected with amebae of nonpathogenic zymodemes were seropositive. Subsequent research using RNA and DNA probes also indicated differences between invasive and noninvasive strains. PCR amplification of genomic DNA, hybridization of cDNA clones, and rRNA probes provided additional evidence for the separation of the invasive *E. histolytica* from the noninvasive *E. dispar*. The inability to morphologically distinguish *E. histolytica* from the nonpathogens *E. dispar* and *E. moshkovskii* underscores the importance of the modern diagnostic tests.

Treatment. Whenever possible, a laboratory diagnosis of *E. histolytica* infection, unless confirmed by visualization of ingested red blood cells in the trophozoite, should be substantiated by (1) presence of red blood cells in the stool, (2) serum antibody titer, and (3) stool *E. histolytica* antigen titer. Treatment varies with the clinical stage of the infection (Table 3-1). For *asymptomatic intestinal amebiasis*, treatment may not be strictly necessary, although it is perhaps imprudent to neglect such infections, which may either become symptomatic or provide a nidus for extraintestinal disease or spread to others. Methods of treatment of the asymptomatic case and of amebic colitis are essentially identical. Mainstays of treatment are metronidazole or the related drug tinidazole for invasive disease and paromomycin for treatment of intestinal (luminal) infection. Diloxanide furoate (Furamide),★ another luminal amebicide, is restricted to patients who only pass cysts. A 14-year study by the Centers for Disease Control and Prevention involving 4371 treatment courses concluded that diloxanide was a safe and effective drug for treating asymptomatic cyst passers and that it was particularly well tolerated in children. The mechanism of action of iodoquinol is unknown. Metronidazole is effective only against anaerobic or microaerophilic organisms. It is activated by reduction by ferredoxin, generating a reactive radical.

★Available at present in the United States only from the CDC Drug Service, Centers for Disease Control and Prevention, U.S. Public Health Service, Atlanta, Georgia 30333; (404) 639-3670.

Metronidazole or tinidazole is recommended for treatment of *acute amebic colitis*. Side effects of metronidazole treatment include nausea, diarrhea, metallic taste, and headache. Other side effects are uncommon, and none is usually so severe as to preclude use of the drug. The patient should be warned to abstain from alcohol during treatment with metronidazole. Reports of increased incidence of tumors in mice fed the drug from birth are a cause of concern; however, no appreciable increase in cancer was observed in a large retrospective study of women treated with metronidazole. It is approved for use during the last two trimesters of pregnancy. Tinidazole is in general better tolerated than metronidazole and requires a shorter course of treatment.

Treatment failures do occur; metronidazole treatment should be followed with a luminal agent (paromomycin or diloxanide) to eliminate intestinal colonization and prevent relapse. Resistance to metronidazole or tinidazole has not been observed. Emetine was formerly used for treatment of amebiasis, but cardiac toxicity (Fig. 3–13) has precluded its routine use.

Metronidazole and tinidazole are first-line agents in the treatment of *hepatic abscess*. Some reports suggest that metronidazole used alone may not effect a cure in all cases and that aspiration may be required. Aspiration of amebic abscesses at one time was a routine procedure. With the advent of metronidazole therapy, this is no longer true. Smaller abscesses may be expected to be resorbed, and their disappearance can be monitored with liver scans, ultrasound, or CT. Drainage of larger abscesses may be necessary in exceptional circumstances. The introduction of percutaneous catheter drainage under the guidance of CT or ultrasonography has greatly facilitated the drainage of amebic abscesses that are resistant to conventional therapy, and even of those that have perforated. For a discussion of these types of treatment see Singh and Kashyap (1989) and Ken et al. (1989).

Prevention. Most amebiasis is acquired through fecal contamination of food and water, and prevention of infection involves measures designed to break the chain of transmission. In North America and Europe, purity of drinking water is generally taken for granted (even though this is not always the case); elsewhere in the world, no such assumption should be made. Water can readily be disinfected by boiling. Treatment with iodine★ is also effective. Ice cubes made with contaminated water may transmit infection, as may fruits and vegetables washed in the water. In many areas these fruits and vegetables may themselves be contaminated by the practice of using human feces (night soil) for fertilizer. In most developing countries, it is best to not eat food sold by street vendors and to avoid salads and fruits that you do not yourself peel.

The importance of food handlers in the spread of enteric diseases, including amebiasis, is brought to our attention by periodic outbreaks of hepatitis, often traced to a particular eating place and sometimes to a single employee. It goes without saying that a food handler found to have amebiasis should not be allowed to resume that occupation until after he or she has been successfully treated. Regulations in this regard may vary from one area to another, but a minimum criterion for cure should be a series of negative results of stool examinations (preferably at least three) taken at least 1 month after completion of treatment.

Entamoeba dispar and E. moshkovskii

Based on evidence accumulated from numerous sources, a redescription of *E. histolytica* has confirmed the hypothesis, originally proposed by Emile Brumpt in 1925, that what was

---

★Place 6 g iodine crystals in a 60-ml (2-oz) amber screw-cap bottle. Fill the bottle with water, shake, and allow to stand at least 2 hours. This solution may then be added to water at the rate of 12.5 ml to 1 L, and if allowed to stand 15 minutes at 25°C (77°F) it is considered safe for drinking. The screw cap may be calibrated initially and used to measure the iodine stock solution. More water is added to stock until all the iodine crystals have gone into solution, making enough of the stock to disinfect several hundred liters of water. The quantity of iodine solution added should be doubled if the water is cloudy.

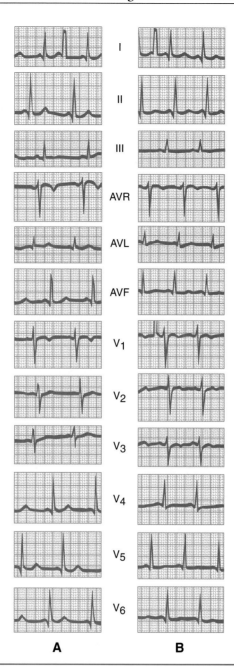

FIGURE 3-13 ▧ Electrocardiographic changes in emetine toxicity. **A,** Pretreatment. **B,** After emetine, 65 mg daily for 10 days. Note T-wave inversion or depression in leads V$_{3-6}$. (Courtesy of Dr. Alfred A. Bolomey, Kaiser Permanente Medical Center, Oakland, CA.)

considered to be a single species is actually a species complex in which *E. histolytica* is the invasive species, and *E. dispar* and *E. moshkovskii* are morphologically identical noninvasive ones. *E. dispar* (dispar = different) and *E. moshkovskii* are then synonymous with what was formerly designated nonpathogenic *E. histolytica*. However, *E. dispar* seems capable of causing focal intestinal lesions in experimental animals such as kittens, gerbils, and guinea pigs. Nonetheless, *E. dispar* does not seem able actually to invade the tissues.

   E. dispar is approximately nine times more prevalent than *E. histolytica*, and together they infect about 10% of the world's population. However, only *E. histolytica* causes disease, which affects some 50 million persons worldwide, with up to 110,000 deaths yearly. As stated earlier,

E. dispar does not cause symptomatic disease, nor does it elicit the production of serum antibodies. The prevalence of *E. moshkovskii* is not known.

Because *E. histolytica*, *E. dispar,* and *E. moshkovskii* are morphologically indistinguishable, one can no longer rely on microscopy alone for the unequivocal detection of *E. histolytica* infection. Microscopic identification of *E. histolytica* can only be made if ingested erythrocytes are present in its trophozoites. However, regardless of symptoms, the presence of what appear to be *E. histolytica*-like forms in the stool, along with a positive serologic response, indicates the presence of true *E. histolytica*. Conversely, a negative serologic test and *E. histolytica*-like amebae in the stool indicates *E. dispar*. Clearly, the development of new diagnostic tests is essential.

The laboratory tests that are being developed to diagnose amebiasis have focused on the detection of parasite antigen in the feces or serum by monoclonal antibodies, or on the detection of parasite DNA by nucleotide probes or PCR amplification. Commercially produced laboratory test kits involving DNA hybridization and PCR amplification undoubtedly will be available in the future. However, the status of current technology favors the development of ELISA tests using monoclonal antibody-based antigen detection. Commercially produced ELISA kits that detect a fecal *Entamoeba* antigen common to both species, and as of the time of this writing (mid-2005) only one kit specific for *E. histolytica*, are presently available (see Chapter 16). A field trial using the commercial kits concluded that they were more sensitive and specific than microscopic identification, but less sensitive than culture, which is generally a research tool and not a clinical tool.

There are no morphologic differences between *E. dispar* and *E. hartmanni*, except for size (see the table below).

Entamoeba hartmanni

E. hartmanni (see Fig. 3-5) has now attained general acceptance as the name for the amebae formerly designated as "small race" *E. histolytica*. The confusion surrounding the relationship between the two forms is based on their morphologic similarity. The only clear-cut distinction between the two species is size. Arbitrarily, but generally satisfactorily, the two species can be separated by considering the upper limits of size of living *E. hartmanni* trophozoites to be 12 μm and of its cysts to be 10 μm (Plate I, 5). These measurements are likewise the lower limits of the size range of *E. histolytica*. Fortunately, most *E. hartmanni* measure well below the dividing point and most *E. histolytica* above it. If but a few 12-μm trophozoites or 10-μm cysts are seen, it may be impossible to make a specific identification.

Rounded trophozoites of *E. hartmanni* measure from 3 to nearly 12 μm (Plate I, 6) in diameter; the cyst size range is from 4 to 10 μm. Nuclear structure shows the same variations seen in *E. histolytica*, and there is no consistent difference between the two species in nuclear-cytoplasmic ratio. The chromatoidal material assumes a similar rod- or cigarlike form in the two species. *E. hartmanni* organisms ingest bacteria but not red blood cells.

Serologic differences between *E. hartmanni* and *E. histolytica* have been measured and are considerably greater than those between different strains of *E. histolytica*. Studies of prevalence in which this ameba has been differentiated from *E. histolytica* indicate roughly similar incidence and distribution for the two. Although there have been reports to the contrary, most authorities consider *E. hartmanni* to be nonpathogenic and accordingly do not treat this infection.

The characteristics shown in the following table are of value in the identification of *Entamoeba hartmanni*.

I. *Trophozoites, unstained*	Not characteristic
II. *Trophozoites, stained*	Diagnostic: nuclear structure similar to that of *E. histolytica*; ingested bacteria; diameter less than 12 μm
III. *Cysts, unstained*	Suggestive: four nuclei; rounded form
IV. *Cysts, stained*	Diagnostic: typical nuclear structure; chromatoidal bars with rounded or squared ends; diameter less than 10 μm

FIGURE 3-14 ■ *Entamoeba coli.* Variations in nuclear structure (some original, others adapted from various sources).

Entamoeba coli

E. coli is a nonpathogenic ameba that closely resembles *E. histolytica*; the two species may be confused, leading either to superfluous treatment for a nonpathogenic parasite or to omission of appropriate therapy for pathogens.

The trophozoites are about the same diameter as those of *E. histolytica* (range 15 to 50 μm); perhaps they average slightly larger than trophozoites of the pathogenic species (see Fig. 3-15; Plate II, 1, 2). The cytoplasm is granular, frequently containing many vacuoles. Red blood cells are not ingested by this ameba except under the most unusual circumstances. *E. coli* is sluggish in its movements in comparison with *E. histolytica*. Pseudopodia are short and blunt, never long and fingerlike as they may be in *E. histolytica*. They are extruded slowly and are not hyaline, and there is no striking differentiation of the cytoplasm into ectoplasm and endoplasm. Motility is not progressive; the pseudopodia appear to function more to ingest food than to produce directional movement. Bacteria are regularly seen in vacuoles in the cytoplasm.★ The nucleus is usually easily discerned. A ring of refractile granules representing the peripheral chromatin encloses another eccentric refractile mass, the karyosome.

When the organisms are stained, the nuclear morphology is more distinct (Fig. 3-14). Peripheral chromatin in *E. coli* is irregular both in size and in arrangement on the nuclear membrane; it is definitely more abundant than is usual in *E. histolytica*. The karyosome is large, frequently irregular in shape, usually eccentric in position, and surrounded by a halo of nonstaining material. Granules of chromatin may be seen scattered between the karyosome and the peripheral chromatin, and sometimes a linin network is visible.

Precystic forms are seen, as in *E. histolytica*, but as in that species the morphology is not very distinctive and identification should never be based on examination of these forms alone, whether stained or unstained.

The cysts of *E. coli* (Figs. 3-15 to 3-17; Plate II, 3, 4) overlap the size range of *E. histolytica*, being 10 to nearly 35 μm in diameter; the average diameter is definitely greater than in cysts of the pathogenic species. The cyst wall is highly refractile and the cytoplasm granular in appearance; food vacuoles are absent. The nuclei are usually readily observed; they vary in number from one to eight. The eccentric position of the karyosome can frequently be distinguished, even in unstained amebae. Chromatoidal bodies are less common than in *E. histolytica* but occasionally may be observed as clear, thin lines or rods of refractile material in the cytoplasm.

With an iodine stain (see Fig. 3-35), glycogen may be seen in the cysts of *E. coli*; often masses of this dark-staining material completely surround the nuclei, which are not, however, entirely obscured. While glycogen may occur in the cysts of *E. histolytica*, the perinuclear disposition of this material is more characteristic of *E. coli*. Eccentric karyosomes may be observed, especially in the mononucleate and binucleate cysts, where they are larger. Permanent stains bring out details of nuclear structure, which is similar to that of the trophozoites. From one to eight nuclei are ordinarily seen; rarely, hypernucleate forms

---

★This ameba seems to be omnivorous, ingesting in addition to bacteria other species of protozoans and even smaller members of its own species.

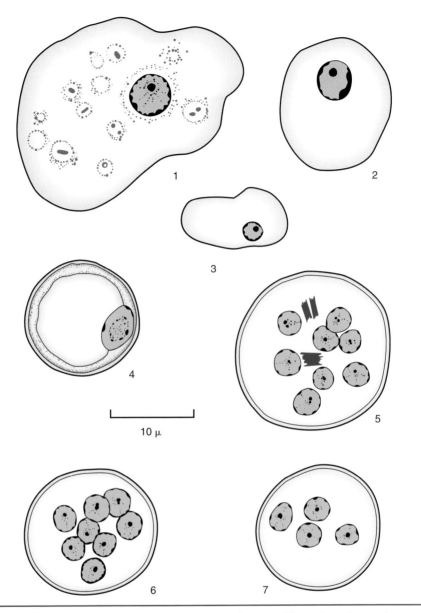

FIGURE 3-15 ■ *Entamoeba coli: 1*, trophozoite with ingested bacteria and granular pseudopodium; *2, 3*, trophozoites; *4*, early cyst with nucleus undergoing division and containing glycogen mass; *5*, octonucleate cyst with chromatoidals; *6*, octonucleate cyst; *7*, quadrinucleate cyst (*2, 3, 5, 6,* and *7* show diagnostic features only).

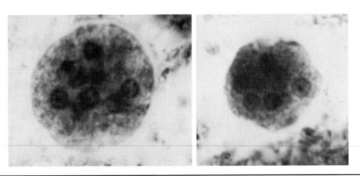

FIGURE 3-16 ■ *Entamoeba coli* cysts. (Photomicrographs by Zane Price.)

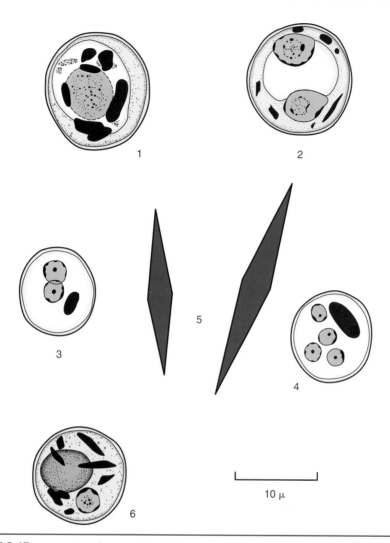

FIGURE 3-17 ■ *1, 2,* Early cysts of *Entamoeba histolytica* and *Entamoeba coli,* respectively; both contain nuclei undergoing division; *3,* binucleate cyst of *Entamoeba hartmanni* with resting nuclei; *4,* quadrinucleate cyst of *E. hartmanni; 5,* Charcot-Leyden crystals; *6, Entamoeba polecki* cyst with inclusion mass and chromatoidals with angular and pointed ends (*3* and *4* show diagnostic features only).

with 16 or 32 nuclei are observed. The chromatoidals are seen to be composed of splinter-shaped or rarely ribbon- or threadlike bodies; heavier bodies with irregular ends are also frequently seen. The cytoplasm of *E. coli* cysts is very granular; areas occupied by glycogen before fixation are marked by empty spaces in the cytoplasm of the fixed and stained cysts.

The following characteristics are of value in the identification of *Entamoeba coli*:

I. *Trophozoites, unstained*	Suggestive: sluggish, nondirectional motility; short, granular pseudopodia; ingested bacteria; visible nucleus
II. *Trophozoites, stained*	Suggestive: granular cytoplasm without much differentiation into ectoplasm and endoplasm; bacteria in food vacuoles
	Diagnostic: nucleus with irregular clumps of peripheral chromatin; large, irregular, eccentric karyosome
III. *Cysts, unstained*	Suggestive: eight nuclei; glycogen mass surrounding nuclei (iodine stains)

IV. *Cysts, stained*	Suggestive: maximum of eight nuclei, having karyosome and peripheral chromatin Diagnostic: typical nuclear structure; splinter-shaped or irregular chromatoidals

Entamoeba polecki

First reported as an intestinal parasite of pigs and monkeys, *E. polecki* has been found occasionally in humans. In parts of Papua New Guinea, it is apparently the most common intestinal ameba of humans. In a survey of 184 children in Papua New Guinea, 35 (19%) were found to be infected with *E. polecki*. Although pig-to-human transmission is considered to be the most likely route of human infection, the possibility of human-to-human transmission exists where the prevalence of infection is high.

E. polecki (Figs. 3-17 and 3-18) resembles *E. histolytica* but can be differentiated from it with comparative ease. Culturally and in its reaction to various therapeutic agents, it behaves somewhat differently from *E. histolytica*. Although few cases of *E. polecki* infection have been reported in humans, it is no more a measure of the possible worldwide importance of this parasite than is the fact that in only some of the reported cases were there any symptoms. How important this ameba may be in areas other than Papua New Guinea is not known. For example, 22 cases of *E. polecki* infection have been diagnosed in Southeast Asian refugees, 14 in Strasbourg, France, eight in Rochester, Minnesota, and 8 cases in Zulia state, Venezuela.

Trophozoites of *E. polecki* resemble those of *E. coli* in their motility, in the granularity and degree of vacuolization of their cytoplasm, and in the ingestion of bacteria. The nucleus is occasionally visible in the unstained trophozoite. Directional motility such as is seen in *E. histolytica* occurs only sporadically if at all; pseudopodia are usually formed slowly but occasionally may be thrust out in the explosive manner characteristic of *E. histolytica*. In stained preparations the nuclear structure appears somewhat intermediate between those of *E. histolytica* and *E. coli*. The karyosome is small in trophozoites and is usually central or nearly so. Normally compact, it is occasionally dispersed. The peripheral chromatin is generally seen in the form of fine granules evenly distributed on the nuclear membrane; sometimes larger granules are scattered among the smaller ones, or the peripheral chromatin may be massed at one or both poles.

The cyst state of *E. polecki* is characterized by a single nucleus (see Fig. 3-18). Very rarely, it is binucleate or quadrinucleate. Chromatoidal material resembling that seen in *E. histolytica* is formed in the cysts and is often abundant. The ends of the chromatoidals are frequently angular and sometimes pointed, rather than regularly rounded or squared off as in *E. histolytica*. Threadlike chromatoidals have also been reported. Glycogen may be present, and in addition approximately half of the cysts contain an "inclusion mass," the nature of which

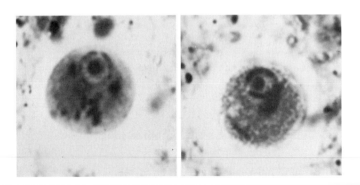

FIGURE 3-18 ■ Cysts of *Entamoeba polecki*. (Photomicrographs by Zane Price.)

is unknown. These masses are spherical or ovoid, without being sharply defined. In hematoxylin preparations they are not dissolved as is glycogen, and they stain much more faintly than chromatoidal material.

Unstained cysts cannot be differentiated with any certainty from mononucleate cysts of the other two species of *Entamoeba*, though the presence in a formed stool of large mononucleate cysts, and the near absence of ones with greater numbers of nuclei, is suggestive. Iodine-stained cysts are likewise not distinctive. The inclusion mass does not take the dark stain characteristic of glycogen and is not seen clearly. In permanently stained preparations, the karyosome is usually large and central in position. It may be spherical or stellate in shape, or it may consist of a group of small granules. A single minute central karyosome is sometimes observed. Peripheral chromatin appears evenly distributed in the form of small spherical granules or flattened plaques, sometimes with interspersed irregular larger granules. As in the trophozoite, the chromatin may be massed at one or both poles. An inclusion mass, if present, stains lightly but uniformly. Chromatoidals may be seen to exhibit the characteristic shape just mentioned.

Entamoeba chattoni, an organism morphologically identical to *E. polecki* and one that frequently is found in apes and monkeys, has been identified in eight human infections. All but one of the infected individuals had close contact with monkeys. Trophozoites were isolated in culture and positively identified as *E. chattoni* by isoenzyme characterization. Apparently, the organisms causes no clinical disease in either simians or humans.

The following characteristics are of value in the identification of *Entamoeba polecki*:

I. *Trophozoites, unstained*	Not characteristic
II. *Trophozoites, stained*	Suggestive: nucleus with minute central karyosome, with peripheral chromatin evenly distributed or massed at one or both poles; ingested bacteria
III. *Cysts, unstained*	Suggestive: uniform mononuclear condition
IV. *Cysts, stained*	Suggestive: mononucleate cysts: large central karyosomes with evenly distributed peripheral chromatin or peripheral chromatin massed at one or both poles
	Diagnostic: inclusion masses, chromatoidal bars with angular or pointed ends

Pathogenesis. Few cases of *E. polecki* infection have been followed for any length of time. One human case was observed for about 3 years without any indication of disease. A few reports describe patients with diarrhea apparently caused by infection with this parasite. Some doubt is cast on the validity of this species by isoenzyme studies of a number of isolates showing the morphologic characteristics of *E. polecki*. In every case, the isoenzyme pattern fell within one or another of what are now recognized as *E. dispar* groupings, whereas that of *Entamoeba moshkovskii*, Huff, Laredo, and other strains did not. Further comparison with *E. dispar* is needed.

Treatment. All of the commonly employed antiamebic drugs, with the exception of diloxanide furoate (Furamide)* and metronidazole (Flagyl), have been used without success in attempts to eradicate this infection. Salaki and coworkers (1979) treated their patient first with metronidazole, 750 mg three times daily for 10 days, and then with diloxanide furoate, 500 mg three times daily for 10 days, and achieved a cure. Whether Furamide alone would have been successful is not known. Metronidazole alone has been used successfully to treat *E. polecki* infection in humans (Chacin-Bonilla, 1980; Gay et al., 1985). The regimens used were metronidazole, 750 mg three times a day for 5, 7, or 10 days.

---

*Available at present in the United States only from the CDC Drug Service, Centers for Disease Control and Prevention, U.S. Public Health Service, Atlanta, Georgia 30333; (404) 639-3670.

Entamoeba gingivalis

Bearing a close morphologic resemblance to *E. histolytica*, *E. gingivalis* (Fig. 3-19) is often found in pyorrheal pockets between the teeth and gums and in the tonsillar crypts. It has been reported to multiply in bronchial mucus and to appear in the sputum, where it might be mistaken for *E. histolytica* from a pulmonary abscess. The cytoplasm of the ameba may contain bacteria and occasional red cells but most frequently is filled with portions of ingested leukocytes. Nuclear fragments from the leukocytes are usually recognizable in stained specimens and serve to identify the ameba, as *E. gingivalis* is the only species that ingests these cells. *E. gingivalis* forms no cysts.

These amebae are most frequently recovered from the mouths of patients suffering from pyorrhea alveolaris. Although numerous attempts have been made to implicate these organisms in the production of periodontal disease, it seems probable that they are most conspicuous under disease conditions simply because they find there a more suitable environment. In a survey made from gingival scrapings, amebae of *E. gingivalis* were found in 59% of 113 dental patients and in 32% of 96 control subjects with good oral hygiene. A few cases of *Entamoeba* infection of the uterus have been described in patients with no intestinal infection who lived in areas of low endemicity. In each case, the patient used an intrauterine device and had an intercurrent bacterial infection. Riboprinting, a technique that compares ribosomal RNA gene sequences, has identified the organism as *E. gingivalis* and infection most likely followed orogenital contact.

OTHER INTESTINAL AMEBAE

It is generally not difficult to distinguish amebae belonging to the genus *Entamoeba* from other amebae occurring in the stool, even before a specific identification is possible. Trophozoites of the various species of *Entamoeba*, if we except *E. hartmanni*, are on average larger than those of *Iodamoeba* or *Endolimax*, but differentiation on this basis alone should not be attempted. Cysts of *Entamoeba* are usually larger than those of *Endolimax* or *Iodamoeba*, although there is somewhat more of an overlap in size range. Cysts of *Entamoeba* are usually spherical; those of *Endolimax* may be spherical but tend more often to be ovoid, whereas *Iodamoeba* cysts are frequently irregular in shape. Nuclear structure in *Entamoeba* is quite different from that seen in the other genera and affords a basis for immediate identification of this genus in stained preparations. Fundamentally, nuclear structure in the species

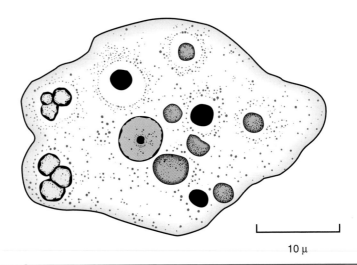

10 μ

FIGURE 3-19 ■ Trophozoite of *Entamoeba gingivalis*. There is no cyst stage. Note ingested leukocytes.

of *Entamoeba* is the same; it is possible to distinguish a karyosome and, in addition, a layer of peripheral chromatin, which typically lies just under the nuclear membrane. Peripheral chromatin forming a distinct layer under the nuclear membrane is not regularly seen in the other two genera.

Like the *E. histolytica–E. dispar–E. moshkovskii* species complex, which is cosmopolitan in distribution, *I. bütschlii* and *E. nana* have prevalence rates roughly equivalent to those of the *Entamoeba* complex. *E. nana* is usually encountered with about the same frequency as *E. coli*; both are somewhat more common than *E. histolytica/E. dispar*. *Iodamoeba* generally has prevalence rates somewhat similar to those of *E. histolytica/E. dispar* and *E. hartmanni*.

There is general agreement that these amebae are nonpathogenic and require no treatment. Their presence in stools is an indication of fecal contamination and may suggest the desirability of a more thorough search for pathogens.

Iodamoeba bütschlii

The ameba *I. bütschlii* (Figs. 3-20 and 3-21) receives its generic name from the characteristic glycogen vacuoles of the cyst stage (see Fig. 3-20; Plate II, 5, 6), which are so prominent that in iodine stains the cysts seem to contain little else (see Fig. 3-35). While glycogen vacuoles occur in other amebae, they are never as regular in outline nor as consistently present an in *Iodamoeba*. Large, somewhat irregular glycogen masses are frequently seen in iodine stains of *E. coli* cysts; in mature cysts they often appear to surround the nuclei. In *Iodamoeba* cysts the single nucleus is seen at one side of the glycogen vacuole. Rarely, hypernucleate forms with two or three nuclei are reported.

Positive identification of unstained trophozoites is difficult. They vary in diameter from 4 to 20 µm, the majority being within the range of 9 to 14 µm. *Iodamoeba* is sluggishly progressive and has hyaline pseudopodia. Bacteria may be seen scattered throughout the cytoplasm, and red blood cells are never ingested. The nucleus is usually not visible. Permanent stains reveal the characteristic nuclear structure (Fig. 3-22). The nuclear membrane is delicate, and if it does not take the stain the karyosome will appear to be contained in a vacuole. The karyosome is large, more or less central in position, irregularly rounded, and surrounded by a layer of small granules. The granules may lie closely applied to the karyosome, in which case they are not visible unless staining and subsequent differentiation have been optimal. In other instances, the small chromatin granules form a ring at some distance from the karyosome, between it and the nuclear membrane.

Cysts range in diameter from 6 to 16 µm (average 9 or 10 µm). The unstained cyst is surrounded by a refractile wall. Instead of having the spherical or ovoid shape of most amebic cysts, the majority of cysts of *Iodamoeba* are irregular in outline, and there is much variation in shape. The glycogen vacuole is prominent even in the unstained cyst because of its refractility. The nucleus is seldom distinct in unstained cysts. When stained with iodine,

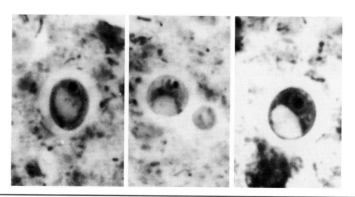

FIGURE 3-20 ■ Cysts of *Iodamoeba bütschlii*.

the glycogen vacuole is a dark brown mass, often more than half the diameter of the cyst (see Fig. 3-35). The nuclear membrane and karyosome appear as highly refractile structures within the pale yellow cytoplasm. The procedures employed in staining with permanent stains dissolve glycogen, but the vacuole is nevertheless characteristic because of its size and clearly demarcated margins. The karyosome is usually quite eccentric and may even be in contact with the nuclear membrane. In the cyst, the chromatin granules, which surrounded the karyosome in the trophic stage, usually form a crescentic aggregate between the karyosome and the nuclear membrane. In particularly well-stained specimens, linin fibrils may be seen running between the karyosome and the chromatin granules. Nuclei exhibiting this struc-ture have been likened to a basket of flowers, the karyosome forming the basket, the linin

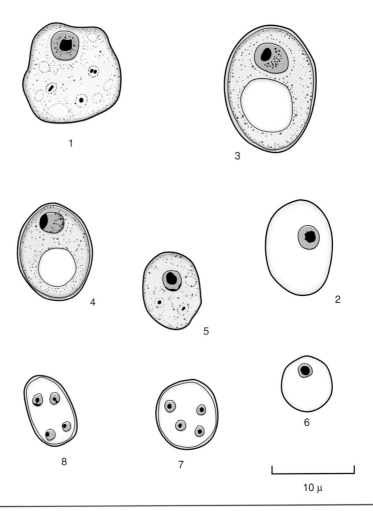

FIGURE 3-21 ■ *1, 2, Iodamoeba bütschlii* trophozoites; *3, 4, I. bütschlii* cysts containing glycogen vacuoles; *5, 6, Endolimax nana* trophozoites; *7, 8, E. nana* cysts (*2, 6, 7,* and *8* show diagnostic features only).

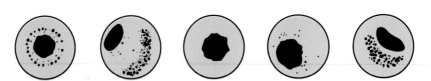

FIGURE 3-22 ■ *Iodamoeba bütschlii*. Variations in nuclear structure.

fibrils the stems, and the granules the blossoms. In other cysts the chromatin granules form a compact crescent closely applied to the nuclear membrane, or they are disposed as in the trophozoite.

Of historical interest, two fatal infections of the CNS were originally attributed to *Iodamoeba*. The first was a case of disseminated amebiasis in a 22-year-old Japanese prisoner of war who previously had been treated for malaria and dysentery. The second case involved a granuloma of the brain in a 6-year-old girl in Arizona who had fallen from a slide a year earlier and bruised the parietooccipital region. In both infections the pathogen was identified as *Iodamoeba* because of the large nuclear karyosome in the amebae in tissue sections, a feature very unlike that of *E. histolytica*, which at the time was the only known pathogenic ameba of humans. What is more likely is that the infections were caused by pathogenic free-living amebae, probably *Naegleria fowleri* in the former and *Acanthamoeba* in the latter, based on the clinical history and histopathological findings. See Chapter 5 for a discussion of infections caused by *Naegleria* and *Acanthamoeba*.

The following characteristics are of value in identification of *Iodamoeba bütschlii*:

I. *Trophozoites, unstained*	Not characteristic
II. *Trophozoites, stained*	Diagnostic: nucleus with large central karyosome surrounded by a ring of small chromatin granules; or nuclear structure as in cyst
III. *Cysts, unstained*	Suggestive: large refractile body in cytoplasm; single nucleus
IV. *Cysts, stained*	Diagnostic: basket nuclei or nuclei as in trophozoite; large glycogen vacuole

Endolimax nana

The most common of the smaller intestinal amebae, *Endolimax* (see Figs. 3-21 and 3-23; Plate III, 1–3) is usually encountered with about the same frequency as is *E. coli*. Both species are considerably more common than other human amebae. The size range for both trophozoites and cysts is similar to that of *E. hartmanni*, with which they may be confused in unstained preparations.

Trophozoites range from 5 to 12 μm in diameter (average size close to 7 μm). Pseudopodia are blunt and hyaline; they are extruded rapidly as in *E. histolytica* but fail to produce the directional locomotion seen in that species. Movement is sluggish and random. The cytoplasm contains food vacuoles with ingested bacteria. When stained, the characteristic nuclear structure (Fig. 3-24) becomes visible. The outstanding feature is a large karyosome, central or eccentric and often irregular in outline (see Fig. 3-23). Smaller extrakaryosomal chromatin granules are sometimes present. When the trichrome stain is employed, the chromatin may at times be seen massed against the nuclear membrane, without formation of a distinct karyosome.

Cysts of *Endolimax* exhibit about the same size range as the trophozoites. They are most frequently ovoid, but sometimes they are spherical or subspherical. A refractile cyst wall is present, which is particularly evident when concentrations are made by the zinc sulfate

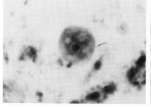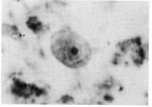

FIGURE 3-23 ■ Trophozoites of *Endolimax nana*.

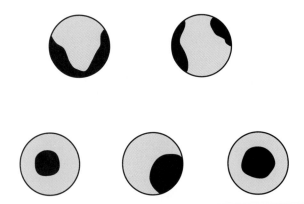

FIGURE 3-24 ■ *Endolimax nana.* Variations in nuclear structure.

technique and the cysts are stained with iodine. Zinc sulfate concentration results in a shrinkage of the cytoplasm of many of the cysts, which pull away from the cyst wall, leaving a clear space on one side of the organisms between the cytoplasm and the undistorted cyst wall. This effect is sometimes seen also in *Giardia*, but rarely in the other species of intestinal protozoa. In unstained cysts, little detail can be seen and an iodine stain (see Fig. 3-35) is seldom more revealing. Occasionally, minute brown masses of glycogen may be seen in the cytoplasm of cysts stained with iodine. When stained with a permanent stain, the cysts are seen to possess one to four nuclei. Rare hypernucleate forms containing eight nuclei have been reported. A large, usually eccentric, karyosome characterizes the nucleus. Other chromatin granules and intranuclear fibrils have been reported but are seldom seen in routine stains. Although bacteria are, of course, not seen in cysts, granules of chromatoidal material that resemble them may be present.

The following characteristics are of value in the identification of *Endolimax nana*:

I. *Trophozoites, unstained*	Not characteristic
II. *Trophozoites, stained*	Diagnostic: a nucleus with large karyosome, generally with little or no peripheral chromatin
	Suggestive: ovoid shape
III. *Cysts, unstained*	Suggestive: ovoid shape
IV. *Cysts, stained*	Diagnostic: four nuclei with large karyosomes and little or no peripheral chromatin

The Flagellates

There are four common species of intestinal flagellates: *Giardia lamblia*, *Chilomastix mesnili*, *Trichomonas hominis*, and *Dientamoeba fragilis*. In addition, two small flagellates, *Enteromonas hominis* and *Retortamonas intestinalis*, are sometimes encountered. There is no evidence that any of these organisms except *Giardia* and *Dientamoeba* can cause disease. A pathogenic trichomonad, *Trichomonas vaginalis*, occurs in the urogenital tract, and the commensal *T. tenax* is found in the mouth.

The flagellates other than *Dientamoeba* are readily recognized by their characteristic rapid motility, and the three larger species can usually be identified in unstained saline mounts. Trichrome stain is generally preferable to iron hematoxylin for staining flagellates. The intracytoplasmic fibrillar structures of these organisms, often of diagnostic importance, are brought out much better by trichrome than by any but the most careful hematoxylin staining.

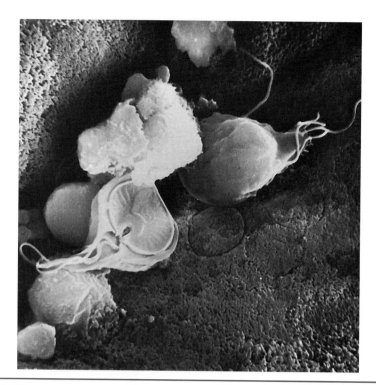

FIGURE 3-25 ▓ Scanning electron micrograph of *Giardia*, showing sucking disk and flagella; imprints of sucking disks are seen on surface of intestinal mucosa. (Courtesy of Dr. Robert L. Owen, San Francisco, CA.)

Giardia lamblia

Trophozoites of *Giardia* are found in the upper part of the small intestine, where they live closely applied to the mucosa. They may penetrate down into the secretary tubules of the mucosa and are found at times in the gallbladder and in biliary drainage. The anterior portion of the ventral surface of the organism is modified to form a sucking disk, which serves for attachment of the organism and which, in relation to its size, may produce a considerable degree of mechanical irritation to the tissues. A scanning electron photomicrograph of the parasitized intestinal mucosa (Fig. 3-25) shows convincing evidence of such damage. Attachment of *Giardia* to the duodenal mucosa also may be facilitated by a lectin produced by the parasite and activated by duodenal secretions. The life cycle of *Giardia* is illustrated in Figure 3-26.

Giardia is one of the most easily recognized intestinal protozoa. The trophozoite is bilaterally symmetrical, each structure being paired (Fig. 3-27; Plate III, 6; Plate IV, 1-3). Like *Dientamoeba*, it possesses two nuclei in the trophic form. Body length ranges from 9 to 21 μm and width from 5 to 15 μm. Motility is somewhat erratic, with a slow oscillation about the long axis. This type of motility has been likened to the motion of a falling leaf. The organism is roughly pear shaped when seen in surface view, having a broad anterior and a very much attenuated posterior end. *Giardia* trophozoites have four pairs of flagella: anterior, lateral, ventral, and posterior. Two nuclei lie in the area of the sucking disk in the anterior portion of the body. Two curved rods are seen posterior to the sucking disk. These rods are known as median bodies. The sucking disk is bordered by the curved intracytoplasmic portions of the anterior flagella, the axonemes. Axonemes of the caudal pair of flagella are straight, closely approximated, and run parallel to each other, dividing the body into halves throughout

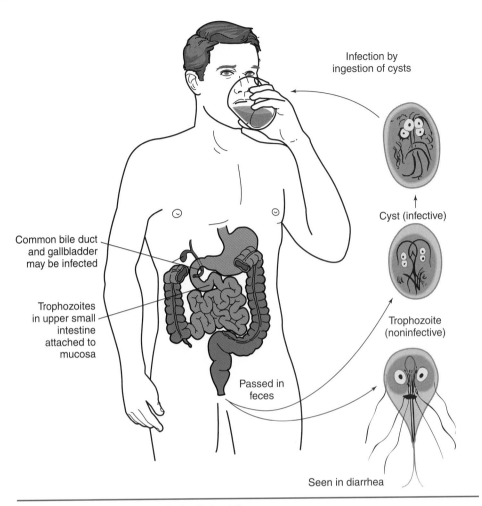

Infection by
ingestion of cysts

Cyst (infective)

Trophozoite
(noninfective)

Common bile duct
and gallbladder
may be infected

Trophozoites
in upper small
intestine
attached to
mucosa

Passed in
feces

Seen in diarrhea

FIGURE 3-26   ■   Life cycle of *Giardia lamblia*.

most of its length. The nuclei are spherical or ovoid and contain a large, usually central, karyosome. There is no peripheral chromatin.

In unstained trophozoites the characteristic body shape and motility may be observed, and some of the flagella can usually be seen. In preparations stained with any of the permanent stains, the most readily observable features are body shape, nuclei, axonemes, and the median bodies.

The cysts are ovoid and measure 8 to 14 μm by 7 to 10 μm. While some of the nuclei or median bodies may occasionally be detected in living specimens, the addition of D'Antoni's iodine usually reveals these structures. In permanent stains of cysts one observes four prominent nuclei and four median bodies, as well as twice the number of intracytoplasmic flagellar structures seen in the trophozoite, all dispersed in a seemingly helter-skelter fashion. The cyst wall is smooth and colorless and is usually well set off from the cytoplasm, owing to shrinkage of the latter at the time of fixation. When stained with trichrome, *Giardia* cysts may appear in varying shades of green or red, or the internal structures may be reddish brown against a green background.

Giardia does not appear consistently in the stools of all patients. Three patterns of excretion have been described: high, with parasites present in nearly all stools; low, with small numbers of parasites present in only about 40% of stool specimens; and a mixed

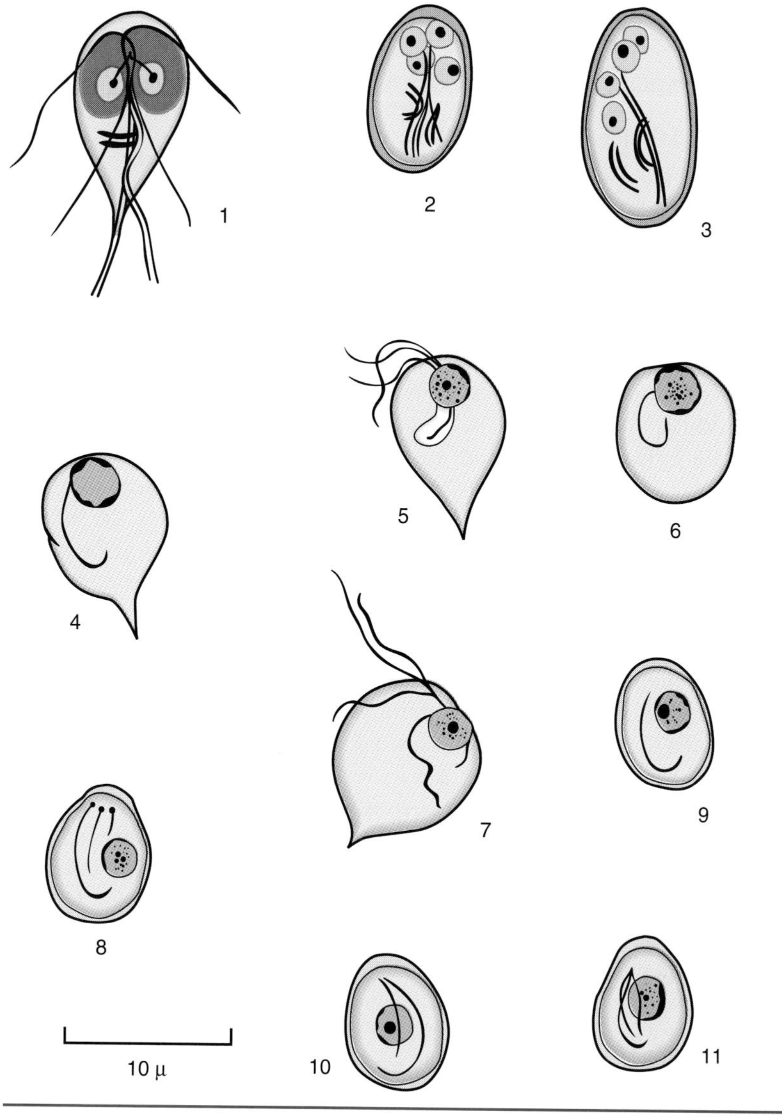

FIGURE 3-27 ■ *1, Giardia lamblia* trophozoite; *2, 3, G. lamblia* cysts; *4, 5, 6, 7, Chilomastix mesnili* trophozoites showing variation in structural detail, which may be seen in permanent preparations; *8, 9, 10, 11, C. mesnili* cysts (*3, 4, 6, 7, 9, 10,* and *11* show diagnostic features only).

pattern, with 1 to 3 weeks of a high excretion rate alternating with a shorter period of low excretion. With this in mind, it is well to collect specimens at intervals some days apart, if initially the results of examinations are negative. Diagnosis may also be made by identifying trophozoites in duodenal fluid obtained by intubation, or string test (Enterotest),★ or by biopsy. In addition, giardiasis may be diagnosed by detecting *Giardia* cysts or trophozoites in fecal specimens by ELISA or immunofluorescence and by detecting *Giardia* fecal antigen by counterimmunoelectrophoresis (CIE) and ELISA.

★Enterotest is available from HDC Corporation, 628 Gibraltar Court, Milpitas, CA 95035; (408) 942-7340; www.hdccorp.com.

The following characteristics are of value in the identification of *Giardia lamblia*:

I. *Trophozoites, unstained*	Suggestive: progressive, "falling leaf" motility; pear-shaped body with attenuated posterior end
II. *Trophozoites, stained*	Diagnostic: nuclei in the area of a sucking disk; the two median bodies posterior to the sucking disk; typical arrangement of axonemes
III. *Cysts, unstained*	Suggestive: ovoid body shape, numerous refractile threads in cytoplasm
IV. *Cysts, stained*	Diagnostic: four nuclei; four median bodies; jumble of axonemes

Symptoms and Pathogenesis. Long considered nonpathogenic and often found in completely asymptomatic persons, there is now abundant evidence of the pathogenic potential of *Giardia*. Children are more frequently affected than adults, although all ages may exhibit symptoms ranging from mild diarrhea, flatulence, anorexia, crampy abdominal pains, and epigastric tenderness to steatorrhea and full-blown malabsorption syndrome. A prepatent period of 10 to 36 days before organisms could be detected in the stools has been observed in groups of students, in whom the mean incubation period before clinical illness was but 8 days. Like celiac disease in children and its adult counterpart, nontropical sprue, severe giardiasis may be marked by the production of copious light-colored, fatty stools, hypoproteinemia with hypogammaglobulinemia, folic acid and fat-soluble vitamin deficiencies, and changes in the architecture of the intestinal villi. In sprue and celiac disease, a gluten-free diet effects a cure, while in giardiasis, administration of quina-crine does the same. Achlorhydria may predispose to symptomatic giardial infections, as may hypogammaglobulinemia, or a relative deficiency in secretory IgA in the small bowel, even in the presence of normal serum immunoglobulin levels. Some reports have indicated an excess of blood group A in children infected with *Giardia*; another study was unable to confirm any such association in adults infected on visits to an endemic area. Others believe that bacterial colonization of the jejunum (as seen in tropical sprue) potentiates the damage done by the giardias and may be responsible for the development of symptomatic malabsorption. Lactose intolerance, apparently precipitated by *Giardia* infection, may persist after eradication of the parasites.

Spontaneous eradication of infection in time seems the general rule in giardiasis. The possible role of T-cell activity in this regard is suggested by the persistence of infection by *Giardia muris* in hypothymic (nude) mice derived from strains that initially were characterized by rapid elimination of this parasite. Lymphoid cells have been shown by scanning electron microscopy to migrate into the intestinal lumen and attach to *Giardia* trophozoites during clearance from the intestine in normal adult mice. Macrophages isolated from intestinal Peyer's patches were able to ingest trophozoites of *Giardia* in vitro, suggesting their role in host defense in giardiasis.

Another report describes the capability of normal human milk to kill trophozoites of *Giardia* and *E. histolytica* in vitro. The killing activity was not dependent on secretory immunoglobulin A (IgA) and co-chromatographed with an unusual lipase that is present in human milk but not in the milk of lower mammals. However, a survey in India of secretory IgA in *Giardia*-infected and noninfected mothers revealed significantly higher titers in the milk of infected mothers and significantly fewer *Giardia*-infected infants (16% versus 63% in noninfected mothers). The killing of *G. lamblia* trophozoites by the lipase of milk from nonimmune humans is due to the release of free fatty acids from milk triglycerides by the action of bile salts. Human milk, therefore, may be instrumental in affording protection against intestinal protozoan parasites to breast-fed babies.

In some patients, biopsy of the jejunum reveals shortening and blunting of the villi, reduction in height of the columnar epithelial cells of the mucosa, and hypercellularity of the lamina propria. Even total villous atrophy has been reported. Others have found these changes primarily in patients with hypogammaglobulinemia. Using the same technique of jejunal biopsy, but with special stains, mucosal invasion by *Giardia* has been noted, and penetration into mucosal cells has been demonstrated by electron micrography. It is by no means clear what relationship mucosal or cellular invasion by the parasite bears to the pathophysiology of giardial infection. Radiographs of the affected small bowel show a picture characteristic of malabsorptive states, with mucosal edema and segmentation of the barium (Fig. 3-28). Giardiasis of the pancreas with reversible pancreatic exocrine dysfunction has been reported in an elderly woman with diabetes.

Epidemiology. *Giardia* is worldwide in distribution. In the United States, it is the most common parasitic infection, and it is considered to be a major cause of diarrheal outbreaks from contaminated water supplies. It is affected by much the same socioeconomic factors that influence the distribution of *E. histolytica*. Giardiasis should be considered in the differential diagnosis of any "traveler's diarrhea." The first recorded waterborne outbreak of giardiasis involved travelers to St. Petersburg, Russia. Numerous less prolonged outbreaks have been reported from the United States and elsewhere. In some of these, it has been possible to recover cysts from the water supply. In an outbreak in the state of Washington, researchers found cysts in the filtered and chlorinated municipal water supply, and on strong epidemiologic grounds they implicated infected beavers in the watershed as the source of this outbreak. *Giardia* has also been found in beavers, muskrats, and water voles from other localities, and these observations may provide an explanation for those infections seen occasionally in backpackers and mountain climbers who have drunk from mountain streams in areas where the possibility of a human source seems remote. Cross-species transmission studies have demonstrated that beavers and muskrats can be infected with *Giardia* cysts obtained from humans. Surveillance for waterborne diseases in Colorado from 1980 to 1983 implicated *Giardia* in 9 of the 18 outbreaks. *Giardia* also was implicated in an outbreak of diarrheal illness in Utah following spring thaw flooding and possible contamination of a public water supply.

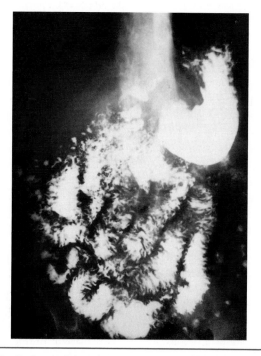

FIGURE 3-28 ■ Giardiasis. Small bowel series showing mucosal swelling, distorted pattern, and fragmentation of barium column. (Courtesy of Dr. Herman Zaiman.)

Day care centers have been implicated as a major site of significant endemic giardiasis and transmission. A report on severe giardiasis in the United States by the Centers for Disease Control and Prevention identified two high-risk groups: children younger than 5 years of age and women of childbearing age. These two groups share an exposure to *Giardia* infection that occurs in children in day care centers. In the United States, approximately 65% of all women with a child younger than 1 year of age are in the workforce, and about 60% of these children are cared for in day care homes or day care centers.

Early isoenzyme studies indicate at least several zymodemes of *G. lamblia*. These may prove to be useful epidemiologic markers. Other studies that have shown that *Giardia* obtained from different mammalian hosts share multiple isoenzymes throw in doubt the validity of assigning *Giardia* species solely on the basis of host. Additional isoenzyme characterizations of *Giardia* isolates in Switzerland suggest that domestic animals (cattle, sheep, dog) may serve as reservoirs for human infection and that cross-transmission between humans and animals is likely to occur.

Sexual practices, particularly anal-oral contact, may favor transmission of this parasite. Several reports document an increased prevalence among homosexual males.

Treatment. Metronidazole (Flagyl) and tinidazole are first-line agents for treatment, and nitazoxanide is recently available in a liquid formulation suitable for children. Additional effective therapies are albendazole (Hall and Nahar, 1993) and mebendazole (Al-Waili and Hasan, 1992).

Prevention. In general, the precautions that were mentioned in connection with the prevention of amebiasis are applicable to giardial infection. Because *Giardia* has been demonstrated to be able to withstand filtration and chlorination of the usual sort, it would seem desirable (though perhaps impractical) to guard against the contamination of municipal watersheds, if not by beavers and other water rodents at least by human carriers. For purification of small supplies of drinking water, a saturated solution of iodine (see footnote page 36), *used double strength*, is effective in killing *Giardia* cysts with a 20-minute exposure at 20°C (68°F). Of the many portable water purification systems available to campers and backpackers, those that use iodine solutions are the most effective, provided the directions are followed precisely.

Chilomastix mesnili

As far as is known, *Chilomastix* is not pathogenic to humans. It must, however, be differentiated from *Giardia* and from the other flagellates occasionally seen in stool specimens. The trophozoites of *Chilomastix* (see Fig. 3-27; Plate IV, 4, 5) are elongate, tapering toward the posterior end. They measure 10 to 20 μm in length. At the anterior, broad end of the body are three flagella, by means of which the animal moves in a directional manner. In fresh specimens one readily distinguishes the flagella and a groove running in a spiral along the length of the body. The stained trophozoites are characterized by a single nucleus near the origin of the anterior flagella; the cytostome, or oral depression, bordered by cytostomal fibrils; and a short flagellum, which is directed posteriorly within the cytostomal area. The most prominent of the cytostomal fibrils, curving posteriorly around the cytostome, resembles a shepherd's crook. The three flagella seldom take a distinct stain. Nuclear chromatin may appear in the form of granules; in addition, it may form plaques applied to the nuclear membrane. A small, central or eccentric karyosome may at times be observed.

Cysts of *Chilomastix* are from 6 to 10 μm long, their width being somewhat less (Plate IV, 6). At the anterior pole of the cyst is a nipplelike protuberance that gives this stage a characteristic lemon shape not seen in any of the other intestinal protozoa. In stained preparations a single, large nucleus may be distinguished, with the chromatin frequently condensed to appear as a large central karyosome. The curved cytostomal fibrils are usually quite prominent and may even be apparent in iodine-stained preparations (see Fig. 3-35);

in specimens particularly well stained with hematoxylin, the recurrent flagellum may be seen between the cytoplasm and the cyst wall at the anterior end of the organism.

The following characteristics are of value in the identification of *Chilomastix mesnili*:

I. *Trophozoites, unstained*	Diagnostic: anterior flagella; a spiral groove
II. *Trophozoites, stained*	Diagnostic: single anterior nucleus; cytostome with curved, shepherd's crook fibril; no costa or undulating membrane (see *Trichomonas*)
III. *Cysts, unstained*	Diagnostic: protuberance at one end of cyst (lemon shape)
IV. *Cysts, stained*	Diagnostic: body shape, as above; single large nucleus; curved cytostomal fibril

Trichomonas hominis

There is little evidence that *T. hominis* is pathogenic for humans. It is, however, indicative of direct fecal contamination, as it does not form cysts. Living trophozoites are 7 to 15 μm long; they move about rapidly, with a jerky and nondirectional motion, and are difficult to observe until slowed down. *T. hominis* (Fig. 3-29) has four anterior flagella plus a recurrent

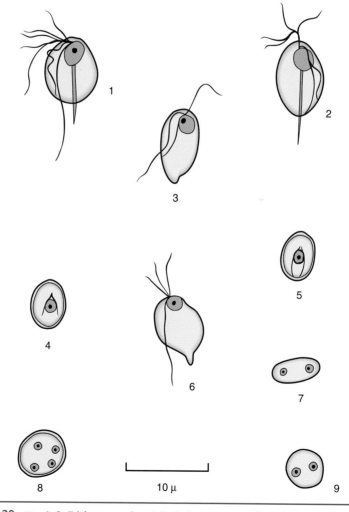

FIGURE 3-29 ■ *1, 2, Trichomonas hominis; 3, Retortamonas intestinalis* trophozoite; *4, 5, R. intestinalis* cysts; *6, Enteromonas hominis* trophozoite; *7, 8, 9, E. hominis* cysts (*2, 4, 5, 7, 8,* and *9* show diagnostic features only).

flagellum that arises anteriorly and parallels the body, running to the posterior end. It forms the outer edge of the undulating membrane, a thin sheet of protoplasm that joins the body along a line marked by the presence of a curved, thin rod called the costa. The costa is about the same length as the undulating membrane and, as it stains well, is an important diagnostic characteristic. The recurrent flagellum, which forms the outer edge of the undulating membrane, projects behind the body as a free flagellum. The undulating membrane imparts a rotatory motion to the organism, while the anterior flagella serve for propulsion. The single nucleus is situated at the anterior end of the body, close to the origin of the anterior flagella. Its chromatin is unevenly distributed, and a small karyosome may be observed. A slender rod, the axostyle, extends through the body from the anterior to the posterior end. It is sharply pointed and protrudes prominently beyond the posterior end of the body.

In living trophozoites, the wavelike motion of the undulating membrane may be observed when the organisms are moving slowly or are at rest. The activity of the anterior flagella may be distinguished even if the individual flagella cannot be seen. The posteriorly protruding axostyle, which may be seen even when other structures are not distinguishable, is diagnostic.

It is more difficult to identify stained organisms than living material. In a routine iron hematoxylin preparation, the flagella and undulating membrane do not stain well, but the single nucleus at the anterior end and the costa are diagnostic. No other intestinal protozoan possesses the latter structure. The costa stains intensely with iron hematoxylin, but careful focusing is needed to demonstrate it. The trichrome stain is superior to hematoxylin to bring out the flagella and axostyle.

The following characteristics are of value in the identification of *Trichomonas hominis*:

I. *Trophozoites, unstained*	Diagnostic: an undulating membrane; an axostyle protruding through the posterior part of the body
II. *Trophozoites, stained*	Diagnostic: the costa; the axostyle

Trichomonas vaginalis

Closely related to *T. hominis*, yet morphologically and physiologically distinct from it, is *T. vaginalis* (Figs. 3-30 to 3-32). The usual size range of this parasite is apparently 5 to 15 μm, but it may reach a length of 30 μm. In general appearance these flagellates are very similar to *T. hominis*, from which they differ in having a short undulating membrane that extends only about half the distance to the posterior end of the body, with no free flagellum. The life cycle of *T. vaginalis* is illustrated in Figure 3-30.

While it is possible to distinguish *T. vaginalis* from *T. hominis* on morphologic grounds, this is not a practical necessity, because the two organisms are site specific. Numerous attempts have been made to introduce *T. hominis* into the vagina, but without success. When *T. vaginalis* is similarly introduced, a high percentage of infections results. Therefore, a specific identification may be made on the basis of finding a trichomonad in the vaginal secretions. Jerky, nondirectional motility characterizes this species, as it does *T. hominis*, and if the organisms are observed under the high dry power of the microscope, when they have become sufficiently slowed down, the undulating membrane is clearly visible.

Symptoms and Pathogenesis. Trichomoniasis is a common sexually transmitted disease that causes an estimated 2 to 3 million symptomatic infections per year among sexually active women in the United States. Vaginal discharge is the most common complaint associated with vaginal trichomoniasis. The discharge is frequently profuse and is often associated with burning, itching, or chafing. When viewed through a speculum, the vaginal mucosa is sometimes diffusely hyperemic, with bright red punctate lesions, sometimes only patchily hyperemic and not infrequently normal in appearance. Frequency of urination and dysuria are the commonest associated symptoms, and urethral involvement is found in a

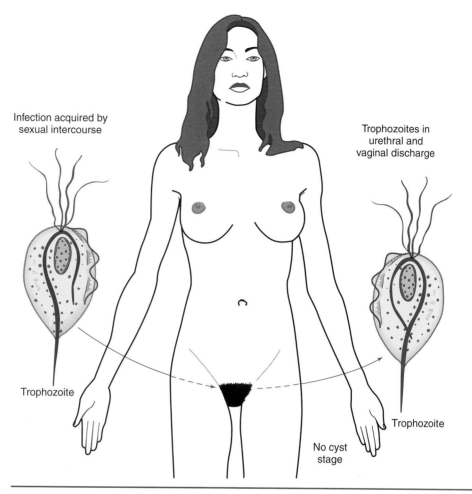

FIGURE 3-30 ▓ Life cycle of *Trichomonas vaginalis*.

large proportion of cases. Cystitis may occur in a small portion of cases. A relationship between this infection and cervical carcinoma has been suggested.

T. vaginalis also may be an important cofactor in amplifying HIV transmission (Sorvillo et al., 2001). The pathology induced by *T. vaginalis* infection in a person co-infected with HIV increases HIV shedding. Studies in Africa have indicated that *T. vaginalis* infection may increase the rate of HIV transmission by approximately twofold.

T. vaginalis has been isolated from the respiratory tract of infants with respiratory disease and from the conjunctivae of several infants with conjunctivitis. Evidence suggests that the infants were infected during vaginal delivery of an infected mother.

In males infection is frequently asymptomatic, but more severe symptoms are likely to be seen when the infection involves the prostate and seminal vesicles or higher parts of the urogenital tract. A thin discharge, frequently containing trichomonads, may be observed, with dysuria and nocturia. The prostate may be enlarged and tender, and there is sometimes associated epididymitis.

Studies in vitro of *T. vaginalis* with mammalian cell cultures have demonstrated a contact-dependent cytopathic effect. Organisms were able to kill target cells by direct contact without phagocytosis. At least four trichomonad surface proteins have been identified in cell adherence. Additional, *T. vaginalis* has been shown to produce a cell-detaching factor that causes detachment of cultured mammalian cells and likely the sloughing of vaginal epithelial cells seen in clinical disease. The amount of cell-detaching factor produced by the flagellates

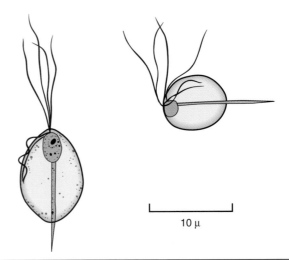

10 μ

FIGURE 3-31   ■   *Trichomonas vaginalis* as seen in permanently stained preparation.

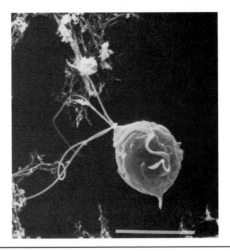

FIGURE 3-32   ■   Scanning electron micrograph of *Trichomonas vaginalis* from culture. Bar is 10 μm. (Photomicrograph by Dr. Thomas B. Cole, Jr.)

appeared to correlate with the severity of the clinical infection and therefore may be a virulence marker in *T. vaginalis* pathogenesis. Experimental evidence also suggests that the symptoms of trichomoniasis may be influenced by the vaginal concentration of estrogens; the greater the concentration the less severe the symptoms. β-Estradiol was shown to decrease the activity of cell-detaching factor and may explain why intravaginal estradiol pellets ameliorate the clinical symptoms of *Trichomonas* vaginitis by providing high local concentrations of estrogens.

Diagnosis. Diagnosis is by demonstration of the trichomonads, most commonly in wet film preparations although they may readily be recognized in Papanicolaou smears. Specimens for examination may best be obtained through a vaginal speculum using a cotton-tipped applicator stick. If the applicator is placed for a short time in a tube containing a small quantity of 5% glucose in normal saline before examination, the organisms are less likely to be rounded up and motionless under the microscope. Phase-contrast microscopy is especially desirable for observing the flagella and undulating membrane of living *T. vaginalis*.

"Rippling" of the undulating membrane can be seen for several hours after the organisms have stopped moving. Examination of urethral discharge in the female may yield positive results when no organisms can be found in the vaginal discharge. In the male, the diagnosis is made by examination of urethral discharge, prostatic secretions, or centrifuged urine. Culture methods may be employed and sometimes increase the percentage of positive identifications. Of the various commercial culture media available, modified Diamond's medium (see Chapter 14) consistently supports growth of *T. vaginalis*.★ Modified thioglycolate medium, supplemented with yeast extract, horse serum, and antimicrobial agents, was found to be as efficient as Diamond's medium in recovering *T. vaginalis* from clinical specimens and may be used as a readily available, low-cost substitute for the standard medium. The combination of wet-mount examination and culture remains the standard approach for detecting *T. vaginalis* in patient samples.

Commercially available kits for the immunodection of *T. vaginalis* antigens in clinical specimens include the following types of tests: enzyme immunoassay (EIA), direct fluorescent antibody (DFA), latex agglutination (LA), and DNA probe.

Treatment. Metronidazole (Flagyl) is generally effective in vaginal trichomoniasis. As the infection can be transmitted by sexual intercourse, treatment of the sexual partner should be considered. Resistance to the drug has been reported from a number of areas but usually responds to higher doses of the drug (Lossick et al., 1986). Metronidazole also might be effective in cases of nonspecific urethritis in which *T. vaginalis* can be demonstrated. Metronidazole should not be used in the first trimester of pregnancy; during the second and third trimesters or for nursing mothers it should be employed only when local palliative measures fail. Infants beyond the fourth week of life with symptomatic trichomoniasis can be treated with metronidazole 10 to 30 mg/kg daily for 5 to 8 days.

Trichomonas tenax

T. tenax, which has also been called *Trichomonas buccalis*, resembles *T. vaginalis* more closely than *T. hominis*. It is a small organism, averaging only 6 to 10 μm in length. Like *E. gingivalis*, it occurs most frequently in pyorrheal pockets and tonsillar crypts, and it is sometimes aspirated to set up a transitory bronchial or pulmonary infection. Since 1942, 36 cases of pulmonary trichomoniasis have been reported. A survey of 38 dental patients in clinical practice revealed six (16%) with oral *T. tenax*. None of the clinical specimens was positive for *E. gingivalis*.

The only treatment necessary is that directed at the underlying condition, if any.

Dientamoeba fragilis

Until fairly recently *Dientamoeba* (Fig. 3-33; Plate III, 4, 5) was considered by most parasitologists to be an ameba, albeit unique among the intestinal amebae in its binucleate condition and in the absence of a cyst stage. Despite the lack of flagella, various protozoologists have recognized its flagellate affinities. It remained for electron microscope studies to confirm the flagellate relationships of this organism, which is classified among the trichomonads.

Dientamoeba is known to live in mucosal crypts of the large intestine and has been seen rarely to ingest red blood cells; apparently it never invades the tissues. The majority of organisms are binucleate. The binucleate form is considered to be in an arrested telophase, and in optimally stained specimens an extranuclear spindle can be seen extending between the two nuclei. Frequently, as many as 80% of them are seen in the binucleate form, although at times the percentage may be considerably lower. Occasional forms are seen with three or four nuclei.

Dientamoeba organisms range in diameter from 3 μm to as much as 18 μm but are generally within the range of 7 to 12 μm. Pseudopodia are hyaline, broad, and leaflike in appearance,

★Available as a freeze-dried medium (ATCC Medium PARA-2154) from the American Type Culture Collection (ATCC), P.O. Box 1549, Manassas, VA 20108; (703) 365-2700; www.atcc.org.

FIGURE 3-33   ■   *1, 2, Dientamoeba fragilis,* mono- and binucleate trophozoites.

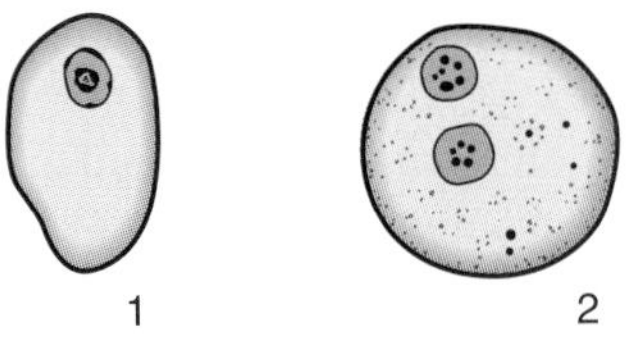

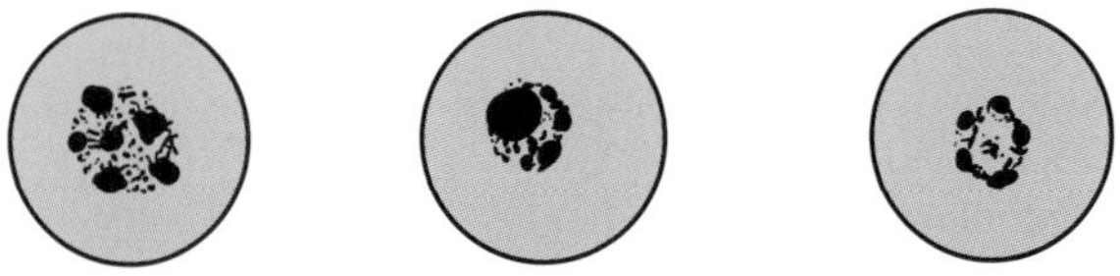

FIGURE 3-34   ■   *Dientamoeba fragilis.* Variations in nuclear structure.

with characteristic serrated margins. Motility is progressive, and organisms are quite active in freshly passed stools but round up quickly on cooling. Unstained, they are inconspicuous, especially if rounded and motionless. Vacuoles containing ingested bacteria may be seen scattered through the cytoplasm; nuclei are not visible in the living trophozoite. When stained, *Dientamoeba* is identified on the basis of a high percentage of binucleate forms and the typical nuclear structure (Fig. 3-34). The nuclear membrane is delicate, and there is no peripheral chromatin. In the center of the nucleus lies a large mass composed of four to eight separate chromatin granules, usually arranged symmetrically. With good iron hematoxylin stains, the separate granules are readily observed. Trichrome stain is less likely to reveal the separate granules of chromatin. Mononucleate forms may be confused with *E. nana* if the individual chromatin granules are not obvious, but binucleate forms are recognized without difficulty.

The following characteristics are of value in the identification of *Dientamoeba fragilis:*

I. *Trophozoites, unstained*	Not characteristic
II. *Trophozoites, stained*	Diagnostic: high percentage of binucleate trophozoites; nuclei without peripheral chromatin and with four to eight chromatin granules in a central mass

Symptoms. A number of reports indicate that *D. fragilis* causes symptoms in some infected persons; estimates of the incidence of symptomatic infection vary from about 15 to as high as 27%. Table 3-2 lists the frequency of various symptoms in patients thought to have pure *D. fragilis* infections, both from a series of 255 patients reported by Yang and Scholten (1977) and from the literature. A number of other symptoms were listed, including anal pruritus and low-grade eosinophilia (perhaps of significance in relation to a current theory about the mode of transmission, discussed below).

Epidemiology. No cyst stage is known for this parasite, and attempts to transmit the infection orally have failed. In 1940 Dobell, one of the first to recognize *Dientamoeba* as a flagellate, suggested (by analogy with the flagellate *Histomonas meleagridis,* transmitted among poultry via the egg of the nematode *Heterakis gallinae*) that transmission might take place by way of the egg of an intestinal nematode. Various workers, including Yang and Scholten (1977), have noted an impressively greater frequency of association between infection with *Dientamoeba* and infection with *Enterobius vermicularis* than would be expected on the basis of chance. Structures resembling *Dientamoeba* have been found in the eggs of *Enterobius,* but only in those from persons infected with both parasites.

TABLE 3-2 ■ **Prevalence of Various Symptoms of *Dientamoeba fragilis* Infection**

Symptom	Percentage of Patients	
	Y. and S. Series	*Y. and S. Literature Review*
Diarrhea	58.4	42.5
Abdominal pain	53.7	46.2
Bloody, mucoid, or loose stools	9.8	22.6
Flatulence	5.9	19.9
Fatigue or weakness	5.9	13.4
Alternating diarrhea, constipation	3.9	13.4
Nausea or vomiting	3.5	20.4
Weight loss	3.1	10.2

Data from Yang J, Scholten T. *Am J Trop Med Hyg.* 1977; *26*:16–22.

The reported prevalence of *Dientamoeba* infection ranges from less than 1.5% to nearly 20%, but it may be much higher in some population groups or among institutionalized persons. Prevalence of *Dientamoeba* was found to be 52.3% among 220 members of a semicommunal group in Los Angeles and 3.1% among a sample of 415 persons surveyed as a part of routine health examination in Oakland, California. Among a series of more than 600 homosexual men from the latter area, the prevalence was found to be about 1%, lending support to the idea that this parasite is not transmitted by the conventional fecal-oral route. It is probable that the true prevalence in most areas is unknown; higher prevalence rates are found when stool specimens are preserved in polyvinyl alcohol (PVA) fixative immediately after passage.

Treatment. Iodoquinol is usually effective. Tetracycline is an alternative. Paromomycin (Humatin) has been found effective in cases refractory to those drugs. Paromomycin is an aminoglycoside antibiotic that inhibits protein synthesis. Gastrointestinal side effects of treatment are not uncommon; eighth nerve and renal damage are rare.

Enteromonas hominis

The small flagellate *Enteromonas* (see Fig. 3-29) is encountered but rarely. Trophozoites are 4 to 10 μm long. The body is broadly oval anteriorly and somewhat attenuated posteriorly. There are three anterior flagella, by means of which the organisms move in a rapid, jerky fashion. The fourth flagellum is directed posteriorly. In living specimens little can be observed other than the general body shape, the anterior flagellar movement, and the trailing flagellum. In stained preparations, the single nucleus is seen near the anterior end. There is a distinct nuclear membrane and a large central karyosome.

Cysts are inconspicuous, usually ellipsoid, and 6 to 8 μm long. In fresh specimens they are likely to be mistaken for yeasts. Stained cysts may be seen to possess one to four nuclei, generally with a predominance of the binucleate condition. Cyst nuclei have the same structure as those of the trophozoites. Cysts of *Enteromonas* are of about the same shape as those of *E. nana*, and the size ranges of cysts of the two species overlap. A predominance of binucleate cysts of small size is highly suggestive of *Enteromonas*.

The following characteristics are of value in the identification of *Enteromonas hominis*:

I. *Trophozoites, unstained*	Diagnostic: anterior flagella; trailing flagellum but no undulating membrane
II. *Trophozoites, stained*	Suggestive: absence of costa, axostyle, or cytostomal fibrils; single nucleus with large central karyosome; small size
III. *Cysts, unstained*	Not characteristic
IV. *Cysts, stained*	Suggestive: oval shape; one to four nuclei; with predominance of binucleate forms; small size

Retortamonas intestinalis

Retortamonas (see Fig. 3-29) is not frequently seen. The trophozoites are ovoid or tear shaped and move rapidly by means of two anterior flagella. Body length ranges from 4 to 10 μm. A cytostome extends from near the anterior end to about half the length of the organism. In unstained trophozoites it is sometimes possible to see the two anterior flagella and cytostome. In stained preparations a relatively large nucleus is seen at the anterior end. The nucleus contains a small, compact central karyosome; there is a layer of fine chromatin granules on the nuclear membrane. A fibril borders the cytostome.

This fibril does not have the shepherd's crook curve characteristic of *Chilomastix*.

The pear-shaped cysts are 4 to 7 μm long and up to 5 μm wide. They contain a single relatively large nucleus, frequently near the center. Two fibrils extend from the nuclear region to the attenuated end of the cyst. This fibrillar arrangement, suggesting a bird's beak, is quite characteristic. Unstained, they are difficult or impossible to identify.

The following characteristics are of value in the identification of *Retortamonas intestinalis*:

I. *Trophozoites, unstained*	Diagnostic: a cytostome; two anterior flagella only; small size
II. *Trophozoites, stained*	Diagnostic: large nucleus with small central karyosome, fine granules of peripheral chromatin; cytostomal fibril (not in form of a shepherd's crook); small size
III. *Cysts, unstained*	Not characteristic
IV. *Cysts, stained*	Suggestive: pear shape; small size
	Diagnostic: bird-beak fibrillar arrangement seen in small, pear-shaped cysts

The appearance of the more common protozoa discussed earlier, and of *Blastocystis hominis* (commonly confused with the intestinal protozoa), as stained with iodine, is illustrated in Figure 3-35.

The Ciliate

Balantidium coli is the only member of its phylum to parasitize humans. The organisms inhabit the large intestine, cecum, and terminal ileum. They are chiefly lumen dwellers, subsisting on bacteria, but they may penetrate the intestinal mucosa to cause ulceration (Figs. 3-36 and 3-37).

Trophozoites of *Balantidium* (Fig. 3-38) have been reported to attain a length of 200 μm. Two size ranges are consistently seen. The smaller organisms average 42 to 60 μm long by 30 to 40 μm wide, while the larger range from 90 to 120 μm by 60 to 80 μm. Conjugation occurs only between "large" and "small" individuals, never between two of the same size range. The body shape is ovoid, somewhat flattened on one side. A funnel-shaped cytostome opens on the flattened side, near the anterior end. The body is covered with cilia, which are especially long and stout near the cytostome. Unstained, the organisms are readily recognized because of their size, ciliary covering, and motility like that of a thrown football. On stained preparations the characteristic two nuclei of a ciliate may be observed. The larger nucleus, or macronucleus, situated near the middle of the body may be spherical, ellipsoid, elongate, curved, or kidney shaped. The micronucleus, involved in genetics and cell division, is spherical and small and lies quite close to the macronucleus. Both nuclei stain intensely with the ordinary stains. Food vacuoles and contractile vacuoles may be seen in the cytoplasm.

The spherical or ellipsoid cysts are about 50 to 75 μm long. There is a thick, refractile cyst wall, within which the organism may be seen. In some specimens, newly encysted, the cilia are still present and the organisms may be seen slowly rotating. After a longer period of encystment, the cilia disappear. In stained specimens the macronucleus can usually be seen within the cyst wall, but other structures usually are not observed.

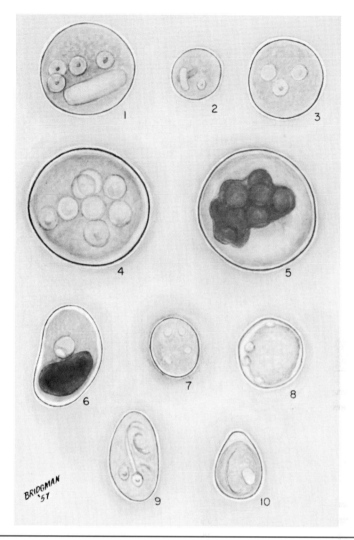

FIGURE 3-35 ■ Cysts of intestinal protozoa and *Blastocystis* stained with iodine.
1, 3, Entamoeba histolytica; 2, Entamoeba hartmanni; 4, Entamoeba coli; 5, E. coli with glycogen
mass obscuring nuclei; *6, Iodamoeba bütschlii; 7, Endolimax nana; 8, Blastocystis hominis;
9, Giardia lamblia; 10, Chilomastix mesnili.*

The following characteristics are of value in the identification of *Balantidium coli*:

I. *Trophozoites, unstained*	Diagnostic: ciliary covering
II. *Trophozoites, stained*	Diagnostic: macronucleus and micronucleus
III. *Cysts, unstained*	Diagnostic: cyst containing ciliated organism
IV. *Cysts, stained*	Diagnostic: macronucleus and micronucleus

Symptoms and Pathogenesis. *Balantidium* produces the enzyme hyaluronidase, which
presumably facilitates its tissue invasion. Secondary bacterial infection may occur following
mucosal invasion by *Balantidium*. After bacterial invasion, a striking inflammatory reaction is
noted around *Balantidium* trophozoites present in tissue. Many patients are asymptomatic
carriers of the infection; clinical balantidiasis may closely simulate severe amebic dysentery,
or there may be only mild colitis and diarrhea. Extraintestinal spread to the mesenteric
nodes, liver, pleura, lungs, and urogenital tract has been reported but is most uncommon.
A case of fatal balantidial infection was reported, in which peritonitis followed perforation

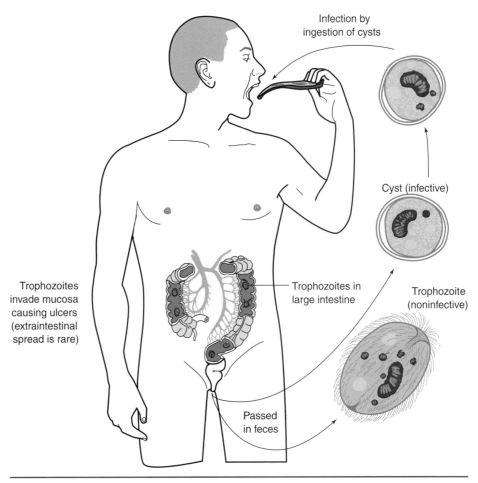

Infection by
ingestion of cysts

Cyst (infective)

Trophozoites in
large intestine

Trophozoite
(noninfective)

Trophozoites
invade mucosa
causing ulcers
(extraintestinal
spread is rare)

Passed
in feces

FIGURE 3-36 ■ Life cycle of *Balantidium coli.*

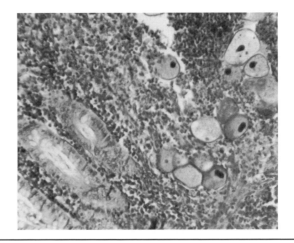

FIGURE 3-37 ■ *Balantidium coli* parasites in intestinal ulcer. (Photomicrograph by Zane Price.)

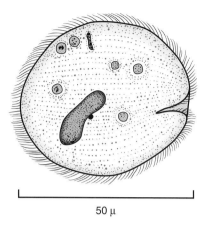

50 μ

FIGURE 3-38 ■ *Balantidium coli* trophozoite, stained specimen.

of the appendix; pulmonary involvement also occurred. An additional case of *Balantidium* appendicitis has been reported in the literature.

Epidemiology. In the United states, balantidiasis is sometimes encountered in epidemic form in mental hospitals, but it is almost unknown in the general population. Worldwide in its distribution, *Balantidium* is rare in most areas, although epidemic outbreaks are occasionally seen. A morphologically identical organism occurs in hogs, and epidemic outbreaks may follow its successful transfer from porcine to human host. This must not be a common occurrence because attempts to infect humans with the porcine strain have not been successful.

Treatment. Oxytetracycline (Terramycin) or iodoquinol, is usually effective in the treatment of this parasite.

The Apicomplexa (Sporozoa)

The intestinal sporozoa of man include *Isopora belli*, two species of *Sarcocystis*, *Cryptosporidium parvum*, and *Cyclospora cayetanensis*. *Toxoplasma gondii* is an intestinal parasite of cats but not of humans. These parasites demonstrate the classic sporozoan alternation of asexual or schizogonic and sexual or sporogonic cycles. All are coccidian parasites.

ISOSPORA

Belonging to the coccidia, *Isospora* is closely related to members of the genus *Eimeria*, which cause disease in various domestic animals, to the ubiquitous *Toxoplasma*, and to *Sarcocystis*. While the life cycle of *Isospora* is not fully known, much can be deduced by analogy with related genera. *Isospora* is a parasite of the epithelial cells of the intestine, in which it may undergo repeated asexual development, with consequent destruction of the surface layer of considerable portions of the intestine. The parasites have been found by small bowel biopsy (Fig. 3-39). In addition to asexual stages, which serve to spread the infection within the bowel wall, sexual stages occur, and these culminate in oocysts passed in the feces.

Three species of *Isospora* have been recognized as human parasites. One of these, *I. natalensis*, has been reported only twice and will not be discussed further. The organisms formerly known as *I. hominis* are no longer considered to belong to this genus at all but to represent sexual stages of two species of *Sarcocystis*, *S. hominis* from cattle and *S. suihominis* from swine,

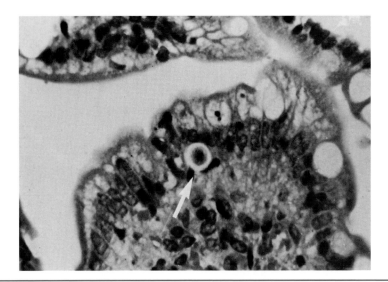

FIGURE 3-39 ■ *Isospora belli (arrow)* in duodenal biopsy. (From Forthal DN, Guest SS. *Isospora belli* enteritis in three homosexual men. *Am J Trop Med Hyg* 1984; *33*:1060–1064.)

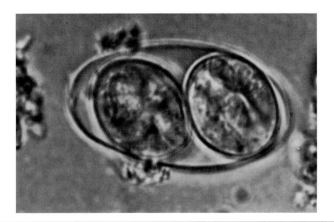

FIGURE 3-40 ■ *Isospora belli.* Oocyst containing two sporocysts with sporozoites. (Photomicrograph by Prof. John Gullberg.)

and are discussed under that heading. *I. belli* is a valid species and probably infects only humans.

Isospora belli

I. belli is characterized by release of immature oocysts from the intestinal wall, so that in this species all stages in development of the oocyst occur in the stool. Immature oocysts are ellipsoid, or at times spindle-shaped, with blunt ends. They average 30 μm in length by 12 μm in width. Contained in the immature oocyst is a spherical mass of protoplasm, which soon divides to form two sporoblasts. The sporoblasts, still within the oocyst, in turn develop heavy cyst walls and are known as sporocysts. Within each sporocyst, four curved, sausage-shaped sporozoites develop (Fig. 3-40). All stages, from immature oocysts containing nothing but an undivided mass of protoplasm to those containing fully developed sporocysts and sporozoites, may be seen in the feces. If in the immature condition when first passed, they will mature within 4 to 5 days to form sporozoites. The sporocysts are rarely seen broken out of the oocysts but measure approximately 11 by 9 μm.

Isospora oocysts may be seen on direct examination of the stool or may be detected in concentrates. They concentrate well with the zinc sulfate technique but are so light that they float even in the customary zinc sulfate–iodine mixture and are seen only if the area directly beneath the coverslip is examined carefully with reduced illumination. The Sheather's sugar flotation procedure, as used with *Cryptosporidium*, has been described as the most sensitive and accurate method for detecting *I. belli* oocysts in the feces. Unless iodine stained, the oocysts and contained material are transparent and very difficult to recognize.

A modified acid-fast procedure and auramine–rhodamine stains have been used to identify oocysts of *I. belli*. The modified acid-fast procedure is especially useful, as it is a simple staining technique and the sporoblasts within the oocysts stain a deep red. Although the oocyst wall itself does not stain, it usually is outlined by a stain precipitate. The duodenal string test (Enterotest) has been used to recover oocysts of *I. belli*.

The following characteristics are of value in identification of *Isospora belli*:

In fresh stool or concentrate, oocysts; either immature, or mature containing two sporocysts; average size 30 by 12 μm

---

Prior to the Second World War, infections with *Isospora* were considered to be exceedingly rare; however, during and since that conflict, large numbers of infections have been described from all parts of the world. It is now realized that while *Isospora* is not easily recognized in the feces and is consequently seldom reported, it is not as rare as it was thought to be. Wherever a systematic search has been made for these parasites, they have been encountered.

Symptoms and Pathogenesis. Infections often are asymptomatic and self-limited, but a number of workers have reported symptoms ranging from mild gastrointestinal distress to severe dysentery with fatal consequences. Chronic diarrhea, vague or crampy abdominal pain, weight loss, weakness, malaise, and anorexia are clinical features of patients with isosporiasis. The infection may evoke eosinophilia, even in asymptomatic patients.

The loose, pale yellow, and foul-smelling stools are suggestive of a malabsorptive process. Fecal fat may be increased, and jejunal biopsy may reveal the villous atrophy commonly associated with the malabsorption syndrome. It will be remembered that this condition is also seen at times in giardiasis. Although infections are generally considered mild, oocysts have been reported to persist in stools for as long as 120 days.

Isospora infection is predominantly an infection of people in the developing world and can be a common presentation of HIV/AIDS.

Treatment. A trimethoprim-sulfamethoxazole combination effectively eliminates chronic *I. belli* infection in immunosuppressed persons, when given for 3 weeks (Whiteside et al., 1984). Combined pyrimethamine and sulfadiazine has also been shown to be an effective treatment. A study involving 32 patients with chronic isosporiasis and AIDS concluded that isosporiasis in patients with AIDS can be treated effectively with a 10-day course of trimethoprim-sulfamethoxazole and that subsequently recurrent disease can be prevented by ongoing prophylaxis with either trimethoprim-sulfamethoxazole or sulfadoxine-pyrimethamine (Pape et al., 1989). An alternative is pyrimethamine alone for treatment and for prophylaxis (Weiss et al., 1988).

SARCOCYSTIS SPP.

Human sarcocystosis remains rare, especially in temperate regions, despite the increasing awareness of human coccidial infection. Humans become infected by ingesting mature intramuscular cysts in pork (*S. suihominis*) or beef (*S. hominis*, referred to by some as *S. bovihominis*). Zoites, released following enzymatic breakdown of the cyst wall, penetrate the intestinal cells and transform into male microgametes or female macrogametes. After fertilization, the zygotes undergo oocyst wall formation and sporogony (formation of sporocysts and sporozoites). Sporulated oocysts contain two sporocysts, each with four sporozoites.

Unlike those of *I. belli*, the oocysts of *Sarcocystis* are usually passed in the feces fully developed and with the sporocysts ruptured out of the oocyst. The sporocysts may occur singly or may be seen in pairs in the feces, apparently held together by some sort of cement substance. Usually no vestige of an oocyst wall is seen. The sporocysts of *S. hominis* measure 13.1 to 17.0 by 7.7 to 10.8 μm. Those of *S. suihominis* measure 11.6 to 13.9 by 10.1 to 10.8 μm. Four sporozoites can be seen within the sporocyst. Humans are also the intermediate host for unknown species of *Sarcocystis* and, as such, harbor intramuscular cysts (see Chapter 5).

Intestinal sarcocystosis generally does not produce clinical symptoms. However, symptoms may occur following ingestion of raw beef or pork containing sarcocysts. Nausea, stomach pains, and diarrhea appeared within 3 to 6 hours after volunteers ingested infected beef, and symptoms were more pronounced in others who ingested infected uncooked pork. Symptoms continued for 48 hours, and in the group who ate the infected pork, mild stomach pains and diarrhea persisted for 2 to 3 weeks when sporocysts were being shed in the feces.

The following characteristics are of value in the identification of *Sarcocystis* organisms:

In fresh stool or concentrate, sporocysts; each containing four sporozoites

CRYPTOSPORIDIUM PARVUM

Accidental human infections with parasites that do not normally infect humans occur from time to time and will probably be seen more frequently as, on the one hand, diagnostic techniques improve and, on the other, we subject more and more people to an artificial depression of their normal immune mechanisms.

Cryptosporidium is a minute coccidian parasite with worldwide distribution. Twenty species of the parasite have been described from a variety of vertebrates including mammals, birds, reptiles, and fish. The species of *Cryptosporidium* that infects humans and most mammals is *C. parvum*. Molecular characterization of *Cryptosporidium* has divided *C. parvum* isolates into two main groups, one containing human isolates and the other containing mostly domestic animal isolates. Genetic analyses have identified an additional species, *C. hominis*, infecting humans (Morgan-Ryan et al., 2002). Human infection by rodent and feline cryptosporidia, *C. muris* and *C. felis*, respectively, has also been reported.

Development of *Cryptosporidium* occurs within the brush border of the epithelial cells of the intestine. Oocysts containing sporozoites are the infective stage. Upon ingestion, sporozoites are released and enter epithelial cells, where they undergo two asexual generations. Gametogony also occurs in the epithelial cells. Sporulated oocysts, containing four sporozoites each (but no sporocysts), are passed in the feces.

Cryptosporidiosis is diagnosed by identifying organisms (meronts containing merozoites and gamonts containing micro- and macrogametes) in intestinal biopsy material and by detecting oocysts in stool specimens. The duodenal string test (Enterotest) has also been used to recover oocysts. Organisms stain lightly with hematoxylin and eosin and appear as small (2 to 4 μm) round bodies on the mucosal surface of biopsy specimens (Fig. 3-41). With Masson's stain, a small red nucleus and blue cytoplasm can be distinguished in many of the organisms.

Oocysts may be concentrated by the modified zinc sulfate centrifugal flotation technique or by Sheather's sugar flotation procedure and examined under phase-contrast microscopy for the best results. Another concentration technique involves formalin–ethyl acetate sedimentation followed by layering and flotation over hypertonic sodium chloride solution to separate oocysts from stool debris. Oocysts appear as highly refractile spherical bodies (4 to 6 μm) containing one to six dark granules. Specimens may be stained using the modified acid-fast method (Fig. 3-42). Oocysts stain red, whereas fecal yeasts stain green. When counterstained

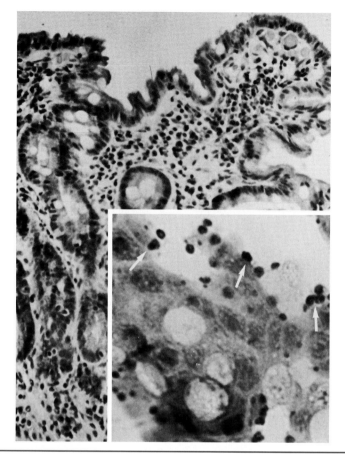

FIGURE 3-41 ▪ *Cryptosporidium* from jejunal biopsy. Inset at higher magnification showing organisms (*arrows*; hematoxylin and eosin stain). (Courtesy of Dr. Milton Bassis, Kaiser-Permanente Medical Center, San Francisco, CA.)

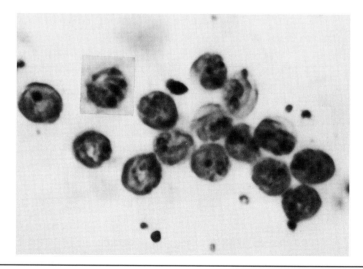

FIGURE 3-42 ▪ *Cryptosporidium* oocysts in feces (modified acid-fast stain).

with methylene blue, *Cryptosporidium* oocysts remain red but yeasts stain blue. With an iodine preparation, oocysts are colorless and yeasts are brown. *Cryptosporidium* can also be detected by staining air-dried, methanol-fixed fecal smears with Giemsa's stain. *Cryptosporidium* oocysts also have been detected in fecal specimens by an indirect immunofluorescence assay, a direct immunofluorescence procedure, and ELISA.

The following characteristics are of value in identification of *Cryptosporidium parvum*:

In duodenal biopsy specimen, gamonts or meronts, either immature or mature, containing four or eight merozoites; average size of gamonts and meronts 2 to 4 μm

In fresh stool or concentrate, oocysts, each containing four sporozoites (without sporocyst); average size 4 to 6 μm

Symptoms. Cryptosporidiosis is both human transmitted and a zoonosis; the first two human cases were reported in 1976. One patient was a 3-year-old child, previously in good health and with no evidence of altered immune status, in whom *Cryptosporidium* apparently produced severe but self-limited enterocolitis. The other was an immunosuppressed 39-year-old man who, in the course of treatment with prednisolone and cyclophosphamide, developed severe diarrhea with malabsorption. His condition cleared 2 weeks after discontinuation of cyclophosphamide treatment. Both cases were diagnosed by identifying organisms in intestinal biopsy specimens.

Symptomatic cryptosporidiosis in immunocompetent persons is characterized by self-limited diarrhea that usually lasts about 2 weeks and, less commonly, is accompanied by abdominal discomfort, anorexia, fever, nausea, and weight loss. Immunodeficient patients typically have severe diarrhea accompanied by these symptoms. In patients with AIDS, *Cryptosporidium* may cause life-threatening disease and has been found in sputum, in lung biopsy material, and in the biliary tract and has been associated with malabsorption. A case of fatal cryptosporidiosis was reported in a child with primary immunoglobulin deficiency. A case of cryptosporidiosis caused by *C. baileyi*, a species of avian hosts, has been reported in a patient with AIDS. Oocysts were found in the stool, and cryptosporidia were detected in autopsy material of the esophagus, entire intestinal tract, trachea, larynx, lungs, gallbladder, and urinary bladder. Oocysts recovered from the patient's feces failed to infect suckling mice but did infect all 1-day-old chicks that were inoculated.

Epidemiology. Cryptosporidiosis is now recognized as a significant cause of diarrhea in humans and, as a zoonosis, may be acquired from domestic animals. A survey in Victoria, Australia, revealed that *Cryptosporidium* was present in 4% of 884 hospital patients with gastroenteritis. Similarly, *Cryptosporidium* oocysts were present in 3% of 100 adults and 10% of 193 children with diarrhea in Rwanda, Central Africa; in 4% of 278 preschool children with diarrhea in Costa Rica; in 17% of 824 Haitian children younger than age 2 years; and in 33% of 84 children and 22% of 18 staff members of a day care center in Florida. A laboratory in Charleston, South Carolina, reported *Cryptosporidium* to be the most frequently encountered intestinal parasite during a year-long survey involving 582 stool specimens. *Giardia* was the second most common intestinal parasite identified. Overall findings have been that children are more commonly infected than are adults and that non–breast-fed infants have more cryptosporidiosis than breast-fed infants. Clinically, cryptosporidiosis appears much like giardiasis.

Environmental studies indicate that *Cryptosporidium* oocysts are present in 65% to 97% of surface water tested throughout the United States. *Cryptosporidium* is highly resistant to the chemicals used to treat drinking water, and its removal by filtration is important in the water treatment process. However, no current water treatment process can guarantee complete removal of oocysts. Consequently, a number of outbreaks of waterborne cryptosporidiosis have occurred in the United States in recent years including the spring 1993 outbreak in Milwaukee, Wisconsin, which affected more than 400,000 persons. The outbreaks have all occurred in communities where water utilities met state and federal standards for acceptable drinking water quality, and all surface water supplies had been filtered. Additional outbreaks of cryptosporidiosis have been associated with swimming in a wave pool in western Oregon, drinking fresh-presented apple cider at an agricultural fair in central Maine, and drinking unchlorinated deep well water in southeastern Washington state.

Because of the risk of acquiring a life-threatening disease, immunocompromised persons, especially those with AIDS, can take the following specific measures to help reduce the risk of waterborne cryptosporidiosis: boil drinking water for 1 minute (for 3 minutes at elevations greater than 6500 feet), or filter drinking water with devices that remove particles 1 μm and larger, or use bottled drinking water, especially water obtained from underground sources (i.e., springs or wells), which are less likely to be contaminated by *Cryptosporidium* oocysts. However, the boiling of water is the most certain method of killing *Cryptosporidium* oocysts. Experimental data show that high-temperature short-time pasteurization (71.7°C for 15 seconds) is sufficient to destroy the infectivity of *C. parvum* oocysts in water or milk.

Treatment. Cryptosporidiosis may be effectively treated with nitazoxanide but is usually a self-limited infection in immunocompetent patients. In AIDS patients there is not an effective treatment for cryptosporidiosis except treatment of the underlying HIV infection.

CYCLOSPORA CAYETANENSIS

Since 1986, cases of prolonged watery diarrhea associated with spherical bodies, 8 to 10 μm in diameter, in the stools of infected persons have been reported worldwide. The organisms, variously referred to as a large *Cryptosporidium*, a coccidian-like body, a cyanobacterium-like body, and a blue-green alga, have been named *Cyclospora cayetanensis* and the spherical bodies are oocysts. Cyclospora is a coccidian parasite that infects a range of vertebrates including reptiles, insectivores, and rodents. The species name recognizes Cayetano Heredia University in Lima, Peru, where the descriptive studies of the parasite were conducted.

Coccidian life cycles are quite varied, with some coccidians, such as *Cryptosporidium*, completing their development in a single host. Others, like *Isospora*, require a period of maturation outside the host, and still others, such as *Toxoplasma*, require a second host. The life cycle of *C. cayetanensis* is not known but appears to be similar to that of *Isospora* because the oocysts are excreted unsporulated and require a period of time outside the host to mature. Under laboratory conditions, sporulation occurs in 5 to 10 days. Mature oocysts contain two sporocysts, each with two crescent-shaped sporozoites. Molecular studies using phylogenetic analysis have shown that *Cyclospora* is closely related to *Eimeria*, more so than it is to *Cryptosporidium*.

The laboratory diagnosis of cyclosporiasis is made by microscopic identification of oocysts in fecal specimens (Fig. 3-43). Stool specimens may be concentrated using the formalin–ethyl acetate procedure; however, some reports claim that concentrated specimens have fewer oocysts than unconcentrated specimens. Oocysts are spherical, 8 to 10 μm in diameter, and, when first passed, unsporulated, with a greenish central morula, or mulberrylike mass, containing 6 to 9 refractile globules. By comparison, *Cryptosporidium* oocysts are spherical and measure 4 to 6 μm in diameter, and *Isospora* oocysts are oval and average 30 μm in length by 12 μm in width. Like the oocysts of *Cryptosporidium* and *Isospora*, the oocysts of *Cyclospora* are acid-fast, although their staining is variable, with some appearing unstained and others pink or dark red. An iodine solution will stain the internal globules brown. Under ultraviolet illumination, the oocysts of *Cyclospora* will autofluoresce and appear as bluish green circles. Asexual stages of *Cyclospora* have also been detected in jejunal biopsy specimens examined by light and electron microscopy.

The following characteristics are of value in identification of *Cyclospora cayetanensis*:

In fresh stool or concentrate, unsporulated oocysts, each with a greenish central morula containing 6 to 9 refractile globules; average size 8 to 10 μm

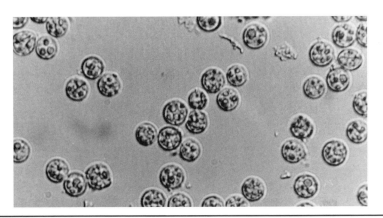

FIGURE 3-43 ■ *Cyclospora cayetanensis* unsporulated oocysts in feces (phase-contrast). (Courtesy of Dr. Ynes R. Ortega and Dr. Charles R. Sterling, University of Arizona, Tucson, AZ.)

Symptoms and Pathogenesis. Cyclosporiasis is clinically indistinguishable from cryptosporidiosis and isosporiasis. Illness is characterized by watery diarrhea that tends to occur in a relapsing or cyclical pattern. The incubation period ranges from 2 to 11 days and the average length of time for the long-lasting diarrhea is more than 3 weeks. Important associated symptoms include abdominal cramping, nausea, vomiting, decreased appetite, weight loss, low-grade fever, and fatigue. Although the illness is self-limited, it may last for weeks with profound fatigue, anorexia, and weight loss overshadowing the persisting diarrheal symptoms.

Among immunocompromised hosts, cyclosporiasis has been reported primarily from AIDS patients, in whom it causes prolonged, severe illness with a high rate of recurrence. Biliary disease has also been described in patients with AIDS.

Histological studies of tissue biopsies have identified the upper small bowel as the site of infection in the immunocompetent host. *Cyclospora* organisms have been observed within the cytoplasm of epithelial cells in jejunal biopsy specimens. Inflammatory changes, villous atrophy, and crypt hyperplasia of jejunal tissue have been reported from patients with diarrhea and *Cyclospora* oocysts in stool specimens. Other *Cyclospora* species of lower vertebrates develop in the intestinal epithelium and produce severe enteritis.

Epidemiology. The first cases of what later would be recognized as *Cyclospora* infection were reported from Papua New Guinea in 1979. Subsequent cases have been described from most parts of the world. Much of the current information on the epidemiology of cyclosporiasis comes from Nepal, Haiti, and Peru.

Epidemiologic evidence indicates that *Cyclospora* infection is acquired by drinking contaminated water. A point source outbreak among employees and housestaff physicians of Cook County Hospital in Chicago in 1990 identified the source as a contaminated water storage tank. However, the ultimate source of contamination of the storage tank was not determined. Another outbreak in 1994 among British soldiers and dependents stationed in Nepal traced the source to a storage tank that delivered chlorinated, filtered water to all the homes in the area. In Nepal, outbreaks of cyclosporiasis have coincided with the rainy season, which occurs from May through October. Prevalence rates of 11% have been reported for adults and children in Kathmandu during the rainy season. A similar prevalence rate was reported for preschool children in a shanty town near Lima, Peru, where peak infection occurred seasonally between April and June. Eleven percent of 450 HIV-infected Haitian adults with chronic diarrhea had *Cyclospora* infection. Contaminated fruit has also been shown to be a source of infection. An outbreak of cyclosporiasis involving 1465 persons in the United States and Canada during the spring and summer of 1996 was traced to raspberries imported from Guatemala. However, the ultimate source of contamination of the raspberries, whether human or animal, was not identified. Additionally, during the early summer months of 1997, at least 1400 persons in the United States were infected with *Cyclospora*. Fresh produce, particularly raspberries and lettuce, and possibly basil, was the source of exposure.

Treatment.   The effective treatment of cyclosporiasis is trimethoprim with sulfamethoxazole (Hoge et al., 1995). HIV-infected patients may need higher doses and long-term mainte-nance (Pape et al., 1994). The laboratory differentiation of *Cyclospora* from *Cryptosporidium* is important because cryptosporidiosis does not respond to trimethoprim-sulfamethoxazole treatment.

The Microsporidia

Microsporidia are obligate intracellular parasites, widely distributed in nature, belonging to the phylum Microspora. Reproduction involves the formation of minute spores, ranging in diameter from 1 to 2.5 μm, that have polar tubules, or filaments. Tubules are used to inject the infective material (sporoplasm) into the host cells. Microsporidia are considered to be primitive eukaryotic organisms because they lack mitochondria, peroxisomes, Golgi mem-branes, and other typically eukaryotic organelles. Additionally, some microsporidia have been shown to possess ribosomes similar to those of prokaryotic cells.

Six genera of microsporidia have been reported in humans: *Encephalitozoon, Trachipleistophora (Pleistophora), Nosema, Brachiola, Vittaforma,* and *Enterocytozoon.* The first human case of microsporidiosis was reported in 1959, and since then, most of the infections have been described in persons infected with HIV. *Enterocytozoon bieneusi* infects the ente-rocytes of AIDS patients. It also invades other epithelial cells and has been recovered from an immunocompetent patient with diarrhea. *Encephalitozoon intestinalis,* formerly known as *Septata intestinalis,* causes enteric and disseminated infections in patients with AIDS. *Encephalitozoon cuniculi* causes disseminated infections in immunocompetent and immuno-compromised persons. *Encephalitozoon hellem,* which primarily causes eye infections, has been exclusively found in AIDS patients. *Vittaforma corneae,* formerly *Nosema corneum,* and *Nosema ocularum* have caused corneal infections in HIV-negative patients. *Nosema connori* produced disseminated infection in an athymic infant. *Pleistophora* sp., recently renamed *Trachipleistophora hominis,* has been identified in the muscles of AIDS patients with myositis. *Brachiola algerae* and *Brachiola vesicularum* cause myositis in immunocompromised patients, and *B. algerae* has been isolated from the cornea of an immunocompetent patient.

Microsporidia multiply within the cytoplasm of their host cells (Fig. 3-44), either in a parasitiferous vacuole as in *Encephalitozoon* spp. or directly in the cytoplasm like *Ent. bieneusi,* undergoing a process of simple binary fission or multiple fission followed by the production of spores. It is the presence of the characteristic polar tubules, or filaments, of the spores that distinguishes the microsporidia from all other intracellular protozoans.

Diagnosis is made by identification of organisms in biopsy material or spores in feces, urine, bile, and duodenal, bronchial, or nasal fluids. Although spores are gram positive and portions of their internal structure are acid fast and periodic acid–Schiff positive, Giemsa-stained organisms are readily seen in histologic sections and in touch preparations of biopsy material (Fig. 3-44). Because of their small size, which approximates that of bacteria, microsporidial spores in the feces and bodily fluids may be easily overlooked by routine lab-oratory procedures. Spores have been detected by Giemsa's stain and by modified trichrome stains. The modified trichrome stains produce a distinct contrast between the minute spores and the background debris. Ryan's modified trichrome method uses reduced phospho-tungstic acid and has an aniline blue counterstain (Ryan et al., 1993). Weber's modification of the trichrome stain includes a fast green counterstain (Weber, 1992). In both procedures,

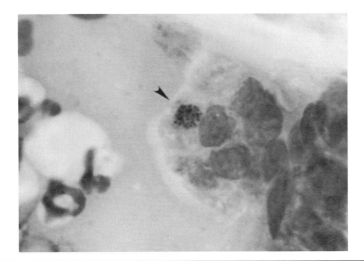

FIGURE 3-44 ■ Spores of *Enterocytozoon bieneusi (arrowhead)* in the cytoplasm of an enterocyte in a Giemsa-stained touch preparation of a duodenal biopsy. (Courtesy of Dr. Murray Wittner, Albert Einstein College of Medicine, Bronx, NY.)

the spores stain pink-red with clear vacuole-like polar or central nonstaining zones, which make the stained portions appear as bands, a feature typical of microsporidial spores. Slides should be examined using oil immersion magnification. Species identification requires transmission electron microscopy.

The standard concentration techniques, whether sedimentation or flotation, reportedly are ineffective in concentrating microsporidial spores. A nonspecific indirect fluorescent-antibody procedure has been described; however, commercial monoclonal or polyclonal reagents are not available. Molecular probes are being developed but at the present are used only in the research laboratory. Several different mammalian cell lines have been used to grow some of the microsporidia, namely, *B. algerae, Enc. hellem, Enc. intestinalis, T. hominis,* and *V. corneae. Ent. bieneusi* has been cultivated only short-term in cell culture. Table 3-3 summarizes some important features of the more common lumen-dwelling protozoan infections of humans.

The following characteristics are of value in identification of microsporidia:

In stool or bodily fluids, minute spores, pink-red when stained by modified trichrome stain, with clear polar or central nonstaining zones, giving appearance of bands; average size 1 to 2.5 mm

Symptoms and Pathogenesis. Clinical manifestations depend on the site of infection, which includes intestinal, ocular, muscular, and systemic. Intestinal infection is the most common form, is seen in AIDS patients infected with *Enterocytozoon bieneusi* or *Encephalitozoon intestinalis,* and is characterized by prolonged diarrhea and wasting. Patients may pass one to several liters of liquid feces per day, which can lead to dehydration and extreme wasting. About half of the patients report abdominal pain, and some have nausea and vomiting. Malabsorption is common in these patients. Although enterocytes of the small intestine are the primary site of infection by *Ent. bieneusi,* it may also spread to other epithelial cells in the biliary tract and nasopharynx and cause cholangitis and rhinosinusitis. In contrast, *Enc. intestinalis,* together with the other species of *Encephalitozoon,* develop in a variety of cells, including macrophages, causing disseminated infections. In immunodeficient patients, inflammatory reaction to microsporidia in infected tissue is often minimal or absent.

TABLE 3-3 ■ Review of Lumen-Dwelling Protozoan Infections of Humans

Disease	Parasite	Means of Human Infection	Location of Parasites in Humans	Other Sites of Infection	Clinical Features	Laboratory Diagnosis
Amebiasis	*Entamoeba histolytica* (ameba)	Ingestion of cysts	Large intestine (causing ulcers)	Liver, lungs, etc. (causing abscesses)	Diarrhea, dysentery, abdominal pain and cramping, tenesmus	Trophozoites or cysts in feces or tissue aspirate, serologic tests
Giardiasis	*Giardia lamblia* (flagellate)	Ingestion of cysts	Small intestine (attached)	Common bile duct, gallbladder	Diarrhea, abdominal cramps, flatulence, steatorrhea, malabsorption	Cysts or trophozoites in feces, duodenal aspirate, or string test
Trichomoniasis	*Trichomonas vaginalis* (flagellate)	Sexual intercourse	Vagina, urethra	Prostate, seminal vesicles	Vaginal or urethral discharge, burning, itching, dysuria	Trophozoites in vaginal or urethral discharge
Balantidiasis	*Balantidium coli* (ciliate)	Ingestion of cysts	Large intestine (causing ulcers)	None	Colitis, diarrhea	Trophozoites or cysts in stool
Isosporiasis	*Isospora belli* (sporozoan)	Ingestion of oocysts	Small intestine epithelium (intracellular)	None	Diarrhea, abdominal pain, anorexia, weight loss	Oocysts in stool or string test
Cryptosporidiosis	*Cryptosporidium parvum* (sporozoan)	Ingestion of oocysts	Intestinal epithelium (intracellular)	Biliary and respiratory tracts of immunodeficient persons	Diarrhea, abdominal pain, anorexia, weight loss	Oocysts in stool or string test, parasites in intestinal biopsy
Cyclosporiasis	*Cyclospora cayetanensis* (sporozoan)	Ingestion of oocysts	Small intestine epithelium (intracellular)	Biliary tract in AIDS patients	Diarrhea, abdominal cramping, anorexia, weight loss	Oocysts in stool
Microsporidiosis (a disease primarily of AIDS patients)	*Enterocytozoon, Encephalitozoon, Trachipleistophora, Nosema, Brachiola, Vittaforma* (microsporidia)	Ingestion and inhalation of spores, ocular and sexual infection possible	Intestinal epithelium (intracellular)	Cornea, biliary tract, muscle, disseminated infection	Chronic diarrhea and wasting	Spores in feces and bodily fluids, organisms in biopsy

Ocular microsporidiosis is caused by *Nosema ocularum* and *Vittaforma corneae* in otherwise healthy persons and by *Enc. hellem* in HIV-infected patients. Infection in immunocompetent patients involves the stroma, with keratitis leading to corneal ulcers. In AIDS patients, infection is restricted to the superficial epithelium of the cornea and conjunctiva.

Microsporidial myositis, caused by *T. hominis*, has been described in patients with severe cellular immunodeficiency. Symptoms include generalized muscle weakness, myalgia, fever, and weight loss. Systemic infections, caused by three species of *Encephalitozoon*—*E. cuniculi, E. hellem,* and *E. intestinalis*—have been found in AIDS patients, especially those with CD4 T-cell counts below 50 cells per microliter. In addition to intestinal, biliary, and ocular infection, these microsporidia have produced hepatic, renal (with renal failure), and respiratory infections. *E. cuniculi* and *N. connori* have caused disseminated infections in HIV-negative, immunocompetent, and immunodeficient persons.

Epidemiology. The microsporidia have an extensive host range, which includes most invertebrates and all classes of vertebrates. They produce significant diseases in commercially important animals such as honeybees, silkworms, fish, laboratory rodents, rabbits and other fur-bearing mammals; and in primates. Nearly 1000 species belonging to over 100 genera have been described in the phylum Microspora.

Microsporidia are emerging as opportunistic pathogens in patients with AIDS. The most common microsporidial disease is prolonged diarrhea with wasting in AIDS patients with CD4 T-cell counts below 50 cells per microliter.

Microsporidia have been reported in up to 39% of AIDS patients with diarrhea. Approximately 30% of AIDS patients with *Cryptosporidium* are also infected with microsporidia. From an intestinal infection, microsporidia may disseminate to produce systemic disease.

The sources of microsporidia infecting humans and the modes of transmission are uncertain. However, infection most likely is acquired by ingestion of spores. The inhalation of spores also may be a route of transmission as may ocular exposure and sexual intercourse. Experiments with laboratory animals suggest that rectal infection, analogous to the sexual transmission of other intestinal protozoa, may lead to disseminated disease.

Treatment. Oral albendazole (Dore et al., 1995; Sobottka et al., 1995) has been effective in treating intestinal and disseminated infection caused by *Encephalitozoon intestinalis*. Albendazole, reduced the number of bowel movements in intestinal disease caused by *Enterocytozoon bieneusi* but did not clear the infection (Dieterich et al., 1994). Disseminated infection by *Encephalitozoon cuniculi* was effectively eliminated by continuous treatment with albendazole, (De Groote et al., 1995). Topical fumagillin has been used successfully in the treatment of ocular infection caused by *Encephalitozoon hellem* (Diesenhouse et al., 1993).

The Myxozoa

The phylum Myxozoa consists of obligate parasites that occur in the tissues and organ cavities of lower vertebrates, primarily fishes and some invertebrates, mainly aquatic oligochaetes, a class of segmented worms. Myxozoans have valved multicellular teardrop-shaped spores, which contain polar capsules with coiled filaments, similar to those found in microsporidia. However, unlike the microsporidia, myxozoans contain mitochondria and Golgi bodies. More than 1200 species of myxozoa have been described.

Myxozoans produce a disease in salmonid fish known as whirling disease. Organisms developing in the cartilage of the head and spine cause the fish to swim erratically and whirl, making it difficult for them to feed and avoid predators. Mortality rates can be very high among young fish.

Myxozoan spores have been identified in the stool specimens of seven patients, two whom were infected with HIV and five who were not immunocompromised. The most recent report is that of Moncada et al. (2001). The patients presented with abdominal pain and diarrhea, with one patient passing more than 30 stools per day. Three of the patients had eaten freshwater golden perch, *Plectroplites ambiguus*, infected with myxozoa. Eating of fish, however, could not be confirmed for the other four patients. Five of the seven patients were also infected with other microorganisms that cause diarrhea. Based on morphology, the spores were identified as *Henneguya salminicola* in two of the patients and *Myxobolus* sp. in the other five.

One of the HIV-infected patients was treated for isosporiasis with trimethoprim-sulfamethoxazole, and at a 2-month follow-up the diarrhea had persisted and spores were still present in stool samples. The proof is not yet there to link the presence of myxozoan spores in the stool to the abdominal pain and diarrhea of the seven patients. Nonetheless, future studies may in fact reveal such an association, especially in immunosuppressed patients.

References

Adam RD. Biology of giardic lamblia. *Clin Micro Rev* 2001; *14*:447–475.

Al-Waili NSD, Hasan NU. Mebendazole in giardial infection: A comparative study with metronidazole. *J Infect Dis* 1992; *165*:1170–1171.

Bailey JM, Erramouspe J. Nitazoxanide treatment for giardiasis and cryptosporidiosis in children. *Ann Pharmacother* 2004; *38*:634–640.

Chacin-Bonilla L. Successsful treatment of human *Entamoeba polecki* infection with metronidazole. *Am J Trop Med Hyg* 1980; *29*:521–523.

Chen XM, Keithly JS, Payer CV, LaRusso NF. Cryptosporidiosis. *N Engl J Med* 2002; *346*:1723–1731.

De Groote MA et al. Polymerase chain reaction and culture confirmation of disseminated *Encephalitozoon cuniculi* in a patient with AIDS: Successful therapy with albendazole. *J Infect Dis* 1995; *171*:1375–1378.

Diesenhouse MC et al. Treatment of microsporidial keratoconjunctivitis with topical fumagillin. *Am J Ophthalmol* 1993; *115*:293–298.

Dieterich DT et al. Treatment with albendazole for intestinal disease due to *Enterocytozoon bieneusi* in patients with AIDS. *J Infect Dis* 1994; *169*:178–183.

Dore GJ et al. Disseminated microsporidiosis due to *Septata intestinalis* in nine patients infected with the human immunodeficiency virus: Response to therapy with albendazole. *Clin Infect Dis* 1995; *21*:70–76.

Gay JD et al. *Entamoeba polecki* in Southwest Asian refugees: Multiple cases of a rarely reported parasite. *Mayo Clin Proc* 1985: *60*:523–530.

Hall A, Nahar Q. Albendazole as a treatment for infections with *Giardia duodenalis* in children in Bangladesh. *Trans R Soc Trop Med Hyg* 1993; *87*:87–89.

Haque R et al. Amebiasis. *N Engl J Med* 2003; *348*:1565–1573.

Hoge CW et al. Placebo-controlled trial of co-trimoxazole for cyclospora infections among travellers and foreign residents in Nepal. *Lancet* 1995; *345*:691–693.

Ken JG et al. Perforated liver abscess: Successful percutaneous treatment *Radiology* 1989; *170*:195-197.

Lossick JG et al. In vitro drug susceptibility and doses of metronidazole required for cure in cases of refractory vaginal trichomoniasis. *J Infect Dis* 1986; *153*:948–955.

Moncada LI et al. *Myxobolus* sp., another opportunistic parasite in immunosuppressed patients? *J Clin Microbiol* 2001; *39*:1938–1940.

Morgan-Ryan UM et al. *Cryptosporidium hominis* n.sp. (Apicomplexa: Cryptosporidiidae) from *Homo sapiens*. *J Eukaryot Microbiol* 2002; *49*:433–440.

Pape JW et al. Treatment and prophylaxis of *Isospora belli* infection in patients with the acquired immunodeficiency syndrome. *N Engl J Med* 1989; *320*:1044–1047.

Pape JW et al. *Cyclospora* infection in adults infected with HIV. Clinical manifestations, treatment, and prophylaxis. *Ann Intern Med* 1994; *121*:654–657.

Ryan NJ et al. A new trichrome-blue stain for detection of microsporidial species in urine, stool, and nasopharyngeal specimens. *J Clin Microbiol* 1993; *31*:3264–3269.

Salaki JS et al. Successful treatment of symptomatic *Entamoeba polecki* infection. *Am J Trop Med Hyg* 1979; *28*:190–193.

Singh JP, Kashyap A. A comparative evaluation of percutaneous catheter drainage for resistant amebic liver abscesses. *Am J Surg* 1989; *158*:58–62.

Sobottka I et al. Disseminated *Encephalitozoon (Septata) intestinalis* infection in a patient with AIDS: Novel diagnostic approaches and autopsy-confirmed parasitological cure following treatment with albendazole. *J Clin Microbiol* 1995; *33*:2948–2952.

Sorvillo F et al. *Trichomonas vaginalis*, HIV, and African-Americans. *Emerg Infect Dis* 2001; 7:927–932.

Tanyuksel M, Petri WA, Jr. Laboratory diagnosis of amebiasis. *Clin Microbial Rev* 2003; *16*:713–729.

Traub RJ, Morris PT, Robertson I, Irwin P, Mencke N, Thompson RCA. Epidemiological and molecular evidence supports the zoonotic transmission of Giardia among humans and dogs living in the same community. *Parasitology* 2004; *128*:253–262.

Weber R. Improved light-microscopical detection of microsporidia spores in stool and duodenal aspirates. *N Engl J Med* 1992; *326*:161–166.

Weiss LM et al. *Isospora belli* infection: Treatment with pyrimethamine. *Ann Intern Med* 1988: *109*:474–475.

Whiteside ME et al. Enteric coccidiosis among patients with the acquired immunodeficiency syndrome. *Am J Trop Med Hyg* 1984; *33*:1065–1072.

World Health Organization. *Amoebiasis*, 52 pp. Report of a WHO expert committee. Technical Report Series, No. 421. 1969, World Health Organization, Geneva.

Yang J, Scholten T. *Dientamoeba fragilis*: A review with notes on its epidemiology, pathogenicity, mode of transmission, and diagnosis. *Am J Trop Med Hyg* 1977; *26*:16–22.

Malaria

Several clinical syndromes now known to be caused by infection by malarial parasites were first recognized centuries before the discovery of their pathogens. Consequently, the diseases were referred to in terms of their outstanding clinical feature, usually the type of febrile cycle. Thus, quotidian, tertian, and quartan fevers are denoted, respectively 24-, 48-, and 72-hour cycles of fever. Other names designated additional clinical features of the disease. The modern tendency is to refer to the various types of malaria by the name of the agent. Thus, benign tertian malaria is now usually called vivax malaria, as it is caused by infection with *Plasmodium vivax*. Similarly aestivoautumnal, malignant tertian, or subtertian malaria is now known as falciparum malaria, from *Plasmodium falciparum*. Quartan malaria may be called malariae malaria after its agent, *Plasmodium malariae*, but for the sake of euphony the old term is usually retained. Fortunately, the fourth type, ovale malaria, was described so recently as to possess only the name derived from *Plasmodium ovale*. These four organisms and the diseases they produce are discussed separately. The many common features of general morphology and life cycle shared by all plasmodia are considered first.

While human malarial parasites were first seen in 1880, and their development both in the anopheline mosquito and in the human bloodstream was well understood by 1900, the entire life cycle was not elucidated until more recently. In the intervening period, many species of *Plasmodium* have been found in other animals, and from those that do not infect humans much information of medical importance has been obtained. Of special interest from the standpoint of drug testing have been those organisms such as *P. berghei* and *P. yoellii*, which cause rodent malaria, and *P. cathemerium*, which causes avian malaria.

Human malaria is thought by some authorities to have originated in Southeast Asia (presumably from simian species, some of which still bear close resemblance to the human malarias), from where it spread first to Africa and then to Europe. It probably was introduced into the Americas no earlier than the 16th century.

The life cycle of *Plasmodium*, in both humans and mosquitoes, is shown in Figure 4-1. Various species of anopheline mosquitoes are definitive hosts of the malarial parasites. When the female mosquito bites an infected person, she draws into her stomach blood that may contain male and female gametocytes. In the mosquito, as the blood temperature falls, the male or microgametocyte undergoes a process of maturation that results in the production of a number of microgametes. The extrusion of these delicate spindle-shaped gametes has been termed exflagellation. At the same time, the female or macrogametocyte matures to become a macrogamete, after which it may be fertilized by the microgamete, forming a zygote. The zygote becomes elongated and active and is called an ookinete. The ookinete penetrates cells of the stomach wall of the mosquito and rounds up just beneath the outer covering of that organ to become an oocyst. Growth and development of the oocyst result in the production of a large number of slender, threadlike haploid sporozoites, which break out and wander throughout the body of the mosquito. Length of the developmental cycle in the mosquito depends not only on the species of *Plasmodium* but on the particular mosquito host and the ambient temperature. It may range from as little as 8 days in *P. vivax* to as long as 35 days in *P. malariae*. Those sporozoites that enter the salivary glands of the mosquito may be inoculated into the next person bitten. Sporozoites injected into the bloodstream leave the

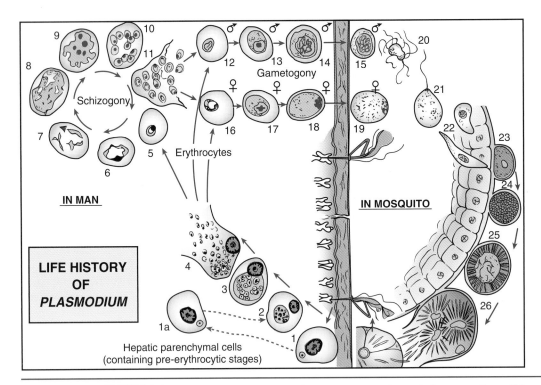

FIGURE 4-1   ■   Life history of *Plasmodium*. *1–4*, Pre-erythrocytic (or exoerythrocytic) asexual stages undergoing schizogony in liver; *1a*, hypnozoite (only in *P. vivax* and *P. ovale* among species infecting humans); *5–11*, erythrocytic asexual cycle; *12–15*, microgametocyte development; *16–19*, macrogametocyte development; *20*, exflagellation to produce microgametes; *21*, fertilization of macrogamete; *22*, ookinete penetrates cells (wall) of mosquito stomach; *23–25*, production of sporozoites within oocyst (sporogony); *26*, release of sporozoites, most reaching salivary glands of mosquito.

blood vascular system within 40 minutes and subsequently invade the parenchymal cells of the liver.

Later development of *P. falciparum* and *P. malariae* differs from that of *P. vivax* and *P. ovale*. In all four species, asexual multiplication takes place within the liver cells, but with *P. vivax* and *P. ovale* a varying proportion of the infecting sporozoites enter a resting stage before undergoing asexual multiplication, while others undergo this multiplication without delay. The resting stage of the parasite is known as a hypnozoite (Fig. 4-2). After a period of weeks or months, reactivation of the hypnozoite initiates asexual division. While hypnozoites have not been observed in human infections (and experimental demonstration in human subjects would be extraordinarily difficult), their presence in *P. vivax* and *P. ovale* is inferred from experimental observations.

These dormant stages have now been demonstrated in the hepatic parenchymal cells of chimpanzees infected by sporozoites of two widely disparate strains of *P. vivax* (Krotoski et al., 1986) and of rhesus monkeys infected with *Plasmodium cynomologi* (Krotoski et al., 1980) or *P. simiovale* (Cogswell et al., 1991), simian analogues of *P. vivax* and *P. ovale*, respectively. Hypnozoite reactivation brings about the relapses* characteristic of these species (Fig. 4-3), producing a wide variation in time of relapse, now considered to be due to differences in

---

Relapse and *recrudescence* have special meanings when applied to malaria. A relapse is a recurrence that takes place after complete initial clearing of the erythrocytic infection and implies reinvasion of the bloodstream by parasites from the dormant pre-erythrocytic stages. A recrudescence is a recurrence of symptoms in a patient whose bloodstream infection has previously been at such a low level as not to be clinically demonstrable or cause symptoms.

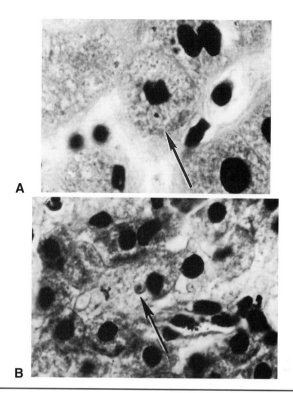

FIGURE 4-2 ▓ *A*, Hypnozoite of *Plasmodium vivax*, Chesson strain *(arrow)*, just below hepatocyte nucleus in chimpanzee's liver, × 1430. *B*, Hypnozoite of *P. cynomolgi bastianelli* in monkey liver *(arrow)*, × 850. Giemsa-colophonium-restained indirect immunofluorescence (IFA) preparations. (From Krotoski WA et al. *Am J Trop Med Hyg* 1982;*31*:218–225, 1291–1293.)

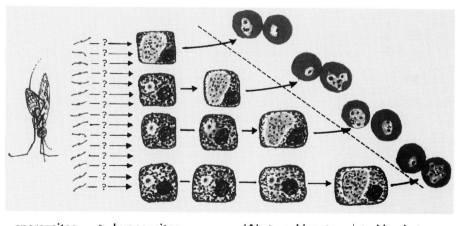

sporozoites ----> hypnozoites --- --- --- (A)--> schizonts ---|-> blood stages

FIGURE 4-3 ▓ Representation of hypnozoite theory of malarial relapse: Activation *(A)* to schizogony of hypnozoites at interals predetermined by intrinsic capability of individual sporozoites, resulting in release of merozoites at species- or strain-determined times. (Original figure drawn by Dr. Steve Ayala. Modified from *Trans R Soc Trop Med Hyg* 1985; *79,* Krotoski WA, Discovery of the hypnozoite and a new theory of malarial relapse, 1–11 with permission from the Royal Society of Tropical Medicine and Hygiene.)

the latency period of hypnozoites produced by distinct subpopulations of sporozoites (Fig. 4-4). Successive relapses in the same patient are the result of infection by a number of sporozoites, each of which produces hypnozoites with a different reactivation time. These subpopulations are grouped characteristically within a given strain, with a distinct tendency to a shorter latency in strains originating from "tropical" areas, and a longer one in those

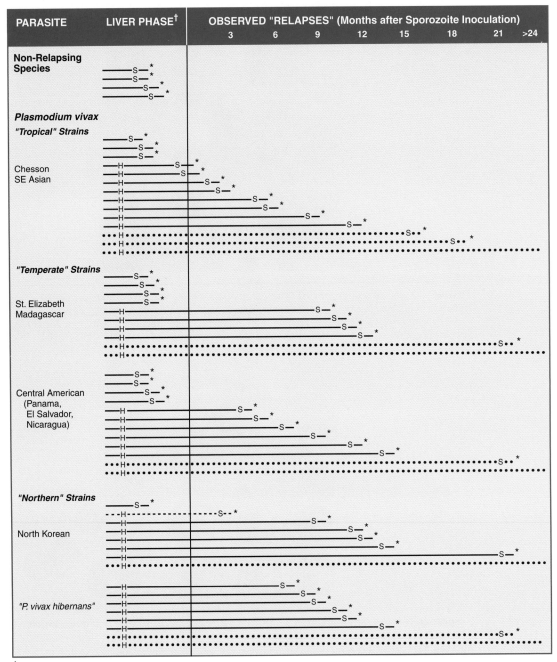

†Except for hypnozoites (when present) this initial phase of the infection lasts only about two weeks

FIGURE 4-4 ■ Schematic presentation of relapse behavior of *P. vivax* strains according to hypnozoite theory. Horizontal lines represent fates of subpopulations of sporozoites of differing development/dormancy potential. *H*, hypnozoite; *S*, onset of schizogony; *, merozoite release. Subpopulations depicted: rare — — —; common ———; unverified clinical or theoretical • • • • • • •. (Adapted from Krotoski WA. *Progr Clin Parasitol* 1989;1:1–19.)

originating in temperate and, especially, colder ("northern") areas (Figs. 4-4, 4-5). In the extreme case of the now-lost *P. vivax hibernans* strain, initial parasitemia reproducibly did not occur until 9 months after the infected mosquito bite. Hypnozoites are not found in the development of *P. falciparum* and *P. malariae*, and true relapses do not occur in disease caused by these species.

Asexual multiplication (schizogony) in the liver results in the production of thousands of tiny merozoites in each schizont (Fig. 4-6). Rupture of the infected hepatic cells releases merozoites into the circulation. In the bloodstream, an asexual cycle takes place within the red blood cells. This process, known as erythrocytic schizogony, results, within a period of 44 to 72 hours, in the formation of from 4 to 36 new parasites in each infected cell. Details of this cycle differ for the various species and are given in more detail when each is described. At the end of the schizogonic cycle, the infected blood cells rupture, liberating merozoites, which in turn infect new red blood cells. Rupture of the red blood cells liberates products of metabolism of the parasites and of the red blood cells, and it is thought that if large numbers of infected cells rupture simultaneously, the volume of toxic materials thrown into the bloodstream may be sufficient to bring about a malarial paroxysm. Generally, in the initial stages of infection, rupture of the infected cells is not synchronous, so fever★ may be continuous or remittent rather than intermittent. It has been theorized that the fever peaks themselves may have a regulatory effect on the development cycle, speeding

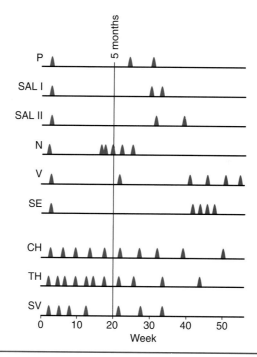

FIGURE 4-5 ■ Relapse patterns observed in *P. vivax* malaria isolates from the Americas ("temperate" strains) and from Oceania/Southeast Asia ("tropical" strains). First peak for each strain represents initial, postinfection parasitemia; all others are relapses seen at indicated intervals after infection. *P*, Panama; *Sal I* and *Sal II*, El Salvador; *N*, Nicaragua; *V*, Venezuela; *SE*, United States (St. Elizabeth Hospital therapeutic strain); *CH*, New Guinea (Chesson strain); *TH*, Thailand; *SV*, South Vietnam. (From Contacos PG et al. *Am J Trop Med Hyg* 1972; *21*[Suppl]:707–712.)

★Fever may be spoken of as *continuous* if it remains elevated with a fluctuation of not more than 1½° F in a 24-hour period; *remittent* fever remains elevated, but the fluctuation is 2° F or more in 24 hours; in *intermittent* fever, the temperature returns to normal one or more times during the 24-hour period.

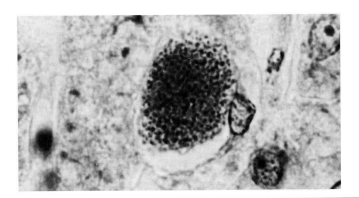

FIGURE 4-6 ■ Pre-erythrocytic schizont of *Plasmodium vivax* in liver.

up those that are out of phase, so that after a number of days the febrile cycle develops a 48- or 72-hour periodicity, depending on the species of parasite. In mixed infections with two or more species, or in the early stages of infection with one species, there may be daily (quotidian) paroxysms, or even double paroxysms in one day. Occasionally, two 48-hour parasite broods may be asynchronous by 24 hours, producing regular, daily fevers in a tertian species. A single case of quadruple infection involving all four human malaria parasites has been reported from Irian Jaya, Indonesia (Purnomo et al., 1999).

Some time after the asexual parasites first appear in the bloodstream, but usually not until after the patient has become clinically ill, gametocytes appear in the red blood cells. These forms, derived from merozoites similar in appearance to those that continue the asexual cycle, grow but do not divide and finally form the male and female gametocytes. Gametocytes continue to circulate in the bloodstream for some time and, if ingested by a mosquito of the genus *Anopheles*, undergo transformation to gametes (gametogony), sexual fusion, and subsequent development to sporozoites (sporogony) in the mosquito.

Morphologic features that distinguish the four species of malarial parasites are presented first, after which details of symptoms, pathogenesis, epidemiology, and treatment are considered for the entire group.

Plasmodium vivax

The predominant malarial parasite in most parts of the world is *P. vivax*. This species is found almost everywhere malaria is endemic and is the only one whose range extends into the temperate regions.

In blood smears from a patient infected with *P. vivax*, a variety of stages in the asexual cycle of the parasite may be seen; gametocytes may also be present. The stages in the asexual cycle that are seen depend on when the blood is taken in relation to the febrile cycle. The paroxysm follows the somewhat synchronous rupture of the majority of infected cells, liberating merozoites, which in turn infect new red blood cells. For the first few hours after the paroxysm, the majority of infected cells contain very early forms of the parasite, referred to as trophozoites or "rings" (Plate V). In a blood film correctly stained with Giemsa's or Field's stain, the parasites appear first as minute blue disks with a red nucleus lying within the pink cytoplasm of the erythrocyte. Sometimes the parasites are first seen as crescentic masses at the periphery of the red blood cell—the so-called accolé (French, *joined together*) forms. Shortly thereafter, an apparent vacuole forms in the blue cytoplasm of the parasite, pushing the nuclear chromatin to a peripheral position. The parasite now resembles a signet ring and has grown to a diameter about one third that of the infected cell. Very active ameboid motility is exhibited during the growth period, and the parasite may assume bizarre and irregular forms within the red blood cell. It was this ameboid activity that suggested the specific name *vivax*, from the Latin for *vigorous*. Between 6 and 24 hours after the beginning of the cycle, the trophozoites grow to approximately half the size of the infected cell and granules of brownish pigment appear within them. At the same time, the infected cell becomes noticeably enlarged and pale, and it may be seen to contain a number of very fine reddish granules known as Schüffner's dots. Schüffner's dots are always seen in a red blood cell infected 15 to 20 hours or longer if the slide has been properly stained. The nature of these dots is not known; if present, they are diagnostic of *P. vivax* or *P. ovale* infection. Increase in size continues during the second 24 hours, and the parasite comes very nearly to fill the infected cell, which may be enlarged to 10 to 12 μm. At about 40 hours, the mature trophozoite largely ceases its ameboid activity and becomes compact, thus sometimes appearing smaller than the actively motile stages that preceded it. The single nucleus divides repeatedly to give rise to 12 to 24 nuclear masses, with average numbers that vary, according to the strain, from 14 to 22. During the stages of division, the parasite is known as a schizont. The cytoplasm finally segments to form separate small masses around each nucleus. The individual parasites thus produced are known as merozoites, and upon rupture of the infected cell at about 44 to 48 hours they are released to infect new red blood cells.

As the cycle is never entirely synchronous, parasites at more than one stage of development are usually seen in the blood smear. In addition to the asexual forms mentioned previously, gametocytes are frequently seen after the first few paroxysms. They mature more slowly than the asexual forms, do not exhibit as much ameboid activity, and develop more pigment. The infected cells enlarge, and Schüffner's granules may be seen. Fully mature gametocytes, in contrast with trophozoites about to undergo schizogony, fill the cell more completely and contain more pigment. One can differentiate the microgametocytes and macrogametocytes morphologically. The nucleus of the macrogametocyte is dense, whereas that of the microgametocyte forms a pale, loose network.

All stages seen in thin films may be found also in thick-film preparations (Plate VII), but the parasites appear somewhat distorted. Young trophozoites may be seen as typical rings, but more frequently they are collapsed. A red dot of nuclear material may have a small wisp of blue cytoplasm at one side, or thin lines of cytoplasm may appear on either side of the nucleus. These distorted early trophozoites are known as comma and swallow forms, respectively; however, if these forms alone are seen, they cannot be distinguished with certainty from similar stages of *P. ovale* or from *P. falciparum* if the infection with the latter parasite is a light one. As the parasites become older, their ameboid activity is reflected by the irregular shapes they assume in thick film. The ghostlike shadows of lysed infected cells may be seen surrounding the parasites, and usually Schüffner's dots are visible within them. Schizonts, if mature can be recognized by the number of merozoites. Gametocytes of *P. vivax*, *P. ovale*, and *P. malariae* are similar in appearance, except those of *P. malariae* are smaller and darker than the other two and do not contain Schüffner's dots. It is best to rely on asexual stages of the parasite for identification.

Plasmodium ovale

P. ovale has been known only since 1922. It seems to be rather widely distributed in tropical Africa, and it apparently supplants *P. vivax* almost entirely on the West African coast. It has also been occasionally reported from South America and Asia.

The morphologic feature that originally led to the establishment of *P. ovale* as a separate species, an ovoid shape of many of the infected red blood cells, has been found to be variable (Plate VI). Thin smears that because of excessive humidity have dried slowly may not show this characteristic at all; however, other criteria may be used to distinguish the two species. The parasite is not as ameboid as *P. vivax*, and the nuclei in all stages are larger than in corresponding stages of that species. Pigment is scanty. In schizogony, typically 4 to 12 merozoites are produced, with an average of 8 as in *P. malariae*. More rarely, 12 to 18 merozoites may be formed, with an average of 14 to 16. The infected cells are enlarged and pale, and if properly stained, they exhibit larger and more distinctly red Schüffner's dots than those of *P. vivax*. The margins of the infected cells are often ragged, and the cells are elongate, ovoid, or irregularly shaped.

Thick films (Plate VII) are similar to those of *P. vivax*. If in such films schizonts larger than those of *P. malariae* but with no more than 12 merozoites are seen to contain distinct Schüffner's dots, a tentative diagnosis of *P. ovale* infection may be made.

Plasmodium malariae

Occurring primarily in those subtropical and temperate areas where other species of malaria are found, *P. malariae* is less frequently seen than *P. vivax* or *P. falciparum*.

The asexual cycle of *P. malariae* occupies 72 hours, as compared with approximately 48 hours for the other species. Ring forms of *P. malariae* (Plate VIII) are not readily distinguished from those of *P. vivax*. As the parasite grows, it exhibits little ameboid activity. It tends to assume an elongate (band or *stab*) form, stretching partway or entirely across the red blood cell. The infected cell is not enlarged. As the parasite grows, it may almost fill the red blood cell prior to schizogony. The cytoplasm of the red blood cell rarely may contain dust-fine, pale pink dots called Ziemann's stippling. This stippling is seen only in heavily stained slides. Pigment is produced in some quantity and is dark. Schizogony results in the formation of 6 to 12 merozoites. The average number of merozoites is eight, an they may be arranged in a rosette, symmetrically around a central mass of pigment, but more typically they are irregularly displaced within the mature schizont.

Gametocytes of *P. malariae* are difficult to distinguish from the growing trophozoites, but when mature they may be slightly larger than the mature trophozoites and tend to be ovoid. They contain proportionately more pigment than the trophozoites at all stages.

In the thick film (Plate VII), trophozoites of *P. malariae* do not assume the ameboid, comma, or swallow forms seen in the other species, but because of their compact nature they usually appear as small dots of nuclear material with rounded or slightly elongate masses of cytoplasm. The older trophozoites of *P. malariae* are also compact, and the predominant color may be that of the abundant pigment. The fully developed schizont, containing an average of eight merozoites, is readily recognized.

Plasmodium falciparum

Falciparum malaria is almost entirely confined to the tropics and subtropics. Clinically, falciparum malaria is quite sharply differentiated from the other malarias in a number of ways. Morphologically, there are certain differences as well. The gametocytes of *P. falciparum* are elongate or sausage shaped, in contrast with the spherical or ovoid gametocytes of the other species. On the basis of the shape of the gametocytes, *P. falciparum* was placed by some workers in a separate genus, *Laverania*.

Schizogony usually does not take place in the peripheral blood in falciparum malaria. Therefore, the only stages of the parasite ordinarily seen are young trophozoites ("rings") and gametocytes. Double and even triple infections of red blood cells are not uncommon, and as *P. falciparum* attacks all stages of red blood cells, the percentage of cell parasitized may be very large. The young trophozoites are minute rings (Plate IX). More frequently than in other species, the ring may have two small chromatin dots. Occasionally the earliest stages do not assume a ring form but lie spread out along the periphery of the red blood cell, in the accolé form previously mentioned for *P. vivax*. The parasites may grow somewhat in size and become irregular in outline, although they still retain the ring form while in the circulating blood. Pigment is rarely seen in the forms normally found in the circulating blood. The infected red blood cells, which retain their original size, may develop a few irregular, dark red, rod- or wedge-shaped markings, known as Maurer's dots or clefts. Gametocytes are characteristic, being crescentic in outline. The ends of the gametocyte may be pointed or bluntly rounded, and the remains of the red blood cell may be seen in the concavity formed by the arched body of the parasite. In heavy infections, generally occurring only in moribund patients, schizonts may be seen in the peripheral blood. The mature schizont forms from 8 to 36 merozoites, with an average of about 24, although varying from 12 to 28 with different strains. Gametocytes, on the other hand, which may continue to circulate after therapy for clinical illness has been completed, have no *clinical* significance if found, unaccompanied by other stages, following clinical resolution.

In the thick film (Plate VII), one is usually impressed by the large number of early trophozoites. As these are delicate, they frequently collapse to assume the comma or swallow shape. Gametocytes are easily recognizable by their shape, which is much the same as in the thin film.

Diagnosis. In the descriptions of the four species of malarial parasites, repeated mention has been made of the use of thick and thin blood films. The proper techniques for preparation of blood films are outlined in Chapter 15, as are stains and staining techniques, equally important to successful identification of the parasites. Of similar importance is the timing of blood examination. It will be appreciated that, depending on the stage of the parasite's developmental cycle at which the blood sample is taken, various stages of the parasite will appear. Immediately after a paroxysm, the merozoite-filled red cells have ruptured and free merozoites are found in the bloodstream. These are difficult to locate and virtually impossible to identify by species; however, gametocytes may be present and readily identifiable. If parasites are not found in the first blood films, it is advisable to take additional thick and thin films every 6 to 12 hours, for as long as 48 hours if necessary. Thick films are best used as a screening procedure; unless the examiner has much experience, painstaking examination of the thin film should be relied upon for specific diagnosis. It should be noted that a first level of diagnosis is the presumptive differentiation of *P. falciparum* from the other species, as the presence of this parasite in a non-native (i.e., in a nonimmune patient) constitutes a medical emergency. A presumptive diagnosis of *P. falciparum* can be made on the basis of finding exclusively "ring" forms, with or without characteristic gametocytes, in a blood film. Various serologic tests are available, as outlined in Chapter 16; however, these tests are not readily obtained, and one is seldom able to use them as a guide to treatment. They may have more value in ruling out malaria in a patient with fever of unknown origin. Molecular biologic approaches to the diagnosis of malaria include the use of recombinant DNA probes and ribosomal RNA probes. Other rapid tests rely on the detection of plasmodial antigens or enzymes (Haditsch, 2004). Undoubtedly, these new methods will become useful in epidemiologic studies or to screen blood for blood banks when perfected.

Symptoms. Some of the features of the four different malarias are compared in Table 4-1. The incubation period is longest in quartan and shortest in falciparum malaria. The last few days of the incubation period may be marked by prodromal symptoms of a nonspecific sort: headache, photophobia, muscle aches and pains, anorexia, nausea, and sometimes vomiting. These symptoms may be seen in all types of malaria; they are at times entirely absent in vivax infections and they are generally mild in ovale malaria. The malarial paroxysm is typically ushered in with a sudden shaking chill, or rigor. This may last 10 to 15 minutes or longer; during this stage the patient complains of extreme cold, although in fact the temperature is elevated at the onset and rises during the period of the chill. The hot stage follows the cold without respite, and the patient who a few moments before was huddled under a pile of blankets now throws them off. The skin, pale and cyanotic in the cold stage, becomes flushed. The patient frequently seems agitated and may be restless, disoriented, or even delirious. Severe frontal headache and pains in the limbs and back are common. The hot stage lasts 2 to 6 hours in vivax and ovale malaria, 6 hours or more in quartan, and considerably longer in falciparum. Following the hot stage, the patient starts to sweat profusely and usually begins to feel better. The sweating stage may last several hours; at its end the patient is usually weak and exhausted and tends to fall asleep. Upon awakening, the temperature is normal or slightly subnormal and the patient usually feels quite well until the onset of the next paroxysm—which, in the case of falciparum malaria, may be only a matter of a very few hours. Acute splenomegaly may occur rapidly, especially in nonimmune patients, and may rarely result in tears of the splenic capsule and intra-abdominal bleeding, requiring surgical intervention.

TABLE 4-1   ▣   **Clinical Comparison of the Types of Malaria**

Feature	Vivax	Ovale	Malariae	Falciparum
Incubation period	10–17 days	10–17 days	18–40 days	8–11 days
	Sometimes prolonged for months to years			
Prodromal symptoms	May be influenza-like in all four types			
Severity	+ +	+	+ +	+
Initial fever pattern	Irregular to quotidian		Usually regular every 72 hours	Continuous, remittent, or quotidian
Periodicity	44–48 hours	48–50 hours	72 hours	36–48 hours
Initial paroxysm				
Usual severity	Moderate to severe	Mild	Moderate to severe	Severe
Average duration	10 hours	10 hours	11 hours	16–36 hours
Duration of untreated primary attack	3–8 + weeks	2–3 weeks	3–24 weeks	2–3 weeks
Duration of untreated infection	5–8 years*	12–20 months*	20–50 + years†	6–17 months
Anemia	+ +	+	+ +	+ + + +
CNS involvement	±	±	±	+ + + +
Nephrotic syndrome	±	–	+ + +	+

*Including relapses.
†Including recrudescences.

Following infection with *P. vivax*, a primary attack may occur early, but with some strains it is delayed for a period of months (Fig. 4-4). Such delay may be seen in areas where a short season of warm weather results in an abbreviated anopheline breeding season. Transmission is better ensured by a primary attack that occurs early in the next mosquito breeding season. Such variation in time of onset of primary attacks and relapses is best explained by strain differences determining the period of hypnozoite dormancy. Figure 4-5 shows such variation in a number of strains from the Americas, contrasted with ones from the South Pacific and Southeast Asia. The Chesson (from New Guinea), Thailand, and South Vietnam strains show a typical *tropical* pattern, with an early primary attack followed quickly by a series of relapses. The other strains shown (and in particular the St. Elizabeth strain, which originated in the United States) also exhibit an early primary attack, but a much longer (latency) period before any relapses occur. It may appear strange that strains from South and Central America show what would be considered a *temperate zone* pattern of relapse, but it must be remembered that malaria is thought to have been introduced from Europe into the Americas no longer ago than the 16th century, and thus might be expected still to exhibit a "temperate" pattern (perhaps showing some indications of selection by the climatic influence on mosquito breeding toward a "tropical" one in the Nicaraguan strain). Although both tropical and temperate strains are characterized by early primary attacks, isolates from North Korea and northern Russia ("northern" strains) have shown marked delays in *initial* parasitemia to as long as 21 months after infection.

Primary vivax attacks, if untreated, may last 3 weeks to 2 months or longer. As the attack wanes, paroxysms may become less severe and irregular in periodicity. In perhaps half of all cases, relapses occur following an asymptomatic period of weeks, months, or even years. In certain strains of vivax malaria there may typically be a series of such relapses, extending over a period of 5 or even 8 years. Early spontaneous recovery is common in ovale malaria and may occur after no more than 6 to 10 paroxysms. When relapse occurs, it is seldom longer than a year after the initial attack. Quartan attacks may terminate in as short a time as 3 weeks or be prolonged for as long as 24 weeks in whites; in blacks the duration is usually shorter. Termination of the quartan attack may mean that the infection has been completely eliminated, or there may be a recrudescence or series of recrudescences over a period of years, denoting a latent infection and persisting low-grade parasitemia. This asymptomatic state of affairs may persist indefinitely or may result in a recrudescence at a time when the patient becomes debilitated, perhaps from intercurrent infection or immunosuppression. However, if at any time blood from such a patient is used for transfusion, the recipient will probably experience a typical attack of quartan malaria. An untreated primary attack of *P. falciparum* malaria tends to run its course quickly and seldom exceeds 2 or 3 weeks in duration; however, complications or death may also occur within this period of time. True relapses do not occur in falciparum malaria; recrudescences may occur over a period of a year or slightly longer but are usually confined to the first 6 months after infection.

Complications. Vivax, ovale, and quartan malaria are relatively benign, and complications that arise during the course of infection with one of these parasites are usually due to preexisting debility or intercurrent disease. Infection with *P. falciparum* can rapidly build up to levels not obtained with the other three species and, because of the physiologic characteristics of red blood cells infected with *P. falciparum*, may lead to localized capillary obstruction, decreased blood flow, tissue hypoxia, infarction, and death. Chronic *P. malariae* infections in children may result in immune-complex deposition on the glomerular walls, leading to the nephrotic syndrome (see Pathogenesis). In general, treatment of malaria complications first depends on vigorous treatment of that infection and then follows the usual procedures for handling the particular problem. For discussions of the treatment of malaria, see Berman (2004) and White (1996, 1997).

Cerebral Malaria. Cerebral malaria is the most serious complication of falciparum infection and a frequent cause of death. Onset may be sudden; it can even be the first sign of the infection. Severe headache is the usual presenting symptom, followed by drowsiness, confusion, and coma. At times coma may be the presenting symptom. Cerebellar ataxia has been reported as the only neurologic involvement and may be significantly delayed. Physical signs of central nervous systems (CNS) involvement may be quite variable or completely absent. Suspicion of cerebral malaria requires prompt administration of quinine or quinidine, usually intravenously at first, and consideration of exchange transfusion. Steroids, previously thought to be useful for reducing cerebral edema in this condition, have been shown to be contraindicated and the edema to be nonexistent. Sequelae of cerebral malaria may include cortical blindness, hemiparesis, generalized spasticity, cerebellar ataxia, and severe hypotonia.

Anemia. Anemia as a consequence of the heavy parasite load in falciparum malaria is to be expected and should be treated, with due care to prevent fluid overload (and overt pulmonary edema) in the process, if the hematocrit falls below 20% or if there is parasitemia of 5% or greater.

Renal Disease. Renal complications are common in severe falciparum malaria and may occur also with repeated *P. malariae* infections, especially in children. Acute renal failure may occur in the course of any severe attack of falciparum malaria, presumably as a result of tubular necrosis resulting from red cell sludging and renal anoxia, but it usually improves as the infection is brought under control. The nephrotic syndrome, due to acute glomerulonephritis and with typical renal biopsy findings by light microscopy, has been reported in quartan as well as falciparum malaria. Proteinuria is common during the period of a clinical attack of quartan malaria, and in children it may be associated with massive edema and other clinical signs of the nephrotic syndrome. Renal lesions are apparently secondary to deposition within the glomeruli of circulating antigen-antibody complexes in the antigen-excess situation that may occur in a chronic low-grade quartan infection. Unlike most forms of the nephrotic syndrome, that associated with *P. malariae* infection is essentially unaffected by the administration of steroids.

Medical management of a malarious patient with renal failure does not differ from standard medical management of malaria. Only some 20% of quinine is cleared through the kidneys, and in oliguric renal failure the quinine doses need not be altered for the first 2 or 3 days of therapy but may need to be lowered thereafter if the patient's condition has not improved.

Blackwater Fever. Blackwater fever is a syndrome that results from massive intravascular hemolysis and consequent hemoglobinuria. It occurs almost exclusively in patients suffering from severe falciparum malaria but has been reported in vivax and quartan malaria as well. Usually there is a history of previous malaria attacks, and occasionally of prior bouts of blackwater fever. The onset generally occurs during a paroxysm of falciparum malaria, but it may take place without any accompanying symptoms, and it is possible for the onset of the condition to be missed, because hemoglobinuria per se does not give rise to symptoms. Destruction of red blood cells, if long continued, may lead to profound anemia. The cause of this condition remains unknown. It has been speculated that it represents an autoimmune phenomenon, with the development of antibodies to the infected erythrocyte. A relationship between blackwater fever and the use of quinine (either sporadically or in inadequate amounts) has long been postulated, but the condition may develop in persons who have not been treated with this drug. Quinine therapy should not be discontinued if blackwater fever develops.

Dysenteric Malaria. Dysenteric malaria is an uncommon but extremely serious complication of falciparum malaria characterized by abdominal pain, nausea, vomiting, and upper gastrointestinal bleeding, which may be related to focal ischemic changes in the intestinal wall capillary bed. At times the liver is enlarged and tender, the skin is icteric, and the urine contains bile (the so-called bilious remittent fever). Both intestinal malabsorption and reduced hepatic blood flow have been demonstrated in severe falciparum malaria.

Algid Malaria. Algid malaria is a term used for falciparum malaria attacks characterized by rapid development of hypotension and impairment of vascular perfusion. The temperature falls rapidly, and the patient may become delirious. Symptoms of generalized vascular collapse and shock develop quickly. This syndrome may be the result of gram-negative septicemia, pulmonary edema, massive gastrointestinal hemorrhage, splenic rupture, or uncorrected dehydration. Initial therapy involves correction of the hemodynamic problems and administration of antibiotics.

Pulmonary Edema. Pulmonary edema may develop rapidly in an oliguric or anuric patient, secondary to overzealous parenteral fluid administration, or it may develop without evidence of fluid retention or cardiac decompensation, possibly as the result of disseminated intravascular coagulation (DIC) or anoxia affecting the pulmonary microcirculation. This frequently fatal complication should receive the same medical management as pulmonary edema or adult respiratory distress syndrome in any critically ill patient.

Tropical Splenomegaly Syndrome. The spleen normally enlarges during an acute attack of malaria but then regresses toward normal, so persistent splenomegaly in adults is not a normal finding. Splenomegaly of unknown cause is a frequent finding in malarious areas of the tropics, and for many years has been referred to as tropical splenomegaly syndrome (TSS). The patient shown in Figure 4-7 was followed for 7 years, until death at age 20 years, at a time before it was realized that long-term antimalarial prophylaxis would reverse the progression of TSS. The syndrome is characterized by chronic splenomegaly and marked elevation of the serum immunoglobulin M (IgM) value as compared with people from the same area who do not have splenomegaly. (This qualification is important, as "normal" IgM levels are generally considerably higher in tropical than in temperate areas.) There may also be lymphocytic infiltration of the hepatic sinusoids. A response to antimalarial treatment is essential to the diagnosis. The spleen may grow to enormous size and cause considerable

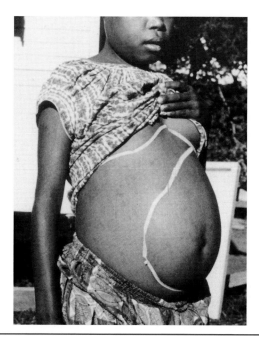

FIGURE 4-7 ■ Tropical splenomegaly. (From Crane GG. Hyperreactive malarious splenomegaly [tropical splenomegaly syndrome]. *Parasitol Today* 1986;2:4–9.)

abdominal discomfort; anemia and reticulocytosis with thrombocytopenia are usual. The majority of patients are only mildly symptomatic.

Most of the work on TSS has been done in two widely separated areas: Papua New Guinea and Africa. The syndrome occurs only in malarious areas, and the condition improves on administration of antimalarials but recurs if treatment is stopped. The basic problem in TSS seems to be related to overproduction of immunoglobulins, especially IgM, and the reduction of T lymphocytes. It has been suggested that the underlying defect may be in the suppressor T cells that control B-cell activation.

The prevalence of TSS varies widely in different areas, from less than 1% to 80% of the adult population. This syndrome may occur in patients who have resided in nonendemic areas for many years and may be diagnosed on the basis of an enlarged spleen, hypersplenism, anemia, and elevated specific immunofluorescent antibody titers to *P. falciparum*. The only effective treatment is lifelong antimalarial suppressive therapy; splenectomy has been tried, but initial improvement is not sustained and hepatomegaly ensues.

Hyperparasitemia. Parasitemias in excess of 10% to 20% of the red blood cells carry a very high mortality rate despite prompt and vigorous treatment, and in cerebral malaria the same seems true of parasite levels as low as 5%. Prompt exchange blood transfusions may be life saving in these circumstances.

Hypoglycemia. Hyperinsulinemia may result from treatment of falciparum malaria in adults with quinine and quinidine, and the subsequent hypoglycemia may be an important cause of fetal distress and death during the third trimester of pregnancy. In African children, profound hypoglycemia leading to death has been noted in the absence of hyperinsulinemia and unrelated to antimalarial treatment; it may be the result of impairment of hepatic gluconeogenesis. Hypoglycemia has also been noted in adults suffering from severe falciparum malaria who did not receive quinine. It has been suggested that quinine be administered in 10% glucose to patients found to be hypoglycemic.

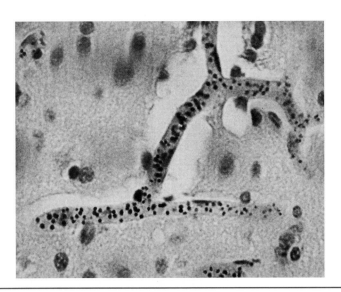

FIGURE 4-8   ■   *Plasmodium falciparum.* Malarial pigment in capillaries of the brain.

Pathogenesis. The pathogenic effects of a malarial infection have been considered to be directly related to hemolysis of infected and uninfected red blood cells, liberation of the metabolites of the parasite and the immunologic response of the host to this antigenic material, and the formation of malarial pigment. Additionally, in falciparum malaria the phenomenon of cytoadherence is basic to the locally diminished tissue perfusion seen in its more severe complications. Cytoadherence is the result of the expression on the surface of the parasitized red cell of strain- and stage-specific parasite-derived ligands (located on the electron-dense "knobs" that appear at about the time the parasite starts to divide), which adhere to a specific receptor complex on the endothelial cells. Some such ligands have been identified, and the glycoprotein thrombospondin may be involved in the specific receptor complex. Small vessels may thus become plugged by masses of parasitized red blood cells (Fig. 4-8). Ischemia consequent to plugging of the vessels produces symptoms that vary with the organ involved and the degree of tissue anoxia. Counts of parasitized erythrocytes in cerebral and other vessels have shown that the proportion of parasitized red blood cells is consistently higher in the brain than in other organs and even higher in patients with cerebral malaria than in patients who do not exhibit this form of the disease. Additional factors may include the dramatic decrease in deformability of the *P. falciparum*-infected red blood cells, once the parasite has matured beyond the ring stage.

In persons (especially children) subjected to repeated attacks of malaria, anemia is disproportional to the numbers of red blood cells infected, and indicates that noninfected red blood cells may become sensitized and be destroyed. The mechanism by which this sensitization takes place is perhaps through the production of autoantibodies to the red blood cell during infection or through the binding of soluble malarial antigen or of circulating antigen-antibody complexes to the cell surface.

The interactions of some of the phenomena discussed earlier, leading to the signs and symptoms characteristic of malaria, are shown schematically in Figure 4-9.

Recent evidence suggests that the symptoms and pathologic changes seen in malaria may be less directly the result of the effect of the parasite on the red blood cell than of proteins (cytokines) secreted by the host's cells in response to the presence of the parasite. Tumor necrosis factor (TNF) and functionally related proteins such as the interleukins are produced as a normal part of the host response to infection. A direct relationship between elevated TNF levels and death from cerebral malaria has been found. Sera from patients with a variety of

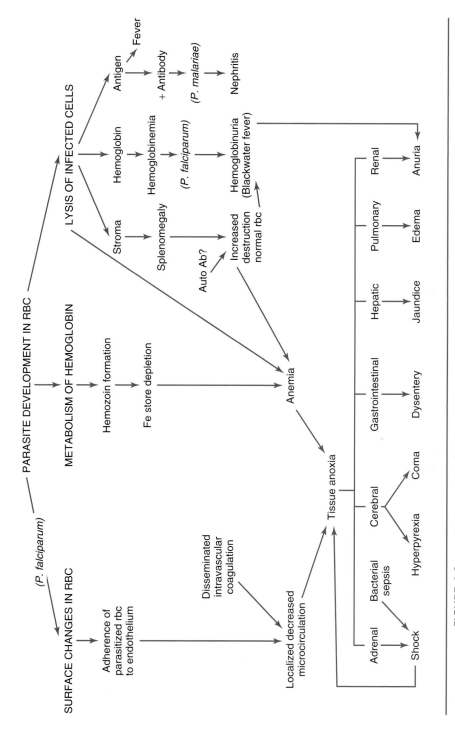

FIGURE 4-9 ■ Pathogenesis of malaria.

infectious and neoplastic diseases contain elevated levels of TNF in two thirds of those with malaria and kala-azar but in fewer than 8% of healthy subjects or persons with neoplastic disease. When these cytokines are present in excess, they may give rise to the nonspecific symptoms of malarial infection. This has been determined in clinical trials, using TNF for the experimental treatment of tumors, and in volunteers by increasing the level of circulating TNF. Antigenic material from murine malarias has been found to trigger the release of TNF. It has also been found that TNF, interleukin-1, and interleukin-2 are all capable of producing neurologic symptoms, which may play some role in cerebral malaria.

The various species of malarial parasites differ in their ability to infect red blood cells. Merozoites of *P. vivax* and *P. ovale* are able to invade only reticulocytes, whereas those of *P. malariae* are limited to senescent cells nearing the end of their life span. Thus, a natural limit is placed on these infections: reticulocytes constitute less than 2% of the total number of red blood cells, and those suitable for infection by *P. malariae*, even less. *P. falciparum* is able to invade all ages of red blood cells indifferently, and consequently infections by this parasite result early in considerable degrees of anemia.

Mechanisms of red blood cell invasion have been studied by means of electron microscopy. The apical end of the simian parasite *Plasmodium knowlesi* is seen to touch the surface of the erythrocyte, which invaginates slightly. A junction forms between merozoite and erythrocyte; it becomes ringlike and expands as the parasite invades the red blood cell and then in turn contracts to seal off the parasite within its vacuole. There is suggestive evidence that anterior organelles within the merozoite, known as rhoptries, play an active part in the invasion process (Fig. 4-10). The entire sequence of attachment and penetration takes only about 30 seconds. Initial recognition and attachment may require specific determinants on the surface of the red blood cell. In the case of *P. knowlesi* and *P. vivax*, the determinant seems related to the Duffy blood group antigen (see Epidemiology). Glycophorin A is apparently involved in the attachment process of *P. falciparum*. Human erythrocyte band 3, a major membrane protein, has also been implicated as a receptor for *P. falciparum* invasion.

Rupture of the infected red blood cells brings on the malarial paroxysm. Both infected and uninfected red blood cells show increased osmotic fragility. Lysis of numerous uninfected cells during the paroxysm, plus enhanced phagocytosis of normal cells in addition to the cell remnants and other debris produced by schizogony, leads both to anemia and to enlargement of the spleen and liver. An increased destruction of normal red blood cells for several weeks after eradication of a malaria infection has been noted and gives evidence that this is caused

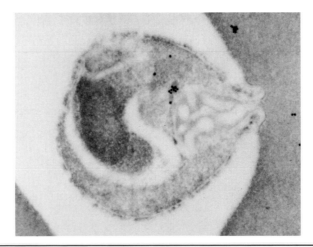

FIGURE 4-10 ■ Transmission electron micrograph showing the apical attachment of a *Plasmodium knowlesi* merozoite to an erythrocyte membrane. (Courtesy of Drs. M. Torii, J. H. Adams, M. Aikawa, and L. H. Miller, National Institutes of Health, Bethesda, MD.)

by a complement-mediated immune process. The spleen enlarges and becomes palpable during the first few weeks of infection, during which time it is soft and subject to rupture. If the infection is treated, the spleen returns to normal size, but in chronic infections it continues to enlarge and hardens. Malarial pigment (hemozoin) collects to give the organ a grayish to dark brown or black color. The liver becomes congested, and the Küpffer cells are packed with hemozoin, which indeed, is seen throughout the viscera. Hemozoin is derived from the hemoglobin of the infected red blood cell, and, as it is insoluble in plasma, its formation depletes the iron stores of the body, thus adding to the anemia.

Leukopenia is generally noted, especially in falciparum malaria, though there may be leukocytosis during the febrile paroxysms. The total plasma protein concentration is unchanged or slightly lower than normal during an attack of malaria; the albumin concentration is generally lower and the globulin concentration is increased. The globulin increase is in the gamma fraction and is associated with the appearance of antibodies measurable by the indirect immunofluorescence technique. Serum potassium may increase with the lysis of red blood cells.

Epidemiology. Falciparum and ovale malaria are primarily diseases of the tropics; quartan malaria is seen in the subtropics and temperate zones as well, while vivax malaria is usually the most common type in all endemic areas. The transmission of all species of malaria parasites depends on the presence both of suitable species of *Anopheles* mosquitoes and of infected (gametocyte-bearing) humans. In many temperate areas where suitable anopheline hosts still abound, endemic malaria has been eradicated, and introduced malaria seldom results in transmission. The suitability of a mosquito as a vector of human disease depends not only on physiologic adaptation to the infection but also on such factors as feeding preferences, hours of biting and flight, resting, and breeding habits. Thus, of more than 200 known species of *Anopheles*, only about 60 are considered to be vectors of malaria.

Gametocytes appear in the circulating blood early in the course of vivax infection and may appear with succeeding clinical relapses, whereas those of *P. falciparum* appear in the circulating blood approximately 10 days after the onset of parasitemia and are not infectious for mosquitoes for another 4 days. Thus, the patient with falciparum malaria is infectious later than the patient with vivax malaria and is less likely already to have infected mosquitoes at the time the infection is discovered and treated. In addition to gametocyte-induced, mosquito-transmitted malaria, transmission by means of transfusion is not unknown, and mechanical transmission through shared syringes is seen among drug users. One such epidemic, reported from California, involved a total of 47 cases. Because sporozoites are not likely to be present in transfused blood, relapse is equally unlikely to occur with transfusion- or syringe-acquired malaria. Congenital transmission is rare. However, pregnant women are more attractive to *Anopheles gambiae* mosquitoes than nonpregnant women, making them more vulnerable to malaria (Ansell et al., 2002).

The various species of malaria parasites have different temperature requirements for development in the mosquito host. Thus, in cooler parts of the endemic areas, development of *P. falciparum* cannot take place in the spring, and attacks of malaria caused by this species occur mainly in the hot weather of summer and early autumn. From this characteristic seasonal appearance comes the old name of aestivoautumnal malaria.

Glucose-6-phosphate dehydrogenase (G-6-PD)–deficient cells are from 2 to 80 times more resistant to invasion by *P. falciparum* than are normal erythrocytes. G-6-PD deficiency involves three alleles, Gd^A, Gd^B, and Gd^{A-}. Clinically, one sees no increased resistance in hemizygous (Gd^A) boys (the gene involved is on the X chromosome) or homozygous (Gd^{A-}/Gd^A) girls, but the resistance of heterozygous (Gd^{A-}/Gd^B) girls is greater. The mechanism whereby this mosaicism offers protection is uncertain, as is that involving hemoglobinopathies. Various hemoglobinopathies, especially the presence of hemoglobin S, have been found to be related to increased resistance to *P. falciparum* infection. Malaria mortality in patients with the sickle cell trait has been found to be less than one twentieth of that expected.

These hemoglobinopathies (as well as thalassemia and hemoglobin C or E, also considered by some to be associated with increased resistance to *P. falciparum* infection) have a geographic distribution that could be readily explained if they confer a selective advantage to their possessors in a hyperendemic malaria zone. Southeast Asian ovalocytosis (a form of hereditary elliptocytosis found in Malaysia, Indonesia, Papua New Guinea, the Philippines, and elsewhere) is associated with increased resistance to malaria, probably because of a structurally and functionally abnormal band 3 protein.

Immunity in malaria is relative and generally strain specific. Infants born to native parents in the regions of Africa in which malaria is hyperendemic (and presumably in other areas of high endemicity) are almost completely free of malaria during the first few months of life. It seems probable that this is due to the passive transfer of maternal immunity. Antibodies to blood stages of the parasites have been detected in such infants, and antisporozoite antibodies to *P. falciparum* in similar titers in mothers and babies; however, the babies lost their titers by age 6 months. Such antisporozoite antibodies (stage- and species-specific for both *P. falciparum* and *P. vivax*) have been noted in adults living in endemic areas of Thailand. Children exposed to repeated infections in hyperendemic areas develop a high degree of immunity, though this immunity does not imply eradication of the infection but rather a balance between parasite and host.

West African blacks and their descendants in the Americas and elsewhere possess relative immunity to *P. vivax* and also to experimental infection with *P. cynomolgi*. An explanation of this remarkable resistance is afforded by observations that Duffy blood group-negative human erythrocytes (Fy/Fy) are resistant to invasion in vitro by *P. knowlesi*, a species of monkey malaria. Duffy-positive erythrocytes (Fy^a or Fy^b) were readily infected. Among black and white volunteers who have been exposed to the bites of *P. vivax*-infected mosquitoes, only the Duffy-negative blacks were immune to infection, thus suggesting that the high prevalence of Duffy negativity in West Africans accounts for the resistance of these peoples, and of approximately 70% of American blacks, to *P. vivax*. Instead of *P. vivax*, *P. ovale* is common in West Africa. In East Africa, where a higher percentage of persons are Duffy positive, *P. vivax* is seen.

A strain of *P. cynomolgi*, usually parasitic in monkeys and morphologically similar to *P. vivax*, has been found to give rise to both natural and experimental human infections. *Plasmodium brasilianum*, a quartan type of parasite, is another species that produces monkey malaria that has been transmitted to humans by the bite of infected mosquitoes. Infection in humans is mild or asymptomatic. Both whites and blacks can be infected with this parasite, in contrast with *P. cynomolgi*, which has been transmitted only to whites. Several monkey malarias may from time to time cause human infections, although simian relapsing species do not appear to relapse in humans; others, probably of human origin, have become established in simian hosts.

A large focus of naturally acquired *Plasmodium knowlesi* infection in humans has been reported in Malaysian Borneo (Singh et al., 2004). *P. knowlesi*, a malarial parasite of long-tailed macaque monkeys (*Macaca irus*), resembles *P. malariae* and originally was described as such by microscopy in the infected humans. Subsequent PCR assays have identified the organisms as *P. knowlesi*. Studies are underway to determine whether the human *P. knowlesi* infections were acquired from macaque monkeys or from other infected humans, indicating that a host switch had occurred.

In the late 1940s and for some years thereafter, authorities spoke with confidence of eradicating the malarias, diseases responsible annually for more deaths than any other infectious diseases. Eradication programs have had some measure of success and in fact have eliminated transmission of these infections in North America, Europe, and Australia. An annual worldwide death rate was estimated at 2.5 million persons in the late 1960s; in Africa 1 million infants still die each year of the disease. As we begin the 21st century, these estimates have changed little, if at all, and the malaria situation appears actually to be worsening. Thus, in some heavily endemic areas such as parts of Africa and Asia, the program objective now is containment, although in certain regions there has been a resurgence of the disease in the past few years.

The reasons for this disappointing lack of success are many, and space does not permit a detailed analysis here. However, important factors have included the development of resistance to previously effective antimalarial drugs, virtually worldwide; the development of resistance to insecticides on the part of the anopheline mosquitoes and a reluctance to use them owing to their side effects; and the sheer magnitude of the task.

Treatment. Proper use of the antimalarial drugs is based on knowledge of their effects on the parasite at various stages of the life cycle. *Suppressive therapy (chemoprophylaxis)* attempts to destroy the parasites as they enter the bloodstream with small doses of drugs effective against the erythrocytic stages. Attempts at *clinical cure* employ larger doses of the same types of drugs or (where suppressive therapy has failed) different ones, to eliminate the large numbers of erythrocytic parasites present in a clinical attack. *Radical cure* implies elimination of not only the bloodstream infection but the tissue stages in the liver as well. Drugs effective against the asexual erythrocytic stages are not necessarily gametocyticidal or active against the pre-erythrocytic stages (including hypnozoites). A clinical cure may then leave the patient infectious because of gametocytes remaining in the circulating blood or subject to relapse after reinvasion of the bloodstream by pre-erythrocytic forms that remain in the liver or (in vivax and ovale malaria) by pre-erythrocytic schizogony initiated by reactivated hypnozoites. A brief synopsis of currently recommended treatment is given on pp. 99–102.

Quinine and its related alkaloids were the only specific antimalarial drugs available prior to World War I. Isolated from the bark of the South American *Cinchona* tree ("Jesuits' bark"), quinine is now grown more extensively in Java; synthesis of the drug has not been commercially practical. Starting in the late 1920s, many synthetic drugs were developed. Quinacrine (Mepacrine, Atabrine) became available in the early 1930s, and with the spread of World War II to the Pacific and the consequent scarcity of quinine, became the drug of choice until it was supplanted by more effective agents (principally chloroquine) developed during that war. Resistance to some of these drugs was noted early but was of little clinical significance until chloroquine resistance appeared in strains of *P. falciparum* from South America and Southeast Asia in the 1950s, subsequently spreading to most areas of intense malaria transmission. *P. falciparum* organisms that are resistant to chloroquine are often resistant to other synthetic antimalarials as well, and quinine has once more emerged as a mainstay of treatment in such cases. Chloroquine resistance has also made its appearance in *P. vivax* in Oceania but as yet is of limited clinical significance. Three grades of resistance are recognized, ranging from RI, in which administration of the drug achieves apparent clinical cure only to be followed by recrudescence, to RIII, in which therapy seems completely ineffective.

Many classes of drugs have either important or ancillary effects on one or more stages of the life cycle of different species of the malaria parasites. Those presently available include the following:
cinchona alkaloids (quinine, quinidine)
4-aminoquinolines (chloroquine, amodiaquine)
8-aminoquinolines (primaquine)
diaminopyrimidines (pyrimethamine)
sulfonamides and sulfones (sulfadoxine, dapsone)
quinoline methanols (mefloquine)
tetracyclines (tetracycline, doxycycline)
biguanides (proguanil)
phenanthrene methanols (halofantrine)
hydroxynaphthoquinones (atovaquone)

In addition, several groups of compounds are undergoing testing in humans or are not available for clinical use in the United States:
sesquiterpene lactones (qinghaosu, artemisinin, artemether, artesunate, and artesunate
     suppositories)
pyronaridine

synthetic endoperoxides (Fenozan B07)
substituted trioxanes
trioxane dimers
nonane endoperoxides
macrolides (azithromycin)
8-aminoquinolines (WR238605)

The known mechanisms of action of these drugs are given in Table 4-2. We first list the drugs in relation to the stage or stages of the life cycle in which they exert their main or only effect and then discuss the more important ones in some detail.

Blood Schizonticides. These drugs may be used for suppression or treatment of an acute attack of malaria. Most have no effect on either the pre-(exo)erythrocytic stages of the parasites or gametocytes. Quinine and its isomer, quinidine, were the first drugs employed to destroy the asexual parasites in the bloodstream. Chloroquine (Aralen, Nivaquine) was the mainstay of blood schizonticidal therapy for all species of malaria except chloroquine-resistant *P. falciparum* (CRPF) through the 1970s; however, rapidly increasing resistance has now markedly reduced its usefulness. Chloroquine resistance (and presumably resistance to other antimalarials as well) may first become evident in nonimmune travelers to areas in which the drug still affords protection to the partially immune native population. Hydroxychloroquine (Plaquenil) and amodiaquine (Camoquin) have virtually the same antimalarial activity as chloroquine, and almost equally reduced usefulness. Pyrimethamine (Daraprim) is a slow-acting blood schizonticide, against which resistance was early developed both by *P. falciparum* and *P. vivax*. Mefloquine (Lariam) is effective against many strains of CRPF as well as the other species of malaria, but resistance to the drug has been reported, especially in Southeast Asia. Tetracycline and doxycycline have some activity against the blood schizonts of all four species of malarial parasites. The efficacy of halofantrine seems generally similar to that of mefloquine. Proguanil (Paludrine) is widely used in East Africa. It is less effective against *P. vivax* than against *P. falciparum*. The herb *Artemisia annua* has been used as a febrifuge and antimalarial for centuries in China, and in 1972 artemisinin (qinghaosu) was isolated from it and shown to have very active antimalarial properties; a number of derivatives of artemisinin have been prepared for treatment of malaria.

Tissue Schizonticides. These drugs act as *causal prophylactics* by destroying the developmental stages in the liver. While a number of the blood schizonticides (proguanil, pyrimethamine, the tetracyclines) have mild tissue schizonticidal activity, only primaquine is effective against tissue stages, including the hypnozoites of *P. vivax* and *P. ovale*.

Gametocyticides. Chloroquine and amodiaquine are effective against the gametocytes of *P. vivax*, *P. ovale*, and *P. malariae* and immature gametocytes of *P. falciparum* but do not affect the mature *P. falciparum* gametocytes. Primaquine is gametocyticidal for all four species of human malaria parasites and thus acts to render the patient noninfectious to the mosquito.

TABLE 4-2 ■ Mechanism of Action of Antimalarial Drugs

Dihydrofolate reductase inhibition: Proguanil.
Folic acid reductase inhibition: Pyrimethamine
Folic acid synthesis inhibition (PABA competition): dapsone, sulfadoxine
Unknown: Artemisinin and related drugs: chloroquine, amodiaquine (binding to DNA, DNA-RNA polymerase? altering pH of parasitophagous vesicles?); halofantrine; mefloquine; primaquine (inhibition of parasite mitochondrial respiration?); quinine, quinidine; tetracyclines; pyronaridine; endoperoxides; trioxanes; macrolides

DRUGS USED IN SINGLE-DRUG THERAPY

Quinine

For many years, quinine was the only effective drug for chemoprophylaxis or treatment of malaria, and with the emergence of resistance to the synthetic antimalarials it and its dextrorotatory stereoisomer, quinidine, have once again become the drugs of choice for treatment of resistant falciparum malaria. Quinine may also be used for chemoprophylaxis in selected individuals. The drug is a potent blood schizonticide against all four species of human malarial parasites, although scattered resistance on the part of *P. falciparum* was described as early as 1908 in Brazil and more recently in Vietnam, Thailand, Irian Jaya, and West Africa. It is somewhat slower acting than the 4-aminoquinolines. The adult suppressive dose is 325 mg taken twice daily with meals and continued for 4 weeks after leaving the endemic area. Smaller daily doses may suppress symptoms without completely eliminating the bloodstream infection, and such a chronic, low-grade infection *may* be the setting in which blackwater fever develops. The potential toxicity of quinine has, perhaps, been over-stated. It is difficult, from the modern literature, to get any appraisal of its toxic effects when used in suppressive doses. Strong (1944) states, "Quinine, except in rare cases of idiosyncrasy, is outstandingly nontoxic in effective doses." Minor side effects of treatment include tinnitus and headache. Cinchonism may also include nausea and vomiting, abdominal pain, blurred vision, transient loss of hearing, vertigo, and tremors; it may be seen during the first 2 or 3 days of treatment, may subside spontaneously during therapy, and always disappears after the drug is withdrawn; it is seldom severe enough to warrant a change in therapy. Serious reactions are rare. Overdose, however, may result in convulsions, hypotension, heart block, ventricular fibrillation, and death. Minor electrocardiographic changes (T-wave flattening with 10% lengthening of the Q-T interval) may be anticipated with either oral or intravenous administration.

The adult treatment dose is 650 mg every 8 hours for 3 to 7 or 10 days. (The shorter course is given if it is administered with another drug or if the patient is known to have partial immunity to malaria). The pediatric dosage is 10–25 mg/kg every 8 hours for the same interval.

Quinine has had popular use as an abortifacient but has often been used to treat severe falciparum malaria during pregnancy; the risk to the fetus of severe maternal malaria greatly outweighs the possible risk of quinine therapy. Quinine may produce maternal and fetal hyperinsulinemia and hypoglycemia, and it is important to monitor blood glucose levels during its administration.

Where quinine resistance is a factor, Looareesuwan's group (1990) suggests increasing the dose of parenteral quinine by 50% or changing to another rapidly acting drug if parasitemia does not fall by 75% within the first 48 hours of treatment. Alternatively, when dealing with infections acquired in areas from which quinine resistance has been reported, another drug such as doxycycline may routinely be added. If initial blood smears indicate a malarial infection but the species cannot be determined, it may be advisable to treat presumptively for falciparum malaria, with appropriate modification when the species is identified.

Quinine dihydrochloride has been used for intravenous administration in patients who are unable to take the oral drug, but it is now being supplanted by intravenous quinidine, which is both more readily available and somewhat more effective.

Quinidine

As with quinine, the mechanism of action of quinidine in malaria is unknown. Its antimalarial activity is slightly superior to that of quinine, though cardiotoxicity is somewhat more pronounced. The great advantage of quinidine is its ready accessibility when intravenous treatment is indicated.

Quinidine gluconate or sulfate is administered intravenously while the patient is monitored electrocardiographically. For this purpose 0.8 g quinidine gluconate or 0.6 g quinidine sulfate is diluted in 250 ml of 5% glucose in water. The initial dose for both adults and children is 24 mg/kg quinidine gluconate or 18 mg/kg quinidine sulfate, given over a 2- to 4-hour period. Subsequent doses, if necessary, are given at the rate of 12 mg/kg gluconate or 9 mg/kg sulfate every 8 hours. Higher dosages have also been recommended to avoid possible undertreatment (White, 1997). If the QRS interval increases more than 25% over baseline, administration is discontinued until this interval becomes shorter. Quinine sulfate or a combination of drugs is given per os as soon as the patient's condition permits.

Chloroquine

Chloroquine-resistant *P. falciparum* (CRPF) may be seen in all areas except the Middle East, Egypt, Central America west of the Panama Canal, Mexico, and Hispaniola (Haiti and the Dominican Republic). *P. vivax* from Papua New Guinea, Indonesia, Myanmar (Burma), India, and the Solomon Islands may also exhibit chloroquine resistance. In areas where resistance is not known to occur, chloroquine is recommended both for chemoprophylaxis and for treatment of uncomplicated malaria.

The mechanism of action of chloroquine is not known, but it may be related to the ability of 4-aminoquinolines to bind to and alter the properties of DNA or through the effects of chloroquine in raising the pH of the parasite vesicle. Resistance to chloroquine often is associated with resistance to other antimalarials; it is thought to mimic the multidrug resistance encountered in cancer chemotherapy and to be related to increased efflux of the drug from resistant forms of the parasite. Verapamil and other calcium channel blockers that reverse drug resistance in cultured cancer cells have been shown to reverse chloroquine resistance, presumably by inhibiting its efflux from the parasite food vacuole. Similar results have been achieved using the tricyclic antidepressant drug desipramine, which presumably works by the same mechanisms. The therapeutic potential of such drug combinations is questionable because of the potential toxicity to normal body cells of increased levels of chloroquine.

In the doses used for prophylaxis or treatment, toxic effects of chloroquine are generally mild and toxicity is infrequent. There may be nausea and vomiting if the pills are taken without food; dizziness, headache, confusion, blurred vision, and fatigue have also been reported. Pruritus, sometimes quite severe, occurs in a substantial percentage of West African blacks after taking chloroquine; it is less common but occurs in other ethnic groups, rarely after a single suppressive dose. Chloroquine is not contraindicated in pregnancy.

As suppressive therapy against all types of malaria except CRPF and resistant strains of vivax malaria (CRPV), the adult dose is 500 mg chloroquine phosphate (300 mg chloroquine base) once weekly starting 1 or 2 weeks before travel to the malarious area and continuing 4 weeks after leaving it. Hydroxychloroquine sulfate (Plaquenil), 400 mg weekly, is an alternative that some tolerate better. For children, hydroxychloroquine may be preferred, as the 200-mg tablets (155 mg hydroxychloroquine base) are more readily divided. The pediatric suppressive dose of either chloroquine or hydroxychloroquine is 5 mg/kg (in terms of the base) once weekly.

For clinical cure in adults, the dosage is 1 g chloroquine phosphate (600 mg chloroquine base) initially, followed by 500 mg (300 mg base) 6 hours later and a single dose of 500 mg (300 mg base) on each of the two following days (total dose = 1.5 g base). Pediatric dosage is 10 mg/kg chloroquine or hydroxychloroquine base initially, followed by 5 mg/kg in 6 hours and on each of the two following days.

Amodiaquine (Camoquin)

Amodiaquine is generally similar to chloroquine in clinical efficacy and toxicity and in development of resistance by *P. falciparum*, though in some areas it may be effective against strains that are resistant to chloroquine. Some cases of severe neutropenia have been associated with its use for suppressive therapy, and the drug is not suitable for routine prophylaxis; it is not commercially available in the United States. For clinical cure in adults and children, the same doses of amodiaquine, in terms of its base, are given at the same intervals outlined above for chloroquine. Amodiaquine may be given during pregnancy.

Pyrimethamine (Daraprim)

Pyrimethamine was once used extensively for chemoprophylaxis, chiefly because of its long half-life and safety in pregnancy, but resistance has become so widespread that it now finds its main use in combination with sulfadoxine as Fansidar and with dapsone as Maloprim.

Mefloquine (Lariam)

Mefloquine was early found to be effective against both chloroquine-sensitive and –resistant strains of *P. falciparum* and *P. vivax*. It is also effective against *P. malariae* and *P. ovale*, though experience in treating these species is limited. It is ineffective against the tissue stages and gametocytes. Resistance has been noted in Southeast Asia (over 50% along the Thailand-Myanmar border), Irian Jaya, the Philippines, and Africa. Resistance to mefloquine in vitro and in vivo has been noted in strains of *P. falciparum* from areas in West Africa in which the drug has never been used.

In prophylactic doses mefloquine usually gives rise to minor side effects similar to those seen with suppressive doses of chloroquine, but there have been isolated reports of acute psychotic episodes and other neuropsychiatric reactions associated with this use of the drug. With treatment doses exceeding 750 mg, side effects may be more pronounced. Neurologic changes, including convulsions, loss of consciousness, and acute psychoses, have been reported following treatment in adults given maximum treatment doses. Mefloquine may also induce sinus bradycardia and should not be given to patients with conduction defects or those taking beta blockers, calcium channel blockers, quinine, or quinidine. It should not be used during the first trimester of pregnancy; the risk of convulsions is increased when it is administered concurrently with chloroquine or quinine. Nevertheless, and despite considerable "bad press" in the popular travel literature, numerous case-control studies have failed to show a causality of mefloquine to reported side effects. Thus, on the basis of a review of more than 1 million European travelers and U.S. Peace Corps volunteers, 90% of whom had used mefloquine continuously for 2 to 3 years—plus an equivalent relative risk (1:13,300) for chloroquine prophylaxis—the U.S. Centers for Disease Control and Prevention (CDC) has concluded that "mefloquine prophylaxis is safe, is well tolerated, and has saved thousands of lives" (Lobel, 1996).

Mefloquine has an extremely long serum half-life of 13 to 24 days, and in some studies even longer. The suppressive dose in adults is 250 mg weekly starting a week before and continuing for 4 weeks after the potential exposure. For children the weekly dose is as follows:
5–10 kg, one-eighth tablet
11–20 kg, a quarter tablet
21–30 kg, a half tablet
31–45 kg, three-quarter tablet
>45 kg, one tablet (250 mg)
The adult treatment dose is 750 mg followed 12 hours later by 500 mg. The recommended pediatric treatment dose is 15 mg/kg followed 12 hours later by 10 mg/kg.

Owing to its lengthy half-life and in case of therapeutic failure of mefloquine, it must be borne in mind that the substitution of quinine or quinidine may expose the patient to increased risk of cardiac conduction problems or convulsions.

Doxycycline

The tetracyclines are blood schizonticides, and while they have some effect on the pre-erythrocytic stages of the malarial parasites, they cannot be relied on to achieve radical cure.

Doxycycline is less effective against *P. vivax* than against *P. falciparum* and so should not be used alone for prophylaxis, or if so used should be followed by a 4- to 6-week course of chloroquine prophylaxis to prevent subsequent development of vivax malaria. The prophylactic dose of doxycycline for adults is 100 mg daily; for children older than 8 years it is 2 mg/kg (maximum 100 mg) daily. As with other chemoprophylactic drugs, it should be continued for 4 weeks after the patient leaves the endemic area.

Proguanil (Paludrine)

Proguanil is a blood schizonticide that initially was effective against all four species of malaria. It is now generally useful against *P. falciparum* in East Africa but not in West Africa, Thailand, or New Guinea, where significant resistance occurs. Strains of *P. vivax* and *P. malariae* that are resistant to this drug have also been found in scattered areas. It is well tolerated in suppressive doses but should not be used for treatment. Paludrine is not available commercially in the United States but may be obtained in Canada and many European and African countries. It is used extensively in East Africa.

The suppressive dose for adults is 200 mg daily, continued for 4 weeks after leaving the malarious area. Some authorities recommend adding a weekly dose of chloroquine at the usual level. To children Paludrine may be given as follows:
before age 2 years, 50 mg daily
2–6 years, 100 mg daily
7–10 years, 150 mg daily
after age 10 years, 200 mg daily

Halofantrine (Halfan)

Halofantrine, a lipophilic phenanthrenemethanol, was released for the treatment of multiple-drug-resistant *P. falciparum* in the United States in 1996. It is not used for suppressive therapy. Field trials in Thailand, with other Southeast Asian strains, and with patients infected in various parts of Africa indicate that the drug is effective in the treatment of multidrug-resistant *P. falciparum* at doses similar to those used with mefloquine, but there have been reports of treatment failures, at least some due to poor and erratic absorption after oral administration. The recommended dosage of halofantrine is 8 mg/kg, repeated after 6 and 12 hours, and, in nonimmune patients, a further three daily doses 1 week later (White, 1996). It should not be given with fatty foods or with drugs known to prolong the Q-T interval. Halofantrine was significantly more efficacious than chloroquine or pyrimethamine-sulfadoxine in Nigeria and Kenya. The French armed forces have found it effective in preventing falciparum malaria in troops returning from Africa.

Artemisinin

Extracts of *Artemisia annua*, a plant known in China as *quinghao*, have been used for centuries to treat malaria in that country, and in 1972, an active component of these extracts (*qinghaosu*) called artemisinin was isolated from that plant. It is interesting that none of some 30 other species of *Artemisia* seems to have antimalarial activity. Artemisinin is effective against both *P. falciparum* and *P. vivax*, and several derivatives, including, among others, artemether, arteether, and sodium artesunate, seem to be even more active, especially in patients with cerebral malaria. Qinghaosu appears to act more rapidly as a blood schizonticide than either quinine or mefloquine, but patients treated with it have a high rate of recrudescences, and it is possible that its chief value will be its use in combination with other antimalarials. Comparative studies of oral artemether alone or followed by mefloquine, and of artesunate in rectal suppository form followed by mefloquine in Thailand and Vietnam have been published and further studies are in progress. However, a potential for neurotoxicity may become a significant concern in artemisinin use. Qinghaosu/artemisinin derivatives may not be suitable for suppressive therapy because of a short half-life. They are not available for clinical use in the United States.

Norfloxacin/Ciprofloxacin

These fluoroquinolone antibacterial agents were found to be effective in vitro against CRPF; however, both were shown to be *ineffective* in clinical trials.

MULTIPLE DRUG PROPHYLAXIS AND TREATMENT OF RESISTANT FALCIPARUM MALARIA

Quinine or Mefloquine and Doxycycline

Although doxycycline alone has been recommended for chemoprophylaxis of malaria in multidrug-resistant areas, it may also be administered in conjunction with mefloquine, quinine, or other antimalarials. When so used, the adult dose is 100 mg daily. If administered for treatment along with other antimalarials, the usual adult dose of doxycycline is 100 mg twice daily, given over a 7-day period. The pediatric treatment dose of doxycycline is 1.5 to 2 mg/kg twice daily. Doxycycline should not be used during the latter half of pregnancy or for children younger than 8 years, because it can discolor tooth enamel.

Side effects include allergic skin reactions, photosensitivity (an important consideration for persons going to tropical areas), and diarrhea. Photosensitivity may be avoided by the use of sunscreens with a sun protection rating of 28 or greater.

Pyrimethamine-Sulfadoxine (Fansidar)

Various combinations of pyrimethamine with sulfonamides or sulfones have proved to be effective antimalarials. A combination of 25 mg pyrimethamine with 500 mg sulfadoxine (Fansidar) is particularly effective because of the long half-life of both components and was widely used for prophylaxis of CRPF until its toxicity became appreciated. Sulfadoxine has the same potential for the production of severe and even fatal cutaneous reactions (such as Stevens-Johnson syndrome, erythema multiforme, or toxic epidermal necrolysis) as the other long-acting sulfonamides, and a number of fatalities have resulted from its use. Granulomatous hepatitis, another complication of sulfonamide therapy, has been reported in patients using Fansidar. Resistance to Fansidar has become a major problem in Thailand and other Southeast Asian countries, New Guinea, sub-Saharan Africa, and Brazil, and it occurs also in other parts of South America and in Indonesia. Indications for its prophylactic use are now limited. Dosage for this purpose is one tablet weekly. It may also be used for presumptive treatment of malaria in situations when medical care is unavailable. Treatment dosage (not usually associated with any severe side effects in patients not allergic to either of its components) is three tablets taken as a single dose for adults. For children, the treatment dose is as follows: 5–10 kg, half tablet; 11–20 kg, one tablet; 21–30 kg, one and one-half tablets; 31–45 kg, two tablets; over 45 kg, three tablets. Resistance to Fansidar used for treatment has been reported from Kenya and from Ghana. There is no agreement about its use in pregnancy.

An absolute contraindication to the use of Fansidar is a history of sulfonamide intolerance. Travelers who use it for suppression should be advised to discontinue it immediately if signs or symptoms of possible intolerance develop, such as itching, redness, rash, oral or genital lesions, or sore throat.

Pyrimethamine-Sulfadoxine-Mefloquine (Fansimef)

This combination was introduced with the hope that it would delay the development of resistance to mefloquine. It consists of the same amounts of pyrimethamine and sulfadoxine found in Fansidar, with the addition of mefloquine, 250 mg per tablet. In studies in Thailand the combination did not appear to be more effective than either mefloquine or Fansidar alone.

Side effects are reported to be similar to those seen with mefloquine but with a higher incidence of nausea and vomiting. The recommended treatment dose for adults is two tablets in areas where Fansidar resistance is not a problem and three tablets where resistance is high. Suppressive use of this combination cannot be recommended because of the potential toxicity of sulfadoxine. Fansimef is not available commercially in the United States or in Canada.

Pyrimethamine-Dapsone (Maloprim)

This combination of pyrimethamine 12.5 mg and dapsone 100 mg is not too effective when given at the adult dose of one tablet weekly and seems to carry an unacceptable risk of agranulocytosis when given in the more effective twice-weekly dosage. Maloprim is not available in the United States or in Canada.

Atovaquone-Proguanil (Malarone)

Atovaquone (Mepron) is a hydroxy-1,4-naphthoquinone that has been used for the treatment of pneumocystosis in patients intolerant to trimethoprim-sulfamethoxazole. It has significant antiplasmodial activity, apparently at the cytochrome bc_1 complex; when used alone in a dosage of 500 to 750 mg daily for 7 days in patients with falciparum malaria, it produced 67% to 76% cure rate (Looareesuwan, 1996). However, when used in combination with proguanil at a dose of 1000 mg atovaquone with 400 mg proguanil (Malarone), once daily for 3 days, a 99.5% cure rate was achieved. The suppressive dose is 250 mg atovaquone/100 mg proguanil daily and continuing for 7 days after leaving the risk area. Malarone should not be taken by pregnant women or children weighing less than 11 kg (25 pounds). A significant drawback for long-term use prospects was the observation that parasites remaining after currently infrequently *un*successful Malarone treatment are totally resistant to virtually any dose of this agent. Also, apparent relapses have occurred following treatment of *P. vivax* malaria. Malarone is well tolerated, and has been approved for use in drug-resistant falciparum malaria.

TREATMENT OF TISSUE SCHIZONTS, HYPNOZOITES, AND GAMETOCYTES

Most of the blood schizonticides have little or no effect on other developmental stages in the life cycle of the parasites, and if these drugs are discontinued when a traveler leaves the malarious area tissue schizonts may continue to develop, producing an attack of malaria a few days or weeks later. Continuing treatment for 4 weeks after the risk of exposure is past should allow the tissue schizonts of *P. falciparum* and *P. malariae* time to complete their development in the liver and enter the bloodstream to be destroyed. The hypnozoite stages of *P. vivax* and *P. ovale* may remain dormant in the tissues long after this period, to produce attacks of malaria weeks, months, or even several years later.

Primaquine

Primaquine is effective against the hypnozoites of *P. vivax*, and probably of *P. ovale,* and is gametocyticidal for all four species of malaria. Routine administration of primaquine after leaving a malarious area safeguard against hypnozoite-induced attacks of *P. vivax* infection and renders patients noninfectious. Primaquine must be given with caution where glucose-6-phosphate dehydrogenase deficiency is common, and is contraindicated in the presence of severe variants of the deficiency.

The treatment dose for adults is 30 mg primaquine base daily for 14 days. It should be given before completion of the suppressive therapy. The dose for children is 0.6 mg/kg of the base daily for 14 days.

The Centers for Disease Control and Prevention recommends the following regimens for the prevention of malaria in travelers★ (recommended dosages are those given in the

---

★Detailed recommendations for the prevention of malaria are available 24 hours a day by calling the CDC Malaria Hotline by phone (770) 488-7788 or for fax information, (888) 232-3299. This information is also available at www.cdc.gov/travel/diseases.htm.

preceding pages):

1. For travel to areas where chloroquine resistance has *not* been reported, chloroquine once weekly.
2. For travel to all other malarious areas, mefloquine once weekly. When mefloquine is contraindicated, alternatives are atovaquone proguanil or doxycycline daily *or* chloroquine once weekly plus a treatment dose of Fansidar for use in case of fever, *if professional medical care is not available within 24 hours.*

Prevention. One aspect of prevention (chemoprophylaxis) has already been discussed. In actuality, this is not a form of prevention, as the person so protected may become infected but fails to manifest disease symptoms while taking the suppressive drugs.

More lasting preventive efforts must be directed at breaking the human-mosquito-human cycle. Mosquito control measures are fundamental to this endeavor, but, as already mentioned, they have been hampered by the rapid emergence of insecticide resistance and by our increasing awareness that these substances are potentially quite harmful in many ways. Ingenious methods of larval and adult mosquito control, such as the use of various types of predators or the breeding and liberation of vast numbers of irradiated and sterile male mosquitoes, have been attempted, sometimes with limited success. Until truly successful methods of mosquito control are available, emphasis must be placed on keeping infected mosquitoes at bay. Mechanical barriers such as proper screening undoubtedly are helpful. Well-controlled studies have demonstrated the efficacy of bed nets (mosquito nets) in the prevention of malaria in hyperendemic areas, particularly when impregnated with permethrin. Space sprays can be used to eliminate mosquitoes from sleeping areas. Mosquito repellents are essential for persons in unprotected areas between the hours of dusk and sunrise, when anopheline mosquitoes bite. Repellents containing *N*,*N*-diethyl-metatoluamide (DEET) are very effective but may be toxic if absorbed through the skin, and fatalities have been reported after oral ingestion. They may be safely applied to clothing. Pyrethroid repellents, such as permethrin, are effective and less toxic and may be applied to clothing, bed nets, or screens for relatively long-lasting protection. Long-sleeved shirts and long trousers also provide protection against mosquito bites.

The development of malaria vaccines would be of immeasurable benefit to the more than 1 billion persons now at risk of developing malaria throughout the world. Three areas of vulnerability on the part of the parasitic life cycle have been focused on the sporozoite, the merozoite, and the developmental stages in the mosquito.

Vaccine candidates based on irradiated sporozoites, recombinant (circum)sporozoite proteins present on the outer surface of the sporozoite, and synthetic polypeptides of merozoites (Spf66) have all shown immunogenic potential in limited clinical trials. However, with the exception of irradiated sporozoites in repeated injection—which is an impractical approach due to the extremely limited availability of these forms, and which, therefore, has not been field tested—none of these have met expectations and/or needs in field trials. Most recently, a pre-erythrocytic vaccine candidate, RTS,S/AS-02A, based on *P. falciparum* circumsporozoite surface antigen, was tested in young African children and demonstrated 58% efficacy against severe malaria (Alonso et al., 2004). Although a malaria vaccine is urgently needed, it seems unlikely that one will be forthcoming in the near future.

References

Alonso PL et al. Efficacy of the RTS,S/AS02A vaccine against *Plasmodium falciparum* infection and disease in young African children: Randomised controlled trial. *Lancet* 2004; *364*:1411–1420.

Ansell J et al. Short-range attractiveness of pregnant women to *Anopheles gambiae* mosquitoes. *Trans R Soc Trop Med Hyg* 2002; *96*:113–116.

Berman J. Toxicity of commonly-used antimalarial drugs. *Travel Med Infect Dis* 2004; *2*:171–184.

Cogswell FB et al. Hypnozoites of *Plasmodium simiovale*. *Am J Trop Med Hyg* 1991; *45*:211–213.

Haditsch M. Quality and reliability of current malaria diagnostic methods. *Travel Med Infect Dis* 2004; 2:149–160.

Krotoski WA et al. Relapses in primate malaria. Discovery of two populations of exoerythrocytic stages. Preliminary note. *Br Med J* 1980; *280*:153–154.

Krotoski WA et al. Observations on early and late post-sporozoite tissue stages in primate malaria. IV. Pre-erythrocytic schizonts and/or hypnozoites of Chesson and North Korean strains of *Plasmodium vivax* in the chimpanzee. *Am J Trop Med Hyg* 1986; *35*:263–274.

Lobel HO. Discussion, in "Update and roundtable on malaria prophylaxis." *Am Comm Clin Trop Med Trav Health*, 45th Annual Meeting American Society of Tropical Medicine and Hygiene, Baltimore, MD, December 4, 1996.

Looareesuwan S et al. Fatal *Plasmodium falciparum* malaria after an inadequate response to quinine treatment. *J Infect Dis* 1990; *161*:577–580.

Looareesuwan S. et al. Clinical studies of atovaquone, alone or in combination with other antimalarial drugs, for treatment of acute uncomplicated malaria in Thailand. *Am J Trop Med Hyg* 1996; *54*:62–66.

Purnomo et al. Rare quadruple malaria infection in Irian Jaya Indonesia. *J Parasitol* 1999; *85*:574–579.

Singh B et al. A large focus of naturally acquired *Plasmodium knowlesi* infections in human beings. *Lancet* 2004; *363*:1017–1024.

Strong RP. Malaria. *Stitt's Diagnosis Prevention and Treatment of Tropical Diseases*, ed 6, p 101, Philadelphia, 1944, Blakiston.

White NJ. The treatment of malaria. *N Engl J Med* 1996; *335*:801–806.

White NJ. The treatment of malaria. *N Engl J Med* 1997; *336*:733–734.

Other Blood- and Tissue-Dwelling Protozoa

Although a strictly taxonomic approach seems unwarranted in a book emphasizing the medical aspects of parasitology, any other is equally arbitrary. In the preceding two chapters we have considered, as lumen dwellers, both those organisms confined to that space as well as the tissue-invasive *Entamoeba histolytica* and the intestinal coccidia and microsporidia that develop within the epithelial cells of the intestine, and as blood parasites, the plasmodia that develop initially in the liver before invading the bloodstream. We now take up a number of flagellates, lumen dwellers in their insect hosts, that invade the tissues or bloodstream of humans. Additionally, we consider the Apicomplexa *Toxoplasma, Sarcocystis,* and *Babesia*, as well as the opportunistic free-living amebae *Naegleria, Acanthamoeba,* and *Balamuthia*.

The Hemoflagellates

The family Trypanosomatidae, which includes the hemoflagellates, contains a number of genera, only two of which parasitize humans. The primitive structure in this group is represented by the genus *Leptomonas*, parasitic in insects. These organisms have a fusiform body, with the nucleus central in position and a single anterior flagellum arising from a kinetoplast near the anterior end (Fig. 5-1, promastigote). In the genus *Trypanosoma*, those forms that are seen in human blood have been rather profoundly modified from the promastigote form. The kinetoplast has assumed a position near the posterior end of the body, and the flagellum passes anteriorly, forming the outer edge of the undulating membrane, a thin protoplasmic sheet running along one side of the organism. Anteriorly in the trypomastigote (see Fig. 5-1), the flagellum may project free of the undulating membrane. One species of trypanosome that parasitizes humans may be found both in the circulating blood and intracellularly in cardiac muscle. It has the typical trypomastigote form as a blood parasite, whereas the stages found in cardiac muscle are more nearly rounded, have lost the undulating membrane and all trace of an external flagellum, and are known as amastigotes (see Fig. 5-1). In these minute parasites, the only structures that can be distinguished are the nucleus and the kinetoplast, with sometimes a remaining short intracytoplasmic portion of the flagellum. This type of organization is also seen in members of the genus *Leishmania*, which are always intracellular parasites, principally in cells of the reticuloendothelial system. They may at times be present in the bloodstream in large mononuclear cells.

The hemoflagellates were in all probability originally parasites of insects. As evidence for this we see that these organisms are transmitted by insects, in which they undergo a

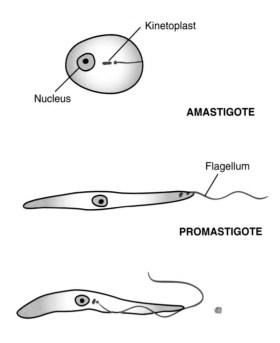

PROMASTIGOTE

EPIMASTIGOTE

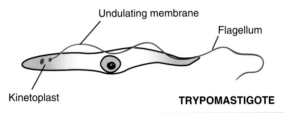

TRYPOMASTIGOTE

FIGURE 5-1   ■   Morphologic types seen in various hemoflagellates of humans.

developmental cycle. Some genera are still exclusively insect parasites. The forms of the parasites that occur in the insect host are often quite different from those found in the vertebrate. In culture, leishmanias assume a promastigote form, whereas trypanosomes also exhibit forms similar to those that occur naturally in the insect host. The Old World forms of leishmaniasis are transmitted by the bite of various species of sandflies of the genus *Phlebotomus*; the South American leishmaniases are likewise carried by sandflies. African sleeping sickness is transmitted by bites of several species of *Glossina*, or tsetse flies; the American forms of trypanosomiasis are carried by reduviid bugs, and transmission occurs when infective feces of the bug contaminate the wound made by the insect's bite or an abrasion of the skin.

TRYPANOSOMA

Two distinctly different forms of the genus *Trypanosoma* occur in humans, represented on the one hand by the species associated with African sleeping sickness, and on the other by Chagas' disease or American trypanosomiasis. In both the Gambian and Rhodesian forms of African trypanosomiasis, the parasites occur as trypomastigotes in the bloodstream,

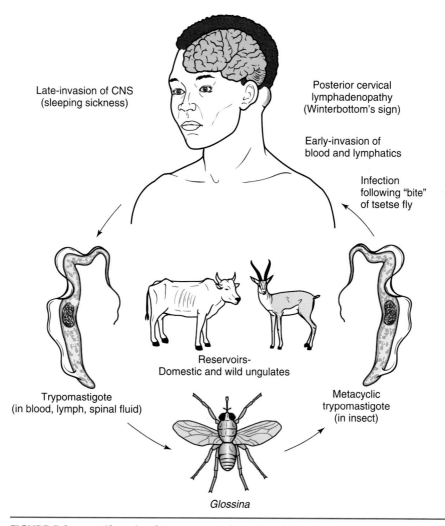

Late-invasion of CNS
(sleeping sickness)

Posterior cervical
lymphadenopathy
(Winterbottom's sign)

Early-invasion of
blood and lymphatics

Infection
following "bite"
of tsetse fly

Reservoirs-
Domestic and wild ungulates

Trypomastigote
(in blood, lymph, spinal fluid)

Metacyclic
trypomastigote
(in insect)

Glossina

FIGURE 5-2 ▪ Life cycle of *Trypanosoma brucei gambiense* and *Trypanosoma brucei rhodesiense.*

lymphatics, and cerebrospinal fluid. They also have been reported to occur as amastigotes in the choroid plexus, and possibly other organs. In Chagas' disease, trypomastigotes are found in the bloodstream, and amastigotes occur intracellularly in cardiac muscle and other tissues.

In Africa, several species of trypanosomes are important parasites of cattle, horses, and other domestic animals; the effects of these diseases on the economy of Central Africa can hardly be overestimated.

Trypanosoma brucei gambiense

African sleeping sickness occurs in what originally must have been two distinctly separate geographic areas and in two clinically distinguishable forms. The causative agents of the two types of disease are not readily differentiated, and there has been considerable controversy over their taxonomic status. Their life cycle is illustrated in Figure 5-2. *T. b. gambiense* (Fig. 5-3) causes the Gambian or West African form of the disease. It is a highly pleomorphic organism, frequently showing in a single blood smear a variety of forms, ranging from slender-bodied organisms with a long, free flagellum that reach a length of 30 μm or more, to fatter,

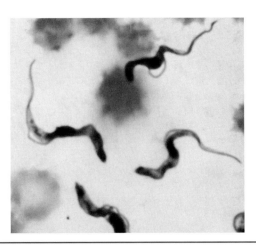

FIGURE 5-3 ■ *Trypanosoma brucei gambiense* trypomastigotes in blood film. (Photomicrograph by Zane Price.)

stumpier forms without a free flagellum that average about 15 µm in length. The same pleomorphism characterizes *Trypanosoma brucei rhodesiense*, the cause of Rhodesian or East African sleeping sickness, and *Trypanosoma brucei brucei*, which produces a relatively mild disease in native game animals and a severe infection in many domestic animals but apparently does not infect humans. These three organisms, morphologically indistinguishable except under special and somewhat debatable circumstances, cannot be differentiated by serologic means with any certainty. As their pathogenicity for humans and laboratory animals is the only criterion for separating them, some authorities prefer to consider all three as varieties of *T. brucei*. Others grant specific status to *T. gambiense* and *T. rhodesiense*. PCR analysis has been used to identify mixed human infection of *T. b. gambiense* and *T. congolense*, a parasite of a variety of domestic and wild mammals, in the West African country of Côte d'Ivoire (Truc et al., 1998).

Symptoms. Following the bite of an infected tsetse fly, most frequently *Glossina palpalis*, there is an asymptomatic incubation period of a few days to several weeks in Africans; an acute onset is usual in non-Africans, and the incubation period is short. Occasionally there is ulceration in the area of the bite, with formation of an indurated, painful "trypanosomal chancre," which slowly disappears. The trypanosomal chancre is much more common in non-Africans. Trypanosomes may be demonstrated in fluid aspirated from the ulcer. At the end of the incubation period, the patient is still in apparent excellent health, but examination of a blood film reveals trypanosomes. Often they are rather scanty and may even be difficult to find on thick-film examination. The essentially symptom-free period of low-grade parasitemia may continue for several weeks or perhaps a number of months. The infection may be abortive and terminate during this period without the development of symptoms, or the parasites may invade lymphatic tissues. There is evidence that macrophages are involved in the elimination of antibody-sensitized trypanosomes.

Invasion of the lymph nodes is usually accompanied by the onset of febrile attacks. The fever is usually rather irregular and may be initiated by a rigor. Malaise and headache usually accompany the fever; there is often anorexia and generalized weakness, and sometimes nausea and vomiting. Night sweats are frequent. A febrile attack lasts a few days to a week and is followed by an asymptomatic interval, usually of some weeks' duration. During the fever, trypanosomes may be found in large numbers in the circulating blood, but in the afebrile periods they are few in number. With the commencement of febrile attacks there is usually some glandular enlargement. Any lymph node may be infected, but those of the

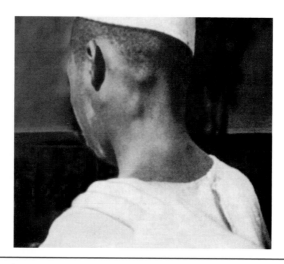

FIGURE 5-4 ▪ Enlargement of posterior cervical lymph nodes—Winterbottom's sign. (Courtesy of Dr. James R. Busvine, London School of Hygiene and Tropical Medicine.)

posterior cervical region are most frequently involved. Enlargement of these nodes is known as Winterbottom's sign (Fig. 5–4). Trypanosomes may be found on aspiration of the enlarged nodes. An irregular erythematous rash, suggestive of erythema multiforme, sometimes with underlying edema and frequently accompanied by pruritus, may appear and disappear during attacks of fever. The rash usually lasts only a few hours. Although congenital transmission is uncommon at any stage of the disease, abortions and stillbirths are frequent.

The infection may terminate without overt nervous system involvement, or this may occur at any time after the patient develops symptoms of infection. The increasing lassitude and apathy common in the later stages of the glandular phase of the disease probably point to beginning nervous system involvement. Usually these symptoms are not sufficiently far advanced to be recognized as a separate phase of the disease for 6 months to a year after the first symptoms are seen. There is steady progression in development of meningoencephalitis, with general deterioration of the patient and increase of apathy, fatigability, confusion, and somnolence. Extreme emaciation is seen in patients who do not have strict nursing supervision. The face, in contrast with the rest of the body, is usually edematous. Neurologic signs develop late. Motor changes may include fibrillation of the muscles of the face, lips, and fingers, and incoordination, leading to slurred speech and an ataxic gait. Sensory changes are frequently less marked; paresthesias and loss of kinesthetic sense sometimes are observed. Pressure on the palms of the hands or over the ulnar nerve may be followed by severe pain a short time after the pressure is removed. This is known as Kerandel's sign.

In the final stages of the disease there may be profound character changes and mental deterioration. Motor involvement may lead to convulsions, hemiplegia or paraplegia, and incontinence of urine and feces; severe paresthesias often occur. The patient is gradually more and more difficult to arouse and finally becomes comatose. The progression of the central nervous systems (CNS) symptoms is usually continuous, but there may be remissions and exacerbations with a course extending over several years. An outline comparison of the evolution of the disease process in African and American trypanosomiasis is given in Figure 5-9; however, it is worth pointing out that the geographic range of these diseases is quite distinct.

Diagnosis depends on demonstration of the trypanosomes in blood, in fluid aspirated from lymph nodes, or in spinal fluid. Examination of the centrifuged sediment of a spinal fluid sample increases the possibility of detection of trypanosomes (Fig. 5-5). A double

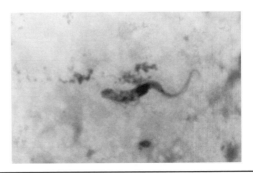

FIGURE 5-5 ■ *Trypanosoma brucei gambiense* trypomastigote in centrifuged spinal fluid (Giemsa stain).

centrifugation technique for trypanosomes in samples of cerebrospinal fluid has been described; it is at least twice as sensitive as single centrifugation and increases the early detection of late-stage cases by some 37%. If parasites cannot be demonstrated in thick or thin blood films, concentration may again be of value. These techniques are described in Chapter 15. Trypanosomes also concentrate in the buffy layer of a hematocrit specimen. Clinical history and physical findings may be of considerable diagnostic value; cell counts and spinal fluid protein determinations are of prognostic interest in evaluating the response to therapy.

T. b. gambiense can seldom be isolated by inoculation into the usual laboratory animals (rats, mice, hamsters), although *T. b. rhodesiense* infects these animals readily. Although several serologic tests have been used experimentally, there is none available commercially or from the Centers for Disease Control and Prevention (CDC). A card indirect agglutination test for trypanosomiasis (*Tryp*Tect CIATT, Brentec Diagnostics, P.O. Box 42477, Nairobi, Kenya) is available in Africa (Asonganyi et al., 1998). Serum and spinal fluid immunoglobulin M (IgM) measurements are of diagnostic value.

Pathogenesis. Until recently, it was believed that trypomastigotes were the only developmental stages of the *T. brucei* complex found in the mammalian host. It is now known that, at least in experimental animals, amastigotes of *T. brucei* are found early in infection in the choroid plexus. There they may block capillaries, causing localized edema and obstruction to the flow of cerebrospinal fluid and possibly by this means producing the headache seen early in human infections. Some of the ependymal cells lining the cerebral ventricles of infected mice contain intracellular *T. brucei*; however, intracellular forms were not found in the ependymal cells in human infection. During the first flush of trypomastigotes in the blood, amastigotes disappear from the choroid plexus to become reestablished there later in the course of infection. They may also occur in the lung.

Overt infection involves particularly the lymphoid tissues early in the disease and the CNS in its later stages. There is generalized lymphoid hyperplasia as the result of proliferation of the parasites in the lymph nodes; aspiration of an enlarged node often reveals trypanosomes when there are too few to be found in blood films. Anemia is usually noted; the white blood cell count is essentially normal, with relative lymphocytosis. Thrombocytopenia, a consequence of hypertrophy of the reticuloendothelial system and of the presence of disseminated intravascular coagulation (DIC), is often seen. Hypergammaglobulinemia is characteristic; immunoelectrophoresis or ultracentrifugation of the serum of infected persons usually demonstrates an IgM level greater than four times that found in pooled normal serum. These sustained IgM elevations are thought to be a result of the antigenic variability chracteristic of these trypanosomes, confronting the immune system with constantly changing antigenic stimuli. Trypanosomes change their surface antigens (glycoproteins) by turning off one gene coding for a variant surface glycoprotein (VSG) and turning on another.

Estimates are that a single trypanosome may have as many as 1000 or more VSG genes. By constantly changing surface proteins (antigens), trypanosomes are able to evade host defense mechanisms. Such an IgM increase, otherwise associated with Waldenström's macroglobulinemia or other dysproteinemias, may, however, be found occasionally in Africans without evidence of these diseases or of trypanosomiasis. *Absence* of an elevated serum IgM level effectively rules out trypanosomiasis, whereas a detectable level in the cerebrospinal fluid is diagnostic for CNS trypanosomiasis.

Invasion of the CNS is marked by a progressive leptomeningitis, with perivascular lymphocyte and plasma cell infiltration of the Virchow-Robin spaces, an increased spinal fluid protein level, and a cell count of 15 to 500 white blood cells per μl. Growth of the parasites in this location is reported to lead to localized antigen-antibody reactions with the release of kinin, disruption of collagen fibers, and destruction of fibroblasts. Trypanosomes may occur outside the bloodstream and spinal fluid and in the gray and white matter of the brain, and they have been reported to invade other organs and tissues as well. The exact mechanism by which these parasites cause death of the host has long been debated and is still uncertain. Both cellular and humoral immunity are depressed in patients with Gambian trypanosomiasis, and such immunosuppression may contribute to the increased susceptibility to secondary infection characteristic of the disease. Exacerbation of a clinically inapparent and unsuspected infection (with the production of ascites and the presence of trypomastigotes in the ascites fluid) has been noted in a patient treated with steroids for an unrelated condition. Microglia and astrocytes have been shown to proliferate in the areas of perivascular infiltration and the surrounding brain parenchyma. Astrocytes, one of the most numerous cell types in the CNS, appear to be the primary antigen-presenting cells regulating immune reactivity in the CNS parenchyma and, as such, would be involved in the production of cytokines, which enhance the immune response, and prostaglandins, which affect immunosuppression. The T lymphocyte suppressor prostaglandin D_2 is elevated in the spinal fluid of patients with advanced sleeping sickness and may in part account for the increased somnolence of these patients.

Epidemiology. *T. b. gambiense* is most frequently transmitted to humans by the bite of the tsetse flies *Glossina palpalis* and *G. tachinoides*. These species dwell on the banks of shaded streams, generally in proximity to human habitation. Consequently, Gambian sleeping sickness is likely to assume an endemic form, affecting persons whose daily activities bring them in contact with such streams. No animal reservoirs are known or suspected for *T. b. gambiense*. Control of the spread of infection is brought about by control of the vector, either by elimination of its breeding grounds through clearing away of streamside underbrush or by means of insecticides, and by case detection and chemotherapy.

Throughout endemic areas, available figures indicate a low prevalence rate, generally well under 1% of the population at present; however, there remain foci with high rates of transmission and areas in which the disease has shown some resurgence in the past few years. An estimated 100,000 deaths a year are occurring in sub-Saharan Africa, the greatest reemergence being noted in southern Sudan, the Democratic Republic of the Congo, and Angola (Welburn and Odiit, 2002).

Treatment. While some authorities recommend the use of melarsoprol (also known as Arsobal, mel B, or melarsen oxide complexed with dimercaprol [BAL]) for treatment of all stages of Gambian sleeping sickness, less toxic drugs may be substituted in the early stages, during which there is no evidence of neurologic involvement. Suramin,* a complex organic compound, is generally effective under such conditions. Suramin is an enzyme inhibitor that

---

*Available at present in the United States from the CDC Drug Service, Centers for Disease Control and Prevention, U.S. Public Health Service, Atlanta, Georgia 30333; (404) 639-3670.

seems to be taken up selectively by trypanosomes (and filariae) and not by mammalian cells. It is a toxic drug, to which a very small percentage of patients exhibit a marked idiosyncrasy consisting of nausea, vomiting, loss of consciousness, and seizures. If a test dose of not more than 200 mg administered intravenously is tolerated well, it is given by the same route in a dose of 20 mg/kg body weight to children, or 1 g for adults, on treatment days 1, 3, 7, 14, and 21. It should not be given as a rapid bolus, or to patients with preexisting renal disease; if proteinuria appears, the course of treatment should be discontinued. Less severe side effects of suramin treatment include fever, hepatitis, rash, pruritus, edema, pains in the palms and soles of the feet, blepharitis, conjunctivitis, photophobia, and tearing. If an early response to suramin is not apparent, consideration should be given to the administration of pentamidine or melarsoprol.

Pentamidine (Lomidine or 4,4-diamidinodiphenoxypentane di[β-hydroxy-ethane-sulfonate]), a diamidine that apparently interacts selectively with kinetoplast DNA to kill trypanosomes, is effective in the hemolymphatic stages of the infection. This drug does not cross the blood-brain barrier and therefore is ineffective during the later stages of the disease. It is administered by intramuscular injection at the rate of 4 mg/kg body weight daily for 10 days. Rather marked toxic reactions have been noted with intravenous administration of the drug; its intramuscular injection may be marked by mild and transient cardiovascular (hypotension, tachycardia) and gastrointestinal (nausea, vomiting) symptoms. Reactions of the Herxheimer type have been reported and, as in treatment with melarsoprol, might be prevented or modified by pretreatment with corticosteroids.

Suramin may be used during pregnancy; if pentamidine is given, it should not be administered prior to the fourth month and is usually prescribed in reduced doses. Arsenicals are contraindicated in pregnancy.

The trivalent arsenical melarsoprol has the trypanocidal activity of melarsen oxide and also has that drug's ability to penetrate the blood-brain barrier; because of its combination with BAL it is considerably less toxic. Melarsoprol interferes with the enzyme systems of the trypanosome by inactivating its sulfhydryl groups. It is the drug of choice for treating Gambian sleeping sickness with neurologic involvement. The drug is given in a dose of 2.2 mg/kg body weight daily for 10 days. Herxheimer reactions are not uncommon, and to prevent them, pretreatment with corticosteroids is suggested. Nausea and vomiting, also common, may be suppressed by administration of prochlorperazine or other antiemetic drugs. Further neurologic complications are seen in about one fifth of patients following melarsoprol therapy.

Reactive encephalopathy, a toxic disorder related to the interaction of the drug, the diseased brain, and the infection, is the more common type of complication and is marked by increased confusion and excitation. This often clears with temporary cessation of therapy and sedation as needed. Therapy may be cautiously resumed a few days after the symptoms abate. Hemorrhagic encephalopathy, fortunately rare, is apparently a direct toxic effect of the arsenical and is usually fatal. Its onset is marked by sudden loss of consciousness and hyperpyrexia. BAL should be administered at the first sign of either type of encephalopathy. Oral prednisolone, 1 mg/kg to a maximum of 40 mg in a single daily dose, given during the melarsoprol treatment period has been shown to reduce significantly the incidence of melarsoprol-induced encephalopathy (Pepin et al., 1989).

Although melarsoprol may be used alone in treatment of patients with minimal CNS symptoms, a longer treatment course is employed in cases of moderately advanced to severe neurologic involvement. Pretreatment with suramin is recommended, at the rate of 0.25 to 0.5 g intravenously on alternate days for two to four doses. Melarsoprol is then given in successive daily or alternate-day doses of 1.5, 2, and 2.2 mg/kg, followed after 1 week by 2.5, 3, and 3.6 mg/kg daily on successive days, and 1 to 3 weeks later by 3.6 mg/kg daily for 3 days. Complete directions for the administration of these drugs are furnished by the CDC Drug Service at the time the drugs are supplied.

DL-alpha-difluoromethylornithine* (DFMO, eflornithine), an inhibitor of ornithine decarboxylase, has been shown to be a highly effective treatment for both early- and late-stage Gambian sleeping sickness. Many of the patients had disease that was refractory to arsenical treatment. The recommended treatment regimen for eflornithine in Gambian trypanosomiasis is 400 mg/kg per day in four doses for 14 days. Trypanosomes are cleared from the blood in 1 to 4 days and from the cerebrospinal fluid by the end of treatment. Tolerance for eflornithine therapy has been generally good. The most frequent side effects have been diarrhea, abdominal pain, and anemia, all of which have been reversible and have not required discontinuation of therapy. Eflornithine is not effective against Rhodesian sleeping sickness. Considerable numbers of *T. b. rhodesiense* infections have been found to be naturally resistant to this drug.

Prevention. After three quarters of a century of effort, African trypanosomiasis is in what has been called a state of controlled endemicity. Large-scale operations involving bush clearing along streams to control breeding sites of the tsetse flies, application of insecticides by airplane to reduce the numbers of flies breeding in inaccessible areas, and surveillance, case detection, and treatment of the people, particularly as they travel from one area to another, are all important. Breakdown of medical surveillance, such as occurred in Zaire between 1960 and 1966, can result in rapid resurgence of the disease. In that country, a prevalence rate of less than 0.02% rose to over 10% before the situation stabilized.

Persons visiting endemic areas should wear protective clothing (long-sleeved shirts and long trousers of reasonably heavy material—flies can bite through thin clothing). The use of screening, bed netting, and insect repellents is advisable. Injections of pentamidine have been used for prophylaxis; this is no longer recommended for individual use because of the possibility that latent CNS infections may develop in persons so treated.

Trypanosoma brucei rhodesiense

In Eastern and Central Africa a more acutely virulent form of trypanosomiasis is seen; it is sporadic in occurrence and generally has a discontinuous distribution. The agent of this type of infection, *T. b. rhodesiense*, is carried by *Glossina pallidipes, Glossina morsitans,* and occasionally other species of game-attacking tsetse flies.

Symptoms. The disease picture is similar to that of Gambian trypanosomiasis but is much more rapidly progressive; patients frequently die before the full development of the meningoencephalitic signs and symptoms seen in the former disease. The incubation period is commonly short, and clinical symptoms may be ushered in with a rigor and fever. Trypanosomes appear in the blood early in the infection and often are present in considerable numbers. There is usually little obvious glandular involvement and Winterbottom's sign may not be present. Weight loss is rapid, and the CNS is involved early. Untreated persons usually die within 9 months to a year after the onset of disease.

The features of imported Rhodesian sleeping sickness as seen in Americans or other expatriates infected on safari or during visits to game parks in East Africa come on shortly after their return and include malaise, confusion, anorexia, and lethargy. Personality changes, headache, fever, and chills are also prominent. Most give a history of tsetse fly bites; most have trypanosomal chancres. All have trypanosomes in the peripheral blood. A majority have organisms in the cerebrospinal fluid.

Diagnosis is made as in Gambian trypanosomiasis. The parasites are more readily found in the peripheral blood in the Rhodesian form of the disease. A differential diagnosis can frequently be made on geographic grounds, but there are some areas, such as Uganda, where the two infections coexist.

---

*Available in the United States from the CDC Drug Service, Centers for Disease Control and Prevention, U.S. Public Health Service, Atlanta, Georgia 30333; (404) 639-3670.

Pathogenesis. Development of the infection in Rhodesian sleeping sickness is similar to that in Gambian, save that in the former the infection is more acute, trypanosomes are numerous in the peripheral blood, and there is little lymphadenopathy. CNS invasion takes place relatively early in the course of the Rhodesian infection.

Glomerulonephritis has been reported both in humans and in experimental animals infected with *T. b. rhodesiense*. A mild proliferative glomerulonephritis, with deposition primarily of IgM in the glomeruli, has been noted in experimentally infects rats. Hypocomplementemia was noted, but C_3 could not be identified in the glomeruli. Electron microscopy demonstrated the presence of mesangial electron-dense deposits.

Electrocardiographic changes similar to those described elsewhere for patients with *Trypanosoma cruzi* infection have been noted in both Gambian and Rhodesian sleeping sickness; the pathophysiologic basis for such changes seems less obvious than in Chagas' disease.

Epidemiology. The vectors of Rhodesian sleeping sickness are game-feeding tsetses. They breed in the lightly covered "bush" rather than along river banks. Control is more difficult than that of *G. palpalis* and its relatives, depending primarily on the elimination of the wild game that is their chief source of food or on the widespread use of insecticides.

Unlike *T. b. gambiense*, the Rhodesian species has a number of animal reservoirs. It has been isolated from the bushbuck, hartebeest, and domestic ox, carried by cyclic transmission through sheep and tsetse flies for many years (with repeated infections of human volunteers), and there is strong circumstantial evidence of natural human infections from game animals in the bush. Identical zymodeme stocks (combinations of isoenzyme patterns exhibited by particular strains) have been identified for *T. b. rhodesiense* isolated from humans, cattle, reedbuck, and tsetse flies (*G. pallidipes*) in western Kenya.

T. b. rhodesiense infection is sporadic, usually affecting only individuals or small numbers of persons, although localized epidemics may occur. Because the infection tends to be acute rather than chronic, asymptomatic carriers do not play the role in transmission of the disease that they do in Gambian trypanosomiasis.

Treatment. The drugs used and the treatment schedules are the same as for Gambian sleeping sickness. However, because of the rapid course of the Rhodesian type of infection, neurologic involvement may be expected to occur very early, especially in non-Africans.

Trypanosoma rangeli

Human cases of an apparently asymptomatic trypanosomal infection have been reported from Brazil, Venezuela, Colombia, Panama, El Salvador, Costa Rica, Honduras, and Guatemala. The organism has been known as *Trypanosoma ariari* and *T. guatemalensis* but seems to be correctly named *T. rangeli*. In Panama, *T. rangeli* is found six times more frequently than *T. cruzi*, in a population in which the average combined infection rate is 3.4%. *T. rangeli* infections are most common in persons less than 16 years old, being encountered in some 75% of that age group. It is transmitted directly by the bite of the reduviid bug *Rhodnius prolixus* and a few related species. No evidence of pathogenicity has been noted in any of the natural infections or in human volunteers. The parasites may be isolated from the bloodstream for some months after infection. They are about 30 μm in length, with a nucleus anterior to the middle of the body and a small kinetoplast. An intracellular amastigote state of *T. rangeli* has been described from the tissues of experimentally infected suckling mice. Natural infections have been found in dogs, and *T. rangeli* will multiply in a number of laboratory, domestic, and wild animals, apparently none of which develop disease. In the Amazon basin of Brazil, *T. rangeli* has been isolated from opossums, anteaters, coati, and the vectors *Rhodnius pictipes* and *Rhodnius robustus*.

The diagnosis of *T. rangeli* infection is made by the identification of trypanosomes in stained blood films. In contrast to the other American trypanosome, *T. cruzi*, in which the kinetoplast is quite large (see Figs. 5-1 and 5-7), that of *T. rangeli* is small and inconspicuous.

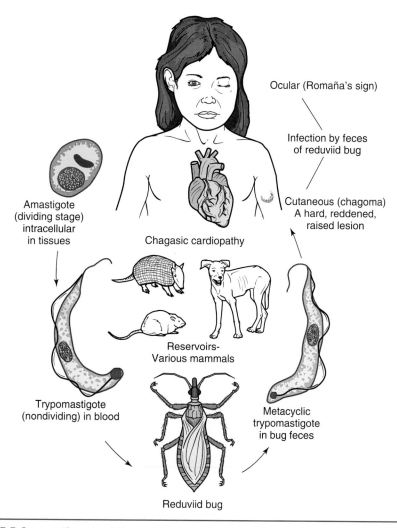

FIGURE 5-6 ▪ Life cycle of *Trypanosoma cruzi.*

Trypanosoma cruzi

From the southern parts of the United States through Mexico and Central America, and in South America as far south as Argentina, various wild rodents, opossums, and armadillos may be found infected with a trypanosome that is also capable of producing disease in humans. The organism was found, first in the reduviid bug *Panstrongylus megistus* and later in humans, by the Brazilian worker Carlos Chagas while he was still a medical student; in his honor the disease received its name. Chagas' disease is caused by *T. cruzi*, an organism that differs from other trypanosomes infecting humans in that it has an intracellular amastigote stage in cardiac muscle and other tissues, as well as trypanosome forms in the circulating blood. Molecular techniques have identified *T. cruzi* DNA in 4000-year-old mummies in the Atacama desert region of coastal southern Peru and northern Chile. The life cycle of *T. cruzi* is illustrated in Figure 5-6.

The trypomastigotes average 20 μm in length, ranging in their proportions from rather short and stubby to long, slender forms. The nucleus is usually positioned centrally and the large oval kinetoplast is located posteriorly. In stained blood films they characteristically assume a **C** or **U** shape (Fig. 5-7). The delicate undulating membrane is best demonstrated by scanning electron microscopy (Fig. 5-8).

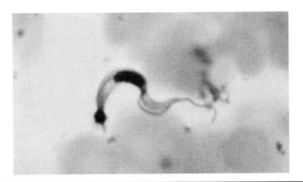

FIGURE 5-7   ■   *Trypanosoma cruzi* trypomastigote in blood film. (Photomicrograph by Zane Price.)

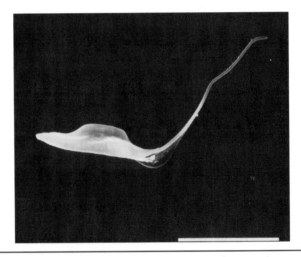

FIGURE 5-8   ■   Scanning electron micrograph of a *Trypanosoma cruzi* trypomastigote. Bar is 10 μm. (Photomicrograph by Dr. Thomas B. Cole, Jr.)

T. cruzi develops successfully in a large number of insects, but it is considered that reduviid bugs are the only vectors of importance and only those species that invade houses and habitually defecate during the process of feeding or immediately thereafter are major vectors of the human disease. The importance of time of defecation lies in the fact that the trypanosomes develop in the hindgut of the insect and are carried in the feces, in contrast to *T. rangeli*, which is transmitted in the reduviid's saliva. Unless the insect deposits infective feces near the bite, it is unlikely that parasites will be introduced into the skin through scratching the intensely pruritic lesions. The infection may also be transmitted congenitally. In Argentina, where congenital transmission constitutes a sizable public health problem, estimates are that approximately 850 cases occur each year (Gürtler et al., 2003).

Symptoms. The disease is seen most commonly, and in its most severe form, in children younger than 5 years, in whom symptoms of central nervous system involvement may predominate. In older children and adults, the disease usually occurs in a milder, subacute or chronic form, which generally follows an acute attack. An outline of the evolution of American trypanosomiasis, as compared with that of African trypanosomiasis, is given in Figure 5-9.

At the site of infection the organisms proliferate, producing an erythematous indurated area known as a chagoma. This lesion occurs most frequently on the face but may appear

COMPARATIVE PATHOGENESIS OF TRYPANOSOMIASIS

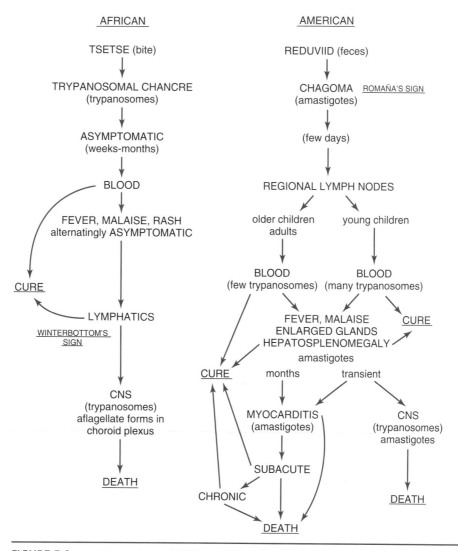

FIGURE 5-9 ■ Comparison of African and American trypanosomiasis.

elsewhere on the body. On the trunk, the chagoma may reach a diameter of several centimeters and become very painful. The lesions reach their full size in a few days and then gradually subside over a period of 2 or 3 months. Trypomastigotes or amastigotes may be aspirated from the chagoma in the early stages of the infection. They spread rapidly to the regional lymph nodes, which become enlarged and palpable within 3 days. The nodes are hard and moderately tender, and they usually contain amastigote forms. Lesions similar to the initial chagoma may appear elsewhere on the body in the first few weeks of infection, apparently by hematogenous spread, and localized areas of hard, nonpitting edema may develop in various parts of the body. These appear suddenly and may subside within a few days or persist for months. While such edematous patches may develop anywhere on the body, they most frequently involve one side of the face. Unilateral edema affecting both the upper and the lower eyelid, usually with conjunctivitis, is known as Romaña's sign. The edema usually spreads to involve the cheek and sometimes the neck of the same side; occasionally the eyelids of the other side may be involved, and rarely there is bilateral facial edema.

Unilateral ocular and facial edema, involving the submaxillary lymph nodes, is also known as the oculoglandular syndrome (ophthalmoganglionary complex).

Symptoms of generalized infection may appear from 4 days to 2 weeks or more after the bite. Organisms appear in the blood at about 10 days and persist during the acute stage; however, they are usually sparse in patients older than 1 year. When the infection occurs in infants, parasites are found in the blood in considerable numbers. Generalized malaise; chills; high fever, which may be continuous, intermittent, or remittent; muscle aches and pains; and increasing exhaustion characterize the acute stage. Epistaxis is common in young children. There is usually a moderate degree of generalized glandular enlargement early in the infection; amastigotes may be found in any enlarged lymph node but are frequently scanty in all but the regional nodes that drain the chagoma. The spleen becomes palpable but generally is not greatly enlarged; the liver may be felt several fingerbreadths below the costal margin. A rash may make its appearance approximately 2 weeks after infection. Pinhead-sized, well-defined red spots appearing on the chest and abdomen are neither painful nor pruritic and fade in 7 to 10 days.

The most severe infections are usually seen in infants and are characterized by high fever (sometimes with the "dromedary" curve, or double daily peak, seen in kala-azar) and the development of generalized lymphadenitis, hepatosplenomegaly, and anasarca. Infected young children may develop signs and symptoms of meningoencephalitis and die of CNS involvement within a few days or weeks. Older children and adults are often said to show no signs of CNS involvement. A study of 11 children admitted to a Brazilian hospital with the diagnosis of acute Chagas' disease yielded the following findings: their ages ranged from 4 months to 15 years; culture of the spinal fluid was positive for *T. cruzi* in 8 of these patients, spanning the entire age range; and the cerebrospinal fluid (CSF) albumin content was elevated in 4 of the 8 patients. The high levels of CSF albumin probably correlate with the presence of amastigotes in meningeal and neuronal tissues, known to occur in acute chagasic meningoencephalitis. Electrocardiographic (EKG) changes are seen in over 40% of acute cases and consist of prolongation of the P-R and Q-T intervals, low voltage of QRS complexes, S-T depression, and T-wave inversion. Tachycardia, various arrhythmias, and cardiac failure may be evident. There is usually a lymphocytosis, though the total white blood cell count may be normal, low, or high. The serum globulin concentration is increased, and the albumin level is decreased.

An acute attack of Chagas' disease may terminate in a few weeks in death or recovery, or the patient may enter the chronic stage of the infection. Variable periods of remission, and exacerbations marked by fever and the appearance of trypanosomes in the circulating blood, may separate the two stages of the disease, or the chronic phase may be initially asymptomatic. Although trypanosomes are seldom seen in the circulating blood, transmission of the disease by means of blood transfusions has been a problem in certain endemic areas. Transmission has occurred after kidney transplantation from an infected donor. Congenital transmission may occur in both the acute and chronic stages of the disease. Most infants with congenital chagasic infection are of low birth weight, and a high percentage are stillborn. Ten cases of pneumonitis have been described among a series of 40 cases of congenital Chagas' disease; amastigotes were found in the lungs in 7 of the patients. Megaesophagus has also been reported in congenital Chagas' disease. A survey in Santa Cruz, Bolivia, identified 25 cases (8%) of congenitally acquired Chagas' disease in 329 newborns examined; serologic prevalence of Chagas' disease in mothers was 51%. Transmission has been shown to occur in breast-fed babies by means of infected mother's milk. Chronic infections may be seen in patients who have no history of the acute stage; and if patients are asymptomatic, at times the infection may be diagnosed by EKG changes. Characteristic alterations in the EKG are seen in a large percentage of patients in the chronic stage of the disease. A majority of such patients will show partial or complete atrioventricular (AV) block, complete right bundle branch block, or premature ventricular contractions, along with abnormalities of the QRS complexes and of the P and T waves (Fig. 5-10). Symptomatic infections exhibit the signs and symptoms of progressive congestive cardiac failure, primarily right-sided failure, and

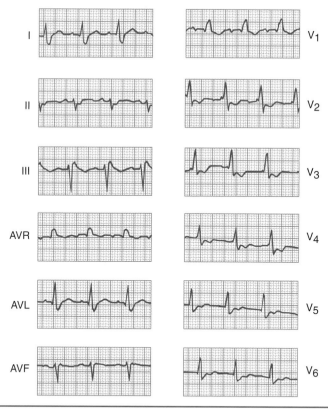

FIGURE 5-10 ■ Electrocardiographic changes in chronic Chagas' disease. Patient is a 21-year-old Brazilian man. See text for discussion of abnormalities. (Tracings courtesy of Dr. A. Prata, University of Bahia Medical School, Bahia, Brazil.)

may occur at any age but are rare in patients under age 25. Syncope is common, probably due to complete heart block, and sudden death is not infrequent.

Less common than the cardiac involvement is dilatation of the digestive tract caused by chronic Chagas' disease. Megaesophagus, usually characterized by dysphagia, and megacolon (Figs. 5-11 and 5-12), with symptoms of prolonged constipation, fecal impaction, or volvulus, are most frequent, though other parts of the digestive tract may be involved. In endemic areas, it is probable that most cases of acquired dilatation of the digestive tract are related to infection with *T. cruzi*. In an area of northeast Brazil where Chagas' disease is endemic, 680 persons were examined, by serologic tests, electrocardiography, and a questionnaire, for esophageal motility disorders. Of these, 40% were seropositive for Chagas' disease, and symptoms of dysphagia occurred 2.5 times more frequently among seropositive than seronegative persons. Among the seropositive ones, 26% with symptoms of dysphagia also had abnormal EKG readings. In addition, some authorities recognize forms of the disease that affect the CNS, thyroid, and so forth. Most of the symptoms ascribed to these forms of the disease are typical of endemic goiter, which is prevalent in many areas where Chagas' disease occurs.

Administration of immunosuppressive drugs to a patient with Chagas' disease may be expected to exacerbate the infection. The administration of cyclophosphamide to mice in the early, the subacute, and the late subacute stages of experimental infections uniformly increased mortality, parasitemia, and severity of the myocarditis. Immunosuppression by HIV can also lead to reactivation of infection. Twenty (87%) of 23 AIDS patients with Chagas' disease are reported to have developed severe meningoencephalitis, with the heart being the second most severely affected site.

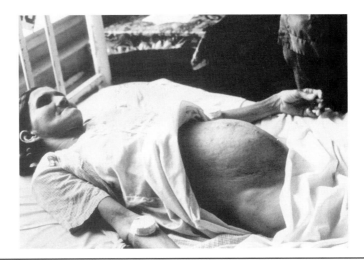

FIGURE 5-11 ■ Patient with chagasic megacolon undergoing xenodiagnosis. Note pillbox, which contains the reduviid bugs, attached to the right forearm.

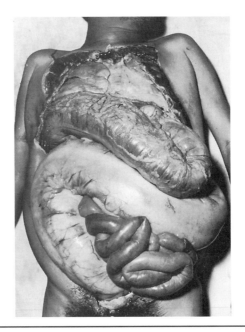

FIGURE 5-12 ■ Megacolon in chronic Chagas' disease. (Courtesy of Dr. Fritz Köberle, Sao Paulo, Brazil.)

Definitive diagnosis of *T. cruzi* infection must be based on demonstration of the parasites. In young children they may be detected in the blood with ease, particularly at the height of the acute stage. In older children and adults, the parasites are frequently very difficult to find. They may be demonstrated by special concentration techniques, by culture, or by the method of xenodiagnosis, which is the feeding of laboratory-reared reduviid bugs on a patient suspected of having Chagas' disease and, after a time, examining the bugs for *T. cruzi* (see Fig. 5-11). Various serologic methods, which are mainly group specific for hemoflagellates, are also available. An indirect immunofluorescence assay (IFA) test is available at the CDC. Several kits are available commercially (see Chapter 16).

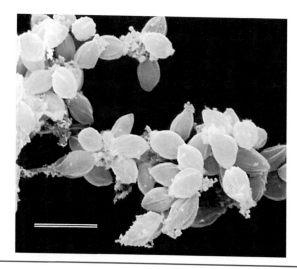

FIGURE 5-13 ■ Scanning electron micrograph of a cluster of *Trypanosoma cruzi* amastigotes from Vero cell culture. Bar is 5 μm. (Photomicrograph by Dr. Thomas B. Cole, Jr.)

The Machado-Guerreiro test is a complement fixation test using *T. cruzi* antigen. A radioimmunoassay (RIA) has been developed for use in the immunodiagnosis of Chagas' disease in humans. The assay is able to discriminate between infection with *T. cruzi* and *T. rangeli* in mice—and presumably in humans. Blood culture, xenodiagnosis, and polymerase chain reaction (PCR) were compared for sensitivity in diagnosing Chagas' disease in 101 Brazilian patients who were seropositive for *T. cruzi*. Blood cultures gave 26% positive results, xenodiagnosis 37%, and PCR 59%. However, PCR kits are not yet available commercially. An ELISA test has been described that detects *T. cruzi* antigens in the urine (antigenuria) of patients with acute, congenital, and chronic Chagas' disease. Biopsy of enlarged lymph nodes may reveal parasites in the amastigote stage. Figure 5-13 shows a cluster of amastigotes by scanning electron microscopy.

Pathogenesis. Upon its entry into the vertebrate host, *T. cruzi* produces an acute local inflammatory reaction. Lymphatic spread then carries the organisms to regional lymph nodes, where upon ingestion by histiocytes or other cells they transform into amastigotes. Alternatively, trypomastigotes may actively invade macrophages and other cells. Evidence suggests that lectinlike carbohydrate interactions are involved in the binding of trypanosomes to the host cell. A protein on the surface of the trypomastigote has been shown to bind to *N*-acetylglucosamine on the host cell. Amastigotes attach to the cell surface, suggesting the presence of receptors, and, although they are usually phagocytosed, they may actively penetrate the cell. After local multiplication, the organisms may assume the trypomastigote form to invade the bloodstream, carrying the infection to all parts of the body. In the amastigote form, parasites can multiply within the cells of virtually every organ and tissue. Cells of the reticuloendothelial system; the cardiac, skeletal, and smooth muscle; and neuroglia cells are preferentially parasitized.

The chagoma consists of an intense inflammatory reaction, with invasion of histiocytes, adipose cells of the subcutaneous tissue and the adjacent muscle cells by the proliferating amastigotes, and of the area by neutrophilic leukocytes and lymphocytes. Eventually a lipogranuloma forms, but not before lymphatic spread of the parasites to the regional nodes has occurred.

As infection spreads beyond the regional lymph nodes, trypanosomes appear in the circulating blood, infecting other organs and tissues as they are carried throughout the body. Küpffer cells of the liver, the macrophages of the spleen, and cardiac muscle are especially

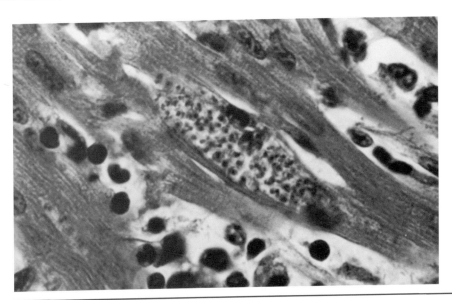

FIGURE 5-14 ■ *Trypanosoma cruzi* amastigotes in heart muscle. (Photomicrograph by Zane Price.)

prone to infection. Within the cardiac muscle (Fig. 5-14) the amastigotes proliferate to form pseudocysts; loss of muscle substance and a diffuse inflammatory exudate and proliferation of interstitial connective tissue are seen. Invasion of the CNS is marked by inflammation of the cortex and meninges, with perivascular lymphocytic infiltrates and small granulomas formed around trypomastigotes or amastigotes in the brain substance around the small vessels.

Early in the chronic stage of infection the heart may be normal in size or only slightly enlarged, although later massive cardiomegaly may develop. There is diffuse inflammation of the myocardium as well as fibrosis and infiltration of lymphocytes, macrophages, and plasma cells. The heart weight increases, and all chambers, especially the right ventricle, become dilated. Damage to the autonomic nervous system of the heart parallels that to Auerbach's plexus in the walls of the digestive tract. Hypertrophy of the muscle layers and diminution in number of the ganglion cells are seen in affected portions of the digestive tract, most frequently in the esophagus and colon.

Levels of IgM rise during an acute infection but decline with treatment. Experimental *T. cruzi* infections are not characterized by the sustained elevations of IgM seen in African trypanosomiasis. In the latter, sustained high IgM levels are thought to be due to antigenic variation, presumably less common in *T. cruzi*.

Circulating antibodies reacting against endocardium, blood vessels, and the interstitium of striated muscle have been found to be present in 95% of patients with chagasic cardiomyopathy and in 45% of asymptomatic patients infected with *T. cruzi*; they are absent in uninfected persons and those suffering from other types of cardiomyopathy. The antibody is known to cross-react with *T. b. rhodesiense*. It has been proposed that the cytokines secreted by *T. cruzi*-infected macrophages may be partly responsible for the proliferation of the lymphocytes that produce the antibodies directed against antigens of parasite origin, and possibly of host origin, resulting in the severe autoimmune pathology observed in Chagas' disease. The parasites may be mimicking host antigens as a strategy for survival.

Host resistance to *T. cruzi* infection involves both humoral and cellular responses. Antibody-mediated immunity has been shown to be associated mainly with the IgG class of immunoglobulins. Lysis of trypomastigotes by complement is related to complement activation by way of the alternative pathway. Cell-mediated resistance includes killing of trypomastigotes by activated macrophages and by neutrophils and eosinophils through antibody-dependent mechanisms. Host intracellular iron pools appear to play a role in protection against *T. cruzi*. *T. cruzi* amastigotes require iron for optimal growth and pathogenicity. Infection of peritoneal macrophages with *T. cruzi* in vitro shows that depletion of iron from within macrophages, using the potent iron chelator deferoxamine (DEF), reduces parasite replication. Therefore, it is suggested that depletion of host intracellular iron stores may protect against *T. cruzi*, whereas host responses that transfer iron to the intracellular sites of *T. cruzi* multiplication may enhance parasite pathogenicity.

Epidemiology. The reduviids (also known as cone-nose bugs or triatomids) that carry *T. cruzi* are widespread throughout the Americas, and the infection has been reported in a variety of mammalian hosts from the United States southward to Argentina and Chile. Human infection occurs in the same areas, but the highest prevalence is in Brazil; the disease is nearly unknown north of the Tropic of Cancer. Dogs and cats are important reservoirs of infection in Brazil. In one endemic area where the rate of infection as judged by seroreactivity was 38%, some 18% of domestic dogs and cats were infected. In households in which infected reduviid bugs were found but dogs and cats were uninfected, the rate of seropositivity among the human occupants was only about half that in households in which both reduviids and domestic pets were infected. *T. cruzi* has been reported in 18 different species of mammalian hosts in the United States in localities extending from California, Arizona, and Utah through the southernmost tier of states, including Oklahoma, to Florida and Georgia and also in Maryland. Only five autochthonous insect-borne cases have been reported in the United States; three from Texas, one from California, and one from Tennessee. The cases were four children, with one death, and one adult. There is also serologic evidence for human infection in Georgia and in northern California. Sporadic infections are, of course, encountered in persons coming from endemic areas. With the millions of people who have emigrated to the United States from areas where Chagas' disease is endemic, it is estimated that there may now be 50,000 to 100,000 immigrants with *T. cruzi* infection living in the United States.

In the endemic areas of South America, the prevalence rate is estimated at about 20% of the population at risk. In Mexico the prevalence rate is unknown, but autopsy figures place it under 0.2% of the general population, and in the United States it is vanishingly small. In South America 20% to 30% of reduviids are infected, and in North America infection rates are similar. However, the loose methods of construction used in human habitations in the endemic areas of South America are much more favorable to domiciliation of the vector than are those methods generally employed in house construction in the United States.

Certain species of reduviids do not ordinarily defecate at the time of feeding, as do the important vectors of Chagas' disease. The lack of domiciliary species of reduviids with the necessary defecation habits may explain the fact that this disease seldom infects humans in North America. In California, woodrat burrows are frequently very heavily infested with the local reduviid, *Triatoma protracta*, an insect that does not ordinarily defecate while feeding, and it is known that the animals can become infected by eating the insects or licking infected feces from their fur. Since the mid-1990s, vector control programs in several Latin American countries have begun to bring Chagas' disease under control. However, 8 million to 9 million people still are infected with *T. cruzi* (WHO Report, 2002).

A developmental cycle of *T. cruzi* involving the multiplication of epimastigotes in the lumen of the anal glands of opossums has been described. The development of the parasite in the anal glands appears to be similar to that in the intestinal tract of the reduviid bug. Mice could be infected by feeding them a mixture of bread crumbs moistened with milk and material squeezed from the glands of an infected opossum. These findings suggest a potential role for opossums in the direct transmission of *T. cruzi* without the aid of the insect vector.

The severity of Chagas' disease also lessens with its northward spread. In South America approximately 10% of infected persons die during the acute stage or develop serious myocardiopathy in the chronic stage of the disease. Some workers consider that the demonstrable strain differences in *T. cruzi* from various areas and hosts are reflected in the apparent difference in incidence of cardiopathy, megaesophagus, and megacolon in different areas. More extensive surveillance is needed before this theory can be confirmed or denied.

Zymodemes have been described for *T. cruzi* isolated in South America: three major zymodemes are reported from Brazil and two from Bolivia. In Brazil, two of the zymodemes are associated with strains involved in the sylvatic transmission cycle, one in arboreal mammals and the other in terrestrial ones. The third *T. cruzi* zymodeme is associated with the domestic transmission cycle in humans or in domestic mammals. The two Bolivian zymodemes both occur in humans; the first is encountered more frequently at high altitudes, whereas the second is more common at low altitudes.

Treatment. The current drug of choice in treatment of Chagas' disease is the nitrofurfurylidine derivative nifurtimox★ (Lampit, also known as Bayer 2502), which has shown promise in the treatment of acute or early chronic cases. It should not be used during pregnancy.

Nifurtimox, 3-methyl-4(5′-nitrofurfurylidenamino-tetrahydro(1,4)-thiazine-1,1-dioxide, inhibits intracellular development of *T. cruzi* in tissue culture. It is given orally over an extended period, and it is better tolerated by young than by older patients. The pediatric dose for children of 1 to 10 years is 15 to 20 mg/kg, and for children 11 to 16 years the dose is 12.5 to 15 mg/kg orally per day in four doses for 90 days. The adult dose is 8 to 10 mg/kg per day orally in three to four doses for 90 to 120 days.

Benznidazole (*N*-benzyl-2-nitro-1-imidazoleacetamide; Rochagan), an imidazole compound, has been used in Argentina, Brazil, and Chile since 1971, where clinical trials have shown consistent antiparasitic activity, in contrast with the variable results obtained with nifurtimox. Benznidazole is used at a dose of 5 mg/kg orally per day in 2 doses for adults, and 10 mg/kg per day in two doses for children, for 60 days. Its main side effects are skin allergy and peripheral neuropathy, both of which are reversible. The mode of action may be similar to that of metronidazole on *Trichomonas vaginalis*, namely inhibition of nucleic acid synthesis. Benznidazole treatment, 7.5 mg/kg orally per day for 60 days, of early *T. cruzi* infection in 64 schoolchildren aged 7 to 12 years, in a rural area of Brazil with endemic Chagas' disease, was found to be safe and 56% effective in producing negative seroconversion of specific antibodies (Andrade et al., 1996). This drug is not available in the United States. Strains of *T. cruzi* isolated from patients and from domestic and sylvatic reservoirs and vectors have demonstrated resistance to both nifurtimox and benznidazole. Verapamil was able to reverse the drug resistance to *T. cruzi* to nifurtimox in vitro.

Allopurinol (4-hydroxy-pyrazolo[3,4-*d*]pyrimidine) appears to be an effective drug for the treatment of *T. cruzi* infection as well as the leishmaniases. Enzyme systems of these organisms, unlike those of humans, transform allopurinol into toxic adenine analogues. In a study involving 307 patients with Chagas' disease in Cordoba, Argentina (Gallerano et al. 1990), allopurinol was found to be as efficacious as either nifurtimox or benznidazole in eliminating parasitemias and in rendering patients seronegative. Adverse reactions, such as generalized pruritic dermatitis, epigastric pain, transient diarrhea, and transient polyneuritis, occurred in 11% of patients receiving allopurinol, compared with 30% for patients receiving nifurtimox or benznidazole. Allopurinol was administered orally 600 or 900 mg per day, in 300-mg doses, for 60 days.

Prevention. Although control of the insect vector must play an important part in any long-range efforts at the control of Chagas' disease, entomologists are no longer optimistic about the control of *any* insect-borne disease by this approach alone, pointing to the "infinite

★Available at present in the United States from the CDC Drug Service, Centers for Disease Control and Prevention, U.S. Public Health Service, Atlanta, Georgia 30333; (404) 639-3670.

resilience" of the vector populations. That such control may be of great importance, at least in certain situations, is shown by studies in the Mexican state of Oaxaca, which found that the use of DDT in malaria control has virtually eliminated household reduviids, with a coincidental dramatic fall in the transmission of Chagas' disease, as judged by serologic tests. The rate of seropositivity was 2% in children younger than 12 years of age and 35% in persons older than 20 years.

About a dozen species of reduviid bugs, belonging to several different genera, are of primary importance as vectors. Many other species can transmit the disease. The ecologies of these different vectors may be of great importance in determining distribution of the disease—as, for example, in Panama, where distribution of the two main vectors seems to correspond with that of a particular species of palm tree in which they live that also shelters reservoir hosts such as opossums and anteaters.

Education and other efforts toward the construction of reduviid-proof housing are being undertaken in areas of high endemicity, where periodic spraying programs are also of value. Antigenic variation does not seem to occur in *T. cruzi* as it does in the African trypanosomes, and prospects for the eventual development of vaccines seem good.

LEISHMANIA

Until recently it had been almost impossible to differentiate among the various leishmanias that cause human disease. Accordingly, differentiating among species was done largely on clinical grounds, and three species of *Leishmania* were recognized, corresponding to the clinical entities of cutaneous, mucocutaneous, and visceral leishmaniasis. In the past few years other criteria have been utilized, such as restriction analysis of kinetoplast DNA, also known as schizodeme analysis, nuclear DNA hybridization, isoenzyme patterns (zymodeme analysis, referred to as zymotaxonomy), and serologic testing. When utilizing isoenzyme profiles to group and identify *Leishmania* isolates, it is essential to use many enzyme systems. Recent reports list from 6 to 25 enzymes, classified into 44 zymodemes, used to identify isolates. These criteria give results that are in surprising agreement and, taken in conjunction with ecological evidence, suggest taxonomic groupings that do not entirely correspond with, and in some cases cut across, clinical groups. However, for clarity of presentation, we consider these diseases under clinical rather than under strictly taxonomic groupings. Table 5-1 lists the various *Leishmania* species and the clinical diseases they cause.

The various species of *Leishmania* are transmitted by sandflies. Amastigotes, liberated from host cells in the insect's gut, transform into promastigotes, which multiply there and finally pass forward into the pharynx and buccal cavity, from which they are introduced into a new host when the sandfly again feeds (see Fig. 5-20 for a generalized life cycle).

Cutaneous Leishmaniasis

Oriental sore, as seen in the Old World (Fig. 5-15), is produced by leishmanias belonging to the *Leishmania tropica* complex. There are three serologically and biochemically distinct species; all are transmitted by sandflies belonging to the genus *Phlebotomus*. *L. tropica* produces chronic disease that, if not treated, lasts for a year or longer; it is characterized by the production of dry lesions that ulcerate only after several months, are usually single, and occur primarily on the face. It is found in urban areas, widely distributed around the Mediterranean littoral, in Armenia, Azerbaijan, Turkmenistan, and Uzbekistan; it is seen also in Afghanistan, India, and Kenya. The dog may be a natural host, but is not thought to be an effective reservoir for humans. A similar chronic disease, seen in the highlands of Ethiopia, in Kenya, and possibly in south Yemen, is caused by *Leishmania aethiopica*. The rock hyrax is a reservoir host of this species.

Leishmania major produces an acute infection with a duration of 3 to 6 months. The lesions occur primarily on the lower limbs, they are moist and tend to ulcerate very early; there may be secondary or satellite lesions. *L. major* occurs in the Kara Kum and Kyzyl Kum

TABLE 5-1 ▨ *Leishmania* Species and the Clinical Diseases They Cause

Clinical Disease	*Leishmania* Species	Geographic Location
Cutaneous leishmaniasis	L. tropica complex	Old World
	L. tropica	
	L. aethiopica	
	L. major	
	L. mexicana complex	New World
	L. mexicana	
	L. pifanoi	
	L. amazonensis	
	L. garnhami	
	L. venezuelensis	
	L. braziliensis complex*	New World
	L. peruviana	
	L. guyanensis	
	L. panamensis	
	L. lainsoni	
	L. colombiensis	
	L. infantum	Old World
	L. chagasi	New World
Mucocutaneous leishmaniasis	L. braziliensis complex*	New World
	L. braziliensis	
	L. guyanensis	
	L. panamensis	
	L. mexicana	New World
	L. tropica	Old World
	L. major	Old World
Visceral leishmaniasis	L. donovani complex	
	L. donovani	Old World
	L. infantum	Old World
	L. chagasi	New World
	L. tropica	Old World
	L. amazonensis	New World

*Members of the *L. braziliensis* complex are considered to be a separate subgenus, *Viannia*, from all other *Leishmania*, which belong to the subgenus *Leishmania*. L. braziliensis complex organisms develop in the hindgut of the sandfly vector (referred to as peripylarian development), whereas other *Leishmania* species develop in the midgut (suprapylarian development).

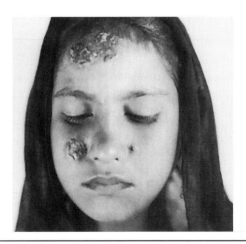

FIGURE 5-15 ▨ Oriental sores on face and forehead. (Armed Forces Institute of Pathology, #80,717.)

deserts of Turkmenistan, Uzbekistan, and Kazakhstan; in Iran, Syria, Israel, and Jordan; and in Africa in Algeria, Egypt, Tunisia, the Sahara, Sudan, Chad, Nigeria, Niger, Burkina Faso, Mali, Senegal, and Kenya. It is primarily a disease of rural areas, and reservoir hosts (gerbils and other rodents) are important sources of human infection.

In the New World, cutaneous leishmaniasis is caused by species of the *Leishmania mexicana* complex, of which *L. mexicana* and *L. pifanoi* are the most important. The chiclero ulcer or Bay sore is caused by *L. mexicana*. It is found in Belize, the Yucatan peninsula, and Guatemala. Twenty-nine cases of autochthonous human cutaneous leishmaniasis have been reported from south central Texas. The disease is believed to be endemic in that area, in which a number of potential reservoir hosts and vectors can be found. Amastigotes of the *L. mexicana* complex have been isolated from dermal lesions of humans and from woodrats and a cat in the same area of Texas. Lesions are usually single, and 40% affect the ear, where they can be quite destructive of cartilage. Rarely the diffuse cutaneous form is seen, with extensive proliferative lesions more or less all over the body. Six cases of diffuse cutaneous leishmaniasis, attributed to infection with *L. mexicana*, have been reported from widely separated geographic regions in Mexico. Three of the patients had evidence of nasopharyngeal mucosal involvement. A number of forest rodents are reservoir hosts of this parasite, and the vector is a sandfly of the genus *Lutzomyia*.

L. pifanoi occurs in the Amazon basin, in Mato Grosso State in Brazil, and in Venezuela. It has been isolated only from patients with the diffuse cutaneous form of the disease. The initial lesion is a single one, and often a period of months or years passes (during which it may ulcerate or even disappear) before the disease spreads both locally and to distant skin areas. The irregularly shaped papules, which bear a resemblance to the lepromatous lesions of leprosy, spread slowly and do not ulcerate or heal. The organisms do not invade the viscera, and the patient remains in general good health.

Leishmania amazonensis is found in the Amazon basin of Brazil and is the cause of cutaneous and diffuse cutaneous forms of leishmaniasis. Reservoir hosts for this species of the *L. mexicana* complex are a number of small forest mammals, including rodents, marsupials, and foxes. The principal vector is a *Lutzomyia* sandfly. Apparently, only a small percentage of the cases of cutaneous leishmaniasis is due to *L. amazonensis*; however, in Belém, Brazil, approximately 30% of cutaneous leishmaniasis cases caused by this parasite have progressed to incurable diffuse cutaneous leishmaniasis, presumably in persons with defective cell-mediated immunity.

Two other described species of the *L. mexicana* complex are *L. garnhami*, which causes Venezuelan Andean cutaneous leishmaniasis, and *L. venezuelensis*, which causes cutaneous leishmaniasis in a forested area along the River Turbio, state of Lara, Venezuela. The identification of these subspecies is based on isoenzyme profiles and monoclonal antibody studies.

A species of the *Leishmania braziliensis* complex, *L. peruviana*, is confined to the western Peruvian Andes and causes a disease in humans known locally as *uta*. There may be one or a small number of skin lesions that are self-healing and similar to those of *L. tropica*; it has, in fact, been suggested that this species is actually imported *L. tropica*. However, isoenzyme profiles show it to be distinct from *L. tropica*. The domestic dog and probably a wild rodent are reservoir hosts, and sandflies of the genus *Lutzomyia* are the vectors. Additionally, a number of isolates from cutaneous leishmanial infections in Brazil and Ecuador have been shown by enzyme electrophoresis, DNA fingerprinting, and monoclonal antibodies to be similar to *L. major*, and not to *L. mexicana*, *L. braziliensis*, or *L. donovani*.

Two other species of the *L. braziliensis* complex, *L. guyanensis* (which occurs in the Guyanas and northern Brazil) and *L. panamensis* (which occurs in Panama, Costa Rica, and Colombia), also produce single skin ulcers, but with both organisms lymphatic spread may occur, resulting in widespread ulceration. *L. panamensis* infection is not uncommon in visitors from North America co Costa Rica, particularly those who travel to the rainforests. Mucocutaneous involvement may occur, but it is rare. The disease caused by *L. guyanensis* is known locally as *pian bois*; reservoir hosts are arboreal sloths and anteaters, and *Lutzomyia* is the sandfly vector. *L. panamensis* has a variety of reservoir hosts, including sloths, rodents, monkeys, and procyonids. *Lutzomyia* and *Psychodopygus* sandflies are vectors.

L. lainsoni, a species belonging to the *L. braziliensis* complex, is another cause of cutaneous lesions. Infections have been reported from Brazil and Peru, where *Lutzomyia* sandflies are the natural vector and the agouti is the wild animal reservoir. The subgenus *Viannia* has been proposed for the *L. braziliensis* complex. Parasites of the subgenus *Viannia* develop in the hindgut of the sandfly vector, whereas organisms of the subgenus *Leishmania* (all non-*L. braziliensis* complex leishmanias) develop in the midgut of the sandfly. The enzyme aconitate hydratase is able to distinguish the subgenus *Viannia* from the other leishmanias.

Another new member of the *L. braziliensis* complex is *L. colombiensis*. It is closely related to *L. lainsonis* causes cutaneous lesions, and has been reported to infect human in Colombia, Venezuela, and Panama. The sandfly vector is *Lutzomyia* and the sloth is a natural reservoir.

Two leishmanias that usually produce visceral disease have been identified as the cause of cutaneous lesions in certain areas. They are *L. infantum* in north Tunisia and *L. chagasi* in Honduras.

Symptoms. The incubation period may be a couple of months or as long as 3 years in *L. tropica* and *L. aethiopica* infections; in *L. major* it is much shorter, as little as 2 weeks. The first sign of infection is a small red papule, which may itch intensely and grows to 2 cm or more in diameter. In *L. major* infections, the papule is covered with a serous exudate and ulcerates early; papules are dry and ulcerate only ofter several months in *L. tropica* and *L. aethiopica* infections.

Although the usual cutaneous lesions heal spontaneously, in certain instances such healing does not occur of itself. These cases may be considered to represent the two poles of the spectrum of response—anergy and hypersensitivity. The anergic patient is incapable of mounting a response to infection, which therefore can proliferate indefinitely, forming many lesions teeming with parasites. This type of disease, known as diffuse cutaneous leishmaniasis, is probably the result not only of deficient cell-mediated immunity but also of some characteristics of the parasite itself, as it is seen primarily in infections caused by *L. aethiopica* and *L. pifanoi*. Such patients generally are not anergic to other infectious agents, react normally to tuberculin, and have normal immunoglobulin levels, but they do not react to the leishmanin (Montenegro) skin test.

The hypersensitive patient is capable of excellent antibody and cellular responses but cannot completely eliminate the parasites, so as the central lesion heals, active peripheral ones continue to form. This type of response, known as leishmaniasis recidiva, may be seen with any of the cutaneous leishmaniases.

Host recovery in cutaneous leishmaniasis depends on the development of cell-mediated immunity. The course of development of cellular immunity was closely monitored in an accidental laboratory infection with *L. tropica*. In vitro bioassays of cell-mediated immunity showed that lymphocyte proliferation and interleukin-2 production, induced by solute *L. tropica* antigens, appeared within 5 weeks of infection and reached maximum levels with ulceration of the skin lesion. Thereafter, interleukin-2 production rapidly decreased, whereas lymphocyte proliferation declined more slowly. Healing was complete after 20 weeks.

Diagnosis of cutaneous leishmaniasis is usually made in endemic areas on clinical grounds, but this requires much familiarity with the disease. It is usually possible to demonstrate the rounded or oval organisms, approximately 4.5 × 3.3 µm in diameter and having a typical amastigote structure, within large monocytic cells obtained by aspiration of fluid from beneath the ulcer bed, especially its active border. Scrapings taken from the ulcer surface do not reveal the organisms, which are destroyed in areas secondarily infected with bacteria. Culture on NNN medium of material obtained by aspiration or biopsy (Chapter 15) may demonstrate promastigote forms. Schneider's *Drosophila* medium supplemented with 30% fetal bovine serum has been useful in isolating organisms from humans with cutaneous leishmaniasis. Aspirate or biopsy material may be inoculated subcutaneously into the nose of a hamster and the animal watched for nasal inflammation. The result of the Montenegro test, involving the intradermal injection of a suspension of killed promastigotes, is positive in a high percentage of *L. tropica* infections and in more than 95% of *L. braziliensis* infections. The CDC offers an indirect fluorescent antibody test. See Chapter 16 for the names of commercial laboratories and commercially available kits.

Pathogenesis. When the bite of an infected sandfly liberates promastigotes into the skin, the parasites proliferate as amastigotes in the macrophages and the endothelium of the capillaries and other small blood vessels of the immediate area. Lysis of the amastigotes occurs following activation of the macrophages by sensitized lymphocytes. A granulomatous reaction results in formation of a localized nodule, which ulcerates when the blood supply to the area is compromised by parasite-induced damage. A pyogenic infection, generally a trivial one, develops in the open ulcer bed, and as host immunity increases, the ulcer heals. Enlarged regional lymph nodes (bubonic leishmaniasis) have been reported to accompany the cutaneous lesions of *L. braziliensis*. A survey in Brazil indicated that 77% of 595 persons with parasitologically confirmed cutaneous leishmaniasis reported lymphadenopathy in addition to skin lesions. *L. braziliensis* should be considered in cases of unexplained lymphadenopathy in endemic areas. Whereas in humans infection with *L. tropica* is confined to the skin and heals spontaneously (Fig. 5-16), the hamster is unable to develop any tissue resistance and is ultimately killed by the infection, which spreads to the viscera. Resistance to reinfection with the same species following a primary infection is nearly absolute. Infection with *L. major* protects the host against subsequent *L. tropica* infection, but infection with *L. tropica* does not confer the same immunity to subsequent challenge with *L. major*.

Epidemiology. Although sandflies are the natural vectors of all types of leishmaniasis, contact infection is possible, and vaccination is practiced in certain areas by inoculating serum from naturally acquired lesions into an inconspicuous location on the body of a nonimmune person. Mechanical transmission through the bites of flies such as *Stomoxys* has also been documented. Infected monocytes may be a source of transfusion-associated leishmaniasis.

The infection produced by *L. tropica* is generally transmitted from one human to another; the other forms of cutaneous leismaniasis are principally zoonoses. Construction work that involves opening the burrows of infected gerbils has caused serious outbreaks of *L. major* infection in humans. Control of the disease in areas where infection is widespread in animals presents special problems.

During an 18-month period in 2002–2004, 522 cases of cutaneous leishmaniasis were confirmed in military personnel deployed to Afghanistan, Iraq, and Kuwait (CDC, 2004). *L. major* was the organism identified by isoenzyme electrophoresis where clinical isolates were cultivated. Patients were treated with sodium stibogluconate at Walter Reed Army Medical Center.

Treatment. Sodium stibogluconate (antimony sodium gluconate; Pentostam),★ less toxic than the earlier pentavalent antimonials, is the most effective compound presently available for treatment of all cutaneous leishmaniasis except the Ethiopian form of diffuse cutaneous leishmaniasis, which is reported to respond best to pentamidine. Pentavalent antimony inhibits glycolytic enzymes and fatty acid oxidation in leishmanial amastigotes. Pentostam is administered either intravenously or intramuscularly; the dosage is 20 mg/kg body weight daily for 20 days. The course may be repeated at 10-day intervals in resistant cases; a maximum of three courses is advised. Pentamidine is administrated as outlined below for the treatment of kala-azar. Coughing, headache, and vomiting are frequent side effects of antimonial drugs.

★Available from the CDC Drug Service, Centers for Disease Control and Prevention, U.S. Public Health Service, Atlanta, Georgia 30333; (404) 639-3670.

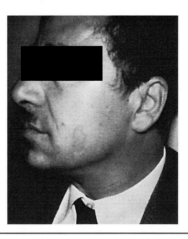

FIGURE 5-16 ▪ Typical depressed, flattened scar left by healed oriental sore. (Courtesy of Dr. Roy Leeper, Kaiser-Permanente Medical Center, Oakland, CA.)

In areas where sodium stibogluconate is not readily available (such as Latin America), meglumine antimoniate (Glucantime) may be substituted. The recommended dose is 20 mg/kg per day intravenously or intramuscularly for 20 days. The course may be repeated or continued, as some patients may need a longer duration. Meglumine antimoniate is not available in the United States. Some authorities recommend continuous administration until healing is complete. EKG abnormalities are rare, but if they occur the drug should be withheld until the EKG returns to normal, at which time the dose is reduced slightly. Antimony-resistant cutaneous leishmaniasis has been successfully treated with suboptimal doses of pentavalent antimonials (Glucantime, 10 mg/kg body weight daily for 30 days) and intramuscular recombinant human interferon gamma, 100 µg/m² of body surface area daily for 30 days (Falcoff et al., 1994). Intradermal injections of interferon gamma around lesions caused by *L tropica* and *L. guyanensis* reportedly promote healing of ulcers (Harms et al., 1989). Apparently, healing was accomplished by cell-mediated immune responses elicited by the interferon gamma.

Amphotericin B has been used in patients unresponsive to pentavalent antimonials, administered by slow intravenous infusion, gradually increasing the dose to 1 mg/kg weight, at which level it should be continued on alternate days until a total of 2 to 3 g has been given. A less toxic alternative is ketoconazole.

Oral ketoconazole, 400 mg daily for 4 to 8 weeks, has been reported to be effective in treating longstanding cutaneous leishmaniasis (Viallet et al., 1986). Itraconazole has been used in India to treat cutaneous lesions. Topical preparations containing chlorpromazine (2%) or paromomycin (15%), used in clinical studies in Israel, have demonstrated considerable potential for the treatment of cutaneous leishmaniasis (El-On et al., 1988). Clotrimazole (1%) cream was an effective topical treatment of cutaneous infection in Saudi Arabia. Oral dapsone, 200 mg daily for 6 weeks, showed an 82% cure rate in a double-blind trial in India (Dorga, 1991). Finally controlled, localized heat, three 30-second treatments of 50° C at weekly intervals, has been used to treat cutaneous leishmaniasis in Guatemala (Navin et al., 1990). The cure rate with heat treatment was the same as with the pentavalent antimonial, 73%.

Steroids may be of value in the initial treatment of leishmaniasis recidiva.

The efficacy of a combined vaccine (heat-killed *L. amazonensis* plus viable bacille Calmette-Guérin [BCG]) in immunotherapy of American cutaneous leishmaniasis was evaluated in a clinical study involving 217 patients (Convit et al., 1989). Clinical cure was observed in more than 90% of those who received the vaccine; the average time for healing was 16 to 18 weeks and it was comparable to that for meglumine antimoniate (Glucantime). The effectiveness of the vaccine in prophylaxis has not yet been tested.

Prevention. Field trials of a vaccine made from cultured promastigotes of several strains of leishmanias from Brazil showed that the use of this vaccine resulted in Montenegro skin-test positivity in 78.4% of the experimental group 3 months after inoculation. The proportion of positive results fell to 73.2 in 1 year, 54.1 after 2 years, and 30.9 after 3 years. Skin test positivity is associated with resistance to superinfection, and these results must be considered promising.

Mucocutaneous Leishmaniasis

In Brazil, eastern Peru, Bolivia, Paraguay, Ecuador, Colombia, and Venezuela, an infection caused by *Leishmania braziliensis* is seen. The outstanding feature of this disease, known in Brazil as *espundia*, is the development, in a variable percentage of patients, of ulcers on the oral or nasal mucosa. In some parts of Brazil, such lesions are said to occur in about one fifth of cases of the disease. The rate of mucous membrane involvement for the endemic area as a whole is considerably lower. The cutaneous lesions develop exactly as does oriental score, but they are more frequently multiple and may become large. Secondary infection plays a prominent role in the persistence of these ulcers and in the size that they may attain. Sometimes ulcerations of adjacent areas extend to involve mucosal surfaces, but more frequently the lesions seem to develop by metastasis. The cutaneous lesions may be completely healed at the time mucosal lesions are first seen, or the two types may coexist. In fact, mucosal lesions sometimes develop many years after the patient has left an endemic area, in persons with no history of cutaneous lesions. The PCR assay has been used to identify *L. braziliensis* in the blood of a woman 30 years after she had been clinically cured of leishmaniasis. If mucosal ulcerations develop, progress of the infection, while slow, is steady. Unless effective treatment is given, the entire nasal mucosa, and that of the hard and soft palates, eventually is affected (Fig. 5-17). The nasal septum is destroyed, but unlike similar syphilitic lesions, the process does not involve the bones. Ulceration may result in loss of all the soft parts of the nose, the lips, the soft palate, and so forth. Death usually occurs from secondary infection. Mucosal disease reportedly is caused by *L. guyanensis* and *L. panamensis* as well.

Various forest rodents and dogs are naturally infected. Sandflies belonging to the genera *Lutzomyia* and *Psychodopygus* are vectors.

A clinically similar disease is seen in Ethiopia and Sudan. It is characterized by ulceration of the lips and mucous membranes of the nose and mouth and sometimes by destruction of the nasal alae. The lesions are not as extensive as those seen in espundia and are believed to results from direct extension of primary cutaneous lesions of the nose or lips. The causative agent is believed to be *L. tropica* and possibly *L. major*.

Treatment. Sodium stibogluconate (Pentostam),★ administered as described for cutaneous leishmaniasis (except that the length of treatment is 28 days rather than 20 days), is also effective in the mucocutaneous form of disease. Cycloguanil pamoate (Camolar), a folic acid inhibitor, is reported effective when administered intramuscularly at the rate of 300 mg for adults, 280 mg for children 1 to 5 years of age, and 140 mg for infants in a single dose. Cycloguanil is not available in the United States. Amphotericin B (Fungizone) is also reported to yield good results when given intravenously at the rate of 0.5 to 1 mg/kg body weight, daily or every other day, for periods up to 8 weeks.

Coughing, headache, and vomiting may be noted with either antimonials or amphotercin; renal damage and bone marrow depression are frequently seen when amphotericin is given for extended periods.

★Available from the CDC Drug Service, Centers for Disease Control and Prevention, U.S. Public Health Service, Atlanta, Georgia 30333; telephone (404) 639-3670.

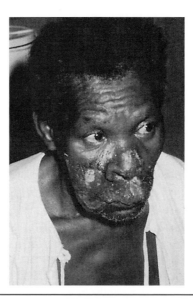

FIGURE 5-17 ■ Patient with mucocutaneous leishmaniasis. (Courtesy of Dr. Q. H. Geiman, Stanford University Medical School, Palo Alto, CA.)

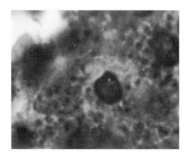

FIGURE 5-18 ■ *Leishmania donovani* amastigotes in Küpffer cells. (Photomicrograph by Zane Price.)

Visceral Leishmaniasis

Widely known by its Indian name of kala-azar, visceral leishmaniasis is no longer considered to be caused by a single agent but by at least three species belonging to the *Leishmania donovani* complex, but clinically and biochemically distinct and with different geographic distributions. As in cutaneous and mucocutaneous leishmaniasis, the causative organisms are parasites of the reticuloendothelial system. Unlike those discussed previously, the parasites that cause kala-azar are not confined to the reticuloendothelial cells of the subcutaneous tissues and mucous membranes but may be found throughout the body (Figs. 5-18 and 5-19). The life cycle of the *L. donovani* complex is illustrated in Figure 5-20.

L. donovani occurs in India, Burma, East Pakistan, Sumatra, and Thailand, and in the Central African Republic, Chad, Ethiopia, Somali Republic, Djibouti, Kenya, northern Uganda, Sudan, Gabon, Gambia, and Niger. It formerly occurred in epidemic proportions in the People's Republic of China but has been brought under control. It affects all age groups. In the Indian area there seem to be no reservoir hosts; the same is possibly true of Kenya, but in the Sudan it is found in various rodents. Dogs are the principal reservoir in China. Vectors are *Phlebotomus* sandflies. It has been suggested that further studies will probably result in the separation of one or more African strains from those seen in the Indian subcontinent.

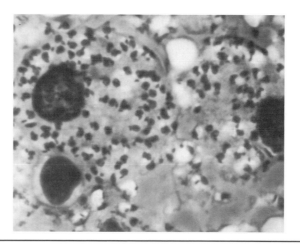

FIGURE 5-19 ▪ *Leishmania donovani* amastigotes in spleen impression preparation from infected hamster. (Photomicrograph by Zane Price.)

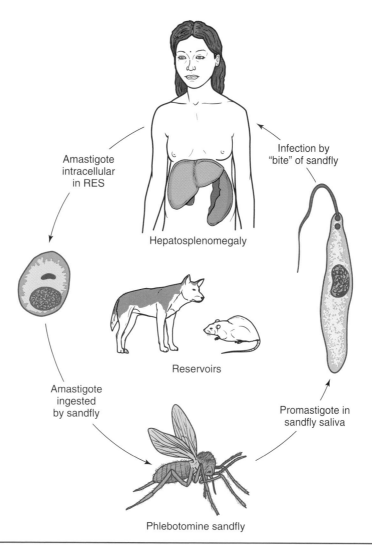

FIGURE 5-20 ▪ Life cycle of *Leishmania donovani* complex.

L. tropica has been the reported cause of visceral leishmaniasis in two patients in Kenya who were unresponsive to treatment with Pentostam, in patients in northeast India, and in veterans returning from the Persian Gulf War.

Leishmania infantum is found along the whole Mediterranean littoral—in Europe, the near East, and Africa. Elsewhere in Europe it occurs in Hungary, Romania, and the former southern USSR. It has also been reported in northern China and southern Siberia. Human infections are confined almost entirely to children; humans are considered to be an accidental host, with natural infections occurring in dogs, other Canidae, and porcupines. Transmission is by *Phlebotomus* sandflies. *L. infantum* has been the cause of an increasing number of cases of visceral leishmaniasis in HIV-infected patients in Italy and other Mediterranean countries.

In Central and South America—Argentina, Bolivia, Brazil, Surinam, Venezuela, Colombia, Ecuador, El Salvador, Honduras, and Guatemala—and in Mexico and Guadeloupe in the West Indies, visceral leishmaniasis is almost always caused by *Leishmania chagasi*. Those affected are primarily children. Foxes and domestic dogs and cats are naturally infected; the vectors are *Lutzomyia* sandflies. However, *L. amazonensis* has been isolated from the bone marrow of a patient with typical visceral leishmaniasis in Brazil.

Symptoms. As in the cutaneous and mucocutaneous leishmaniases, the parasites that cause visceral leishmaniasis are transmitted by various species of sandflies. Promastigote forms of the parasite multiply in the gut and migrate anteriorly to escape from the proboscis when the fly feeds. The onset of the disease is gradual, after an incubation period that may vary between 2 weeks and 18 months. Frequently the patient may present with a complaint of abdominal swelling, which has taken place without any definite illness. On examination, hepatomegaly and splenomegaly are found. Sometimes there is acute onset, which may closely mimic an attack of malaria, even to the tertian or quartan periodicity. There is sometimes diarrhea and an onset resembling typhoid fever. If the onset is insidious, there may be only an indefinite feeling of ill health during the earlier stages of the disease. Fever may be continuous, intermittent, or remittent, and recur at irregular intervals. A double (or "dromedary") or even triple fever peak daily is characteristic but is not always seen, as the temperature must be taken every 3 hours day and night to detect the sometimes transitory peaks. Anemia is generally present. There is progressive weight loss as the disease pursues its course. The body becomes emaciated, with the abdomen hugely swollen by the enlarged liver and spleen. Both organs are frequently soft and generally not tender. Ascites may occur in advanced stages of the disease. Kala-azar means, literally, black fever, having reference to a characteristic darkening of the skin, which has been most often noted in light-skinned Indians and is difficult to distinguish in persons with either very dark or very light skin. It is most marked on the forehead, over the temples, and around the mouth.

L. donovani does not in most areas cause skin lesions, although an initial papule (presumably at the site of the infecting bite) has rarely been noted. A condition known as dermal leishmanoid (Fig. 5-21) is sometimes seen in patients who have been treated for visceral leishmaniasis and may occur in persons who deny any history of disease. In light of the insidious course that kala-azar may exhibit, it is difficult to rule out the possibility of earlier, abortive visceral disease in such cases. The dermal lesions may be erythematous or depigmented macules, distributed over the entire body or in patches. A butterfly distribution over the nose is not uncommon. Later the lesions tend to become nodular and at this stage may be mistaken for leprosy nodules. Organisms may be found in the dermal lesions, and it has been suggested that patients with such lesions represent an important source of infection for the sandfly.

Neurologic changes in visceral leishmaniasis are rarely reported. However, 46% of 111 patients with visceral leishmaniasis in Khartoum, Sudan, had neurologic signs or symptoms. The most common symptom was a sensation of burning feet, followed by deafness, foot drop, and multiple cranial nerve palsies. *L. donovani* amastigotes have been recovered from the cerebrospinal fluid of a 10-year-old boy with kala-azar in India.

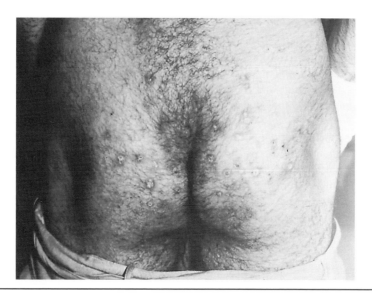

FIGURE 5-21   ■   Dermal leishmanoid lesions on buttocks. (Armed Forces Institute of Pathology, #384,447.)

The clinical picture may be suggestive, but a definitive diagnosis rests on demonstration of the parasites. Splenic puncture is undoubtedly an effective method for securing reticuloendothelial cells for study but is a somewhat risky procedure. Liver puncture is safer but possibly not as productive. Sternal marrow aspiration may likewise reveal the parasites and is considered by some the diagnostic procedure of choice. Buffy coat films, prepared from venous blood, are sometimes of value. It appears that in certain forms of visceral leishmaniasis parasites frequently are found in the blood. For example, parasitemia was detected in 15 of 20 patients with Kenyan visceral leishmaniasis. Similar results have been reported for visceral leishmaniasis in India. Culture of venous blood or of specimens of sternal marrow, liver, or spleen may reveal the parasites when they are scanty in the original material. Three culture media and Giemsa-stained smears have been compared for their ability to detect *Leishmania* organisms in splenic aspirates from patients with visceral leishmaniasis. Microscopy and culture were equally sensitive in detecting parasites before treatment. However, during and after treatment, culture on Schneider's *Drosophila* medium was the most sensitive method for detecting organisms, followed by microscopy and culture on RPMI medium 1640 and NNN medium (see Chapter 15). Hamsters are very susceptible to the disease and can be infected by intraperitoneal inoculation (see Fig. 5-19). Interestingly, the result of the Montenegro (leishmanin) test is negative in active kala-azar, but it becomes positive within 2 months following successful treatment. Presumably it likewise is positive after spontaneous cure; in surveys a leishmanin-positive rate of over 5% is considered evidence of endemic kala-azar. Enzyme immunoassay, immunoblot, and indirect fluorescent antibody tests are the serologic tests available in the United States. Details of the more important diagnostic procedures are given in Chapters 15 and 16.

Pathogenesis. The various species that cause visceral leishmaniasis parasitize cells of the reticuloendothelial (RE) system occur throughout the body. The disease is progressive, and the mortality rate in untreated cases ranges from 75% to 95%; death usually occurs within 2 years. In a relatively mild form, the disease may persist for many years; spontaneous cures undoubtedly occur.

Proliferation of the RE cells, particularly of the spleen and liver, leads to massive hypertrophy of these organs, which may return essentially to normal size after successful treatment.

The bone marrow may be involved, resulting in anemia and leukopenia. The white blood cell count is generally below 4000 per μl, often ranging from 2000 to 3000, accompanied by a progressive monocytosis. In kala-azar and trypanosomiasis, gamma globulins may constitute 60% to 70% of the serum proteins. Splenomegaly with stasis of blood in the sinusoids may result in increased destruction of both red and white blood cells. Glomerular involvement, with deposition of subendothelial and mesangial immune complexes resembling those found in the kidney in human cases of hepatosplenic schistosomiasis, has been desribed. IgA, IgG, IgM, complement, and fibrinogen have been identified from these glomerular complexes. Interstitial nephritis, with infiltration of lymphocytes and plasma cells, has been described in human infection. Ocular complications of kala-azar are rare. They includes retinal hemorrhage, keratitis, central retinal vein thrombosis, papillitis, iritis, and uveitis. Amastigotes have been demonstrated in eye lesions of patients with anterior uveitis in southern Sudan. Death usually is the result of intercurrent infection.

Mechanisms that are involved in recovery from leishmanial infection are generally believed to involve interactions between T lymphocytes and macrophages; however, recent studies have demonstrated a role for humoral factors in human resistance to reinfection with *L. donovani*. Normal human serum and serum from patients with kala-azar are cytotoxic for amastigotes of *L. donovani*, killing parasites via the alternate pathway of serum complement. Cytotoxicity of normal serum was enhanced by factors present in patient serum characterized as parasite-specific IgG.

Epidemiology. Various clinical forms of visceral leishmaniasis are characteristic of different localities. In general, two different forms of transmission are observed. In the urban form, transmission is primarily from human to human. A rural form of transmission, seen in other areas, is primarily a zoonosis. The infection is epizootic in rodents or other wild animals; humans are sporadic and somewhat accidental victims. In the semiarid Transcaucasian areas, wild jackals serve as a reservoir of infection, which in rural areas occurs primarily in adults. In Africa a rural form of transmission is generally seen; rats in Sudan and gerbils and ground squirrels in East Africa carry the infection, which sporadically infects humans. Epidemics have occurred in these areas, however. The African forms of kala-azar differ in several ways from those seen elsewhere. Primary skin lesions (leishmaniomas) are characteristic; they generally occur on the legs and represent healed ulcerations at the site of infection. The Montenegro tests is often positive in the early stages of the disease, a consequence presumably of the dermatotrophic nature of *L. donovani* strains in this area.

The ground squirrel strain of *L. donovani* isolated in Kenya is apparently not viscerotropic in humans. Introduced into the skin, it gives rise to a leishmanioma but does not extend to produce a visceral infection. At least a temporary immunity is produced against viscerotropic strains of *L. donovani* by this means.

In Tuscany, Italy, where human and canine leishmaniases are endemic, rats have been shown to carry *L. infantum*, suggesting their role as wild reservoirs of infection.

Clinical visceral leishmaniasis has been described in foxhounds in central Oklahoma. The dogs, all from the same private kennel, had never traveled to areas of known leishmaniasis or associated with known infected animals, suggesting that infection was acquired locally. Ticks have been proposed as possible vectors. Ultrastructural studies show the organisms to be morphologically similar to *L. donovani*.

Treatment. Sodium stibogluconate (Pentostam),★ administered as described for *L. tropica* infections, except that the suggested length of treatment is 28 rather than 20 days, is the drug of choice for initial therapy in all but Sudanese infections. Strains acquired in Sudan are generally resistant to antimonials, and treatment should be initiated with pentamidine at the

★Available from the CDC Drug Service, Centers for Disease Control and Prevention, U.S. Public Health Service, Atlanta, Georgia 30333; (404) 639-3670.

rate of 2 to 4 mg/kg body weight, given in daily intramuscular doses for 10 to 15 days. Resistance to Pentostam has also been reported in Kenya. Meglumine antimonate (Glucantime), not available in the United States, may be used as described for cutaneous leishmaniasis, except it is administered for 28 days.

Animal experiments suggest that liposomal encapsulation may be utilized to deliver antimonial drugs to the reticuloendothelial system, allowing treatment with much smaller doses than is now the case. Liposomal amphotericin B has been effective in treating anti-mony-resistant case of visceral leishmaniasis in the Mediterranean, France, India, and Brazil, as has amphotericin B.

Allopurinol, 20 mg/kg three times a day, has been used in the treatment of visceral leish-maniasis in patients with AIDS. Allopurinol plus sodium stibogluconate has been found effec-tive in treating antimony-resistant cases of visceral leishmaniasis in Kenya. Patients with visceral leishmaniasis have also been treated with a combination of interferon gamma and pentavalent antimony. Interferon gamma may enhance the intracellular killing of *Leishmania* amastigotes.

Miltefosine (Impavido), an alkylphosphocholine, has been used in India to treat visceral leishmaniasis (Sundar et al., 2002). The drug was administered orally at a rate of 2.5 mg/kg daily in two doses for 28 days. The cure rate was 94% for the miltefosine-treated group as compared to 97% for the amphotericin B-treated standard treatment group. The drug appears to be an effective and safe oral treatment for visceral leishmaniasis. It is not available in the United States.

NONHUMAN TRYPANOSOMATIDS

There have been two reports of HIV-positive patients who were infected with nonhuman trypanosomatids, members of the family Trypanosomatidae, which parasitize a wide variety of plants, insects, and vertebrates. Trypanosomatids that infect plants and insects are referred to as lower trypanosomatids. The first individual, a male from Martinique, initially was diag-nosed as having diffuse cutaneous leishmaniasis, but biochemical and transmission electron microscope characterization of skin lesion isolates, amastigotes in the lesions, and promastig-otes in culture showed them to be monoxenous (single host) trypanosomatids of insects. The second person, a female living in Spain, was suspected of having visceral leishmaniasis because of clinical and laboratory findings. Organisms were isolated from a bone marrow aspirate, and isoenzyme analysis and DNA hybridization of the cultured promastigotes failed to identify them as *Leishmania*. All that could be determined was that the isolate was of non-human origin, possibly a lower trypanosomatid of insects. It is likely that additional cases of nonhuman trypanosomatid infection will be described from AIDS patients and from other severely immunocompromised persons.

Another isolate was described from the skin lesions of a patient also living in Martinique (Noyes et al., 2002). Isoenzyme analysis found it to be identical with the first Martinique isolate, although the patient in the second case was HIV-negative and immunocompetent.

The Tissue Coccidia

Isospora, discussed in Chapter 3 with species that are intestinal parasites of humans and various other animals, is a typical coccidian. Two other genera, *Toxoplasma* and *Sarcocystis*, were not until recently recognized as coccidia, because the stages seen in humans did not suggest coccidian affinities.

While oocysts essentially identical in appearance are produced by all three genera, details of life cycles of the three genera and the appearance of the tissue stages may vary considerably. In *Isospora*, the enteric stages are of greatest importance, and oocysts readily infect members of the species in which they developed. *Toxoplasma* oocysts, on the other hand, more readily infect a variety of other species (including humans); they may also infect the

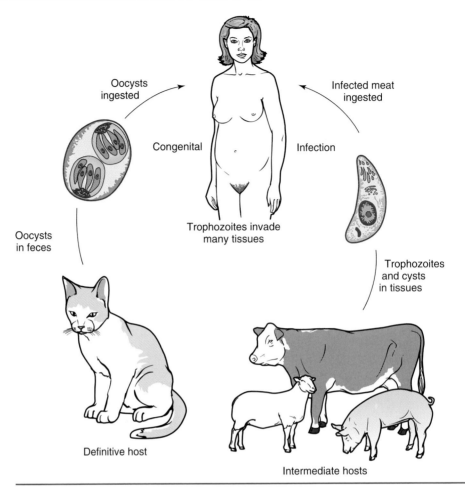

Oocysts
ingested

Infected meat
ingested

Congenital

Infection

Trophozoites invade
many tissues

Oocysts
in feces

Trophozoites
and cysts
in tissues

Definitive host

Intermediate hosts

FIGURE 5-22   ■   Life cycle of *Toxoplasma gondii.*

definitive hosts (cats), but with a long prepatent period. *Sarcocystis* is obligatorily heteroxenous, as its oocysts are not infectious for the host of origin.

Toxoplasma gondii

Toxoplasma is a parasite of cosmopolitan distribution, able to develop in a wide variety of vertebrate hosts, but its definitive host is the house cat and certain other Felidae. It was originally described in a North African rodent called the gundi, from which it derives its specific name. Serologic evidence indicates that human infections are common in many parts of the world, but most are of a benign nature or are completely asymptomatic. The life cycle of *T. gondii* is illustrated in Figure 5-22.

Within the epithelial cells of the small intestine of the cat, the organisms develop first to produce schizonts and gametocytes (Fig. 5-23, *A*) and finally oocysts, which are passed in the feces. These oocysts, 9 to 11 μm in width by 11 to 14 μm in length, similar in appearance to those of *Isospora belli* but smaller, contain two sporocysts, each of which encloses four sporozoites (Fig. 5-23, *B*).

Toxoplasma trophozoites (tachyzoites) may be found in the mesenteric lymph nodes and in other organs of the cat, whereas in other vertebrates these nonintestinal forms are the only stages seen. They are crescentic in shape and, as seen apparently free in the peritoneal exudate of experimentally infected mice (Fig. 5-24), vary in length from 4 to 6 μm and in breadth from 2 to 3 μm. Intracellular forms are somewhat smaller and tend to be less pointed at the ends. Many different tissues, especially lung, heart, lymphoid organs, and the

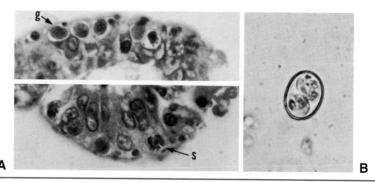

FIGURE 5-23 ■ *Toxoplasma gondii* in intestine of cat (× 1000). **A,** Gametocytes *(g)* and schizonts *(s)*. **B,** Oocyst containing two sporocysts with sporozoites (× 1600). (Courtesy of Dr. J. K. Frenkel, University of Kansas School of Medicine, Kansas City, KS.)

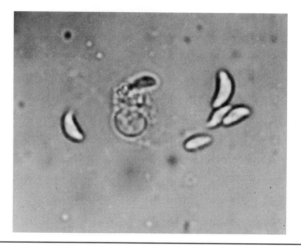

FIGURE 5-24 ■ *Toxoplasma gondii* tachyzoites from peritoneal exudate of mouse. (Photomicrograph courtesy of Dr. Leon Jacobs, National Institutes of Health.)

cells of the CNS, may be parasitized by these organisms. Multiplication of the parasites within an infected cell usually leads to death and rupture of the cell, freeing the parasites to spread the infection to new cells, or it may lead to formation of a cyst. Two terms are used for the trophozoites of *Toxoplasma*. The quickly multiplying forms, tachyzoites (Fig. 5-25), are responsible for initial spread of infection and tissue destruction, while the slower-developing bradyzoites form cysts. Although cysts (Fig. 5-26) are more characteristic of older infections, perhaps forming as a consequence of increased host immunity, they are present at least in small numbers early in the course of experimental infections.

In trophozoites stained by any routine method, a spherical nucleus is seen, situated closer to the rounded than to the pointed end (Fig. 5-27). A smaller, dark-staining mass may be visible at the end opposite the nucleus in organisms stained with certain silver stains, giving a superficial resemblance to the amastigote form of hemoflagellates. The small mass is part of the apical complex and is referred to as the conoid.

Symptoms. It has been mentioned that the majority of human infections with *Toxoplasma* are benign. In adults and in children past the neonatal period, the disease is usually asymptomatic. Nevertheless, a generalized infection probably occurs. In a small percentage of cases, symptoms ranging from mild to severe result. When symptoms are seen, they are most frequently mild. The disease picture may simulate infectious mononucleosis, with chills, fever,

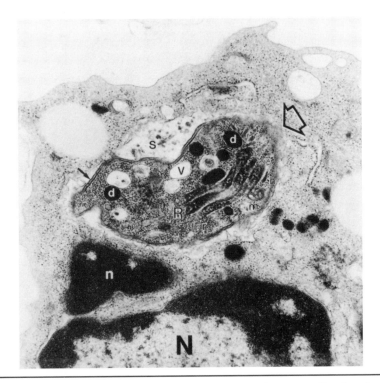

FIGURE 5-25 ■ Transmission electron micrograph of *Toxoplasma gondii* tachyzoite within parasitophorous vacuole of neutrophil. Large open arrow points to apical complex; small solid arrow points to multi-layered pellicle; *(d)* dense body; *(m)* mitochondrion; *(N,n)* segmented nucleus of neutrophil; *(R)* rhoptries; *(S)* secretory granules of parasitophorous vacuole; *(V)* vesicle. (From Tang TT et al. *Am J Clin Pathol* 1986: *85*:104–110.)

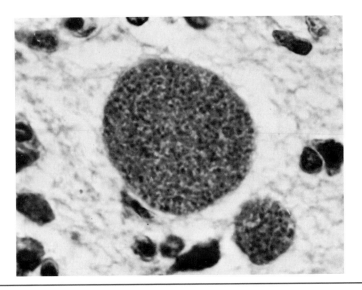

FIGURE 5-26 ■ *Toxoplasma gondii* cysts containing bradyzoites in brain of mouse.

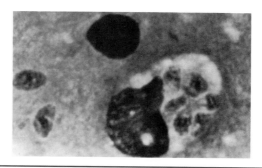

FIGURE 5-27 ■ Trophozoites of *Toxoplasma gondii* in brain impression film (Giemsa stain).

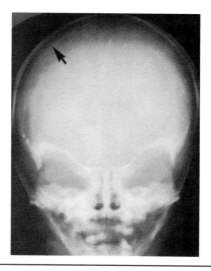

FIGURE 5-28 ■ Radiograph of skull with congenital toxoplasmosis showing calcifications and hydrocephalus. Curvilinear calcific plaque is seen in the right parietal area *(arrow)*. (From Tucker A. *Am J Roentgenol Rad Ther* 1961; *86*:458, © by American Roentgen Ray Society.)

headache, myalgia, lymphadenitis, and extreme fatigue. A chronic toxoplasmic lymphadenitis has been described. Rarely the infection may be severe, with a maculopapular rash in addition to the above symptoms, and sometimes evidence of hepatitis, encephalomyelitis, or myocarditis. In a very few cases retinochoroiditis occurs, which may progress to produce blindness. In intrauterine infections, however, the picture is the reverse of that seen in older patients. Instead of there being a majority of asymptomatic infections, most infections contracted during this period are quite severe, and in only a small percentage is there complete recovery. Retinochoroiditis, encephalomyelitis, and hydrocephalus or microcephaly are such common sequelae of infection at this stage as to be highly suggestive of toxoplasmosis when seen in very young children. Many of those infected in the last trimester are normal at birth but develop retinochoroiditis later; only about 20% are symptomatic. *Toxoplasma* encephalomyelitis may result in cerebral calcifications demonstrable in radiographs (Fig. 5-28). Infection in newborns is marked by fever, pneumonitis, and often the development of hepatosplenomegaly. Convulsions are common. There is seldom complete recovery; most infections result in blindness or severe visual impairment and mental retardation. In a small percentage of cases there appears to be a milder systemic infection with complete recovery, but even these patients develop retinochoroiditis in subsequent years. Additional reports suggest a causal relationship between polymyositis and toxoplasmosis, with improvement of the polymyositis after treatment of the infection and coincident with serologic improvement.

Reactivation of cerebral toxoplasmosis is a major cause of encephalitis in patients with AIDS. Toxoplasmic encephalitis occurs in 10% to 50% of AIDS patients who are seropositive for *Toxoplasma* and have CD4$^+$ T lymphocyte counts of less than 100/μl. Clinical features may include headache, confusion, ataxia, hemiparesis, and retinochoroiditis; spinal fluid lymphocytic pleocytosis, detectable *Toxoplasma*-specific IgG antibodies in serum, and lesions on the brain revealed by computed tomography (CT) are suggestive. Necrotic foci, with *Toxoplasma* organisms in brain biopsy, or organisms demonstrable in spinal fluid are diagnostic, as may be a rise in spinal fluid IgG antibodies in the absence of a similar response in serum IgG. For the majority of patients, the lack of IgM antibody or a change in IgG antibody titers suggests that the disease is due to reactivation of a chronic latent infection rather than an acquired primary infection. In immunocompromised patients with cerebral toxoplasmosis, it is the tachyzoite form rather than the bradyzoite form and cysts that commonly are seen. Toxoplasmosis of the spinal cord with myelopathy has been reported in patients with AIDS.

Toxoplasma orchitis has been described in a 27-year-old man with HIV infection. The infection, which produced a nontender testicular mass, occurred several days before the onset of *Toxoplasma* encephalitis. Other forms of infection in AIDs patients have included pulmonary toxoplasmosis and *Toxoplasma* myocarditis and myositis of colonic muscularis propria.

Primary infection may be promoted by immunosuppression. Such infections in cardiac transplant patients have been described. One patient had a brain abscess, diagnosed by CT, with the organisms identified in Wright-Giemsa stains of the aspirate. Another patient had acute disseminated toxoplasmosis with involvement of many organs, including the transplanted heart. Both recipients had negative serologic tests for toxoplasmosis prior to surgery, and both donors had serologic evidence of acute *Toxoplasma* infection. The importance of screening potential donors for such infection is obvious, at least in retrospect.

Reactivation of toxoplasmosis is also seen in medically immunosuppressed or otherwise compromised hosts. Of 81 such patients who developed reactivation of a latent toxoplasmosis, 32 had Hodgkin's disease, 9 non-Hodgkin's lymphoma, and 15 leukemia. Most of the remainder had some type of malignancy, but six had collagen-vascular diseases, and seven had received organ transplants. In 45 of the patients, the presenting symptoms of *Toxoplasma* infection were neurologic, most frequently consistent with diffuse encephalopathy, meningoencephalitis, or cerebral mass lesions. Of the patients who received anti-*Toxoplasma* chemotherapy, 80% showed marked clinical improvement or complete remission.

Diagnosis is seldom made by recovery of the organisms, although intraperitoneal inoculation of tissues into suitable laboratory animals such as mice may demonstrate the infection. Cell cultures such as Vero or MRC5 fibroblasts may be used instead of mice to isolate and cultivate *Toxoplasma*. Whereas mouse inoculation may require as long as 30 days, *Toxoplasma* organisms may be isolated within a few days in cell culture. The only laboratory tests of value are the various serologic procedures that have been employed for diagnostic purposes (see also Chapter 16). The first of these techniques to be employed was the Sabin-Feldman dye test, a reaction based on the fact that serum from a patient who has had toxoplasmosis affects *Toxoplasma* organisms in such a manner that they become refractory to staining with a solution of methylene blue. This test requires the use of living *Toxoplasma* organisms obtained from the peritoneal fluid of infected mice and is not adapted for use in the average laboratory. The dye test, like the toxoplasmin skin test, which is prepared from a saline extract of mouse peritoneal exudate, does not necessarily indicate current infection. As in the tuberculin skin test, positive reactions may denote either previous exposure or active disease. Enzyme immunoassay (EIA) and indirect fluorescent antibody (IFA) tests are available from the CDC and are available in kit form, including IgG and IgM kits, from many companies (see Chapter 16). As might be expected, the reactivated latent infections seen in patients with AIDS generally do not react to these or other serologic tests. A comparison of the Abbott Toxo IgG and IgM IMx tests, which are enzyme immunoassays, with the dye test and an IgM ELISA revealed high overall agreement.

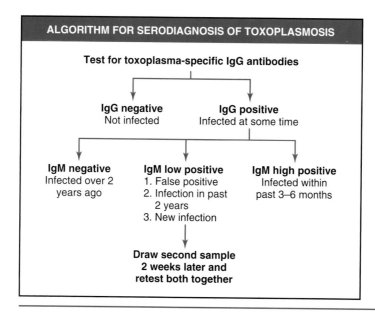

Adapted from Wilson M *et al.* Clinical immunoparasitology, Chap. 67. *In* Rose NR (ed). *Manual of Clinical Laboratory Immunology,* 5th ed, 1997. ASM Press, Herndon VA.

Indirect fluorescent and dye test antibodies are demonstrable within the first 2 weeks after infection and may rise to levels of 1:4096 or greater early in infection, falling slightly thereafter but persisting at an elevated level for many months before declining to low levels after many years. The indirect fluorescent and hemagglutination antibodies appear slightly later than the dye test but parallel it in titer and duration.

Prenatal diagnosis of congenital toxoplasmosis may be made by detecting specific anti-*Toxoplasma* IgM antibodies in fetal blood, isolating organisms in mice or cell culture from fetal blood or amniotic fluid, and ultrasound examination of the fetus to detect enlargement of the cerebral ventricles. Additionally, a polymerase chain reaction (PCR) test has been used to detect a gene sequence specific for *Toxoplasma* in samples of amniotic fluid, and has also been used to detect *Toxoplasma* in the urine of congenitally infected infants.

Pathogenesis. These obligate intracellular parasites disseminate via the bloodstream to many organs and tissues, throughout which they invade the cells, multiply, and finally disrupt them. Focal areas of necrosis, surrounded by lymphocytes, monocytes, and plasma cells, result from death of the infected cells. Cysts form in many organs but particularly in the muscles and brain, probably as a response to developing host immunity. *Toxoplasma* infection in most immunocompetent adults is asymptomatic because of effective protective immunity involving extracellular antibody and intracellular T-cell factors. Endogenous interferon gamma appears to be an important mediator of host resistance to *Toxoplasma*.

In the CNS, including the eye, an active infection may persist much longer than elsewhere. In the brain, minute scattered necrotic areas may later calcify, producing a characteristic x-ray picture. Retinochoroiditis may be either a hypersensitivity response to cyst rupture (the more sporadic and evanescent attacks) or a chronic progressive effect of the proliferation of tachyzoites in the retina, an immunologically deficient tissue.

Epidemiology. Toxoplasmosis occurs in a wide variety of both carnivorous and herbivorous mammals and in birds. In humans, evidence of infection has been found in all population groups investigated. Prevalence rates vary from place to place for reasons that remain largely obscure. The highest recorded rate (93%) occurs in Parisian women who prefer under-cooked or raw meat; at least 50% of their children (in infancy often fed the juices expressed

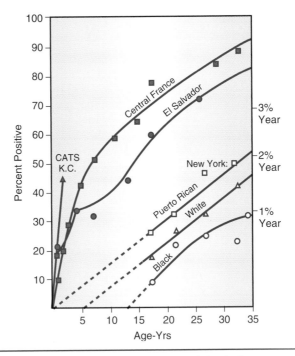

FIGURE 5-29 ■ Prevalence rate of *Toxoplasma* antibody in the human population. (From Frenkel JK. *BioSci* 1973; *23*:343–352.)

from raw meat) are likewise infected. (Figure 5-29 shows this rate as compared with that in El Salvador and in three ethnic groups in New York City.) At yearly seroconversion rates of 3% to 5%, such as are seen in central France, fetal risk is highest because more mothers in the childbearing range of 20 to 30 years become infected. In areas having such rates, more than 40 fetuses are at risk per 10,000 pregnancies. Lower seroconversion rates, such as are seen in the United States, or considerably higher ones are both associated with less fetal risk (Fig. 5-30). It is estimated that in the United States at least 3000 babies are born each year with congenitally acquired toxoplasmosis. A small epidemic among medical students in New York apparently resulted from the consumption of undercooked meat, presumably beef. Contamination of the beef with pork or mutton, from which *Toxoplasma* has been more commonly isolated, could not be excluded. A national survey of *Toxoplasma* in pigs in the United States showed the seroprevalence to be 42% in breeder pigs and 23% in market pigs. An outbreak involving a household of several members, all presumably infected through the ingestion of undercooked lamb, was reported; five persons developed fever and lymphadenopathy, which cleared spontaneously over several weeks. One of the five developed toxoplasmic retinochoroiditis, for which he received specific treatment during the course of the illness. All five developed serologic evidence of acute infection, as did one of the two asymptomatic household members; the other was not tested.

An outbreak of acute toxoplasmosis among 10 members of a large family in northern California appeared to be associated with drinking raw milk from infected goats. One person had retinochoroiditis; the other nine had asymptomatic infections, detected by IFA-IgM antibody tests. Experimental studies have shown that infected animals are able to transmit tachyzoites to their suckling young by way of milk.

Whereas ingestion of cyst-containing meat may be a common means of infection among carnivores, herbivorous animals must acquire the infection by ingesting oocysts. Oocysts shed in the feces are immature, becoming infective in 1 to 5 days. They are resistant to acids, alkalis, and common laboratory detergents but are killed by drying or by exposure to temperatures of 55° C for 30 minutes. Sporulated oocysts will survive a temperature

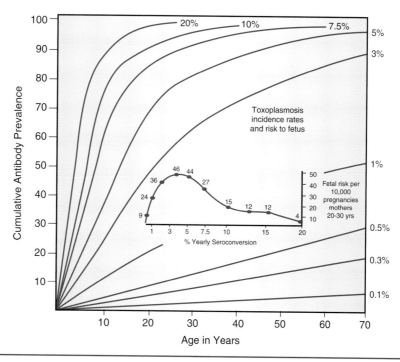

FIGURE 5-30 ■ Toxoplasmosis incidence rates in mothers and risk to fetus. (From Frenkel JK. *BioSci* 1973; *23*:343–352.)

of − 21° C for 28 days, though the muscle cysts are killed by freezing at − 6° C for 1 day or immediately at − 21° C. Of perhaps great epidemiologic significance is the observation that oocysts in cat feces survived for a year in the soil in Costa Rica and for up to 18 months (including two winters) in Kansas.

Toxoplasma has been isolated from the soil, using mouse and cat inoculation, during an outbreak of human toxoplasmosis in a rural area of Brazil. Oocyst-transmitted toxoplasmosis, acquired by drinking contaminated water, occurred in soldiers of an infantry battalion undergoing jungle training in Panama. Thirty-nine of 98 soldiers in one company developed a febrile illness and had positive *Toxoplasma* IFA and IFA-IgM titers. Epidemiologic investigation implicated a jungle stream, presumably contaminated by feces from infected jungle cats. An outbreak of toxoplasmosis associated with municipal drinking water has been reported in the Greater Victoria area of British Columbia, Canada.

Toxoplasma encephalitis is an important cause of sea otter mortality along the California coast (Miller et al., 2002). Coastal freshwater runoff appears to be a risk factor, and the source of infection may be filter-feeding benthic invertebrates, such as clams and mussels, which serve as food for sea otters. Experimental studies have shown that oysters can readily remove and concentrate *T. gondii* oocysts from seawater by their filter-feeding activity, and the oocysts can survive for several months, a possible source of infection not only for marine mammals but also humans (Lindsay et al., 2004).

Transplacental transmission usually takes place in the course of an acute but inapparent or undiagnosed maternal infection. In some domestic animals, chronic toxoplasmosis may lead to abortion, and it has been suggested that this may take place in women. If so, it is probably quite rare. In England and in New Zealand it is estimated that toxoplasmosis accounts for about half of the spontaneous abortions of sheep.

In addition to transplacental transmission, transmission by means of tachyzoites in blood transfusions has been observed on rare occasions, and that via other body fluids is a theoretical possibility. However, this mode of transmission is of little importance in comparison with that by means of cysts and oocysts.

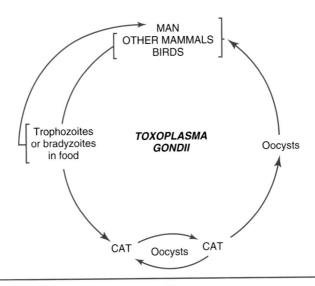

FIGURE 5-31 ■ Life cycle of *Toxoplasma gondii.*

Although the complete life cycle of *Toxoplasma* is believed to occur only in felines (Fig. 5-31), the role of domestic and other cats in dissemination of the infection has not been fully assessed. On Pacific atolls, serologic evidence of infection in the rat population depends on the presence of cats. On islands devoid of cats, there is no evidence of infection among the rats. A similar correlation between *Toxoplasma* antibodies in humans and the presence of cats was noted in New Guinea. Neotropical Felidae are also involved in the spread of infection among Colombian Indians. It is interesting that in the cat, the period that must elapse between ingestion of toxoplasmas and their appearance as oocysts in the feces varies considerably with the stage at which they are ingested. This period is short (3 to 10 days) when the cat ingests cysts from a chronic infection and longer (21 to 24 days) when the infection is initiated with oocysts. Oocysts are as effective in producing a generalized infection as are cysts in a variety of animals.

Cats eliminate oocysts for about 2 weeks following a primary infection; however, on reinfection, because of developing immunity cats shed fewer oocysts, or none at all, and for a shorter time. Kittens that were fed bradyzoites in cysts developed the greatest immune response, as measured by oocyst production. Decreasing levels of immunity occurred in kittens fed tachyzoites and sporozoites, respectively. Interestingly, natural infection occurs primarily through the consumption of bradyzoites in prey animals.

Prevention. Human infection with *Toxoplasma* may come either from consumption or handling of infected meat or from contact with cat feces in litter pans or soil. Meat should be heated throughout to 150° F (66° C) before consumption, and hands should be washed with soap and water after handling uncooked meat. Indoor cats fed on dry, canned, or boiled food are unlikely to be infected, whereas those that can hunt or are fed uncooked food are liable to infection. Such cats' litter pans should be cleaned daily and the pans disinfected with boiling water. Pregnant women, unless they have evidence of old *Toxoplasma* infection, should avoid contact with cats whose source of food is not controlled and should not empty litter pans. Disposable gloves should be worn to clean litter boxes or work in soil that may have been contaminated with cat feces. Children's sandboxes should be made cat proof.

Treatment. The only accepted treatment for toxoplasmosis is a combination of pyrimethamine at the rate of 25 to 100 mg daily for 1 month, with trisulfapyrimidines, 2 to 6 g daily, for the same period. This drug combination acts synergistically to inhibit the

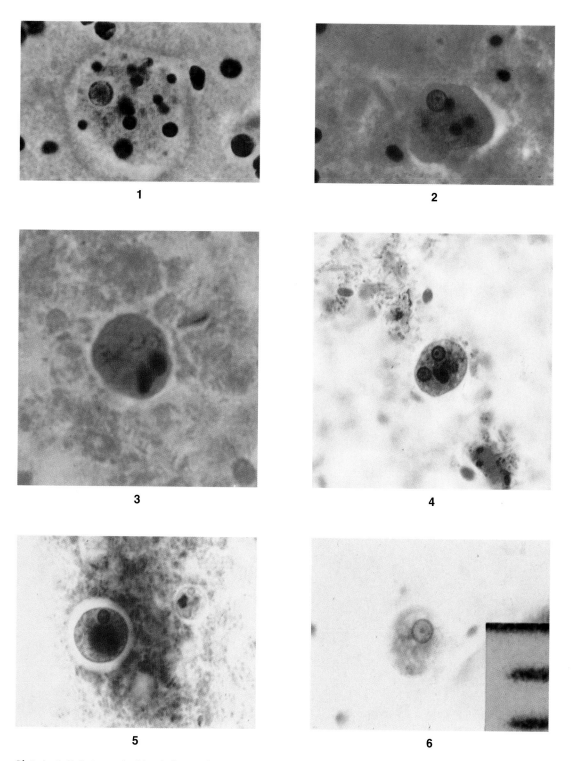

Plate I *1, 2, Entamoeba histolytica* trophozoites; *3, 4, E. histolytica* cysts; *5, E. histolytica* and *E. hartmanni* cysts; *6, E. hartmanni* trophozoite. (All color photographs taken at same magnification; total scale shown equals 20 μm.)

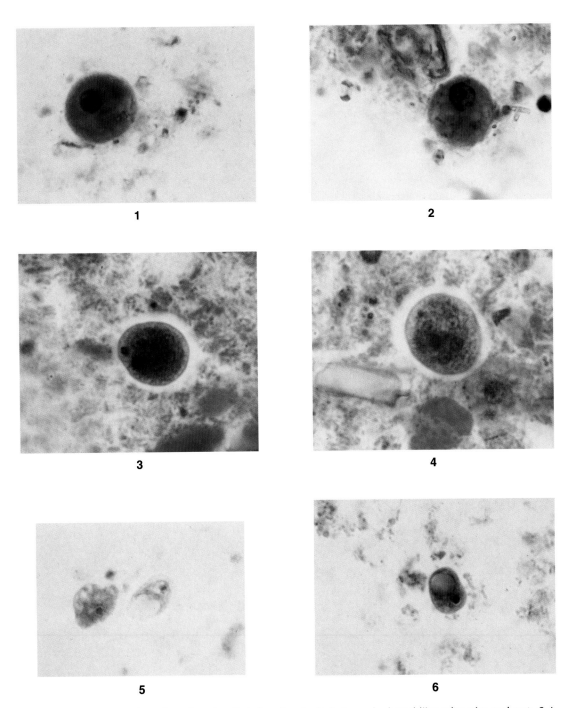

Plate II *1, 2, Entamoeba coli* trophozoite; *3, 4, E. coli* cysts; *5, Iodamoeba bütschlii* trophozoite and cyst; *6, I. bütschlii* cyst.

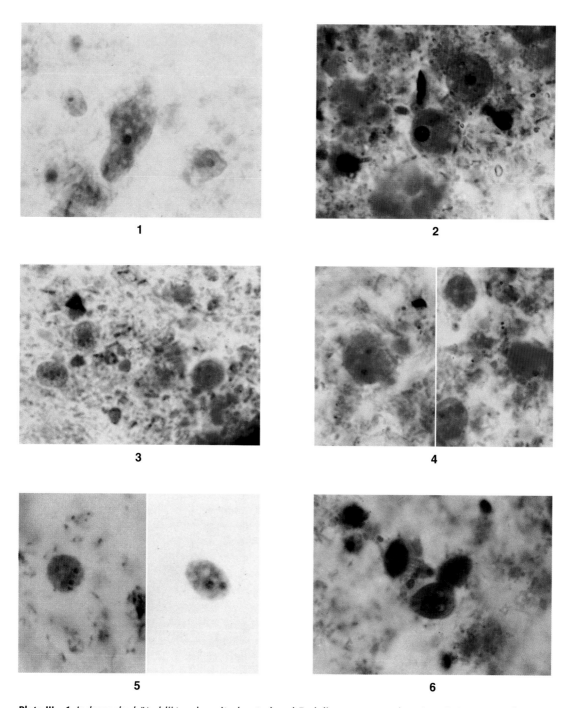

Plate III   *1, Iodamoeba bütschlii* trophozoite (center) and *Endolimax nana* trophozoites; *2, E. nana* trophozoite (top) and *Entamoeba hartmanni* trophozoite; *3, E. nana* cysts; *4, 5, Dientamoeba fragilis; 6, Giardia lamblia* trophozoite.

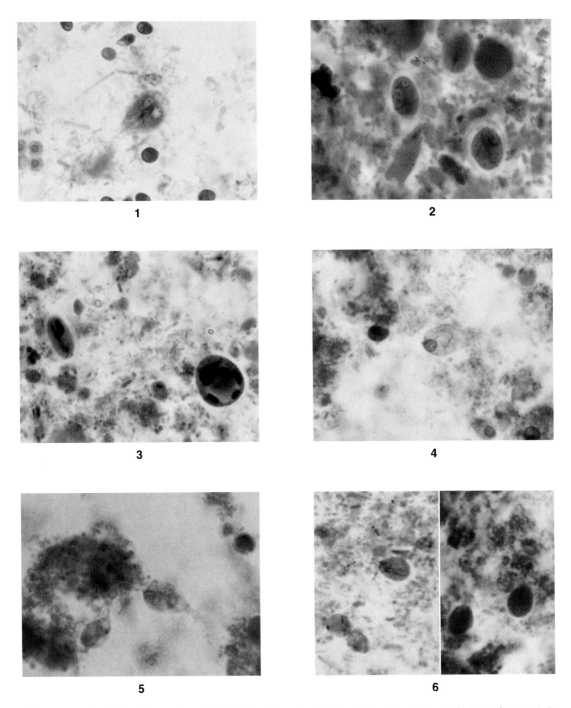

Plate IV *1, Giardia lamblia* trophozoite; *2, G. lamblia* cysts; *3, G. lamblia* cyst and *E. histolytica* early cyst; *4, 5, Chilomastix mesnili* trophozoites; *6, C. mesnili* cysts.

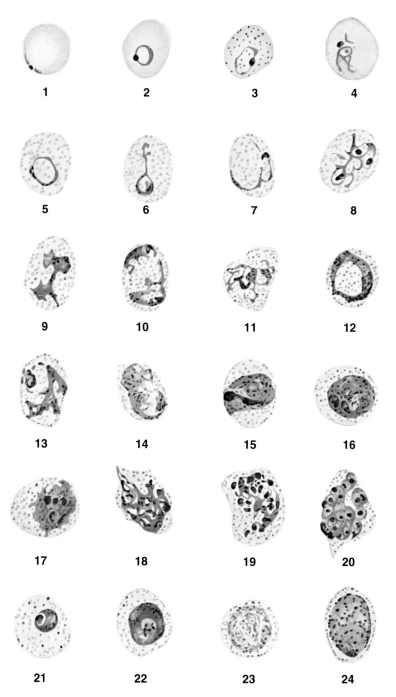

Plate V *Plasmodium vivax: 1,* normal-sized red cell with marginal ring form trophozoite; *2,* young signet ring form trophozoite in a macrocyte; *3,* slightly older ring form trophozoite in red cell showing basophilic stippling; *4,* polychromatophilic red cell containing young tertian parasite with pseudopodia; *5,* ring form trophozoite showing pigment in cytoplasm, in an enlarged cell containing Schüffner's stippling (Schüffner's stippling does not appear in all cells containing the growing and older forms of *P. vivax* as would be indicated by these pictures, but it can be found with any stage from the fairly young ring form onward); *6, 7,* very tenuous medium trophozoite forms; *8,* three ameboid trophozoites with fused cytoplasm; *9–13,* older ameboid trophozoites in process of development; *10,* two ameboid trophozoites in one cell; *14,* mature trophozoite; *15,* mature trophozoite with chromatin apparently in process of division; *16–19,* schizonts showing progressive steps in division ("presegmenting schizonts"); *20,* mature schizont; *21, 22,* developing gametocytes; *23,* mature microgametocyte; *24,* mature macrogametocyte. (Courtesy of the National Institutes of Health, USPHS[AU2].)

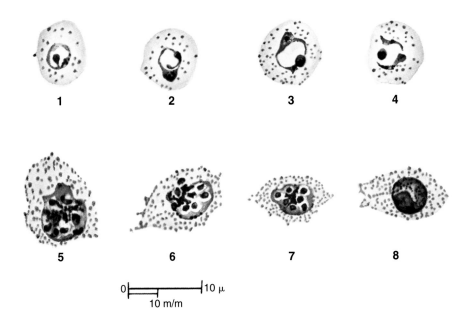

1   2   3   4

5   6   7   8

0 ├───────┤ 10 μ
    10 m/m

Plate VI *Plasmodium ovale: 1,* young ring-shaped trophozoite; *2–4,* older ring-shaped trophozoites; *5–7,* schizonts, progressive stages; *8,* mature gametocyte. Free translation of legend accompanying original plate in "Guide pratique d'examen microscopique du sang appliqué au diagnostic du paludisme" by Georges Villain. (Reproduced with permission from "Biologie Medicale" supplement, 1935. Courtesy Aimee Wicox. National Institutes of Health Bulletin no. 180.)

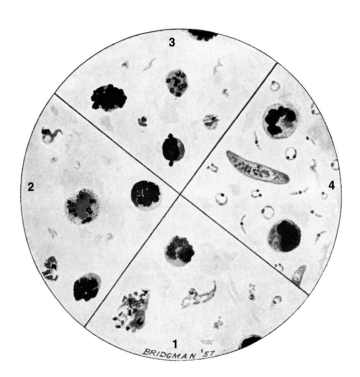

BRIDGMAN '57

Plate VII The human plasmodia as seen in thick film: *1, Plasmodium vivax:* young and older trophozoites and schizont; *2, P. ovale:* developing trophozoite and schizonts, one within a "ghost cell'; *3, P. malariae:* trophozoites and schnizont; *4, P. falciparum:* young trophozoites and gametocyte.

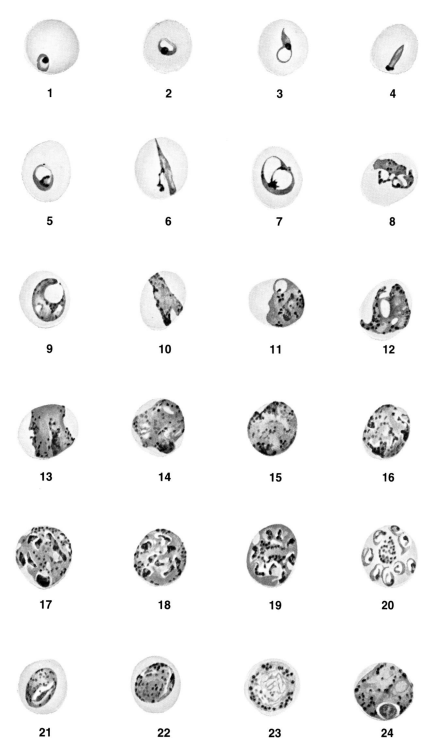

Plate VIII *Plasmodium malariae:* *1,* young ring form trophozoite of quartan malaria; *2–4,* young trophozoite forms of the parasite showing gradual increase of chromatin and cytoplasm; *5,* developing ring form trophozoite showing pigment granule; *6,* early band form trophozoite-elongated chromatin, some pigment apparent; *7–12,* some forms that the developing trophozoite of quartan may take; *13, 14,* mature trophozoites-one a band form; *15–19,* phases in the development of the schizont ("presegmenting schizonts"); *20,* mature schizont; *21,* immature microgametocyte; *22,* immature macrogametocyte; *23,* mature microgametocyte; *24,* mature macrogametocyte. (Courtesy National Institutes of Health, USPHS.)

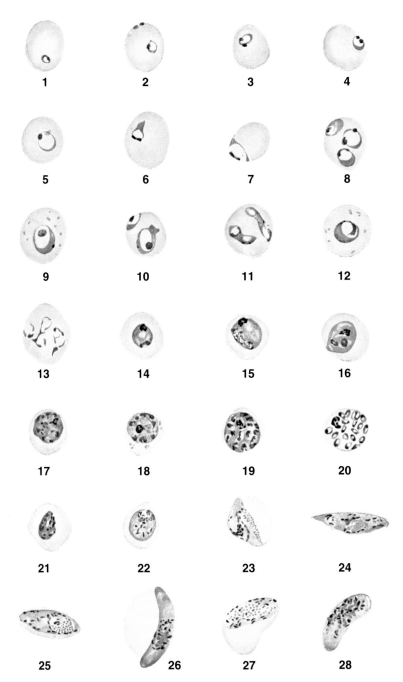

Plate IX *Plasmodium falciparum: 1,* very young ring form trophozoite; *2,* double infection of singled cell with young trophozoites, one a "marginal form," the other "signet ring" form; *3, 4,* young trophozoites showing double chromatin dots; *5–7,* developing trophozoite forms; *8,* three medium trophozoites in one cell; *9,* trophozoite showing pigment, in a cell containing Maurer's dots; *10, 11,* two trophozoites in each of two cells showing variation of forms that parasites may assume; *12,* almost mature trophozoite showing haze of pigment throughout cytoplasm; Maurer's dots in the cell; *13,* estivo-autumnal "slender forms"; *14,* mature trophozoite, showing clumped pigment; *15,* parasite in the process of initial chromatin division; *16–19,* various phases of the development of the schizont ("presegmenting schizonts"); *20,* mature schizont; *21–24,* successive forms in the development of the gametocyte-usually not found in the peripheral circulation; *25,* immature macrogametocyte; *26,* mature macrogametocyte; *27,* immature microgametocyte; *28,* mature microgametocyte. (Courtesy National Institutes of Health, USPHS.)

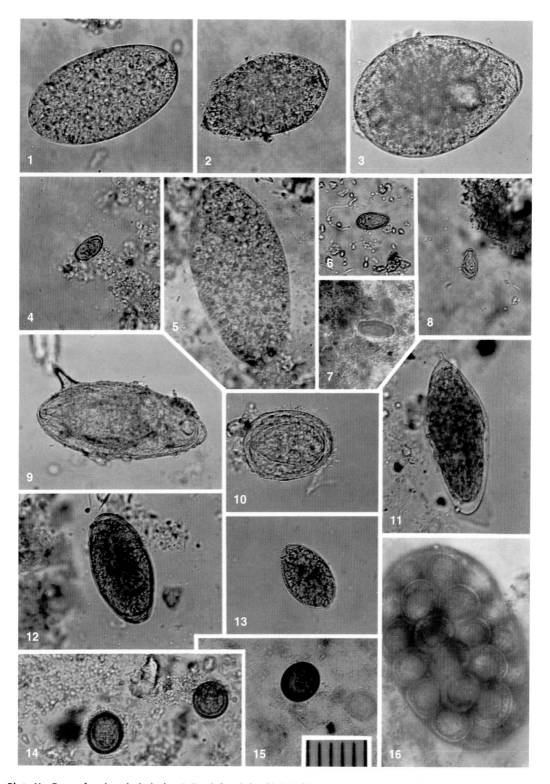

Plate X Eggs of various helminths: *1, Fasciolopsis buski; 2, Echinostoma* sp.; *3, Gastrodiscus aegyptiacus* (similar to *Gastrodiscoides); 4, Metagonimus yokogawai; 5, Fasciola gigantica; 6, Clonorchis sinensis; 7, C. sinensis* (trichrome stain); *8, Opisthorchis viverrini; 9, Schistosoma mansoni; 10, S. japonicum; 11, S. haematobium; 12, Paragonimus westermani; 13, Diphyllobothrium latum; 14, Taenia* sp.; *15, Taenia* sp. (trichrome stain); *16, Dipylidium caninum* egg packet. Scale equals 50 μm. (*Gastrodiscus* egg courtesy of Dr. Lawrence Ash.)

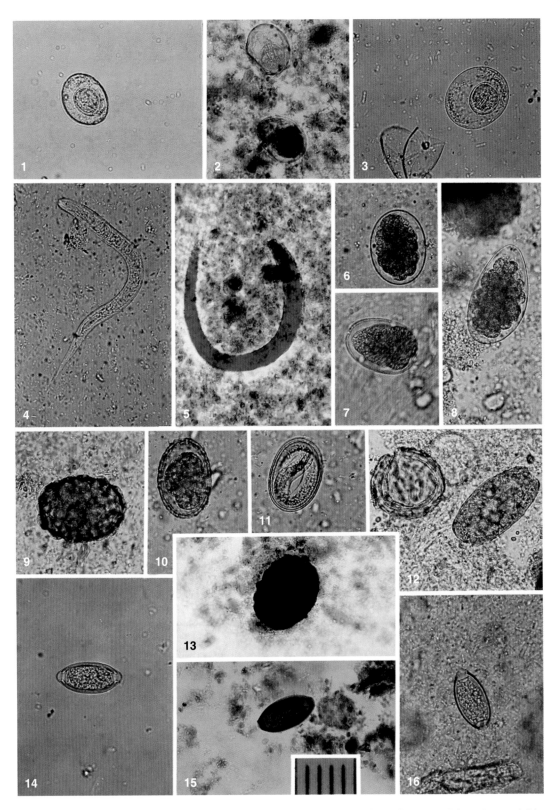

Plate XI Eggs and larvae of various helminths: *1–3, Hymenolepis nana* (*2,* trichrome stain); *4, Strongyloides stercoralis* larva (unstained); *5, S. stercoralis* larva (trichrome stain); *6, 7,* hookworm; *8, Trichostrongylus orientalis; 9–13, Ascaris lumbricoides* (*10,* cortex thin; *11,* decorticated; *12,* hatched and unfertilized eggs; *13,* trichrome stain); *14–16, Trichuris trichiura* (*15,* trichrome stain). Scale equals 50 μm.

production of dihydrofolate reductase by the parasite and the synthesis of DNA, RNA, and protein. Folinic acid may be administered to counteract the bone marrow depression caused by pyrimethamine. In acute retinochoroiditis, a loading dose of 75 mg pyrimethamine daily may be used for 3 to 5 days. Corticosteroids may have value for their antiinflammatory action. Intravenous clindamycin has been used to treat *Toxoplasma* encephalitis in patients with AIDS, with promising results. In France, spiramycin has been used for many years to treat toxoplasmosis during pregnancy, apparently preventing transmission in utero. However, spiramycin does not appear to be effective therapy for preventing relapse of neurotoxoplasmosis in immunosuppressed patients. Spiramycin is available in the United States on a case-by-case basis for toxoplasmosis.* Plastids, nonphotosynthetic chloroplast-like organelles that occur in several apicomplexan parasites, including *Plasmodium* and *Toxoplasma* (Lang-Unnasch et al., 1998), have been the target of drugs such as clindamycin, used as salvage treatment for toxoplasmosis in a sulfur-allergic patient.

Sarcocystis spp.

Parasites belonging to the genus *Sarcocystis* were first described in mice by Miescher in 1843 and since that time have been reported from numerous other mammals, especially sheep, cattle, and pigs, and rarely horses. They occur as elongated cylindrical bodies referred to as Miescher's tubules, sometimes large enough to be visible to the naked eye, in striated muscle (including cardiac muscle) and sometimes in unstriated muscle.

Human sarcosporidia were originally named for Lindemann, who was credited with the first description of the parasite in humans. It is interesting that the organisms described by Lindemann are not now believed to be *Sarcocystis*. In 1979, Beaver and coworkers reviewed the reported human cases, recognized 40 of them as valid, and distinguished seven morphologic types, each of which they believed represented one or more different species. Humans are an accidental intermediate host, then, of several species of *Sarcocystis*. The scarcity of reported cases is not thought to reflect the true prevalence of this parasite, as many cases are believed to be asymptomatic, and pathologic examination of "normal" muscle tissue is not frequently performed. In Malaysia, examination of the tongue tissue in 100 routine autopsies revealed an infection rate of 21%.

Details of cyst morphology and size make it possible to differentiate *Sarcocystis* from *Toxoplasma* cysts in many, though not in all, cases. Some sarcocysts may measure less than the 100 μm considered to be the upper limit of size for the cysts of *Toxoplasma*, but others may attain a length of 5 cm. The limiting membrane may show radial striations (Fig. 5-32) not seen in *Toxoplasma*, and septa may divide the cyst into compartments. Neither of these characteristics is uniformly seen in *Sarcocystis*, however. The contained trophozoites (bradyzoites) are considerably larger than those of *Toxoplasma*, measuring 4 to 9 μm in breadth and 12 to 16 μm in length.

It is thought that most human cases are asymptomatic. In some cases local symptoms such as myositis seemed associated with presence of the parasite. Myositis in laboratory animals accompanies cyst degeneration and is characterized by infiltration of lymphocytes, plasma cells, and eosinophils. More generalized symptoms have been described in human cases, including pain and swelling of an isolated muscle, dyspnea, and wheezing, associated with eosinophilia. An outbreak of acute eosinophilic myositis among seven members of a 15-person U.S. military team operating in rural Malaysia was attributed to tissue parasitism by *Sarcocystis*.

It will be recalled that the organism previously known as *Isospora hominis* (see Chapter 3) has been found to be the sporocyst stages of *Sarcocystis hominis* and *Sarcocystis suihominis*, from cattle and swine, respectively. Humans are the definitive hosts of these two species; male and female gametes develop in the lamina propria of the small intestine, producing oocysts that sporulate and are passed in the feces. There are at least three *Sarcocystis* species in cattle, one

---

*Available from the Food and Drug Administration

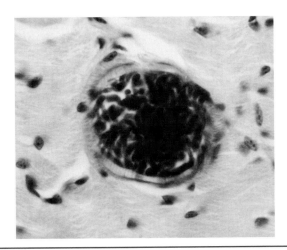

FIGURE 5-32 ▪ *Sarcocystis* in section of muscle. Note radial striations of limiting membrane. (Photomicrograph by Zane Price.)

of which develops in the intestine of dogs and coyotes, and another in cats. Another species of *Sarcocystis*, which develops in the cat intestine, produces sarcocysts in the muscles of mice. Much remains to be learned concerning the interrelationships of the *Isospora-Toxoplasma-Sarcocystis* group, the complexities of which have only been touched on here.

Other Apicomplexa (Sporozoa)

Babesia spp.

Apicomplexan parasites belonging to the genus *Babesia* have long been known as parasites of domestic and wild animals, causing at times inapparent infections but also causing such economically important disease as Texas cattle fever and malignant jaundice in dogs. Human infections have been reported from North America, Europe, Taiwan, and Japan. The organisms infect the red blood cells, in which they appear as somewhat pleomorphic ringlike structures (Fig. 5-33). Most resemble ring stages of plasmodia. Infection is transmitted by various species of ixodid ticks, in which a sexual multiplicative cycle occurs.

Human infection is diagnosed by identifying the intraerythrocytic parasites in Giemsa-stained blood films. The small parasites, several of which may infect a single red blood cell and which appear much like *Plasmodium falciparum*, can be differentiated from malarial parasites by the absence of pigment (hemozoin) in the infected erythrocytes. The organisms frequently occur in pairs, or as tetrads (also known as "Maltese cross" forms). Hamsters are susceptible to the disease and can be infected by intraperitoneal inoculation of blood specimens. Parasitemia can be detected within 2 to 4 weeks after inoculation. The indirect immunofluorescence (IFA) test is performed by the Centers for Disease Control and Prevention (CDC). An immunoblot (IB) serologic kit is available (see Chapter 16). The polymerase chain reaction (PCR) test has also been used to detect infection.

Symptoms and Pathogenesis. Human babesiosis was first recognized and reported from Europe in 1957. In most of the European cases, disease occurred in persons who had been splenectomized prior to infection with *Babesia*. It is likely that splenectomy affected their susceptibility to infection and the severity of the illness. Five of the seven patients reported to have contracted the infection in Europe died after a rapidly progressive illness characterized by fever, anemia, jaundice, and renal failure.

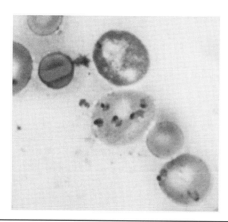

FIGURE 5-33 ■ *Babesia* in red blood cells. (Photomicrograph by Zane Price.)

Most of the cases of human babesiosis in North America have occurred in persons with intact spleens. The incubation period varies from 1 to 4 weeks. For the most part, infection is self-limited and characterized by the gradual onset of malaise followed by fever, headache, chills, sweating, arthralgias, myalgias, fatigue, and weakness. The fever shows no periodicity, such as seen in malaria. Mild hepatosplenomegaly has been reported, as has mild to moderately severe hemolytic anemia. Serum bilirubin and transaminase levels are slightly elevated. Fatal infections in the United States have also occurred primarily in asplenic patients, but self-limited infection has been reported in at least one splenectomized patient (a child).

Asymptomatic infections have also been reported, primarily from a serologic survey for *Babesia* in Mexico. Transfusion-induced babesiosis from an asymptomatic donor with an intact spleen contributed to the death of a patient with disseminated intravascular coagulopathy. The donor's infection was so light that parasites could not be detected in thick or thin blood films, although his serum had an IFA titer of 1:4096 to *B. microti*, and blood inoculated into hamsters produced a heavy parasitemia.

Epidemiology. The European cases of human babesiosis have been caused by *Babesia divergens (bovis)*, a parasite of cattle. All of the patients have been associated with land grazed on by cattle with babesiosis. Of the seven described cases, five had a fatal outcome. PCR analysis of recent human isolates in Italy, Austria, and Switzerland has identified the organisms as *B. microti* and non-*B. divergens*, possibly *B. odocoilei*, a parasite of deer (Foppa et al., 2002; Herwaldt et al., 2003).

Human babesiosis in North America usually is not fatal and is caused by *B. microti*, a parasite of rodents. The majority of infections have been acquired in southern New England, specifically Nantucket, Martha's Vineyard, Shelter Island, Long Island, and Connecticut. However, babesiosis has been reported from a number of other areas—40 cases in New Jersey; 10 cases from Wisconsin, with three deaths; one fatal case in a splenectomized patient from Missouri; one case from Georgia; and serologic evidence of foci in North Carolina and in Mexico.

A new focus of infection appears to be emerging in the western United States, wherein the organism may be a different species of *Babesia*. The parasite, first isolated from the blood of a patient in Washington state, and designated WA1, is morphologically indistinguishable from *B. microti* but antigenically and genotypically distinct. The patient's serum had very strong IFA reactivity with WA1, strong reactivity with *B. gibsoni*, a canine pathogen, but weak reactivity with *B. microti*. DNA hybridization clearly differentiated WA1 from *B. gibsoni* and *B. microti*. Similarly, organisms isolated from four asplenic patients in California were more closely related to *B. gibsoni* than to *B. microti*. Convalescent sera from three of the patients tested were reactive to WA1 but not to *B. microti*. Another isolate from Washington state appears to be closely related to *B. divergens*, based on PCR analysis.

Ixodes dammini is considered to be the tick vector of human babesiosis on Nantucket Island, where about 5% of the nymphal ticks are infected in nature. *I. dammini* is also the vector for the spirochetes that cause Lyme disease, and simultaneous human infections of babesiosis and Lyme disease have been reported. Approximately 10% of patients with Lyme disease in southern New England are co-infected with babesiosis in sites where both diseases are zoonotic. Patients with concurrent Lyme disease and babesiosis had a great number of symptoms and longer duration of illness than patients with either infection alone. White-footed mice (*Peromyscus leucopus*) have been identified as the principal reservoir host of *B. microti* on Nantucket Island. Patients with co-infections of babesiosis, Lyme disease, and human granulocytic ehrlichiosis have been reported.

Other members of the family Babesiidae have been found infecting humans on rare occasions, generally in splenectomized persons or those with impaired T-cell function.

Treatment. Treatment for babesiosis is a combination of clindamycin and oral quinine. The dosage for adults is clindamycin, 1.2 g intravenously twice a day or 600 mg orally three times a day, plus quinine, 650 mg orally three times a day, both for 7 to 10 days. Combination therapy using atovaquone, 750 mg twice a day, and azithromycin, 600 mg daily for 7 to 10 days, has also been used.

Chloroquine, perhaps because of its antiinflammatory properties, affords symptomatic relief in most cases of babesiosis but seems to have no effect on the degree of parasitemia or its duration. The aromatic diamidines pentamidine and diminazene (Berenil) have been found to suppress the parasitemia but not to eliminate infection in experimental animals. One patient who failed to respond symptomatically or parasitologically to chloroquine was treated with diminazene; the parasitemia cleared completely, but the patient subsequently developed an acute Guillain-Barré polyneuritis thought to be related to the use of the drug. Pyrimethamine and quinine, either alone or in combination, failed to eliminate experimental *B. microti* infections in hamsters.

Most cases of human babesiosis occur in later summer and early fall, and the only recommended control measure is to avoid tick-infested areas. Persons who frequent such areas are advised to use an effective repellent and to examine the body for ticks after leaving. Apparently, ticks must feed for at least 12 hours before they transmit infective organisms. Transmission of the pathogens of babesiosis and Lyme disease has been prevented by killing immature ticks (*I. dammini*). This was accomplished by distributing permethrin-treated cotton in wooded areas, which the rodents then use as nesting material. After such distribution, only 28% of all mice (*P. leucopus*) captured in the treated areas were infested with ticks, compared with virtually 100% infestation of mice captured in untreated areas.

The Opportunistic Free-Living Amebae

Several species of ordinarily free-living amebae have been observed as human symbionts. In some instances the association seems to be without pathologic consequence; in others it may result in devastating disease.

The free-living amebae comprise a large group, inhabiting fresh, brackish, and salt water, moist soil, and decaying vegetation. Some are coprozoic. The taxonomy of this large and diverse group is involved; for convenience, they may be separated into two groups on the basis of their ability to undergo transformation from an ameba to a flagellate stage. *Naegleria* belongs to the family Vahlkampfiidae, members of which are characterized as amebo-flagellates, able temporarily to assume a flagellate form while being completely devoid of flagella in the ameboid stage. *Acanthamoeba* organisms, belonging to the family Acanthamoebidae, never produce flagella. The invasive potential of these normally free-living

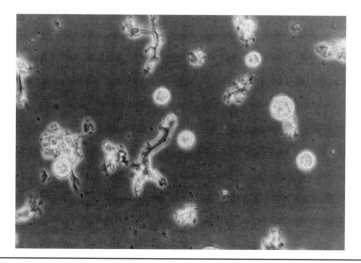

FIGURE 5-34 ■ Phase-contrast micrograph of *Balamuthia mandrillaris* trophozoites and cysts in culture, originally isolated from human brain. Note extensive branching of trophozoites and wavy appearance of cysts. (Courtesy of Dr. Govinda S. Visvesvara, Centers for Disease Control and Prevention, Atlanta, GA.)

organisms has been recognized since 1959; human infections were first reported in 1965. Most cases of primary amebic meningoencephalitis (PAM) can be ascribed to *Naegleria*; less commonly *Acanthamoeba* organisms are involved.

A new agent of amebic meningoencephalitis in humans and animals has been described, a free-living ameba, *Balamuthia mandrillaris*, belonging to the family Leptomyxidae (Fig. 5-34). Sixteen fatal human cases, previously identified as being caused by *Acanthamoeba*, and fatal infections in a baboon, a gorilla, and a sheep have been attributed to this organism. Additional cases continue to be described. Two other cases of fatal meningoencephalitis attributed to free-living amebae have been described in which the organisms could not be identified positively as *Naegleria, Acanthamoeba*, or *Balamuthia*, and *Vahlkampfia* has been suggested as the cause. *Vahlkampfia* reportedly causes disease in farm animals.

Another free-living ameba, *Sappinia diploidea*, has been identified as the cause of amebic encephalitis in a patient who recovered following treatment with azithromycin, pentamidine, itraconazole, and flucytosine (Gelman et al., 2001, 2003). The patient lived on a small farm in Texas and often handled domestic animals. He was otherwise healthy and not immunosuppressed. Prior to treatment, he had experienced some loss of consciousness, headache, photophobia, and blurred vision. MRI revealed a mass in the posterior left temporal lobe, which was excised surgically. The patient was treated for 25 weeks and recovered completely. Much remains to be learned of the role of the opportunistic amebae in disease production.

Naegleria fowleri

This genus of ameboflagellates has an ameboid phase that alternates with one possessing two flagella (Figs. 5-35, 5-36, and 5-37). The forms found in the tissues are ameboid, and in the tissues they are distinguished with difficulty from the genera to be discussed next; however, in *Naegleria* infection only trophozoites occur in the tissue, whereas with *Acanthamoeba* and *Balamuthia* infections both trophozoites and cysts are found in the tissues. While fatal intracerebral infections of this type are now thought to be caused primarily by *Naegleria*, amebae found in the earlier cases were erroneously identified as belonging to the genus *Hartmannella* (now *Acanthamoeba*).

Since the first reports of PAM in Australia and America, a number of similar infections have been documented in the United States, Europe, Asia, New Zealand, Africa, Central

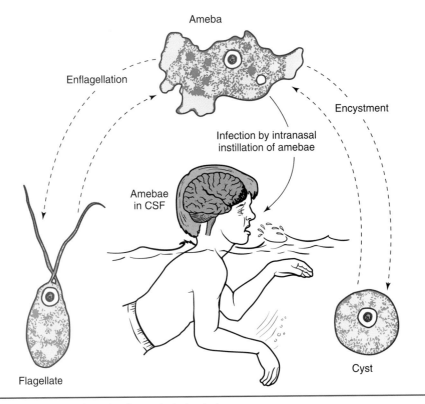

FIGURE 5-35 ■ Life cycle of *Naegleria fowleri.*

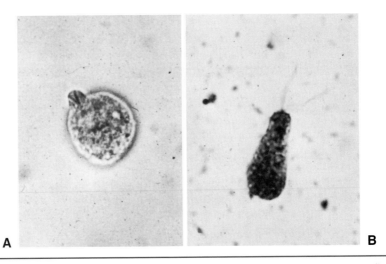

FIGURE 5-36 ■ *Naegleria fowleri.* Ameba transforming to flagellate form, **A,** and flagellate form, **B.**

America, and South America. Both epidemiologically and clinically, a characteristic pattern is seen. Most cases have occurred during the hot summer months in young persons who within the preceding week swam or dived in fresh or brackish water. Lakes, streams, hot springs, and swimming pools have been apparent sources of the infection.

That the source of infection is not always aquatic is illustrated by a case report from Nigeria, where the organisms were apparently inhaled during a dust storm by an 8-month-old infant, from whose nasal mucosa and spinal fluid they were recovered prior to death.

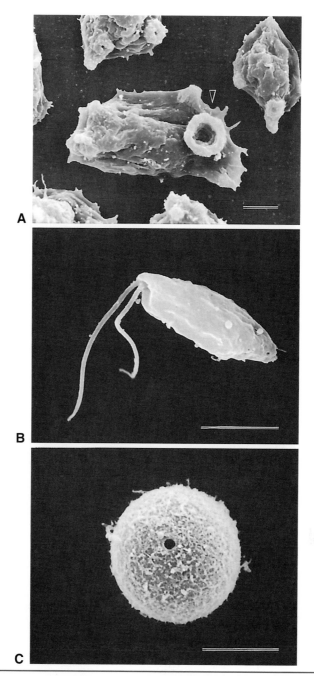

FIGURE 5-37   ■   Scanning electron micrographs of stages in the life cycle of *Naegleria fowleri*. **A,** Ameba with a single amebostome *(arrowhead).* **B,** Flagellate with two flagella emerging from beneath the anterior rostrum. **C,** Cyst with a single pore, or ostiole, through which the ameba escapes. Bars are 5 μm. (Photomicrographs by Dr. Thomas B. Cole, Jr.)

Another interesting report from Nigeria concerns a Muslim farmer thought to have become infected during the ritual washing before prayer, which involved sniffing water up his nose.

The diagnosis of PAM is made by microscopic identification of living or stained amebae in the patient's CSF. Amebae can be distinguished from other cells by their "limax" (Latin, sluglike) shape and progressive movement. It is not necessary to warm the slide, because these amebae are fully active at room temperature. Refrigeration of the spinal fluid is not recommended. See Chapter 15 for cultivation procedures. The flagellate form of *N. fowleri* may be induced by suspending amebae in distilled water. At 37°C, maximum enflagellation occurs in 4 to 5 hours.

Symptoms and Pathogenesis. The clinical course is dramatic. A day or so of prodromal symptoms of headache and fever is followed by the rapid onset of nausea and vomiting accompanied by the signs and symptoms of meningitis with involvement of the olfactory, frontal, temporal, and cerebellar areas. Meningeal irritation may be accompanied by stiff neck, generalized seizures, and Kernig's sign. Olfactory lobe involvement is perhaps most characteristic; disturbances in the sense of smell or taste may be noted early in the course of the disease but are not always seen. Patients often become irrational before lapsing into coma. Death occurs early; the entire clinical course seldom extends beyond 3 to 6 days. There is serologic evidence that infection in humans is caused by a single species, distinct from the nonpathogenic *Naegleria gruberi* isolated from soil and water. The causative organism is referred to as *N. fowleri*, named in honor of Dr. Malcom Fowler, who first recognized the disease it caused.

Spinal puncture reveals a cloudy to frankly purulent or sanguinopurulent fluid, usually under increased pressure. The cell count ranges from a few hundred to more than 20,000 white blood cells per microliter, predominantly neutrophils, and the failure to find bacteria in such a purulent spinal fluid should alert physicians and laboratory technologists to the possibility of PAM. Spinal fluid protein is generally, though not invariably, increased, and glucose levels are low. Red blood cells are frequently present, and motile amebae may be found in unstained preparations of spinal fluid. Their activity is characterized by the explosive formation of blunt pseudopodia, like those of *E. histolytica*, rather than the tapering, spiky projections (acanthopodia) seen on the pseudopodia of *Acanthamoeba*. Characteristically, these amebae do not stain well with the usual bacterial staining procedures. Iron hematoxylin stains of impression smears reveal a nucleus with a large karyosome that extends nearly to the delicate nuclear membrane. The nuclei can be distinguished in Wright's stain and in hematoxylin and eosin-stained tissues (Fig. 5-38). Novel phagocytic structures referred to as amebostomes (see Fig. 5-37) have been described for amebae of *N. fowleri*. Used for engulfment, their role in pathogenesis is unclear. Red blood cells may be seen within the amebae.

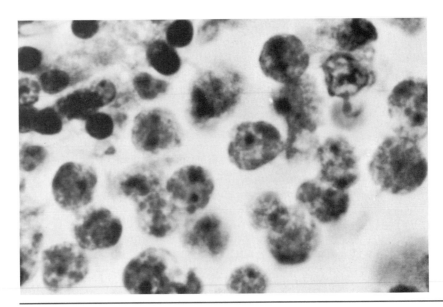

FIGURE 5-38 ■ Trophozoites of *Naegleria fowleri* in human brain. (Photomicrograph by Zane Price.)

On autopsy, signs of acute meningoencephalitis are seen: an exudate of neutrophils and monocytes is found in the subarachnoid space, and hemorrhage and an inflammatory exudate extend into the gray matter. Rounded amebae, 10 or 11 μm in diameter, are seen in the gray matter (see Fig. 5-38), ahead of the advancing margin of hemorrhage or necrosis. They are particularly prominent in the Virchow-Robin spaces. Focal demyelination of the white matter of the brain and spinal cord has been described. Curiously, demyelination has occurred in the absence of amebae or cellular infiltrate. It has been suggested that demyelination may have been caused by a phospholytic enzyme or enzymelike substance produced by actively growing amebae in the adjacent gray matter.

Epidemiology. PAM is a relatively rare disease with a worldwide distribution. Compared to protozoan diseases such as malaria, African sleeping sickness, and amebic dysentery, infections caused by free-living amebae seem inconsequential. Yet, because of their pervasiveness, their extreme virulence, and the lack of effective therapy, these organisms have an impact far greater than the number of cases suggests. *Naegleria* infection is seen most often in active, healthy, young persons, the majority of reports coming from developed rather than developing nations, probably because of greater awareness and not because of greater incidence.

Australia, Czechoslovakia, and the United States have reported 75% of all cases of PAM. In the United States, the greatest number of reported cases have been from the coastal states of Virginia, Florida, and Texas, accounting for 67% of the U.S. cases.

The majority of patients with *Naegleria* infection have a history of recent swimming in fresh water during hot summer weather. In Richmond, Virginia, infection in 14 of 16 cases probably was acquired in two artificial lakes located within a few miles of each other. Over a 3-year period, 16 young people died in Czechoslovakia after swimming in the same heated, chlorinated, indoor swimming pool. Similar fatal cases have been reported following swimming in pools in Belgium, England, and New Zealand; in hot springs in California and New Zealand; in lakes in Arkansas, Florida, Missouri, Nevada, South Carolina, and Texas; in streams in Belgium, Mississipi, and New Zealand; and in an irrigation ditch in Mexico.

Another pathogenic species of *Naegleria, N. australiensis*, has been recovered from environmental sources in Australia, Europe, Asia, and the United States. Although human infection with *N. australiensis* has not yet been described, the species is pathogenic to mice (via intranasal instillation) and, therefore, should be considered a potential human pathogen.

Treatment. At present there is no satisfactory treatment for PAM. The antibiotics used to treat bacterial meningitis are ineffective, as are the antiamebic drugs. Amphotericin B, a drug of considerable toxicity, is the anti-*Naegleria* agent for which there is evidence of clinical effectiveness. All known survivors of PAM have been treated with amphotericin B given intravenously and intrathecally.

Amphotericin B is a polyene compound that acts on the plasma membrane, disrupting its selective permeability and causing leakage of the cellular components. It is administered intravenously in large doses: 1 to 1.5 mg/kg body weight daily for 3 days, followed by 1 mg/kg daily for 6 days. Additionally, amphotericin B may be given intrathecally.

Seidel and colleagues (1982) successfully treated a 9-year-old girl with proven *Naegleria* infection with the following regimen:

Amphotericin B intravenously, 0.75 mg/kg twice daily × 3 days, then 1.0 mg/kg daily × 6 days

Amphotericin B intravenously via lumbar catheter, 1.5 mg daily × 2 days, then 1.0 mg every other day × 8 days

Miconazole intravenously, 117 mg/m² body surface three times daily × 9 days

Miconazole intrathecally via lumbar catheter, 10 mg daily × 2 days, then 10 mg every other day × 8 days

Rifampin by mouth, 3.3 mg/kg three times daily × 9 days

In retrospect, the amphotericin B is thought to have been the effective drug. Its efficacy has been demonstrated to be markedly potentiated by tetracycline in the delayed treatment of mice experimentally infected with *N. fowleri*. Similarly, amphotericin B and rifampin have been found to be synergistic in mice.

Goswick and Brenner (2003) have described the effective treatment of experimental PAM in mice with azithromycin. Treatment was initiated 72 hours after infection and was continued for 5 days, with protection being 100% and greater than for the amphotericin B-treated mice. Interestingly, the patient who recovered from *Sappinia diploidea* encephalitis, described at the beginning of this section, also was treated with azithromycin (Gelman et al., 2001).

Prevention. Because of the swimming-related nature of *Naegleria* infection, swimming areas have been subjected to intensive investigation. Although *N. fowleri* has been isolated from many such areas, not all sampling efforts have yielded the organism. Obviously, there are factors that favor the development of *N. fowleri* in swimming areas: warm temperature, the presence of an adequate food supply, minimal competition from other protozoans, and probably optimal pH and oxygen levels.

Given the present limited understanding of the ecology of *N. fowleri*, practical measures for the prevention and control of *Naegleria* infection include public education, awareness in the medical community, and adequate chlorination of public water supplies, including swimming facilities. Adequate chlorination is a continuous free chlorine residual of 0.5 mg/L water. This level of chlorination has effectively controlled the *N. fowleri* problem in the public water supplies of South Australia.

Acanthamoeba spp. and Balamuthia mandrillaris

The majority of the infections previously described were first thought to be caused by amebae variously classified as *Hartmannella* or *Acanthamoeba*. These two genera are similar in appearance to the ameboid stage of *Naegleria* but have no flagellate stage. *Hartmannella* has been reported to be associated with human infection on only two occasions, once with a CNS infection and once with a corneal infection. A fatal case of meningoencephalitis was reported from Mexico in a malnourished 18-year-old male patient with chronic meningoencephalitis and bronchopneumonia. Although *Hartmannella vermiformis* was isolated three times from the spinal fluid, it was thought that the amebae were not the cause of the disease but were opportunistic colonizers that may have worsened the patient's condition. As stated previously, cases originally attributed to *Acanthamoeba* were later redescribed as *Balamuthia*, which in tissue is virtually indistinguishable from *Acanthamoeba*. The characteristic spiky acanthopodia of *Acanthamoeba* are seen in Figures 5-39 and 5-40. *Balamuthia* and *Hartmannella* do not have spiky pseudopodia.

Acanthamoeba was first noted as a contaminant in tissue cultures and subsequently was found to produce lethal meningoencephalitis on nasal instillation into mice and other animals. *Hartmannella* has been reported as a transient member of the changing fauna and flora of the upper respiratory tract of humans, but it has not been noted to produce disease in that location. It is possible that these isolations represent inhaled cysts; these and other free-living amebae have been collected by means of a slit sampler in random air samples.

Acanthamoeba may produce a chronic CNS infection (which is known as granulomatous amebic encephalitis [GAE] to distinguish it from the fulminant disease caused by *N. fowleri*) or a serious eye infection referred to as *Acanthamoeba* keratitis. Other forms of *Acanthamoeba* infection include chronic granulomatous infection of the skin and other tissues and invasion of bone with subsequent osteomyelitis. *Balamuthia* causes a chronic CNS infection similar to that produced by *Acanthamoeba*, also termed GAE. Skin lesions are the most commonly reported clinical condition caused by *Acanthamoeba* and *Balamuthia* in patients with AIDS.

GAE is not associated with swimming, as is *Naegleria* infection, and invasion of the CNS is secondary to infection elsewhere in the body. Amebae reach the brain by way of the

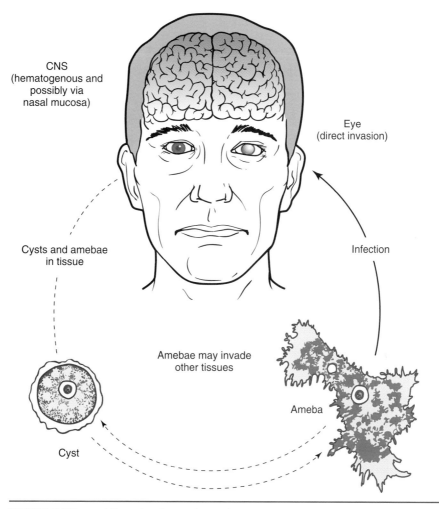

CNS
(hematogenous and
possibly via
nasal mucosa)

Eye
(direct invasion)

Cysts and amebae
in tissue

Infection

Amebae may invade
other tissues

Ameba

Cyst

FIGURE 5-39   ■   Life cycle of *Acanthamoeba* organisms.

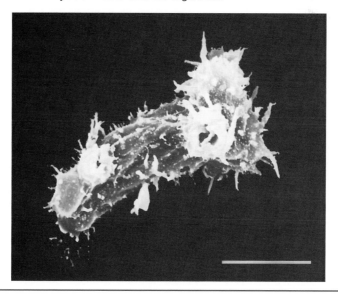

FIGURE 5-40   ■   Scanning electron micrograph of a trophozoite of *Acanthamoeba culbertsoni*. Note characteristic thorn- or spikelike acanthopodia. Bar is 10 μm. (Photomicrograph by Dr. Thomas B. Cole, Jr.)

TABLE 5-2   ■   *Acanthamoeba* Species Causing Human Disease

Acanthamoeba Species	CNS Infection	Eye Infection	Other Tissues
A. castellanii*	X	X	Skin, lung, prostate, bone, muscle, sinus
A. culbertsoni	X	X	Skin, liver, spleen, uterus
A. rhysodes	X	X	
A. astronyxis	X		Skin, lymph node, adrenal, thyroid sinus
A. divionensis	X		
A. healyi	X		
A. griffini		X	
A. hatchetti		X	
A. lugdunensis		X	
A. polyphaga		X	

*A. castellanii is the species identified most frequently in cases of CNS and ocular infection.

bloodstream, most likely from the lower respiratory tract or through ulcers of the skin or mucosa. The disease tends to be chronic, with a prolonged course, and occurs most often in debilitated or immunocompromised persons. Infection by *Balamuthia* may also occur in the immunocompetent. In contrast, *Acanthamoeba* keratitis affects healthy persons. The first cases of *Acanthamoeba* keratitis were reported in the mid-1970s from Great Britain and the United States and were associated with trauma to the eye. A dramatic increase in the number of cases since 1985 has been linked to the wearing of contact lenses, especially soft ones. *Hartmannella* and *Vahlkampfia* have also been isolated from cases of amebic keratitis.

Ten species of *Acanthamoeba* have been identified from human infections (see Table 5-2). *A. castellanii* is the species most often seen in cases of GAE and ocular infection, followed by *A. culbertsoni* for GAE and *A. polyphaga* for ocular infection.

The laboratory diagnosis of GAE is made by identifying trophozoites of *Acanthamoeba* or *Balamuthia* in CSF or trophozoites and cysts in brain tissue (see Fig. 5-42). Differentiation of the organisms in tissue is made by using the indirect immunofluorescent antibody technique and antisera to *Acanthamoeba* or *Balamuthia*. Whereas *N. fowleri* is readily cultured from spinal fluid, *Acanthamoeba* and *Balamuthia* are not. On just a few occasions have *Acanthamoeba* or *Balamuthia* been isolated in GAE. In such infections, characteristic cysts (Figs. 5-41 and 5-42, *B*) may be found in the tissues. Cysts are never seen in the tissues in *Naegleria* infections.

Acanthamoeba keratitis is diagnosed by identifying amebae cultured from corneal scrapings or by histologic examination of infected corneal tissue. As with PAM, *Acanthamoeba* may be cultivated from corneal scrapings on nonnutrient agar spread with gram-negative bacteria and later transferred to liquid medium (see Chapter 15) with antibiotics for axenic growth. Cultures of corneal material should be incubated at 30°C rather than 37°C. Species identification is based on indirect immunofluorescent antibody staining. Calcofluor white staining also has been used to identify *Acanthamoeba* cysts in corneal scrapings.

Herpes simplex keratitis is the disease most commonly mistaken for *Acanthamoeba* keratitis. The single most consistent clinical symptom of *Acanthamoeba* keratitis is severe ocular pain, which is not characteristic of an infection limited to the cornea and generally not of herpes simplex keratitis.

Symptoms and Pathogenesis. Although GAE usually occurs in debilitated or chronically ill persons, some of whom may be undergoing immunosuppressive therapy, not all victims of GAE have been debilitated or immunocompromised; some have been otherwise healthy.

GAE is not as well defined as disease caused by *N. fowleri*. The course of infection is subacute or chronic, lasting from weeks to months, in some instances perhaps even years, and is characterized by focal granulomatous lesions of the brain. The onset of GAE, unlike that of

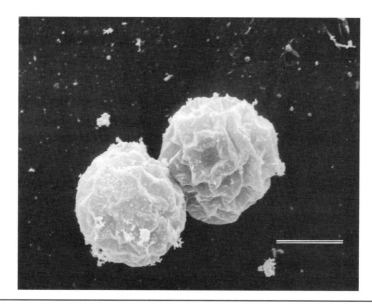

FIGURE 5-41 ■ Scanning electron micrograph of cysts of a pathogenic environmental isolate of *Acanthamoeba castellanii*. Note the characteristic wrinkled appearance of *Acanthamoeba* cysts in contrast to the smooth appearance of *Naegleria* cysts (Fig. 5-37, **C**). Bar is 10 μm. (Photomicrograph by Dr. Thomas B. Cole, Jr.)

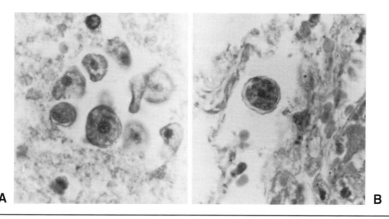

FIGURE 5-42 ■ *Acanthamoeba castellanii.* **A,** Trophozoites and **B,** cyst in human brain. (Photomicrographs from material furnished by Dr. A. Julio Martinez.)

PAM, is insidious, with a prolonged clinical course. GAE most probably occurs by way of the lungs or through skin and mucosal ulcers, with invasion of the CNS by hematogenous spread. The incubation period in GAE is not known but probably takes weeks or months, during which single or multiple space-occupying lesions develop. An altered mental state is a prominent feature of GAE. Headache, seizures, and stiff neck occur in about half the cases. Nausea and vomiting may also be noted. In contrast to *Naegleria* infection, characterized by diffuse meningoencephalitis, GAE is focal.

Since amebae reach the brain via the bloodstream, invasion of the CNS tends to become established first in the deeper tissues, from which it may extend toward the brain surface.

Trophozoites and cysts (see Fig. 5-42) occur in most infected tissues and around blood vessels. Within the infected primary tissues (the site of initial invasion) occurs a chronic granulomatous reaction like that seen in the brain, with trophozoites, cysts, and multinucleate giant cells. Similar lesions have been described from other tissues as well, including prostate, kidneys, uterus, and pancreas, probably the result of hematogenous dissemination of amebae from the primary focus in skin or lungs, or possibly even from a secondary CNS lesion. Cases of disseminated acanthamebiasis have been described in patients with AIDS.

Acanthamoeba keratitis is a chronic infection of the cornea caused by several species of *Acanthamoeba* (see Table 5-2). Infection is by direct contact of the cornea with amebae, which may be introduced through minor corneal trauma or by exposure to contaminated water or to contact lenses that have become contaminated. Keratitis in contact lens wearers has also been associated with infection by amebae of *Hartmannella* and *Vahlkampfia*.

Keratitis usually develops over a period of weeks or months and is characterized by severe ocular pain, often out of proportion to the degree of inflammation observed, affected vision, and a stromal infiltrate that frequently is ring shaped and composed predominantly of neutrophils. *Acanthamoeba* keratitis is a serious ocular infection and if not properly managed can lead to loss of vision and of the eye. Ocular infections are characterized by a chronic progressive ulcerative keratitis. Corneal ulceration may progress to perforation. A case of endophthalmitis, in which *Acanthamoeba* was recovered from aqueous and vitreous specimens, has been reported in a patient with AIDS. Topical propamidine, clotrimazole, and neomycin could not control the infection. Trophozoites and cysts of *Acanthamoeba* are found in the infected corneal tissue.

Epidemiology. Fewer cases of *Acanthamoeba* or *Balamuthia* CNS infection have been reported than of *Naegleria* infection, more than half from the United States. Unlike *Naegleria* infection, GAE is not associated with swimming. Infections often occur in persons who are debilitated or immunosuppressed and fatal cases have been reported in patients with AIDS. In one of the AIDS patients, the features of the disease were more like PAM than GAE, presumably because of the immunosuppression.

Acanthamoeba has been reported to cause disease in domestic and wild animals, including beavers, cattle, dogs, rabbits, turkeys, and water buffaloes. Just as in GAE, *Acanthamoeba* may produce a fatal CNS infection in immunocompromised animals. A case of meningoencephalitis caused by *A. castellanii* was described in a young immunodeficient dog. *Balamuthia* also causes disease in animals. Most cases of *Acanthamoeba* keratitis have been reported from the United States. One survey of 208 cases reported that 85% of the patients wore contact lenses.

Treatment. As with *Naegleria* infection, there is no satisfactory treatment for GAE, partly because most cases have been diagnosed after death and there has not been adequate opportunity to evaluate therapeutic regimens. There are three reports of persons having recovered from *Acanthamoeba* CNS infections. A 7-year-old girl with a single *Acanthamoeba*-induced granulomatous brain tumor recovered following total excision of the mass and treatment with ketoconazole. *A. healyi*, formerly identified as *A. palestinensis*, was cultured from brain biopsy material (Ofori-Kwakye et al., 1986). The second report concerned a 40-year-old man with *Acanthamoeba* meningitis who recovered following treatment with penicillin and chloramphenicol. *A. culbertsoni* was repeatedly cultured from the patient's cerebrospinal fluid (Lalitha et al., 1985). The third case, a partial recovery because the patient returned home and was lost to follow-up, was a 30-year-old man with chronic meningoencephalitis who was treated with sulfamethazine and from whose cerebrospinal fluid *A. rhysodes* was cultured (Cleland et al., 1982).

There are two reports describing the recovery of three immunocompetent patients from *Balamuthia* infection. In the first (Deetz et al., 2003), two patients received flucytosine,

TABLE 5-3 ■ Review of Other Blood- and Tissue-Dwelling Protozoan Infections of Humans

Disease	Parasite	Means of Human Infection	Location of Parasites in Humans	Clinical Features	Laboratory Diagnosis
African trypanosomiasis (sleeping sickness)	*Trypansoma brucei gambiense, T. b. rhodesiense* (flagellates)	"Bite" of infected tsetse fly (*Glossina*)	Blood lymphatics, CNS (extracellular)	Winterbottom's sign, fever, headache, "sleeping sickness," increased IgM	Trypanosomes in blood, lymph, CSF; culture, serologic tests
American trypanosomiasis (Chagas' disease)	*Trypanosoma cruzi* (flagellate)	Feces of infected reduviid bug (*Triatoma* and other) entering "bite"	Blood (extracellular); reticuloendothelial system, heart, brain, (intracellular)	Romaña's sign, fever, hepatosplenomegaly, myocarditis, meningoencephalitis	Trypanosomes in blood; culture, xenodiagnosis, biopsy, serologic tests
Cutaneous leishmaniasis	*Leishmania tropica, L. mexicana, L. braziliensis* complexes (flagellates)	"Bite" of infected sandfly (*Phlebotomus, Lutzomyia*)	Skin (intracellular)	Skin ulcers (single or multiple; self-healing to incurable)	Parasites in smears and culture of ulcer aspirate, skin test, serologic tests
Mucocutaneous leishmaniasis	*Leishmania braziliensis* complex (flagellates)	"Bite" of infected sandfly (*Lutzomyia, Psychodopygus*)	Skin and adjacent mucous membranes (intracellular)	Ulcers of skin and oral and nasal mucosa	Parasites in smears and culture of ulcer material, skin test, serologic tests
Visceral leishmaniasis (kala-azar)	*Leishmania donovani* complex (flagellates)	"Bite" of infected sandfly (*Phlebotomus, Lutzomyia*)	Liver, spleen, lymph nodes, bone marrow (intracellular)	Hepatosplenomegaly, anemia, fever, weight loss	Parasites in smears and culture of bone marrow, hamster inoculation, serologic tests
Toxoplasmosis	*Toxoplasma gondii* (apicomplexan)	Ingestion of infected meat or oocysts in cat feces (congenital infection)	Cells of reticuloendothelial system, lungs, eye, brain (intracellular)	Lymphadenopathy, fever, pneumonia, eye and brain damage	Parasites in biopsy or fluids, serologic tests
Babesiosis	*Babesia microti* in North America, *B. divergens* in Europe (apicomplexa)	"Bite" of infected *Ixodes* tick	Erythrocytes (intracellular)	Chills and fever, headache, fatigue, anemia	Parasites in blood films, hamster inoculation, serologic tests
Primary amebic meningoencephalitis	*Naegleria fowleri* (free-living ameba)	Intranasal instillation of ameba	Brain tissue, meninges	Severe frontal headache, fever, nausea, vomiting, stiff neck	Trophozoites in CSF
Granulomatous amebic encephalitis	*Acanthamoeba* spp. and *Balamuthia mandrillaris* (free-living amebae)	Through lungs or skin ulcers	Lungs, skin, hematogenous spread to brain (disseminated in AIDS patients)	Altered mental state, headache, seizures, stiff neck	Trophozoites in CSF, trophozoites or cysts in brain tissue
Acanthamoeba keratitis	*Acanthamoeba* spp. (free-living amebae)	Eye trauma, contaminated contact lenses	Cornea	Severe ocular pain, corneal ulceration, CNS abscess	Trophozoites or cysts in corneal scraping or biopsy

pentamidine, fluconazole, sulfadiazine, and azithromycin or clarithromycin. The third patient received pentamidine, fluconazole, and clarithromycin (Jung et al., 2004).

Most of the earlier cases of *Acanthamoeba* keratitis required corneal transplants to manage the disease. The first successful medical cure, reported by Wright and coworkers (1985), involved the use of a combination of dibromopropamide ointment (Otamidyl), propamide isethionate drops (Brolene), and neomycin drops. The success of this treatment regimen has been confirmed by others. Another report describes the successful treatment of three patients with oral itraconazole (Sporanox), a new antifungal agent, in addition to topical miconazole and surgical debridement of the lesions (Ishibashi et al., 1990). Additional successful treatment regimens have been propamidine isethionate, neomycin sulfate, and clotrimazole (D'Aversa et al., 1995), 0.02% topical polyhexamethylene biguanide, a polymeric biguanide disinfectant (Elder and Dart, 1995), and 0.02% chlorhexidine digluconate, propamidine isethionate, and oral itraconazole (Mathers et al., 1996). Propamidine remains the best documented treatment for *Acanthamoeba* keratitis.

For a thorough discussion of the treatment of the diseases caused by the opportunistic amebae, including PAM, GAE, and *Acanthamoeba* keratitis, see the review by Schuster and Visvesvara (2003).

Prevention. Factors that have been associated with *Acanthamoeba* keratitis in contact lens wearers include the use of nonsterile, homemade saline; disinfection of lenses less frequently than recommended; and wearing lenses while swimming. Persons who wear contact lenses should follow closely the manufacturer's recommendations for wear, care, and disinfection of the lenses. Homemade saline solutions remain an important risk factor associated with *Acanthamoeba* keratitis. Table 5-3 summarizes some important features of the more common blood- and tissue-dwelling protozoan infections of humans.

References

Andrade ALSS et al. Randomized trial of efficacy of benznidazole in treatment of early *Trypanosoma cruzi* infection. *Lancet* 1996; *348*:1407–1413.

Asonganyi T et al. A multi-centre evaluation of the card indirect agglutination test for trypanosomiasis (TrypTect CIATT). *Ann Trop Med Parasitol* 1998; *92*:837–844.

CDC. Updated: Cutaneous leishmaniasis in U.S. military personnel–Southwest/Central Asia, 2002–2004. *MMWR* 2004; *53*:264–265.

Cleland PG et al. Chronic amebic meningoencephalitis. *Arch Neurol* 1982; *39*:56–57.

Convit J et al. Immunotherapy of localized, intermediate, and diffuse forms of American cutaneous leishmaniasis. *J Infect Dis* 1989; *160*:104–115.

D'Aversa G et al. Diagnosis and successful medical treatment of *Acanthamoeba* keratitis. *Arch Ophthalmol* 1995; *113*:1120–1123.

Deetz RT et al. Successful treatment of *Balamuthia* amoebic encephalitis: Presentation of 2 cases. *Clin Infect Dis* 2003; *37*:1304–1312.

Dorga J. A double-blind study on the efficacy of oral dapsone in cutaneous leishmaniasis. *Trans R Soc Trop Med Hyg* 1991; *85*:212–213.

Elder MJ, Dart JKG. Chemotherapy for acanthamoeba keratitis. *Lancet* 1995; *345*:791–793.

El-On J et al. Topical chemotherapy of cutaneous leishmaniasis. *Parasitol Today* 1988; *4*:76–81.

Falcoff E et al. Clinical healing of antimony-resistant cutaneous or mucocutaneous leishmaniasis following the combined administration of interferon-γ and pentavalent antimonial compounds. *Trans R Soc Trop Med Hyg* 1994; *88*:95–97.

Foppa IM et al. Entomologic and serologic evidence of zoonotic transmission of *Babesia microti*, Eastern Switzerland. *Emerg Infect Dis* 2002; *8*:722–726.

Gallerano RH et al. Therapeutic efficacy of allopurinol in patients with chronic Chagas' disease. *Am J Trop Med Hyg* 1990; *43*:159–166.

Gelman BB et al. Amoebic encephalitis due to *Sappinia diploidea*. *JAMA* 2001; *285*:2450–2451.

Gelman BB et al. Neuropathological and ultrastructural features of amebic encephalitis caused by *Sappinia diploidiea. J Neuropathol Exp Neurol* 2003; *62*:990–998.

Goswick SM, Brenner GM. Activities of azithromycin and amphotericin B against *Naegleria fowleri* in vitro and in a mouse model of primary amebic meningoencephalitis. *Antimicrob Agents Chemother* 2003; *47*:524–528.

Gürtler RE et al. Congenital transmission of *Trypanosoma cruzi* infection in Argentina. *Emerg Infect Dis* 2003; *9*:29–32.

Harms G et al. Effects of intradermal gamma interferon in cutaneous leishmaniasis. *Lancet* 1989; *1*:1287–1292.

Herwaldt BL et al. Molecular characterization of a non-*Babesia divergens* organism causing zoonotic babesiosis in Europe. *Emerg Infect Dis* 2003; *9*:942–948.

Ishibashi Y et al. Oral itraconazole and topical miconazole with debridement for *Acanthamoeba* keratitis. *Am J Ophthalmol* 1990; *109*:121–126.

Jung S et al. *Balamuthia mandrillaris* meningoencephalitis in an immunocompetent patient. *Arch Pathol Lab Med* 2004; *128*:466–468.

Lalitha MK et al. Isolation of *Acanthamoeba culbertsoni* from a patient with meningitis. *J Clin Microbiol* 1985; *21*:666–667.

Lang-Unnasch N et al. Plastids are widespread and ancient in parasites of the phylum Apicomplexa. *Internat'l J Parasitol* 1998; *28*:1743–1754.

Lindsay DS et al. Survival of *Toxoplasma gondii* oocysts in eastern oysters (*Crassostrea virginica*). *J Parasitol* 2004; *90*:1054–1057.

Mathers WD et al. Outbreak of keratitis presumed to be caused by *Acanthamoeba. Am J Ophthalmol* 1996; *121*:129–142.

Miller MA et al. Coastal freshwater runoff is a risk factor for *Toxoplasma gondii* infection of southern sea otters (*Enhydra lutris neresis*). *Internat'l J Parasitol* 2002; *32*:997–1006.

Navin TR et al. Placebo-controlled clinical trial of meglumine antimonate (Glucantime) vs. localized controlled heat in the treatment of cutaneous leishmaniasis in Guatemala. *Am J Trop Med Hyg* 1990; *42*:43–50.

Noyes H et al. A previously unclassified trypanosomatid responsible for human cutaneous lesions in Martinique (French West Indies) is the most divergent member of the genus *Leishmania ss. Parasitol* 2002; *124*:17–24.

Ofori-Kwakye SK et al. Granulomatous brain tumor caused by *Acanthamoeba. J Neurosurg* 1986; *64*:505–509.

Pepin J et al. Trial of prednisolone for prevention of melarsoprol-induced encephalopathy in gambiense sleeping sickness. *Lancet* 1989; *1*:1246–1250.

Schuster FL, Visvesvara GS. Opportunistic amoebae: challenges in prophylaxis and treatment. *Drug Resistance Updates* 2004; *7*:41–51.

Seidel JS et al. Successful treatment of primary amebic meningoencephalitis. *N Engl J Med* 1982; *306*:346–348.

Sundar S et al. Oral miltefosine for Indian visceral leishmaniasis. *N Engl J Med* 2002; *347*:1739–1746.

Truc P et al. *Trypanosoma brucei* ssp. and *T. congolense*: mixed human infection in Côte d'Ivoire. *Trans R Soc Trop Med Hyg* 1998; *92*:537–538.

Viallet J et al. Response to ketoconazole in two cases of long-standing cutaneous leishmaniasis. *Am J Trop Med Hyg* 1986; *35*:491–495.

Welburn SC, Odiit M. Recent developments in human African trypanosomiasis. *Curr Opin Infect Dis* 2002; *15*:477–484.

WHO Expert Committee. Control of Chagas disease. WHO Technical Report Series 2002; *905*:1–109.

Wright P et al. *Acanthamoeba* keratitis successfully treated medically. *Br J Ophthalmol* 1985; *69*:778–782.

CHAPTER
6

The Trematodes

The Trematoda, or flukes, constitute one class of the phylum Platyhelminthes. Adult trematodes are parasites of vertebrates. Most are hermaphroditic, and many are capable of self-fertilization. All have complex life cycles, requiring one or more intermediate hosts. Eggs laid by the adult within the vertebrate host pass outside, and a larva develops within them. This larva, called a miracidium, may hatch and swim away, or in some species, emergence may have to wait upon ingestion of the egg by the next host. In either case, development cannot proceed unless the proper first intermediate host—a mollusk (snail or clam)—is available. Each species of trematode requires certain species of molluscan intermediate hosts for development, lacking which it dies. A complex series of generations follows within the mollusk, resulting finally in the liberation of large numbers of larvae known as cercariae. In some species, the cercaria must penetrate directly through the skin of the vertebrate host; in others it enters an insect, fish, or other second intermediate host; in still others it must attach to vegetation and secrete a resistant cyst wall, waiting to be eaten by the final host. The forms found in a second intermediate host or encysted on vegetation are known as metacercariae. Life cycles of trematodes are complex and varied; they illustrate an extraordinary range of evolutionary adaptations. A "typical" life cycle is shown in Figure 6-1.

Most trematodes are described as leaf shaped, but they vary considerably in form (see Figs. 6-5, 6-12, 6-13, and 6-17). The largest human parasite belonging to this group is *Fasciolopsis buski*, which may attain a length of 75 mm and a breadth of 20 mm but is not over 3 mm thick. *Heterophyes heterophyes*, the smallest, is under 2 mm in length and 0.5 mm in breadth. The body of a trematode is covered with a resistant cuticle, which may be smooth or spiny. There are two suckers or attachment organs: an anterior one (the oral sucker) surrounding the mouth and a more posterior one (the acetabulum or ventral sucker) on the ventral surface. The oral cavity leads to a muscular esophagus, from which the intestine branches to form two intestinal ceca, which run parallel to each other, ending blindly near the posterior end of the worm. Most of the rest of the body is taken up with reproductive organs and associated structures. There are usually two testes leading to the genital pore, which usually lies in the region of the ventral sucker. There is a single ovary. A series of glandular structures called vitellaria, usually in two masses lying lateral to the intestinal ceca, produce the shell material. Vitelline ducts lead inward to the region of the ovary where the shell is formed over the ovum. The uterus winds forward to the genital pore. In most trematodes, it is the largest organ in the body, filled with thousands of eggs.

Trematode eggs have a smooth, hard shell that is transparent and generally yellow-brown or brown. They range in length from under 30 μm to as much as 175 μm, depending on the species. The majority have close to what would be considered a conventional egg shape. Most have an operculum or lid at one end, an "escape hatch" through which the miracidium emerges. This operculum may be difficult to detect, but it can usually be seen by careful focusing with reduced illumination. The miracidium is covered with cilia, and in some species it is fully developed when the eggs are passed in the feces. The shell may be smoothly continuous in outline, or there may be a slight flare, marking the line of cleavage between shell and operculum, known as the opercular shoulders. Possession of these shoulders is characteristic of the eggs of certain species. Spines may be present, either very small and

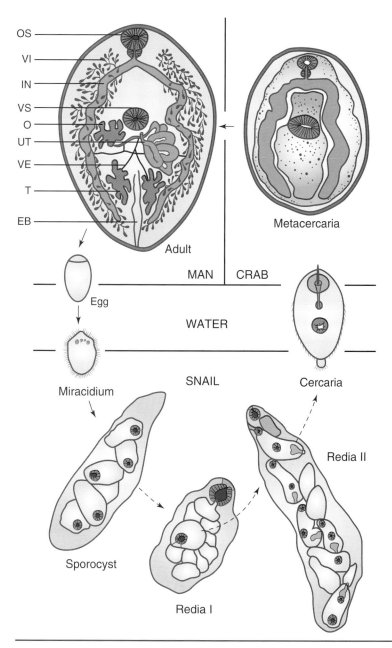

OS
VI
IN
VS
O
UT
VE
T
EB

Adult

Metacercaria

Egg

MAN | CRAB

WATER

Miracidium

SNAIL

Cercaria

Redia II

Sporocyst

Redia I

FIGURE 6-1 ■ *Paragonimus,* an example of a trematode life cycle: *(EB)* excretory bladder; *(IN)* intestine; *(O)* ovary; *(OS)* oral sucker; *(T)* testis; *(UT)* uterus; *(VE)* vas efferens; *(VI)* vitellaria; *(VS)* ventral sucker. (Adapted from Porter in Burrows, Textbook of Microbiology.)

inconspicuous as in *Clonorchis* or *Opisthorchis*, or large and striking as in certain species of *Schistosoma*. Eggs of the schistosomes are nonoperculate, and the egg is irregularly ruptured in hatching. Trematode eggs cannot successfully be concentrated by the zinc-sulfate technique, as both the operculate and the nonoperculate forms rupture and fail to float. Formalin-ether concentrates are quite satisfactory, or the sediment of the zinc-sulfate concentrate may be examined for the eggs, which are still recognizable even when ruptured.

Eggs of the flukes, as well as of the tapeworms, and eggs or larvae of the intestinal nematodes are shown in color in Plates X and XI.

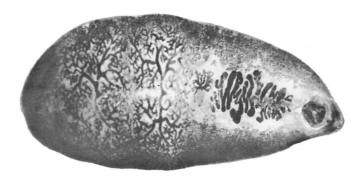

FIGURE 6-2   ■   *Fasciolopsis buski.* (Photomicrograph by Zane Price.)

The Intestinal Flukes

Fasciolopsis buski

The giant intestinal fluke *F. buski* (Fig. 6-2) is found in China (including Taiwan), Vietnam, and Thailand, and in parts of Indonesia, Malaysia, and the Indian subcontinent. Adult worms live attached to the bowel wall, primarily in the duodenum and jejunum; in heavy infections they may be found throughout the intestinal tract. Their life span seldom exceeds 6 months. An estimated 10 million infections occur annually.

Infection is acquired by ingestion of the metacercariae, encysted on fresh-water vegetation (Fig. 6-3) such as bamboo shoots or water chestnuts, which may be consumed raw or peeled with the teeth. Reservoir hosts include pigs, dogs, and rabbits.

Adult worms are seen only following purgation after specific anthelminthic treatment. They are fleshy worms, 2 to 7.5 cm long by 0.8 to 2 cm wide. The ellipsoid eggs (Fig. 6-4, *A*; Plate X) are yellow-brown in color. The shell is transparent, with a small operculum at the more pointed end. Eggs are unembryonated when first passed, containing early cleavage stages; they measure 130 to 140 μm by 80 to 85 μm.

Symptoms and Pathogenesis. Attachment of these large worms to the mucosa of the bowel causes local inflammation and ulceration, sometimes accompanied by hemorrhage. A few worms do not give rise to any recognizable symptoms, but with heavier infections there may be abdominal pain, at times suggestive of duodenal ulcer disease, and diarrhea. In heavy infections (with hundreds or perhaps thousands of worms in the bowel) the stools are profuse, light yellow in color, and contain much undigested food; they are suggestive of a malabsorptive process such as is seen in giardiasis. Vitamin B_{12} absorption has been found to be impaired in some infected persons. Intestinal obstruction may occur. Edema and ascites, which may develop in severe infections, have traditionally been considered to be secondary to the absorption of worm toxins, but these symptoms can perhaps more rationally be ascribed to a hypoalbuminemia resulting from long-continued malabsorption or from a protein-wasting enteropathy. Marked eosinophilia is usually seen.

Treatment. The drug of choice is praziquantel (Biltricide), an isoquino-linepyrazine derivative, which seems an almost idea platyhelminthicide. It is administered orally, 25 mg/kg body weight three times in 1 day. The mode of action of praziquantel is uncertain, but it seems to work by altering the permeability of cell membranes to mono- and divalent cations, especially calcium. Causing a massive influx of calcium, it initiates a tetanic contractile process on the part of the worm. It also leads to disruption and vacuolization of the tegument (covering) of the worm, with subsequent eosinophil attachment. The mammalian host metabolizes the drug rapidly and tolerates it well. Side effects, including epigastric pain, dizziness, and

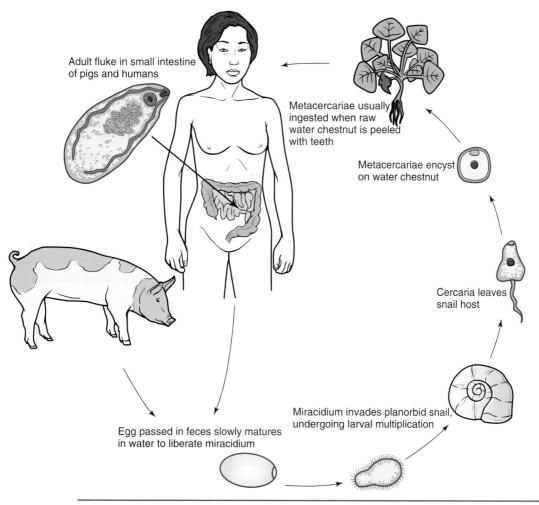

Adult fluke in small intestine of pigs and humans

Metacercariae usually ingested when raw water chestnut is peeled with teeth

Metacercariae encyst on water chestnut

Cercaria leaves snail host

Miracidium invades planorbid snail, undergoing larval multiplication

Egg passed in feces slowly matures in water to liberate miracidium

FIGURE 6-3 ■ Life cycle of *Fasciolopsis buski*.

drowsiness, are minimal and disappear within 48 hours. Experimental testing has failed to reveal evidence of teratogenicity, mutagenicity, or other adverse effects. At the time of this writing, praziquantel is approved by the United States Food and Drug Administration (FDA) only for the treatment of clonorchiasis, opisthorchiasis, and schistosomiasis.

The Echinostomes

A number of medium-sized intestinal flukes belonging to the genus *Echinostoma* and to several related genera have been reported from Japan, the Philippines, Malaysia, Sumatra, Java, Sulawesi, India, and a few other localities in Asia. There is suggestive evidence that echinostomes may also occur in East Africa. They live attached to the wall of the small intestine, where they may produce an inflammatory reaction and ulceration, leading to diarrhea. They average under 1 cm in length and 0.2 cm in width and are distinguished by a collarette of spines on a disk surrounding the oral sucker (Fig. 6-5). The life cycle (Fig. 6-6) involves not one but two snail intermediate hosts; metacercariae encyst in the second. The most important species is *Echinostoma ilocanum*, which occurs in the Philippines. Human infections are generally inadvertent, except in the Philippines, where the second snail host is customarily eaten raw; the worms are found in a variety of mammals whose food habits promote infection.

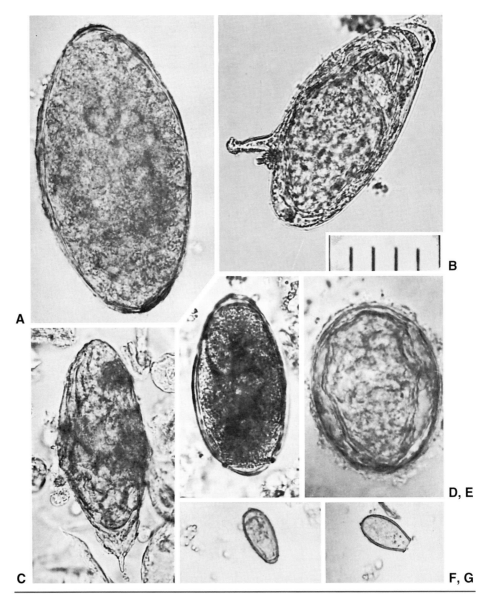

FIGURE 6-4   ■   Some trematode eggs; **A,** *Fasciolopsis buski.* **B,** *Schistosoma mansoni.*
C, *Schistosoma haematobium.* **D,** *Paragonimus westermani.* **E,** *Schistosoma japonicum.*
F, G, *Clonorchis sinensis.* All eggs photographed at same magnification; scale equals 50 μm.

The adult worms are seen only after treatment but can be recognized by the circumoral spines. The unembryonated eggs are similar in shape to those of *Fasciolopsis* and vary in size in the different species (Plate X). Some species overlap the size range of *Fasciolopsis,* and therefore an exact identification cannot be made from examination of the eggs. Frequently a diagnosis can be established on the basis of the patient's history or the clinical findings.

Symptoms and Pathogenesis. Little damage is caused to the intestinal mucosa by attachment of these flukes. Heavy infections may produce inflammation and mild ulceration, with diarrhea and abdominal pain, while light ones are probably asymptomatic.

Treatment. The drug of choice is praziquantel, 25 mg/kg body weight three times in a single day. Tetrachloroethylene is also known to be effective. The dose is 0.1 ml/kg, taken on an

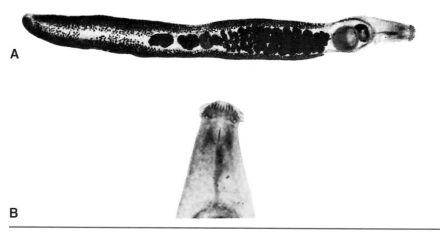

FIGURE 6-5 ■ **A,** *Echinostoma* sp. **B,** Anterior end of *Echinostoma,* showing circumoral spines. (Photomicrographs by Zane Price.)

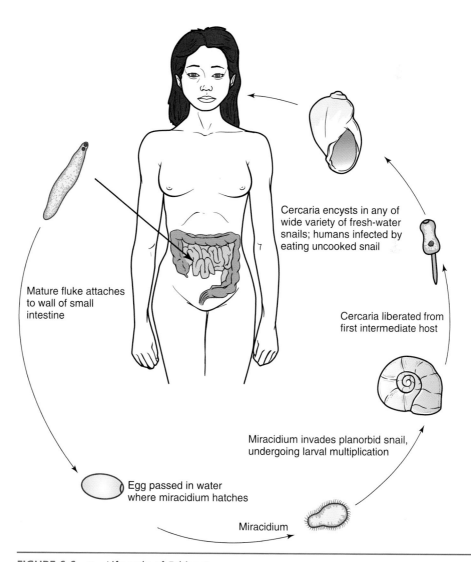

Cercaria encysts in any of wide variety of fresh-water snails; humans infected by eating uncooked snail

Mature fluke attaches to wall of small intestine

Cercaria liberated from first intermediate host

Miracidium invades planorbid snail, undergoing larval multiplication

Egg passed in water where miracidium hatches

Miracidium

FIGURE 6-6 ■ Life cycle of *Echinostoma.*

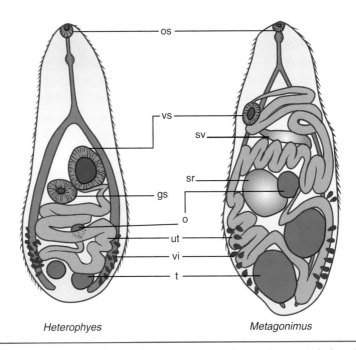

Heterophyes   *Metagonimus*

FIGURE 6-7 ■ *Heterophyes heterophyes* and *Metagonimus yokogawai: (gs)* genital sucker; *(o)* ovary; *(os)* oral sucker; *(sr)* seminal receptacle; *(sv)* seminal vesicle; *(t)* testis; *(ut)* uterus; *(vi)* vitellaria; *(vs)* ventral sucker. Drawings made with the aid of a camera lucida (approximately × 40).

empty stomach after a light meal the preceding night. The maximum adult dose is 5 ml. Alcohol and fats should be avoided for 24 hours before and after treatment, and nothing other than water should be taken for 3 hours after ingestion of the medication.

The Heterophyids

Two minute flukes, *Heterophyes heterophyes* and *Metagonimus yokogawai* (Fig. 6-7), occur in Japan, Korea, China (including Taiwan), the Philippines, and western India. *Heterophyes* has also been reported from Egypt and Israel, and *Metagonimus* from the Balkans, Spain, Israel, the former USSR, and Indonesia. The parasites live attached to the wall of the small intestine. *Metagonimus* is somewhat larger than *Heterophyes* but does not exceed 2.5 mm in length by 0.75 mm in width. *Heterophyes* has a third sucker, surrounding the genital pore; this structure is not present in *Metagonimus*.

Many other species of heterophyids have been found as occasional human parasites; it has been stated that all heterophyids have this potential. In one area of Laos, serologic techniques indicated the probable presence of heterophyids (*Haplorchis* spp.) in 75% of persons tested (Giboda et al., 1991).

Heterophyids are acquired by ingesting raw or pickled fresh-water fish of many kinds. The life cycle is similar to that of the opisthorchids (see Fig. 6-10), except that heterophyids parasitize the small intestine. Metacercariae of the heterophyid flukes encyst under the scales or in the flesh of fish. They are not killed by the various pickling processes to which fish is sometimes subjected. Thorough cooking will, of course, kill them. A variety of fish-eating mammals serve as reservoir hosts for both of the heterophyids that infect humans. Human infections outside the endemic area may result from the consumption of pickled fish or of sushi made from fish imported from the endemic areas. Such infections are known to have occurred in the United States.

Only following anthelminthic treatment are the adult worms seen in the feces. The eggs, which contain fully developed miracidia and possess prominent opercular shoulders, are brownish yellow (Plate X). Those of *Heterophyes* are, on average, slightly larger than those of *Metagonimus*, but differences are too slight to be of value. The size range for the two species is 26.5 to 30 μm by 15 to 17 μm. The eggs closely resemble in size and shape those of worms belonging to the genera *Clonorchis** and *Opisthorchis*. Some morphologic differences have been described, but these are slight and not constant.

Symptoms and Pathogenesis. Attached to the intestinal wall, the adult worms produce no symptoms unless present in large numbers. Chronic intermittent diarrhea, nausea, and vague abdominal complaints have been reported. Occasionally the worms invade the mucosa, and their eggs deposited in the tissues may gain access to the circulation to embolize to the brain, spinal cord, or heart. Seizures, neurologic deficits, and cardiac insufficiency have been ascribed to granulomas that form around these eggs.

Treatment. The drug of choice is praziquantel, administered as indicated for treatment of fasciolopsiasis (again unapproved for this indication by the FDA). An alternative drug is tetrachloroethylene, as used in treatment of the echinostomes.

Gastrodiscoides hominis

Gastrodisciasis is commonly seen in Assam and other parts of India, where it also occurs in pigs. It has also been reported from Southeast Asia and Malaysia; in the latter area the reservoir host is the mouse deer *Tragulus napu*. The worm is pear shaped, the flattened ventral surface of the enlarged posterior end being composed of a much enlarged ventral sucker, or acetabulum. Worms range in size from 5 to 14 mm by 4 to 6 mm. The ovoid, greenish brown eggs measure about 150 μm by 60 to 72 μm (Plate X). The life cycle is not known, but by analogy with related worms, infection of the mammalian host is probably contracted by ingesting metacercariae encysted on vegetation.

Symptoms and Pathogenesis. The worms live attached to the mucosa of the cecum and ascending colon, where they produce local inflammation and mucous diarrhea.

Treatment. Tetrachloroethylene, administered as outlined for echinostomiasis, is said to be effective. It is probable that praziquantel, given in the usual dose of 25 mg/kg three times in 1 day, would be preferable, as it is less toxic.

The Liver Flukes

Several trematodes are parasites of the biliary passages of humans. Three of them, *Clonorchis*, *Opisthorchis*, and *Dicrocoelium*, are relatively elongate and narrow-bodied worms that tend to localize in the smaller, more distal parts of the biliary tree. Only in heavy infections are these worms found in the common bile duct or gallbladder. *Fasciola*, a much larger worm, is confined by its size to the larger passages.

These worms all produce hyperplastic changes in the epithelium of the bile ducts and fibrosis around them. Massive infection by any of them may lead to portal cirrhosis, with all its associated manifestations.

The eggs of the opisthorchid flukes are similar in appearance to those of the heterophyids, while those of *Fasciola* closely resemble both *Fasciolopsis* and the echinostomes. If eggs of one of these forms are found in the stool, and the diagnosis of hepatic or intestinal infection cannot be made on clinical grounds, examination of bile obtained by duodenal

---

*Most modern authorities consider *Clonorchis* to be a synonym of *Opisthorchis*; however, *Clonorchis* is entrenched in the medical literature, and we refer to the Chinese liver fluke as *Clonorchis sinensis*.

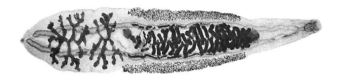

FIGURE 6-8 ■ *Clonorchis sinensis.* (Photomicrograph by Zane Price.)

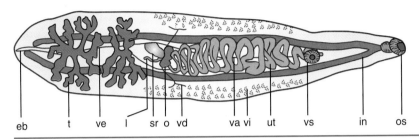

FIGURE 6-9 ■ *Clonorchis sinensis; (eb)* excretory bladder; *(in)* intestine; *(l)* Laurers' canal; *(o)* ovary; *(os)* oral sucker; *(sr)* seminal receptacle; *(t)* testis; *(ut)* uterus; *(va)* vas deferens; *(vd)* vitelline duct; *(ve)* vas efferens; *(vi)* vitellaria; *(vs)* ventral sucker. Drawing made with the aid of a camera lucida.

drainage will provide the correct answer. If uncontaminated bile is obtained and eggs are found in this material, they must have been produced by worms in the liver or gallbladder.

Clonorchis sinensis

The Chinese liver fluke, *C. sinensis* (Figs. 6-8 and 6-9), occurs in large areas of China (including Taiwan), Japan, Korea, and Vietnam. It is of moderate size, from 1 to 2.5 cm by 0.3 to 0.5 cm. It is broadest in the midportion of the body, tapering toward both ends. Adult worms live in the bile ducts and apparently localize first in the more distal portions, just under the capsule of the liver. In more massive infections, they occupy most of the bile passages and may even be found in the gallbladder and pancreatic duct. Worms are known to live as long as 30 years.

Human infection results from the consumption of fresh-water fish containing the encysted metacercariae (Fig. 6-10). Fish may be eaten raw, pickled, smoked, or dried. The disease has been reported in native Hawaiians as a result of the consumption of infected fish imported from the Orient. Dogs and cats are the most important reservoir hosts; their wholesale slaughter in the People's Republic of China has probably reduced transmission of the disease in that area.

The adult worms are seen only at autopsy, or rarely upon surgical removal. Eggs are found in the feces, and as the average daily output per worm is probably more than 2400 eggs, they may be very numerous. Eggs of *C. sinensis* (Plate X; see also Fig. 6-4 *F, G*) resemble very closely those of *Heterophyes* and *Metagonimus* but may have a small comma-shaped process at the abopercular end. The average length is 29 μm, and breadth is 16 μm, which falls within the *Heterophyes-Metagonimus* range. The extreme measurements are significantly larger than those of the heterophyid worms, about 35 μm in length and 19.5 μm in breadth for eggs of *C. sinensis.*

Diagnosis is by recovery of the eggs from the feces or from duodenal aspirates, or the enteric capsule or EnteroTest. Complement fixation and intradermal tests have been described but are not generally available.

Symptoms. Light infections, which are the rule, are generally asymptomatic. Heavier infections, if acquired over an extended period, seldom cause early symptoms. The ingestion

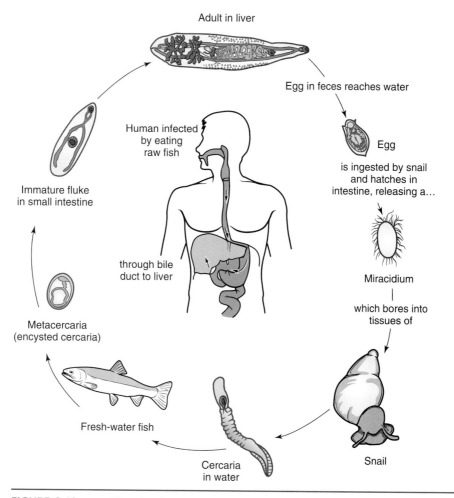

FIGURE 6-10 ■ Life cycle of *Clonorchis sinensis*.

of large numbers of metacercariae over a short period of time may produce symptomatic early infections. The acute phase lasts less than a month and may be characterized by fever, diarrhea, epigastric pain, anorexia, enlargement and tenderness of the liver, and sometimes jaundice. There may be leukocytosis, and eosinophilia is generally present. Eggs appear in the feces about a month after infection takes place, and the acute symptoms subside. Once this has happened, persons not subject to repeated reinfection generally do not have any recognizable symptoms from a chronic low-grade infection. An epidemic of early-onset symptomatic clonorchiasis occurred among Jewish refugees, unaware of the dangers of eating uncooked fish, living in Shanghai at the end of World War II. Treatment at that time was not very effective, and many of those persons still harbored an asymptomatic infection 20 years later.

Heavy worm burdens—the result of repeated infection over a period of years—may result in a degree of functional impairment of the liver; this impairment is secondary to localized biliary obstruction (Fig. 6-11) and is at times aggravated by intrahepatic stone formation, cholangitis, and the formation of multiple liver abscesses. Cholecystitis and cholelithiasis may be the result of invasion of the gallbladder by these worms, which have also been considered to cause acute pancreatitis. Such symptoms may come on after years of asymptomatic infection. Cirrhosis is probably a rare complication, related more to chronic malnourishment than to the parasitic infection.

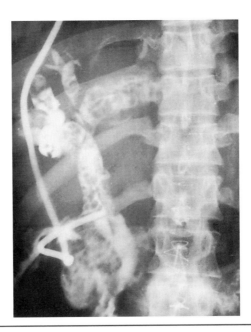

FIGURE 6-11 ■ Clonorchiasis. T-tube cholangiogram demonstrates dilated bile ducts filled with flukes. (Courtesy of the Armed Forces Institute of Pathology. #69–5522–3.)

Pathogenesis. Thickening and localized dilatation of the bile ducts are seen in heavy infections, accompanied by moderte to marked hyperplasia of the small mucinous glands of the duct mucosa. The degree to which both of these changes may take place bears a direct relationship to the intensity of infection. However, these adenomatous changes may persist for many years in patients whose infections have become very light. Adenocarcinomas arising from the hyperplastic bile duct mucosa in persons chronically infected with *C. sinensis* have long been considered to be related to that infection, although dietary and other factors may also play a role.

Treatment. The drug of choice is praziquantel, with cure rates in the neighborhood of 100% when administered at 25 mg/kg three times daily for 1 day. Albendazole,[*] a member of the benzimidazole group of drugs that includes thiabendazole and mebendazole, seems equally effective (Liu et al., 1991) when given at 10 mg/kg daily for 7 days. Both drugs have minimal toxicity.

Opisthorchis felineus

As the name suggests, *O. felineus* parasitizes cats. In central and eastern Europe and in Siberia, it is prevalent in both cats and dogs; in various sectors where the human population eats raw or pickled fish, humans are also infected. It is particularly prevalent as a human parasite in East Prussia, Poland, and parts of Siberia. Human infections have also been reported from the Philippines, Korea, Japan, North Vietnam, and India, although there is a question whether or not the parasite is indigenous to all of these areas. Like *C. sinensis*, *O. felineus* inhabits the bile ducts, and much the same disease picture is produced by both parasites. The life cycle of the two parasites is likewise similar.

The adult *O. felineus* differs from *C. sinensis* only in some relatively minor details of structure. Eggs of *O. felineus* are narrower than those of *C. sinensis*, averaging 30 μm by only 11 to 12 μm. They are otherwise indistinguishable.

[*]Albendazole may be obtained from the manufacturer, Glaxo SmithKline, on a case-by-case basis; (215) 751-4000.

Praziquantel is effective if administered at the rate of 25 mg/kg three times daily for 1 or 2 days.

Opisthorchis viverrini

A third species of liver fluke, *O. viverrini*, is a major health problem in northern Thailand and Laos. The overall prevalence is reported to be from 80% to 90% in rural people, and 55% in urban dwellers, increasing with age up to 10 years, after which it remains fairly constant. The infection is acquired by the consumption of uncooked fresh-water fish. Mild to moderate infections seem to produce few symptoms, but heavier ones are associated with abdominal distress, epigastric pain, and generalized malaise. As in clonorchiasis, there seems to be a strong relationship between long-standing heavy infections and the development of cholangiocarcinoma (Chiu et al., 1996). *O. viverrini* also occurs in Cambodia and Malaysia, and it is quite possible that opisthorchid infections, reported from neighboring areas such as North Vietnam, and attributed to *O. felineus*, may in reality be caused by *O. viverrini*.

The adult *O. viverrini* differs only slightly in structure from the other two opisthorchids. The eggs are relatively short and broad, with an average length of 26.7 μm and breadth of 15 μm (Plate X).

Praziquantel is reported to have had an almost 100% efficacy when given as a single dose of 40 mg/kg to a large group of mildly to moderately infected Thais studied over a 2-year period (Pungpak et al., 1994). Alternatively, praziquantel may be administered at 75 mg/kg in 3 doses for 1 day. However, because of the efficacy of this therapy, many Thais continue the consumption of raw fish, interspersed with periodic praziquantel treatments!

Dicrocoelium dendriticum

A common parasite of the biliary tree of herbivores in many parts of the world is *D. dendriticum* (Fig. 6-12), a fluke of about the same size and shape as *Clonorchis*. Many apparent human infections with this parasite have in fact been spurious, the result of the consumption of infected liver with subsequent appearances of the ingested eggs in the feces. Other reported cases, from many parts of the world, have been true *Dicrocoelium* infections. As a consideration of the life cycle will show, such human infections must be uncommon. *Dicrocoelium* is similar to *Clonorchis* as regards both localization and the pathologic lesions it produces. After ingestion, the metacercariae excyst in the duodenum and pass through the common bile duct to invade the biliary system.

The life cycle of this parasite is most unusual. Eggs, fully embryonated when passed in the feces, are ingested by land snails, in which they undergo a developmental cycle. Cercariae are liberated from the snails during rainy periods and become massed in "slime balls" shed on vegetation as the snail crawls. These slime balls, each of which contains a large number of cercariae, are eaten by ants. In this host, the cercariae become encysted to form metacercariae. For humans to acquire this disease, they must ingest an infected ant! Drabick and associates (1988) report a case, considered by them *not* to be a spurious infection, acquired through ingestion of bottled water contaminated by ants.

The adult worm is easily distinguishable from *Clonorchis* in that its testes are slightly lobed and situated in the anterior third of the body, while in *Clonorchis* they are highly

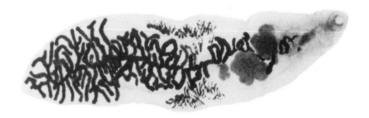

FIGURE 6-12 ■ *Dicrocoelium dendriticum.* (Photomicrograph by Zane Price.)

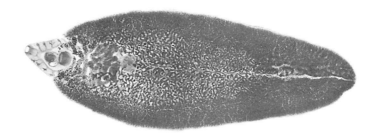

FIGURE 6-13 ■ *Fasciola hepatica.* (Photomicrograph by Zane Price.)

branched and in the posterior third. The eggs, passed in the feces, are dark brown in color, are thick shelled, and have a large operculum. They measure 38 to 45 μm in length by 22 to 30 μm in breadth.

Symptoms and Pathogenesis. Human infections are almost invariably light and often asymptomatic. Biliary colic and digestive disturbances have been described. With the heavy infections sometimes seen in animals, enlargement of the bile ducts and hyperplasia of biliary epithelium may occur, with periductal fibrosis and eventual portal cirrhosis.

Treatment. The patient previously referred to (Drabick et al., 1988) was treated with praziquantel, 20 mg/kg body weight three times in 1 day, with apparent success.

Fasciola hepatica

The sheep liver fluke *F. hepatica* (Figs. 6-13 and 6-14) is a common parasite of herbivores and one that is cosmopolitan in its distribution. Human infections have been reported from many areas of the world and are of considerable importance in parts of South America. A minimum of 350,000 human infections is estimated for the highlands of Bolivia, with similarly high rates of infection in corresponding areas of Peru; in other South American countries human infections are sporadic, though the disease is prevalent in cattle in Uruguay, Argentina, and Chile (Hillyer and Apt, 1997). In Cuba, southern France, and Algeria, human infections are not uncommon.

Fasciola is a large fluke, measuring as much as 3 cm long and nearly 1.5 cm in width. It has a characteristic "cephalic cone" at the anterior end. The adult worms reside in the larger biliary passages and the gallbladder. Infection follows consumption of aquatic vegetation upon which metacercariae of *Fasciola* have encysted (Fig. 6-15), which presupposes exposure of such vegetation to the feces of infected animals. Human cases can usually be traced to watercress or similar plants, taken from water to which herbivores have access. Spurious infections, in which eggs ingested during the consumption of infected liver appear in the stools, may be detected by reexamination of the stools at a time when such food has not been ingested. Most human infections reported from this country are seen in immigrants or travelers (Price et al., 1993).

Unlike the opisthorchids, which enter the biliary tree by passing through the ampulla of Vater and ascending the common bile duct, *Fasciola* metacercariae burrow into and through the duodenal wall, migrate actively across the peritoneal cavity, and enter the bile ducts by way of Glisson's capsule and the liver parenchyma. It is not surprising that some are lost on the way and occasionally may develop in the peritoneal cavity or other ectopic foci. Eggs of *Fasciola* are found in the feces but cannot readily be differentiated from those of *fasciolopsis* (see Fig. 6-4) and the echinostomes. They are operculated and measure 130 to 150 μm in length and 63 to 90 μm in breadth. Use of the enteric capsule (EnteroTest) may be helpful in recovering eggs and making a differential diagnosis.

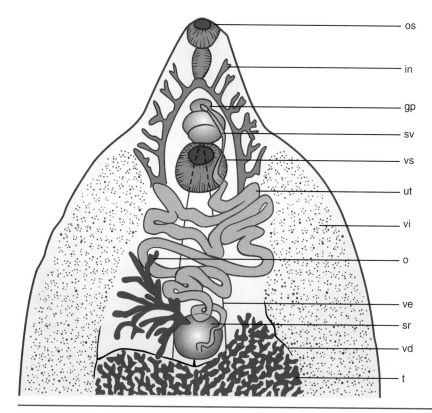

FIGURE 6-14 ■ *Fasciola hepatica,* anterior end of worm: *(gp)* genital pore; *(in)* intestine; *(o)* ovary; *(os)* oral sucker; *(sr)* seminal receptacle; *(sv)* seminal vesicle; *(t)* testis; *(ut)* uterus; *(vd)* vitelline duct; *(ve)* vas efferens; *(vi)* vitellaria; *(vs)* ventral sucker. Drawing made with the aid of a camera lucida but somewhat diagrammatic.

Symptoms. Because of the size of these worms, even light infections (though often asymptomatic) may produce signs and symptoms of biliary obstruction and cholangitis. Fever, chills, right-upper-quadrant pain with radiation to the scapula, jaundice, an enlarged tender liver, and eosinophilia may appear and prove puzzling unless eggs are found in the stool or biliary aspirate. The adult worms may be visualized in the liver by means of ultrasonography. Computed tomography with enhancement may demonstrate the burrow tracts made by worms migrating in the liver parenchyma, and dilatation of the bile ducts; endoscopic retrograde cholangiopancreatography may show the worms in the pancreatic duct (Han et al., 1993).

A pharyngeal form of the disease, known as halzoun, has been described in the Middle East and results from eating raw animal liver infected with *Fasciola.* Young adult worms attach to the pharyngeal mucosa, causing pain, bleeding, and edema that sometimes interfere with respiration.

Pathogenesis. In human infections, symptoms are occasionally seen that suggest that there may be considerable local irritation during the migration of the young worms to the liver. In sheep, migration through the liver parenchyma gives rise to such massive tissue destruction that the disease at this stage is known as liver rot. Once established in the bile ducts, the worms may produce both mechanical and toxic effects, which differ from those seen with infection by the opisthorchids or *Dicrocoelium* only inasmuch as *Fasciola* is a larger and more powerful worm. Mechanical irritation, the effects of toxic metabolites of the worms on host

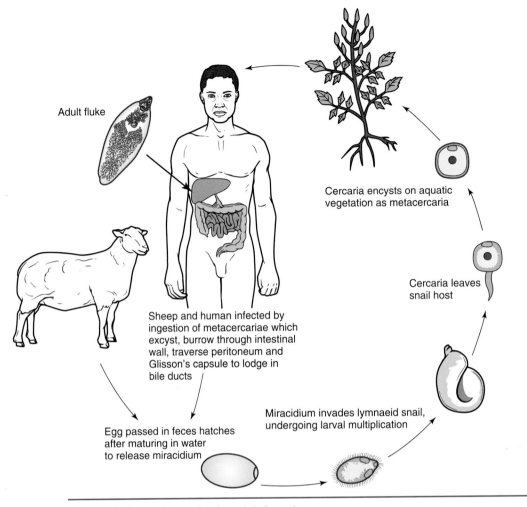

Adult fluke

Cercaria encysts on aquatic
vegetation as metacercaria

Cercaria leaves
snail host

Sheep and human infected by
ingestion of metacercariae which
excyst, burrow through intestinal
wall, traverse peritoneum and
Glisson's capsule to lodge in
bile ducts

Miracidium invades lymnaeid snail,
undergoing larval multiplication

Egg passed in feces hatches
after maturing in water
to release miracidium

FIGURE 6-15 ■ Life cycle of *Fasciola hepatica.*

tissue, and mechanical obstruction may bring about hyperplasia of the biliary epithelium, proliferation of connective tissue around the ducts, and partial or total biliary obstruction. The adult worms may erode through the walls of the bile ducts to invade once again the liver parenchyma. Secondary bacterial infection may occur; portal cirrhosis is usually the final outcome in severe infections.

Treatment. Bithionol,* administered orally at the rate of 30 to 50 mg/kg every other day for 10 to 15 doses, is recommended for treatment of fascioliasis. Its use is associated with frequent photosensitivity skin reactions, urticaria, vomiting, diarrhea, and abdominal pains (see further discussion under treatment of *Paragonimus*). Praziquantel, even when given at the rate of 25 mg/kg three times daily for 5 to 7 days, seems only to lessen the severity of infection. Dehydroemetine and albendazole have likewise been found to give unsatisfactory results. A more promising drug is triclabendazole, unfortunately approved only for veterinary use in the United States. The drug is well tolerated, and doses of 10 mg/kg body weight twice in 1 day produce cure rates approaching 100% (Apt et al., 1995; Rictiter et al., 2002) Triclabendazole (Egaten; Novartis) is available from Victoria Pharmacy, Zurich, Switzerland.

---

*Available from the CDC Drug Service, Centers for Disease Control and Prevention. U.S. Public Health Service, Atlanta, Georgia, 30333; (404) 639-3670.

Control. Infection follows consumption of aquatic vegetation upon which metacercariae of *Fasciola* have become encysted (see Fig. 6-3). Human cases can usually be traced to infected watercress, which should never be grown for human use in water to which herbivores have access. Spurious infections, in which eggs ingested by the consumption of infected liver appear in the stool, may be detected by reexamining the patient's stools at a time when he or she has not consumed such food.

Fasciola gigantica

The giant liver fluke *F. gigantica* may attain a length of 7.4 cm. It has a more attenuated shape than has *F. hepatica*, from which it also differs in some details of structure. *F. gigantica* is a parasite of herbivores, particularly camels, cattle, and water buffalo in Africa and the Orient. It has been introduced into other areas, and human cases have been reported from several regions, including Hawaii.

The life cycle of the parasite is very similar to that of *F. hepatica*, and the clinical picture in the two infections is also much alike. The eggs of *F. gigantica* (Plate X) are large, measuring 150 to 190 μm by 70 to 90 μm.

The Blood Flukes

Three species of schistosomes that parasitize humans are of major importance: *Schistosoma mansoni, S. japonicum,* and *S. haematobium*. Less common are *Schistosoma intercalatum* in Africa and *Schistosoma mekongi* in the Mekong Basin. Although the adult worms live in the blood vascular system, the eggs of *S. mansoni, S. japonicum, S. intercalatum,* and *S. mekongi* are generally found in the feces. Eggs of *S. haematobium* are occasionally seen in the stool but usually occur in the urine.

The schistosomes differ in a number of ways from other trematodes. They are diecious (i.e., the sexes are separate), and the two sexes are dissimilar in appearance. Female worms are long (1.2 to 2.6 cm) and slender, with a body almost circular in cross section and 0.3 mm or less in diameter. Male worms (Fig. 6-16) are 0.6 to 2.2 cm long, and although the body is flattened behind the ventral sucker, it looks cylindrical, as it is characteristically incurved ventrally to form a gynecophoral canal in which the female reposes (Figs. 6-17 and 6-18).

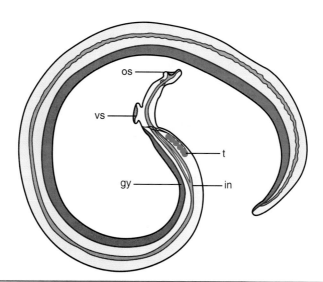

FIGURE 6-16 ■ *Schistosoma mansoni,* male: *(gy)* gynecophoral canal; *(in)* intestine; *(os)* oral sucker; *(t)* testes; *(vs)* ventral sucker.

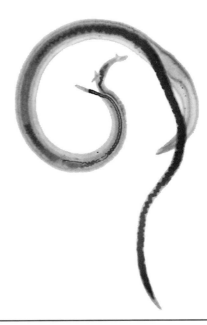

FIGURE 6-17 ■ *Schistosoma mansoni, male and female in copula.* (Photomicrograph by Zane Price.)

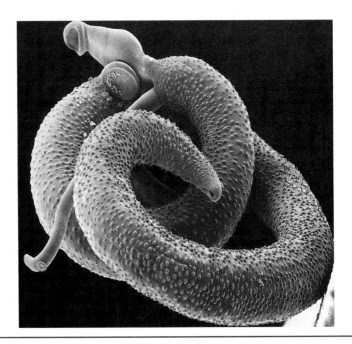

FIGURE 6-18 ■ Scanning electron micrograph of male and female *Schistosoma mansoni.* (Courtesy of Dr. Ming-Ming Wong.)

The body structure of the schistosomes, and particularly that of the long, thin females, seems clearly an adaptation to an intravascular existence. The females leave the male worms to deposit their eggs in small venules close to the lumen of the intestine or bladder. The worms dilate the vessels when they penetrate into them for oviposition and withdraw as the eggs are laid, so that the eggs are wedged firmly into the small vessels. Sharp spines on the

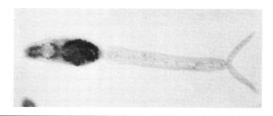

FIGURE 6-19 ■ Cercaria of *Schistosoma mansoni* showing penetration glands. (Courtesy of Dr. David Bruckner, University of California Los Angeles School of Medicine.)

eggs of *S. mansoni* and *S. haematobium* probably assist in their retention in the blood vessels. An enzyme elaborated by the miracidium diffuses through the egg shell and helps to digest the overlying tissue. The action of this enzyme, together with necrosis of the tissue caused by pressure and the effect of the spine, works to liberate the egg from the tissues into the lumen of the intestine or bladder. Schistosome eggs are not operculated, and they hatch by rupture if liberated into fresh water. The miracidium that escapes swims in search of an appropriate snail host. If successful, it penetrates the snail, where it undergoes a cycle of development, giving rise to a large number of cercariae infective for humans.

All other trematode parasites of humans are acquired through ingestion of metacercariae, but infection with schistosomes follows exposure to water in which infected snails have liberated their cercariae. Human infection takes place by direct penetration of the cercariae through the skin to invade the circulatory system. Cercariae of the schistosome parasites (Fig. 6-19), both of humans and of other animals, have a forked tail and glands at the anterior end that assist penetration through the skin. During this process, the tail is lost, and profound metabolic changes take place (e.g., an almost instantaneous change from aerobic to anaerobic respiration). The immature fluke, referred to as a schistosomulum, remains in the subcutaneous tissues for about 2 days. After invasion of a blood vessel, the young flukes are carried to the lungs and thence to the liver sinusoids, where they begin their growth. Two weeks or longer after infection, the maturing worms commence a migration against the flow of the blood in the portal system to their final location in mesenteric or vesicular veins. Their final locations in the host differ in the different species and will be discussed separately for each.

Schistosoma mansoni

A consequence of the African slave trade was the establishment of *S. mansoni* (Fig. 6-20) in the Western Hemisphere. This fluke, which occurs over extensive areas of Africa and in the Arabian peninsula and Malagasy, has also become well established in Brazil, Surinam, and Venezuela, as well as in parts of the Caribbean. Of special interest is infection in Puerto Rico. The influx of people from this island into New York and other larger cities has resulted in a more frequent diagnosis of schistomiasis mansoni in this country. It does not seem to present a public health problem, however, and there is little reason to expect that the infection could become successfully established in North American snail hosts.

Adults of *S. mansoni* usually live in the smaller branches of the inferior mesenteric vein in the region of the lower colon. They may be found elsewhere in the portal system, in the vesical venous plexus, or in other ectopic foci on occasion. They subsist on ingested blood. *S. mansoni* is the smallest of the schistosomes that infect humans: males attain a length of only 1 cm and females an extreme length of 1.6 cm. Although they have been found on rare occasions infecting both African and West Indian monkeys and rodents in Africa and South America, it is not thought that any of these animals is of importance as a reservoir host.

Diagnosis during the acute period of the disease is based on the recovery of the characteristic eggs in the stool. The light yellowish brown eggs (Plate X; see Fig. 6-4, *B*) measure 114 to 118 µm by 45 to 73 µm. They are elongate, regularly ovoid, and possess

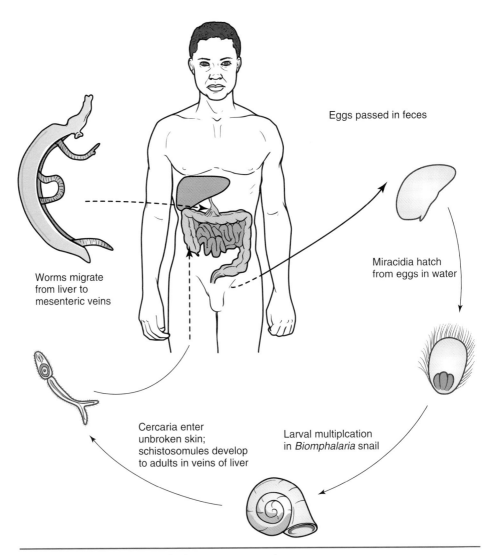

Eggs passed in feces

Worms migrate
from liver to
mesenteric veins

Miracidia hatch
from eggs in water

Cercaria enter
unbroken skin;
schistosomules develop
to adults in veins of liver

Larval multiplcation
in *Biomphalaria* snail

FIGURE 6-20 ■ Life cycle of *Schistosoma mansoni.*

a large lateral spine, shaped rather like a rose thorn, which projects from the side of the egg near one pole. In the chronic stage of the disease, eggs may not be found in the stools. Rectal biopsy may be of value in such cases, as eggs can be demonstrated in the tissue (Fig. 6-21) by flattening between two glass slides and examination under the microscope. Adequate sampling involves taking four snips, on the anterior, posterior, and both lateral walls. Various specialized techniques employed in the laboratory diagnosis of schistosmiasis are described in Chapter 14. Serologic tests are discussed in Chapter 16.

Schistosoma japonicum

The Oriental blood fluke *S. japonicum* (Fig. 6-22) is confined to the Far East, where it occurs in parts of China (including Taiwan), Japan, the Philippiness, and Indonesia (Sulawesi). Unlike *S. mansoni*, which rarely infects other animals, *S. japonicum* is found in virtually all mammals exposed to infected water. During World War II, larger numbers of American and Australian troops serving on the island of Leyte in the Philippines acquired the infection. Vigorous control measures, involving both patient treatment and snail eradication, have resulted in marked reduction in prevalence of this infection in recent years.

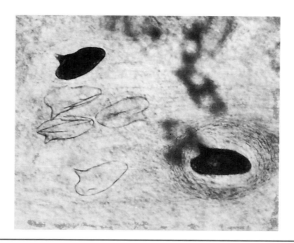

FIGURE 6-21 ■ *Schistosoma mansoni* eggs, as seen in rectal biopsy. (Courtesy of Dr. W. Jann Brown, University of California Los Angeles School of Medicine.)

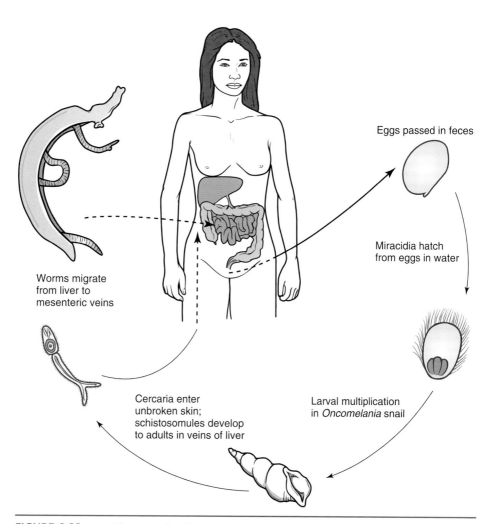

FIGURE 6-22 ■ Life cycle of *Schistosoma japonicum.*

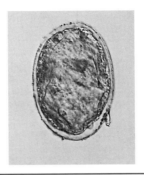

FIGURE 6-23 ■ Egg of *Schistosoma japonicum*. Material for this figure courtesy of the Shanghai Institute for Parisitic Diseases, the People's Republic of China. (Photomicrograph by Zane Price.)

S. japonicum adults inhabit the branches of the superior mesenteric vein adjacent to the small intestine; the inferior mesenteries and caval system may also be invaded, as the worms tend in time to migrate farther and farther from the liver. The males may reach a length of 2.2 cm and the females 2.6 cm. This species produces more eggs than the other two schistosomes, and the eggs are smaller and more nearly spherical. For a combination of these reasons, more eggs become free in the general circulation, to be filtered out in the liver, lungs, or other organs. Infection with even a few worms of this species may be very serious. Hepatic and pulmonary cirrhosis are commonly seen in the chronic stage of this infection, and CNS symptoms may occur following lodgment of eggs in or near nerve tissue.

Diagnosis may be made by identification of the eggs in the stool. The eggs are spherical to oval in shape (Plate X; see Fig. 6-4, *E*). They may have a minute lateral spine (Fig. 6-23), but this structure may be absent in some strains. The size range is from 55 to 85 μm by 40 to 60 μm. Examination for eggs should be carried out as indicated for *S. mansoni*. Rectal biopsy is sometimes helpful in making the diagnosis in chronic cases, as are serologic tests (see Chapter 16).

Schistosoma haematobium

Urinary schistosomiasis is generally caused by *S. haematobium* (Fig. 6-24) although, as has been mentioned, the other two species may sometimes inhabit the vesical plexus. The original focus of this disease was apparently the Nile Valley, where it is highly endemic. From there it has spread widely throughout Africa and now occurs also in the islands off the east coast of that continent, in Asia Minor, on the island of Cyprus, and in southern Portugal. There is an isolated focus in India, and it has recently been introduced into Jordan.

After the worms mature in the sinusoids of the liver, they migrate from that organ, and in the case of *S. haematobium* the majority of them reach the vesical, prostatic, and uterine plexuses by way of the hemorrhoidal veins. Adult male worms may reach a length of 1.5 cm, and the females 2 cm. The eggs are deposited in the walls of the bladder or to a lesser extent in the uterus, vaginal wall, prostate, or other organs. Those deposited in the wall of the bladder may break through into the lumen and escape with the urine.

Diagnosis is most readily made by recovery of the characteristic eggs (Plate X; see Fig. 6-4, *C*) by centrifugation or sedimentation of the urine. Containers used for collection of urine specimens must not contain preservatives if the hatching test is to be done (see Chapter 14). The eggs contain a fully developed miracidium when deposited and are from 112 to 170 μm in length and 40 to 70 μm in breadth. They have a conspicuous terminal spine and are a light yellowish brown color. Terminal hematuria in a patient from the endemic areas should make one highly suspicious of this infection. It may be possible to find the eggs in biopsy material from the bladder wall, the uterine cervix, or the vagina. See Chapter 16 for serologic tests.

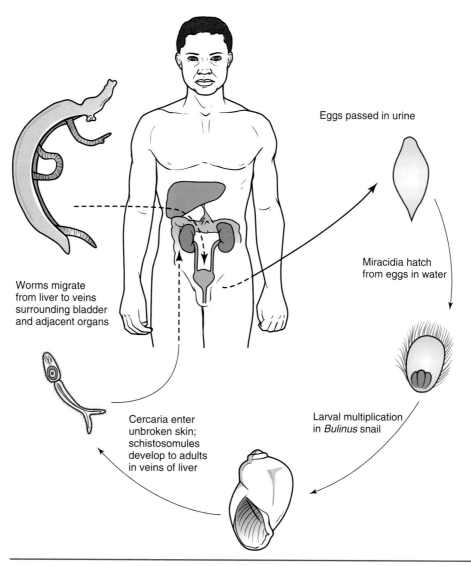

Eggs passed in urine

Miracidia hatch from eggs in water

Worms migrate from liver to veins surrounding bladder and adjacent organs

Larval multiplication in *Bulinus* snail

Cercaria enter unbroken skin; schistosomules develop to adults in veins of liver

FIGURE 6-24   ■   Life cycle of *Schistosoma haematobium*.

Schistosoma mekongi

A schistosome from the Mekong River basin in southern Laos and Cambodia resembles *S. japonicum* in adult structure and in its ability to infect vertebrate hosts other than humans, but it has a different snail intermediate host and seems to produce a milder disease in humans. Domestic pigs have been shown to be reservoir hosts for *S. mekongi* in Laos (Strandgaard et al., 2001). The eggs of *S. mekongi* are consistently smaller than those of *S. japonicum*, having a size range of 30 to 55 μm by 50 to 65 μm. Those of *S. japonicum* show regional size differences, but the overall size range is 40 to 60 μm by 55 to 85 μm. Human infections with a schistosome having eggs of a similar size have also been reported from Malaysia. The identity of this latter schistosome remains to be determined.

Schistosoma intercalatum

This species occurs in humans in Western and Central Africa. Adult worms are found in the mesenteric vessels, and eggs are voided in the feces. The eggs of *S. intercalatum* closely resemble those of *S. haematobium* but can be differentiated by a slight bend in the terminal spine

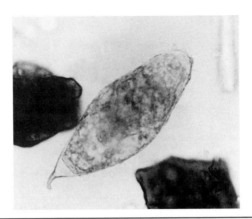

FIGURE 6-25 ■ Egg of *Schistosoma intercalatum.* Note curvature of terminal spine. (From Odongo-Aginya et al. *Am J Trop Med Hyg* 1994; *55*:724. Courtesy of the authors.)

(Fig. 6-25); the egg shell is Ziehl-Neelsen positive, whereas those of the other schistosomes are not. A cross-sectional survey of more than 1200 persons in the city of Bata, Equatorial Guinea, revealed an overall prevalence of 21% *S. intercalatum* infection. This was the only schistosome found in stools or urine in this area. Peak prevalence and highest parasite load were in 5- to 14-year-old children.

The disease produced by this infection is relatively benign, and hepatomegaly is usually not marked. There may be severe digestive disturbances accompanied by pain and bloody stools.

SYMPTOMS

Before we discuss symptoms in detail, it must be emphasized that many patients with brief exposure to schistosomiasis (i.e., travelers) may have either no symptoms or symptoms that do not differ materially from those of noninfected control travelers. This seems to be more true of those infected with *S. mansoni* than of those who acquire *S. haematobium*, although acute symptoms, occurring in a small percentage of patients, are more likely to been seen in *S. mansoni* infections. As even a mild infection may lead to serious complications, it is good to perform serologic tests on all travelers who give a history of possible exposure to infection and to treat all those who prove to be infected.

Following penetration of the skin by cercariae of a schistosome that infects humans, a transient reaction may be seen. Petechial hemorrhages occur at the site of penetration, with some localized edema and pruritus, which reach a maximum in 24 to 36 hours and disappear in 4 days or less. During the succeeding 3 weeks there may be transient toxic and allergic manifestations. These may be mild and may pass unnoticed, or there may be generalized malaise, fever, giant urticaria, vague intestinal complaints, and so forth, partly depending on the intensity of infection. Migration of the worms throughout the lungs may cause cough or hemoptysis. Soon after the developing schistosomes reach the liver, acute hepatitis may develop.

When the flukes reach the mesenteric or vesical venules and egg laying commences, the acute stage of the disease is seen. The onset of this stage may occur 1 to 3 months after infection. Symptoms of the acute stage may range from mild to severe, and the degree of reaction is not necessarily proportional to the number of parasites involved. Clinical disease at this stage is usually seen only in relatively heavy infection or in persons recently arrived in an endemic area. With the extrusion of eggs through the wall of the intestine or bladder, there may once again be generalized malaise, fever, urticaria, abdominal pain, and liver tenderness. In *S. mansoni* or *S. japonicum* infections there may be diarrhea or dysentery at this stage, while in *S. haematobium* infections there is often hematuria at the end of micturition, and sometimes dysuria.

In schistosomiasis japonicum the early symptoms tend to be quite severe in heavily infected persons, with abrupt onset of fever, chills, and the other signs and symptoms mentioned previously coming from 4 to 6 weeks after infection. There is often a significant mortality rate at this stage of the disease, which is called Katayama fever for the locality in Japan from which it was first described. A Katayama-like syndrome may be seen with the other types of schistosomiasis, but is not as common.

The chronic stage of the disease comes on gradually. Egg deposition takes place in the smaller vessels, close to the lumen of the intestine or bladder. Many eggs remain where deposited; secretions of the contained miracidia evoke the formation of minute abscesses around them, and they are liberated into the lumen of the affected organ. Other eggs are dislodged and swept into the circulation; it is these embolic eggs that produce most of the pathologic changes seen in chronic schistosomiasis.

Hepatosplenic schistosomiasis, the most common form of chronic infection in patients with *S. mansoni* or *s. japonicum*, also occurs regularly in *S. haematobium* infections, but tends to be subclinical or mild in schistosomiasis japonicum. Hepatic parenchymal damage, unresolved after successful treatment with praziquantel, may be found in approximately 50% of patients with *S. japonicum* infections (Watt et al., 1991). Eggs, carried back through the mesenteric vessels, lodge in the liver, where granulomas form around them. Over a period of time, which may range from as little as 18 months in heavy infections to many years in lighter ones, the liver becomes grossly enlarged and the left lobe disproportionately so. The chronically enlarged liver is not tender. The spleen may be barely palpable or massively enlarged. Portal hypertension, resulting from the obstructive liver disease, leads to esophageal varices, which may bleed, and finally to massive ascites (see Fig. 6-26).

Intestinal schistosomiasis is also more common in *S. mansoni* and *S. japonicum* infections, although not unknown in schistosomiasis haematobium. The disease may involve the entire intestinal tract but is more likely to be confined to the large bowel. It may present a picture suggestive of granulomatous colitis, with abdominal cramps and tenderness and intermittent

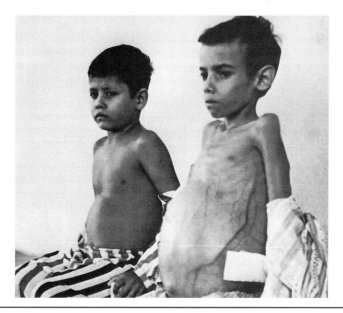

FIGURE 6-26 ■ Schistosomiasis mansoni. Note development of collateral circulation secondary to severe hepatic involvement. (Photograph by F. Etges. From Zaiman H [ed.]. *A pictorial presentation of parasites.*)

bloody mucoid stools. Intestinal polyposis is not uncommon in schistosomiasis mansoni, and in such patients the diarrhea is more pronounced, and the protein-losing enteropathy results in marked weight loss and anemia. Colonoscopy is often the most successful means of diagnosing this condition.

Hepatosplenic and intestinal involvement are present in every case of *S. mansoni* or *S. japonicum* infection, but clinically one or the other almost always predominates. In their more advanced forms, they are usually readily diagnosed, although the hepatosplenic form of the disease can be confused with other conditions such as chronic viral hepatitis and protein malnutrition, and the intestinal form with granulomatous colitis.

Urinary schistosomiasis is seen with *S. haematobium* infections, and as with the other two types of disease, light infections are usually asymptomatic. Dysuria, urinary frequency, and hematuria are early symptoms and signs, but in endemic areas they are so frequent as to be in large measure disregarded—in fact, hematuria is so common among adolescent boys in the Nile River valley as to have been widely considered a phenomenon analogous to the menarche in girls. Terminal hematuria is usually the first sign of infection. Eosinophiluria (see Chapter 12) is a constant finding in urinary schistosomiasis. Chronic bacteriuria is common. Obstructive uropathy occurs primarily in persons with high total egg burdens. Bladder cancer, usually a squamous cell carcinoma, is seen much more frequently in patients with heavy *S. haematobium* infections than in the general population, and occurs primarily in areas of the bladder where there has been heavy egg deposition. It is thought that these heavy egg concentrations promote urothelial carcinogenesis. A nephrotic syndrome is occasionally seen in both *S. mansoni* and *S. haematobium* infections; immune complex nephropathy has occasionally been demonstrated.

Pulmonary involvement may be seen in all forms of schistosomiasis but is more common with *S. haematobium* infections. Egg deposition in the lungs leads to fibrosis of the pulmonary bed and resultant cor pulmonale, characterized by exertional dyspnea, cough, and occasional hemoptysis. Dilatation of the pulmonary arteries and right ventricular enlargement may be evident on x-ray examination, and there may be electrocardiographic evidence of right ventricular hypertrophy and strain.

Cerebral manifestations of schistosomiasis are most commonly seen in *S. japonicum* infections but may also be caused by *S. haematobium* and *S. mansoni*, which more frequently affect the spinal cord. Early in the course of the disease, more generalized neurologic symptoms, such as lethargy and confusion, may occur and have been thought to have a toxic cause. Later, focal neurologic symptoms are probably due to egg deposition in the cerebral or spinal cord vasculature and subsequent inflammatory reaction around them. Focal and generalized seizures, speech difficulties, and optical field defects characterize the cerebral infection.

Transverse myelitis, usually in the lumbar area, is seen in spinal cord involvement. That such involvement may come on very early is seen in a report concerning 18 American students participating in a travel-study program in Kenya. The students were exposed to schistosomiasis by bathing in a small stream, which they dammed for that purpose. Within 2½ to 3 months, 2 of the students developed rapidly progressive weakness and flaccid paralysis of the lower limbs, and another 12 had fever, diarrhea, malaise, and weight loss. These 14 and 1 asymptomatic student were found to have *S. mansoni* infections.

IMMUNOLOGY AND PATHOGENESIS

Immunologic processes have been more exhaustively studied in schistosomiasis than in any other worm disease. They are complex and not fully understood, and they will be discussed in brief outline. In part, the complexity results from profound antigenic differences among the various stages of the life cycle within the human host: cercaria, schistosomulum, adult worm, and egg.

A mild localized reaction, perhaps mediated by cercaria-provoked histamine release by mast cells, may be seen on initial infection though a marked dermal reaction is unusual in persons who had no previous exposure. When such a local reaction occurs, it subsides within about a week. In previously infected, immunocompetent hosts, schistosomula are subject to two kinds of antibody-dependent cell-mediated cytotoxic assault. Antischistosomular antibodies cover the parasites, and the Fc portions of the IgG antibodies attach to the Fc receptors of eosinophils, which degranulate with the release of eosinophilic major basic protein, with consequent damage to the schistosomular membrane and possible death of the parasite. Macrophages may also contribute to elimination of the parasites at this stage, through the action of specific IgE, effecting the release of lysosomal enzymes from these cells.

After a few days within the host, the schistosomules either become covered with host antigens or produce antigens that so resemble those of the host that the antibody-related responses mentioned above no longer are effective. The maturing schistosomule and the adult worm do not evoke a measurable protective response on the part of the host, although it is possible to detect in vitro antibodies produced against the adult worms. This may be something of a trade-off; although the host is not well protected against the adult worms, these worms do not cause any apparent damage to the host; however, the "immunologic camouflage" that protects the adult worm does not extend to its eggs.

Early in *S. mansoni* infections, local damage caused by egg deposition and abscess formation may give rise to schistosomal dysentery, accompanied by abdominal pain, cramping, and frequent bloody or blood-flecked stools. There may be considerable hypertrophy of the affected sections of bowel (Fig. 6-27) with polyp formation. Fibrosis of the submucosa in areas of egg deposition has long been advanced to explain the decrease in egg passage that is noted as the infection progresses.

Eggs swept back to the liver with the portal blood flow lodge in the finer branches of the portal system. Around them granulomas develop. Granuloma formation is responsible for

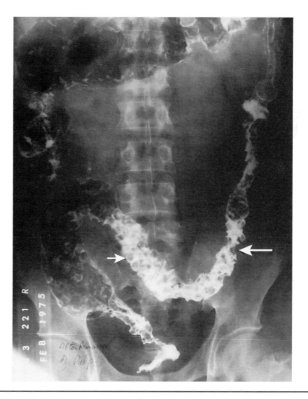

FIGURE 6-27 ■ Schistosomiasis mansoni from the Nile delta. Multiple strictures *(large arrow)* in ascending colon and rectum, with multiple polyps *(small arrow)* and much altered mucosal pattern. (Courtesy of Dr. N. Avad El-Nasry, U.S. Naval Medical Research Unit 3, Cairo, Egypt.)

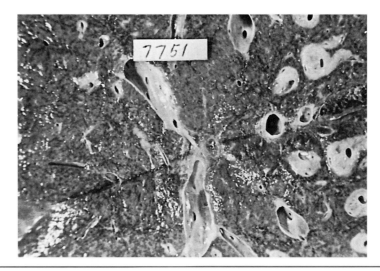

FIGURE 6-28 ▪ *Schistosoma mansoni.* Human liver showing "pipestem" fibrosis. (Photograph by L. Millman. From Zaiman H [ed.]. *A pictorial presentation of parasites.*)

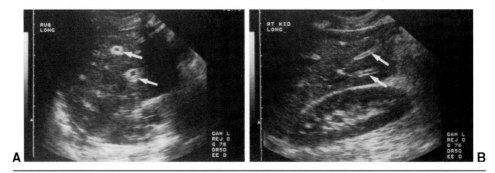

FIGURE 6-29 ▪ Sonogram of liver shows schistosomal periportal fibrosis. **A,** Liver. **B,** Liver above normal kidney. Both show dense echogenic bands *(arrows)* surrounding intrahepatic portal radicles. (Courtesy of Dr. Lester Hollander, Kaiser Foundation Hospital, Oakland, CA.)

much of the pathology associated with schistosomiasis, which would be worse were it not for the fascinating though incompletely understood process of immunologic modulation, which results (in the *S. mansoni*-infected mouse model and presumably in humans) in a reduction, after some weeks, in the granulomatous reaction around the eggs. Modulating mechanisms have been shown to include both cellular and humoral elements and to be T-cell dependent. They are not exhibited by athymic (Nu/Nu) mice. If the infection is heavy enough, periportal fibrosis may develop as well. This fibrous tissue may finally come to surround the branches of the portal vein in a thick white layer, visible grossly as the "clay pipestem" fibrosis of Symmers (Fig. 6-28). Ultrasonograms of the liver (Fig. 6-29) clearly and characteristically demonstrate periportal fibrosis, the severity of which can be graded and which (at least in the Sudan) may occur in children younger than 8 years. Such periportal fibrosis has been reported in about 20% of patients who die of schistosomiasis or its complications. The majority of patients exhibit granuloma formation around eggs in the liver and fibrosis of small portal tracts but no generalized liver involvement. Cirrhosis is no more common than in uninfected controls. On the other hand, cirrhosis is very commonly seen in Egyptian patients with this disease, possibly because of nutritional factors. Even if cirrhosis does not develop, evidence of marked portal hypertension (splenomegaly, esophageal varices) is seen in nearly all patients with Symmers' fibrosis. Cor pulmonale (Fig. 6-30) has

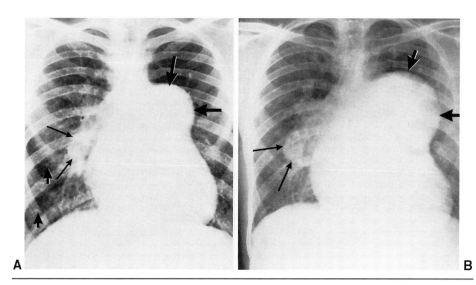

FIGURE 6-30 ▪ Pulmonary schistosomiasis: Progressive pulmonary hypertension and cor pulmonale. **A,** There are numerous linear and nodular densities in the pulmonary parenchyma *(short broad arrows).* The heart is enlarged, and the right pulmonary arteries are greatly enlarged *(slender arrows).* The main pulmonary artery *(large broad arrows)* is almost aneurysmal. **B,** Three years later, the main pulmonary artery *(short broad arrows)* has increased further in size; the heart and right pulmonary artery *(slender arrows)* are also much larger. The pulmonary markings are considerably decreased, owing to obliteration of the peripheral pulmonary vasculature. The extreme dilatation of the pulmonary artery caused by pulmonary schistosomiasis is unequaled by almost any other disease. (Courtesy of Z. Farid, Cairo, Egypt.)

been reported in over 15% of patients with periportal fibrosis. The collateral circulation that develops in severe hepatosplenic schistosomiasis mansoni and japonicum carries eggs past the hepatic bed and into the pulmonary capillaries, where they lodge and granuloma formation takes place. Eggs of *S. haematobium* may bypass the liver entirely. Venous blood from the vesical, prostatic, and uterine plexuses enters the hypogastric vein, from whence it goes by way of the common iliac vein to the vena cava, the right heart, and the lungs.

Eggs of *S. japonicum* may be deposited at any point along the distribution of the microvascular tributaries to the superior mesenteric vein and those of *S. mansoni* in the corresponding venules leading to the inferior mesenteric vein. The eggs that escape into the lumen of the intestine cause permanent damage, but those that are unable to escape provoke the formation of granulomas and an intense inflammatory reaction, with fibrosis and patchy ulceration. Adhesions to other loops of bowel and to mesentery and constrictions secondary to the fibrosis compound the functional problems. Polyps may form from masses of eggs deposited in the submucosa, with their surrounding granulomas, and if in the rectum may prolapse through the anal sphincter.

Urinary symptoms usually are not seen for 3 to 6 months after infection with *S. haematobium* and may not develop for a year or more. As the bladder wall becomes increasingly infiltrated with eggs that have become entrapped, and around which granulomas form, papillomas appear, and there may be areas of ulceration. Ultrasonography detects bladder wall irregularities and polyps (but not calcification) and congestive changes in the kidneys. Obstruction of the ureteral openings or of the neck of the bladder may lead to back pressure and a predisposition to ascending bacterial infection. The subsequent involvement of ureters and kidneys is similar to that seen in urinary tract obstruction from any source (Fig. 6-31). The uterine cervix is the most common site of *S. haematobium* infection in women, and granulomatous inflammation of the cervix is a common manifestation (Poggensee et al., 2001). In males, heavy infections may involve the urethra, prostate, seminal vesicles, and even

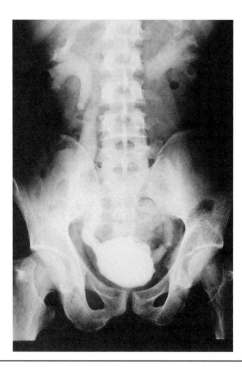

FIGURE 6-31 ■ Hydronephrosis and hydroureter in patient with schistosomiasis haematobium.

the spermatic cord and penis. Elephantiasis of the penis may follow blockage of scrotal lymphatics by egg deposition and subsequent granuloma formation. Both *S. haematobium* and *S. mansoni* may invade the placenta to give rise to a granulomatous placentitis, with adults and eggs of *S. mansoni* in the intervillous spaces and decidual vessels.

Neurologic involvement is facilitated by anastomoses among mesenteric, pelvic, and spinal veins, the means by which both the worms and their eggs can reach the central nervous system. Inflammatory reactions around them may produce focal lesions. Symptoms of spinal cord schistosomiasis may occur early in the course of the infection, particularly in immunologically naive persons, and the rapidly progressive myelopathies are believed to represent hypersensitivity reactions to the deposited eggs. Transverse myelitis is generally rare, and eggs have been found on autopsy in the spinal cord of persons who had no symptoms of spinal cord involvement.

An association between chronic salmonellosis and schistosomiasis has been reported from many areas, involving all three of the major species of human schistosomes. There is usually a long history of a mild febrile illness, with frequent isolation of one or another species of *Salmonella* from the blood. *Salmonella* has on occasion been cultured from the treatment of adult schistosomes removed surgically from patients with chronic salmonellosis.

EPIDEMIOLOGY

Even though *S. mansoni* is widely distributed throughout the world, humans are apparently the only important host in most areas of high endemicity. In Africa, nonhuman primates, insectivores, and wild rodents are found to harbor the schistosomes, whereas in Brazil several species of marsupials and rodents carry the infection. The importance of these reservoir hosts in maintaining and spreading the disease to humans probably varies from one area to the next.

Extension of the disease into new areas still occurs with the migration of infection people and the agricultural development of virgin land where the snail vector is present. Irrigation and the establishment of artificial bodies of water, combined with unsanitary practices, may quickly result in new foci of high endemicity. Since the snail intermediate host is entirely aquatic, the aqueous environment (water flow, vegetation, water temperature, and pH) determines snail density and distribution.

As far as is known, humans are the only important host for *S. haematobium*. The snail intermediate host apparently has less stringent requirements for water temperature than the snail host of *S. mansoni*. This may partly explain the relatively wide distribution of *S. haematobium* on the African continent. In some areas of high endemicity in East Africa, the snail lives in relatively small bodies of water that may dry up during part of the year. The snails then estivate while buried in the mud but retain the infection and resume shedding of cercariae when the rainy season begins. Thus, special adaptations of the snail host may be of prime importance in maintaining and perpetuating the disease in foci where water is not at all times plentiful.

The complexity of the epidemiologic problems of schistosomiasis is further enhanced in *S. japonicum* because so many domestic animals are efficient reservoirs of the infection. Cats, dogs, cattle, horses, and pigs, as well as some wild mammals, are susceptible and may show a high infection rate in certain areas. Prevention of the disease is further complicated by the semiaquatic habits of the snail intermediate hosts, which visit water only for the purpose of egg laying, so that molluscicides applied to the water are virtually useless. Rice, the staple crop in almost all areas where *S. japonicum* is endemic, grows in water, so infection of the agricultural population is a constant occupational hazard. It is estimated that about 80 million people are infected with *S. japonicum*.

TREATMENT

Praziquantel is the drug of choice for treatment of all schistosome infections. For infection with *S. mansoni*, *S. haematobium*, and *S. intercalatum*, a single dose of 40 mg/kg body weight produces cure rates of 63% to 90%, while three doses of 20 mg/kg body weight in a single day give rates that approach 100% in schistosomiasis mansoni and haematobium. This higher dose is required for successful treatment of *S. japonicum* or *S. mekongi*. Administration of the drug while the worms are in the schistosomula or immature stages seems to have little effect and may actually worsen acute-stage symptoms. In severe Katayama fever, steroids may be required initially, with definitive treatment postponed until the acute symptoms subside. Both periportal fibrosis and bladder wall thickening and polyps respond to praziquantel therapy as evaluated by ultrasonography. Yearly retreatment may be necessary in advanced cases. Praziquantel has been used in mass distribution programs and is shown to be safe to use during pregnancy (Adam et al., 2004).

Praziquantel in standard doses seems effective in cerebral schistosomiasis japonicum, and has proved so in the less common cerebral form of schistosomiasis haematobium (Pollner et al., 1994). Schistosomal transverse myelitis, seen most commonly in infections with *S. mansoni* and *S. haematobium*, does not respond well to praziquantel therapy alone; large doses of steroids may be needed, and laminectomy may be necessary for decompression.

Oxamniquine (Vasnil), 6-hydroxymethyl-2-isopropylamino-methyl-7-nitro-1,2,3, 4-tetrahydroquinoline, is effective for treatment of *S. mansoni* infections. Considerably less expensive than praziquantel, it may be preferred for mass treatment programs when dual infections do not exist. The effective dose depends on the origin of the infection. A single dose of 15 mg/kg body weight is suggested for adults who acquire their infection in South America, the Caribbean islands, and West Africa; for children from these areas, two doses of 10 mg/kg, at an interval of 3 to 8 hours, is suggested. In East and Central Africa and the Arabian peninsula, 15 mg/kg twice in 1 day is required. This must be increased to 20 mg/kg twice in 1 day in Ethiopia, Zaire, and the West Nile. Elsewhere in Egypt and in the Sudan and South Africa, 20 mg/kg daily for 3 days is recommended. Generalized seizures have been reported after the use of this drug but seem to be rare.

Metrifonate★ (Bilarcil), an organophosphorus compound, is an alternative to praziquantel for treatment of *S. haematobium* infections. It seems equally effective against any *S. mansoni* that are located in the perivesical plexus but not those in the mesenteric venules. The drug is administered orally, 10 mg/kg body weight, once every other week for a total of three doses. Side effects are transient and mild and include abdominal pain, diarrhea, vomiting, weakness, headache, and dizziness. A cure rate of about 90% is achieved 5 to 6 months after treatment.

CONTROL

Education is the prerequisite for all control measures, since without an understanding of the life cycle of the parasite, attempts at its eradication are doomed to failure. With education programs brought to the people, it has been demonstrated in areas such as China that progress can be made. Differences in the snail hosts of the various schistosome species in some cases dictate different control measures, which may involve mollusciciding, biologic control by means of snail-eating fish or birds (or even competing species of snails, as has been done with some success in Puerto Rico and Brazil [Giboda et al. 1997]), environmental modification, or various combinations of these measures. Proper disposal of urine and feces keeps eggs from hatching to initiate the cycle, but such measures are difficult to enforce if foreign to the cultural (and at times the religious) practices of the people and in places where human excrement is of great economic importance as fertilizer.

Teaching people to avoid snail-infested waters is impractical in areas where their economic livelihood depends on planting crops such as rice in these waters and where potentially snail-infested water is the only kind available for bathing, washing clothes, and so forth. Niclosamide, a chloronitrosalicylanilide, applied as a 1% lotion to the skin before contact with snail-infested waters, seems to have some value in preventing penetration of cercariae (Abu-Elyazeed et al., 1993). This agent was first developed as a molluscicde, and only later was found to have antiparasitic activity. Topical N,N-diethyl-*m*-toluamide (DEET), when applied as a 50% solution to the skin, has been shown to provide protection against cercarial penetration (Jackson et al., 2003). Mass treatment programs of infected humans are costly, both in terms of drugs and the personnel necessary to carry them out. Efforts to control *S. japonicum* by treatment are further complicated by its many reservoir hosts. Cobalt-irradiated cercariae of *Schistosoma bovis* have been used with promising results to protect cattle from this parasite. Several schistosome proteins have good potential for vaccines, and one of these has been cloned and found to be immunogenic in humans and to have some protective power in baboons.

SCHISTOSOMAL DERMATITIS

Many schistosome cercariae that ordinarily infect birds and semiaquatic mammals are capable of penetration into human skin but not of producing a permanent infection. A dermatitis may be produced from penetration by the cercariae of the human species of schistosomes; dermatitis caused by species that are not ordinarily human parasites is frequently more severe. Fresh-water lakes as well as some marine beaches are plagued by the presence of cercariae of the blood flukes of aquatic birds, which cause a dermatitis known as swimmer's itch (Fig. 6-32).

There is suggestive evidence that exposure to the schistosome cercariae of nonhuman species, many of which are present in the endemic areas of human schistosomiasis, may increase humans' resistance to infection with the human species.

★Not available in the United States or Canada.

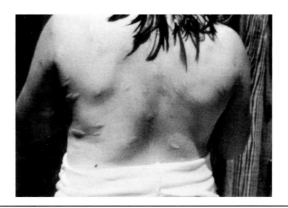

FIGURE 6-32 ■ Swimmer's itch. Papular eruption caused by penetration of skin by cercariae of various schistosome parasites of lower animals.

The Lung Flukes

At least eight different species of lung flukes, all belonging to the genus *Paragonimus*, are known to infect humans. It is probable that others may do so from time to time. Worldwide, at least 28 species of *Paragonimus* have been identified. These are primarily parasites of wild felines such as tigers, lions, leopards, and civet cats; of canines such as dogs, foxes, and wolves; and of a variety of other mammals, including wild pigs, badgers, mongooses, opossums, raccoons, minks, and others that eat fresh-water crabs and crayfish. Humans, then, are accidental hosts of these parasites, to some of which they seem better adapted than others.

Paragonimus spp.

Paragonimus westermani (Fig. 6-33) is the best known of the lung flukes affecting humans, and the one with the widest geographical range. It also behaves in humans much as in its feline and other wild hosts, and we can assume that the host-parasite relationship is good. *P. westermani* is a common human parasite in the Far East, including Japan, Korea, Manchuria, the People's Republic of China (including Taiwan), Southeast Asia, and Papua New Guinea. In the Pacific area it is found in the Solomons and Samoa. In the Indian subcontinent it occurs in Bengal, Madras, Manipur, Assam, the area around Bombay, and in Sri Lanka. In Africa it has been reported from the Congo, Nigeria, and the Cameroon. Two other species are reported as human parasites in Africa, and two have been reported in Japan (one of which occurs also in Korea and Taiwan). At least two other species infect humans in China and Southeast Asia. The identity of the species infecting humans in the Philippines is in question, but at any rate it is closely related to *P. westermani.*

Paragonimus kellicotti is enzootic throughout the eastern and midwestern United States, affecting a wide variety of animals that from time to time eat crayfish. There have been only two reported human cases of presumed *P. kellicotti* infection—one in 1934 and the other in 1984 (Pachucki et al., 1984). The latter case involved a young man who ate raw river crayfish in Missouri, developed pulmonary infiltrates and eosinophilia, and had eggs in his sputum. He was successfully treated with praziquantel. Refugees from Southeast Asia may be infected with *P. westermani* (Yee et al., 1992) and possibly other species. *P. mexicanus* occurs from Mexico down through most of South America; human infections with this parasite are sporadic in most areas. In Ecuador human paragonimiasis is endemic; in Peru it is focally important, and at least two different (as yet unidentified) species infect humans (Hillyer and Apt, 1997).

Adult worms are reddish brown and thick bodied. They measure 0.8 to 1.6 cm in length, 0.4 to 0.8 cm in width, and 0.3 to 0.5 cm in thickness. Typically they are encapsulated in cystic structures adjacent to the bronchi. The eggs are discharged into the bronchi or bronchioles; they may be expectorated or, if swallowed, appear in the feces.

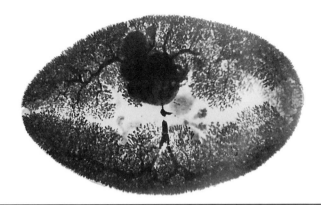

FIGURE 6-33   ■   *Paragonimus westermani.* (Photomicrograph by Zane Price.)

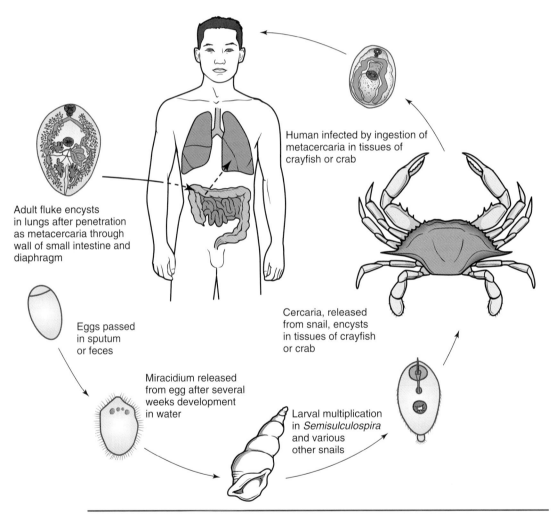

Human infected by ingestion of
metacercaria in tissues of
crayfish or crab

Adult fluke encysts
in lungs after penetration
as metacercaria through
wall of small intestine and
diaphragm

Eggs passed
in sputum
or feces

Cercaria, released
from snail, encysts
in tissues of crayfish
or crab

Miracidium released
from egg after several
weeks development
in water

Larval multiplication
in *Semisulculospira*
and various
other snails

FIGURE 6-34   ■   Life cycle of *Paragonimus westermani.*

Infection results from the ingestion of raw or insufficiently cooked crayfish or fresh-water crabs (Fig. 6-34), in which the encysted metacercarial stage occurs. Humans acquire paragonimiasis in a variety of ways. Some eat infected crabs or crayfish uncooked or pickled, either as food or as folk remedies. In much of the Orient, live crabs are immersed in wine and the "drunken crab" is eaten as a delicacy. Crab soup is boiled and safe for the consumer, but in its preparation live crabs are crushed, and living metacercariae may contaminate the fingers and utensils of the person preparing the meal. Metacercariae excyst in the small intestine, penetrate through its wall into the peritoneal cavity, and normally make their way to the diaphragm, through the esophageal hiatus, and pleura into the lungs. A cystlike capsule surrounds the developing parasite, which grows to maturity in a period of 6 weeks. Rupture of the cyst capsule into a bronchiole leads to a discharge of eggs but not of the parasite, which continues to produce eggs for a long time. Chronic infections may persist for many years after the patient leaves an endemic area.

Diagnosis depends on identification of the characteristic dark golden-brown eggs (Plate X; see Fig. 6-4, *D*) in sputum or feces, although the clinical picture may be suggestive. The ovoid eggs have a flattened operculum, distinctly set off from the rest of the shell by raised opercular shoulders. They measure 80 to 120 μm by 48 to 60 μm and are immature when found in the sputum or feces. Various serologic tests have been developed (see Chapter 16).

The chest film (Fig. 6-35) may show a patchy infiltrate with nodular cystic shadows or calcification; pleural effusion may be seen. Cerebral calcifications may also occur. Eosinophilia is generally present.

Symptoms. No recognizable symptoms attend the migration of the parasites. As they grow in the lungs there is an inflammatory reaction, which may be sufficient to produce fever. When the cysts rupture, a cough develops, and there may be increased production of sputum. The sputum is frequently blood tinged and may contain numerous dark brown eggs and Charcot-Leyden crystals. The appearance of the eggs in sputum has suggested iron filings to some observers. Hemoptysis may occur after paroxysms of coughing. There may be severe chest pain. The severity and progression of symptoms depend on the number of parasites present and on whether or not the infection is treated successfully, but as time goes on there is increasing dyspnea, and chronic bronchitis develops. Bronchiectasis may result, and pleural effusion is sometimes seen. Increasing fibrosis of the lungs occurs with longstanding infection. The clinical picture may closely resemble that of pulmonary tuberculosis.

Humans may not be as suitable a host as the normal one for many of these parasites, and as is often the case under such circumstances, the worm may behave in an abnormal manner. Instead of taking its usual migratory path to the lungs, it may enter other parts of

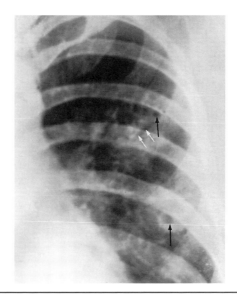

FIGURE 6-35 ■ Pulmonary paragonimiasis with ring shadows *(black arrows)* and linear lucency *(white arrows)* representing burrow tract. (Courtesy of R. Suwanik, Dhonburi, Thailand.)

the body such as brain, spinal cord, or abdominal cavity, or wander through the subcutaneous tissues. The most serious consequence of such migration is cerebral paragonimiasis, in which the fluke enters the cranial cavity through the jugular foramen and invades the brain tissue. The onset of symptoms is usually insidious, with fever and headache, nausea, vomiting, visual disturbances, and motor weakness culminating in convulsive seizures, especially focal (Jacksonian) ones, and often with meningeal signs as well as motor and sensory disturbances. Cutaneous paragonimiasis seems characteristic of certain species such as *Paragonimus skrjabini* (also known as *Paragonimus szechuanensis*) in China, which may also invade and severely damage the liver. These abnormal wanderings may be characteristic of the behavior of a parasite in an unfamiliar host.

Pathogenesis. Migration of larval *Paragonimus* though the intestinal wall and into the pleural cavity is generally accomplished in experimental animals within 5 to 10 days. Some young flukes wander about in the peritoneal cavity for 20 days or more, growing considerably in size and penetrating into various organs en route. Those reaching sexual maturity in ectopic sites apparently remain there. Worms that reach the brain do so by way of the soft tissues of the neck and the cranial foramina. Passage of worms through the tissues produces local hemorrhage and leukocytic infiltration of a transitory nature and without clinical significance except for rare cases in which they wander subcutaneously.

When the worms settle down, either in the lungs or in ectopic foci, more pronounced tissue reactions occur. In the lungs a leukocytic infiltrate forms around the parasite, and fibrous tissue surrounds the infiltrate to form a cyst wall. Communication of the cyst with the respiratory tree may result from inclusion of a bronchiolar branch within the cyst or from erosion of the cyst into adjacent bronchioles. Eggs may infiltrate the surrounding pulmonary tissues (Fig. 6-36) or may be carried by the circulation to other parts of the body, in which they evoke a granulomatous reaction similar to that surrounding schistosome eggs in tissues. Such lesions have been observed in many organs and tissues, including both pericardium and myocardium, but they are apparently rare in the central nervous system.

Worm cysts in the peritoneal cavity or other sites outside the lungs are similar to pulmonic cysts. Peritonitis and abdominal adhesions resulting from infection have been reported, although there is usually little or no inflammatory reaction, and suppurative and ulcerative lesions are uncommon.

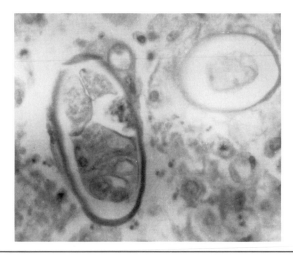

FIGURE 6-36 ■ *Paragonimus westermani* eggs in section of lung tissue; note operculum (hematoxylin and eosin stain).

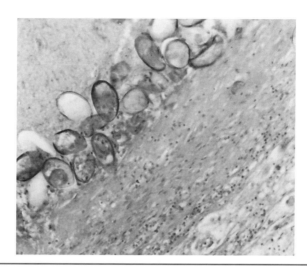

FIGURE 6-37 ■ Eggs of *Paragonimus westermani* in human brain; note extensive collagen scar beneath the eggs. (Courtesy of Dr. W. Jann Brown, University of California Los Angeles School of Medicine.)

In the brain (Fig. 6-37) lesions may occur in both gray and white matter, and sometimes they are connected by passageways. Lesions in the gray matter may cause a thickening of the pia and adhesive arachnoiditis. In older lesions a more or less definitive cyst wall develops.

Since the majority of worms migrate to the lungs, and since most infections are light, extrapulmonary paragonimiasis is rarely seen in humans. Cysts, in whatever location, may contain living or dead worms; a yellow to brownish, thick fluid, sometimes hemorrhagic; eggs; and Charcot-Leyden crystals. If the worms die or escape, the cysts gradually shrink as their contents are absorbed, eventually leaving a nodule of fibrous tissue and eggs, which may partly calcify.

Epidemiology. In some areas human paragonimiasis may be common enough that human-to-human transmission (via the appropriate snail and crab intermediate hosts) occurs. In most areas the disease is principally one of the local crab-eating mammals, and humans enter into the life cycle accidentally. Many different species of crabs and crayfish may be infected in various parts of the world, and only seldom are these part of the human diet. Thus, endemicity of the disease rests on dietary habits, methods of food preparation, and the presence of appropriate snail hosts, fresh-water crustaceans, and the reservoir host.

Paratenic (transfer) hosts may play an important role in the life cycle of *Paragonimus* in the wild and may also contribute to human disease. In southern Kyushu, Japan, hunters customarily eat thinly sliced raw wild boar meat, which may contain migrating larvae of *Paragonimus*. These larvae can pass through the intestinal wall of their new host and continue their development in humans. Tigers in Sumatra are heavily infected, and this infection is believed to result from infected paratenic hosts such as wild boar, wild pigs, monkeys, and other small mammals.

Treatment. Praziquantel, 25 mg/kg three times daily for 2 days, is the drug of choice for treatment of pulmonary paragonimiasis and presumably for cutaneous forms of the disease. Smaller daily doses, even when administered over a longer period to achieve the same cumulative dose, have been found ineffective. We have seen no reference to its use in cerebral paragonimiasis but suspect that (as in cerebral cysticercosis) it might have to be administered over an extended period.

An alternative drug for the treatment of pulmonary paragonimiasis is bithionol,* administered orally at the rate of 15 to 25 mg/kg body weight twice daily on alternate days for a total of 10 to 15 days. Bithionol was formerly used in the formulation of medicated soaps but is no longer used for this purpose because of its association with contact dermatitis. Skin rashes and urticaria are not infrequently seen in the course of bithionol treatment. Abdominal cramps, nausea and vomiting, and diarrhea are rather frequent side effects, as are dizziness and headache. Hepatic and renal involvement, hypertension, extrasystoles, and first-degree heart block have all been reported to occur during the course of treatment but are apparently transient. Bithionol is contraindicated in patients with a clear history of sensitization to preparations containing this drug. A list of such preparations is given in the informational leaflet supplied by the CDC Drug Service.

Reports indicate that triclabendazole (approved by the FDA only for veterinary use) in one or two oral doses of 10 mg/kg body weight is effective in treatment of pulmonary paragonimiasis (Calvopiña et al., 2003; Ripert et al., 1992), as in human fascioliasis.

Uncommon Trematode Parasites of Humans

Humans are incidental hosts to a variety of flukes, usually acquired by eating uncooked or undercooked meats. A few examples follow.

Acanthoparyphium

Originally described as an echinostomatid intestinal parasite of ducks in Korea, *Acanthoparyphium tyosenense* has also been reported as an intestinal parasite of humans in the Republic of Korea (Chai et al., 2001). The patients were nine adults, ages 35 to 66, and one 7-year-old child, all of whom resided in two coastal villages. Patients were treated with 10 mg/kg praziquantel in a single dose, and worms were recovered following purgation with magnesium salts. An epidemiological investigation of intermediate hosts determined that brackish water mollusks were the source of human infection.

Alaria

Mammalian hosts of adult *Alaria* in the United States and Canada are foxes and other canids, which become infected by eating frogs and other small game containing the metacercariae of this parasite. Human infections, including at least one fatality, are reported following ingestion of such undercooked meats (Kramer et al., 1996).

Gymnophalloides

The minute trematode *Gymnophalloides seoi*, belonging to a family of worms ordinarily infecting shore birds, was first discovered in the stools of a patient complaining of epigastric pain and diarrhea, from a small island village off the southwest coat of Korea. Subsequent investigation revealed eggs of this parasite in 49 of 98 inhabitants of the village, and worm burdens averaging more than 3000 worms per individual. The life cycle is unknown, but other gymnophallids infect marine bivalves, and raw oysters are a common food in this village. Worms are broadly flattened, less than 0.5 mm in length; operculate eggs measure 20 to 23 μm by 13 to 15 μm (Lee et al., 1994).

Haplorchis taichui

A focus of human infection by the heterophyid trematode *Haplorchis taichui* has been reported in Mindanao Island, southern Philippines (Belizario et al., 2004). Previously, occasional cases had been reported from Thailand and the Philippines. In the present study, the

*Available from the CDC Drug Service, Centers for Disease Control and Prevention, Atlanta, Georgia 30333; (404) 639-3670.

prevalence of infection was 36%. An intestinal fluke, *H. taichui*, lives attached to the wall of the small bowel, producing symptoms of abdominal discomfort or pain, nausea, diarrhea, and borborygmi. Praziquantel, 75 mg/kg divided in three doses in 1 day, was an effective treatment. The source of infection likely was fresh-water fish, which serve as second intermediate hosts harboring metacercariae. Dogs, cats, and swine have been reported as definitive hosts for *H. taichui* in the Philippines.

Metorchis conjunctus

An important cause of death in sled dogs, this opisthorchid fluke infects a wide range of carnivores in the United States and Canada. Metacercariae are found in various fresh-water fish, notably the white sucker, *Cataostomus commersoni*. Seventeen of 20 persons consuming sashimi prepared from these fish, caught in a river north of Montreal, developed an acute febrile illness with epigastric pain and eosinophilia. Eggs similar to those of *Opisthorchis* were found in the feces. Identification of the parasite was accomplished by feeding metacercariae from the fish to hamsters. Symptoms responded promptly to treatment with praziquantel (MacLean et al., 1996).

Nanophyetus (Troglotrema) salmincola

A minute intestinal fluke less than 1 mm long, *N. salmincola* has long been associated in the Pacific northwest coast of North America and in Siberia with a disease of dogs, wolves, and foxes that, if untreated, is frequently fatal. The disease, "salmon poisoning," is caused not by the parasite itself but by rickettsiae of which it is the vector. Cercariae of *Nanophyetus* liberated from their snail hosts encyst in the tissues of salmonid fish. Numerous fish-eating mammals, including humans and some fish-eating birds, become infected upon ingesting the metacercariae, but apparently only canids (dogs, wolves, foxes) are affected by the rickettsia, *Neorickettsia helminthoeca*, that it carries, and can develop severe or fatal enteritis from this infection. Until recently, it was thought that human infection with *Nanophyetus* was asymptomatic, and it seems that this is usually so; however, some patients present with gastrointestinal complaints, otherwise unexplained eosinophilia, weight loss, or fatigue. Fish handlers may become infected by hand-to-mouth transmission of the metacercariae.

Praziquantel, 20 mg/kg body weight, three times in 1 day, has been found effective in treatment.

Eggs of *N. salmincola* are light brown, ovoid, and operculate at one end, with a small blunt projection at the aboperculate end. They mesure 64 to 97 μm by 34 to 55 μm (Fig. 6-38).

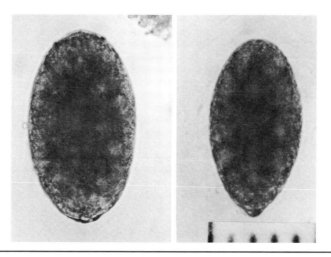

FIGURE 6-38 ■ Eggs of *Nanophyetus salmincola*. The egg on the left shows the operculum; that on right show the blunt aboperculate projection. Scale, 50 μm. (Eggs courtesy of Dr. Thomas R. Fritsche, University of Washington, Seattle, WA.)

TABLE 6-1 ■ **Review of Trematode Infections of Humans**

Disease	Parasite	Means of Human Infection	Location of Larvae in Humans	Location of Adults in Humans	Clinical Features	Laboratory Diagnosis
Fasciolopsiasis	*Fasciolopsis buski* (intestinal fluke)	Ingestion of larvae encysted on aquatic plants	Small intestine	Small intestine (attached)	Abdominal pain, diarrhea, edema, ascites, eosinophilia	Undeveloped operculate eggs in stool
Clonorchiasis	*Clonorchis sinensis* (Chinese liver fluke)	Ingestion of larvae encysted in fresh-water fish	Duodenum, bile ducts	Bile ducts, gallbladder	Hepatomegaly, diarrhea, jaundice, eosinophilia (carcinoma of biliary tract)	Embryonated operculate eggs in feces or duodenal aspirate
Fascioliasis	*Fasciola hepatica* (sheep liver fluke)	Ingestion of larvae encysted on aquatic vegetation	Intestinal wall, peritoneal cavity, liver (biliary tree)	Bile ducts, gallbladder	Hepatomegaly, eosinophilia, jaundice, portal cirrhosis	Undeveloped operculate eggs in stools, serologic tests
Schistosomiasis (bilharziasis)	*Schistosoma mansoni, S. japonicum, S. haematobium* (blood flukes)	Penetration of skin by larvae in water	Subcutaneous tissues, liver (sinusoids)	Mesenteric veins (vesical, prostatic, or uterine veins: *S. haematobium*)	Hepatosplenomegaly, diarrhea, portal fibrosis, hypertension (hematuria bladder cancer with *S. haematobium*)	Embryonated nonoperculate eggs in stool (urine or feces for *S. haematobium*), serologic tests
Paragonimiasis	*Paragonimus westermani* (lung fluke)	Ingestion of larvae encysted in fresh-water crabs or crayfish	Intestinal wall, peritoneal cavity, lung tissue	Lungs (in fibrous capsule)	Hemoptysis, cough, fever, eosinophilia (cerebral paragonimiasis)	Undeveloped operculate eggs in sputum or feces, serologic tests

Phaneropsolus

Members of the genus *Phaneropsolus* are intestinal parasites of reptiles, birds, and mammals. *P. bonnei* has been reported as a human parasite in Indonesia and Thailand and *P. spinicirrus* similarly from Thailand. A single dose of praziquantel was used to treat the 44-year-old female patient with *P. spinicirrus* (Kaewkes et al., 1991) and presumably is an effective form of treatment for other species of *Phaneropsolus* as well.

Philophthalmus

Species of *Philophthalmus*, referred to as eyeflukes, infect the eyes of wild and domestic birds. A total of 24 human cases have been reported worldwide from Europe, Asia, Israel, Mexico, and the United States. The patient from Mexico (Lamothe-Argumendo et al., 2003), a healthy 31-year-old male, experienced a foreign-body sensation in his left eye lasting for 2 months. Examination revealed a small, approximately 6 mm, elongated worm in the conjunctiva. The patient's symptoms ceased shortly after surgical removal of the worm, which was identified as *Philophthalmus lacrimosus*.

Table 6-1 summarizes some important features of the more common trematode infections of humans.

References

Abu-Elyazeed RR et al. Field trial of 1% niclosamide as a topical antipenetrant to *Schistosoma mansoni* cercariae. *Am J Trop Med Hyg* 1993; *49*:403–409.

Adam I et al. Is praziquantel therapy safe during pregnancy? *Trans R Soc Trop Med Hyg* 2004; *98*:540–543.

Apt W et al. Treatment of human chronic fascioliasis with triclabendazole; Drug efficacy and serologic response. *Am J Trop Med Hyg* 1995; *52*:532–535.

Belizario VY et al. A focus of human infection by *Haplorchis taichui* (Trematoda: Heterophydiae) in the southern Philippines. *J Parasitol* 2004; *90*:1165–1169.

Calvopiña M et al. Comparison of two single-day regimens of triclabendazole for the treatment of human pulmonary paragonimiasis. *Trans R Soc Trop Med Hyg* 2003; *97*:451-454.

Chai JY el al. *Acanthoparyphium tyosenense*: The discovery of human infection and identification of its source. *J Parasitol* 2001; *87*:794–800.

Chiu A et al. Late complications of infection with *Opisthorchis viverrini*. *West J Med* 1996; *164*:174–176.

Drabick JJ et al. Dicrocoeliasis (lancet fluke disease) in an HIV-seropositive man. *JAMA* 1988; *259*:567–568.

Giboda M et al. Human *Opisthorchis* and *Haplorchis* infections in Laos. *Trans R Soc Trop Med Hyg* 1991; 85:538–540.

Giboda M et al. Human schistosomiasis in Puerto Rico: Reduced prevalence rate and absence of *Biomphalaria glabrata*. *Am J Trop Med Hyg* 1997; *57*:564–568.

Han JK et al. Radiologic findings in human fascioliasis. *Abdom Imaging* 1993; *18*:261–264.

Hillyer GV, Apt W. Food-borne trematode infections in the Americas. *Parasitol Today* 1997; *13*:87–88.

Jackson F et al. Schistosomiasis prophylaxis *in vivo* using N, N-diethyl-m-toluamide (DEET). *Trans R Soc Trop Med Hyg* 2003; *97*:449–450.

Kaewkes S et al. *Phaneropsolus spinicirrus* N. sp. (Digenea: Lecithodendriidae), a human parasite in Thailand. *J Parasitol* 1991; *77*:514–516.

Kramer MH et al. Respiratory symptoms and subcutaneous granuloma caused by mesocercariae. A case report. *Am J Trop Med Hyg* 1996; *55*:447–484.

Lamothe-Argumedo R et al. The first human case in Mexico of conjunctivitis caused by the avian parasite, *Philophthalmus lacrimosus*. *J Parasitol* 2003; *89*:183–185.

Lee S-H et al. High prevalence of *Gymnophalloides seoi* infection in a village on a southwestern island of the Republic of Korea. *Am J Trop Med Hyg* 1994; *51*:281–285.

Liu Y-H et al. Experimental and clinical trial of albendazole in the treatment of clonorchiasis sinensis. *Chin Med J* 1991; *104*:27–31.

MacLean JD et al. Common-source outbreak of acute infection due to the North American liver fluke *Metorchis conjunctus*. *Lancet* 1996; *347*:154–158.

Pachucki CT et al. American paragonimiasis treated with praziquantel. *N Engl J Med* 1984; *311*: 582–583.

Poggensee G et al. Diagnosis of genital cervical schistosomiasis: Comparison of cytological, histopathological and parasitological examination. *Am J Trop Med Hyg* 2001; *65*:233–236.

Pollner JH et al. Cerebral schistosomiasis caused by *Schistosoma haematobium*: Case report. *Clin Infect Dis* 1994; *18*:354–357.

Price TA et al. Fascioliasis: Case reports and review. *Clin Infect Dis* 1993; *17*:426–430.

Pungpak S et al. *Opisthorchis viverrini* infection in Thailand: Symptoms and signs of infection—a population-based study. *Trans R Soc Trop Med Hyg* 1994; *88*:561–564.

Richter J et al. Fascioliasis. *Curr Treat Opt Infect Dis* 2002; *4*:313–317.

Ripert C et al. Therapeutic effect of triclabendazole in patients with paragonimiasis in Cameroon: A pilot study. *Trans R Soc Trop Med Hyg* 1992; *86*:417.

Strandgaard H et al. The pig as a host for *Schistosoma mekongi* in Laos. *J Parasitol* 2001; *87*:708–709.

Watt G et al. Hepatic parenchymal dysfunction in *Schistosoma japonicum* infections. *J Infect Dis* 1991; *164*:1186–1192.

Yee B et al. Pulmonary paragonimiasis in Southeast Asians living in the Central San Joaquin valley. *West J Med* 1992; *156*:423–425.

The Cestodes

The cestodes, or tapeworms, constitute a class of the phylum Platyhelminthes. The adult tapeworms found in humans all have a flat and ribbonlike body. Living worms are white or yellowish. The cestode body consists of an anterior attachment organ, or scolex, followed by a chain of segments, proglottids (Fig. 7-1), also known as a strobila. The strobila grows throughout the life of the tapeworm by continuous proliferation of new segments or proglottids in the region immediately posterior to the scolex, referred to as the neck. The new segments are referred to as immature because they do not yet contain fully developed internal structures. The mature segments are larger and are found near the middle of the chain, and each may contain either one or two sets of both male and female reproductive organs. The terminal portion of the strobila contains the ripe or gravid segments, usually filled with eggs. The eggs are enclosed in the uterus, a structure that varies in shape and size in different cestode species. The form of the uterus is quite characteristic and serves as an important diagnostic feature. Terminal proglottids of some species may become detached in the intestine and pass out with the stool; some types may be too small to be seen in gross examination.

Adult tapeworms inhabit the small intestine, where they live attached to the mucosa. Tapeworms do not have a digestive system; their food is absorbed from the host's intestine. Attachment is accomplished by means of the scolex, an organ that varies in morphology from species to species; however, with the exception of *Diphyllobothrium latum*, the broad or fish tapeworm, and related species, all cestodes of humans have four muscular, cup-shaped suckers on the scolex. In addition to suckers, the scolex may have an elongate and protrusible structure, the rostellum, situated in the center of the scolex. In some species the rostellum bears hooks and is referred to as armed. While precise identification of the tapeworms of humans is usually made on the basis of eggs or proglottids, the scolex of each species is quite characteristic and is sufficient for specific diagnosis.

Cestodes that parasitize humans have complex life cycles that generally involve both a definitive and an intermediate host. Some species utilize humans only as the definitive hosts, growing to adulthood in the intestine after ingestion of the infective larvae (e.g., *D. latum, Taenia saginata, Hymenolepis diminuta*). For some species, humans are equally acceptable as definitive or intermediate hosts (e.g., *Taenia solium, Hymenolepis nana*). Still others, such as *Echinococcus*, utilize humans as one of their possible intermediate hosts but never as the definitive host. In general, extraintestinal infection with the larval forms is a much more serious matter than infection with the adult worm.

Unlike the trematodes, the eggs of which are usually operculate, human tapeworms, with few exceptions, do not have operculate eggs. Cestode eggs vary considerably in the appearance of the external shell as well as in the number and thickness of the embryonic membranes. These membranes serve as protective coverings of the embryo, which is called an oncosphere and bears six elongate hooks (see Fig. 7-10; Plates X and XI).

Diphyllobothrium latum

The broad or fish tapeworm of humans is almost worldwide in distribution, occurring in northern temperate areas of the world where pickled or insufficiently cooked fresh-water fish

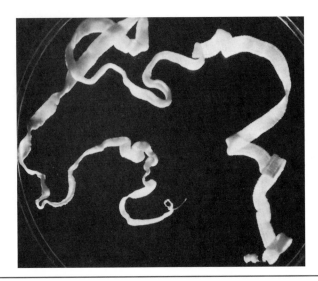

FIGURE 7-1 ■ Entire tapeworm—*Hymenolepis diminuta.* (Photograph by Zane Price.)

are prominent in the diet. A high prevalence of *D. latum* in humans is seen in Scandinavia and Finland as well as in Alaska and Canada. In the United States, *D. latum* once occurred in the lake region of Minnesota and Michigan but it is apparently no longer endemic there. Although infection with *D. latum* is, in many instances, relatively harmless, it may produce in some persons a condition closely resembling pernicious anemia. One of the reasons for this may be the relatively high vitamin B_{12} content of the adult worm. This vitamin is selectively absorbed from the host's intestinal tract by *D. latum*.

The life cycle of this tapeworm requires not one but two intermediate hosts (Fig. 7-2). Eggs passed in the feces hatch into small ciliated coracidium embryos, which swim about until ingested by copepods, in which growth and development of the first larval stage (the procercoid) are completed. When these infected fresh-water crustaceans are ingested by fish, the larvae continue growing in the flesh of the fish, developing to a second larval stage called the plerocercoid. Often, the fish ingesting an infected copepod is small and unlikely prey for a mammal of any size. If in its turn this fish is ingested by a larger fish, the plerocercoid may infect the larger fish but will not continue to grow in this transport (or paratenic) host. However, by this mechanism the transport host may become heavily infected. If the infected fish is then eaten by a human or other suitable mammalian host, the plerocercoid larva is not digested but remains in the small intestine and grows to adulthood.

The adult worm may be several meters in length. The scolex of *D. latum* (Fig. 7-3) is elongate, spoon shaped, and characterized by two longitudinal grooves. Mature and gravid segments (Fig. 7-4) are wider than they are long. In freshly passed or formalin-preserved segments, one frequently observes a pronounced central elevation, which marks the site of the egg-filled uterus. The uterus of *D. latum* is a coiled tube confined to a relatively small area in the center of the segment. This arrangement of the uterus is unlike that of the other tapeworms of humans; it has been frequently likened to a rosette.

Ripe eggs escape through a uterine pore and are discharged into the intestine. Both eggs and proglottids may be found in the stool. Eggs of *D. latum* (Plate X; see also Fig. 7-10, *E*) are ovoid and possess an operculum for the escape of the embryo. Eggs are about 70 μm long and 50 μm wide. The shell is smooth, of moderate thickness, and yellowish brown.

Symptoms. The presence of adult worms in the intestinal tract causes no symptoms in most infected persons. Some rather nonspecific abdominal symptoms have been ascribed to this infection, but the only significant consequence is the result of chance localization of the

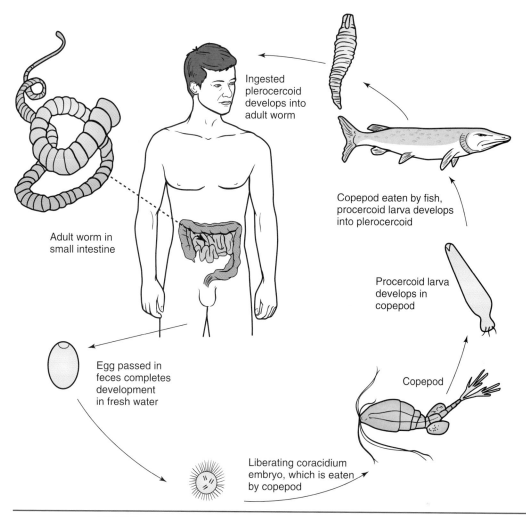

FIGURE 7-2 ■ Life cycle of *Diphyllobothrium latum*.

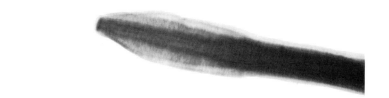

FIGURE 7-3 ■ *Diphyllobothrium latum,* scolex. (Photomicrograph by Zane Price.)

parasite in the proximal portion of the jejunum. If the worm attaches in this area, clinical vitamin B_{12} deficiency develops in a small percentage of those parasitized. Such tapeworm anemia, indistinguishable from genuine pernicious anemia, is seen most frequently in areas such as Finland, where many persons have a genetic predisposition to pernicious anemia, suggesting that B_{12} deprivation through *D. latum* infection is seldom sufficient to produce clinical symptoms in an otherwise normal patient.

Epidemiology. Various species of fresh-water fish and ones that live in brackish waters may be infected with the plerocercoid larvae, as may salmonids that spawn in fresh water.

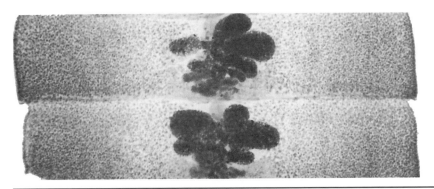

FIGURE 7-4 ■ Gravid proglottids of *Diphyllobothrium latum*. (Photomicrograph by Zane Price, from material furnished by Dr. Justus F. Mueller.)

Both humans and a variety of fish-eating mammals, such as wild and domestic members of the dog and cat families, bears, minks, pigs, walruses, and seals, may become infected. Peoples such as Jews, Russians, Finns, Scandinavians, and Japanese, whose dietary customs include eating raw or insufficiently cooked fish, are more vulnerable, as are campers who cook their catch over an open fire. In the coastal areas of Peru, another species, *Diphyllobothrium pacificum*, is the most common tapeworm infecting humans. It is a natural parasite of seals, which acquire the infection from eating fish. These same fish, marinated in lime juice but not cooked, are *ceviche*, a delicacy in Peru and other Latin American countries. *Diphyllobothrium nihonkaiense*, not *D. latum*, is the common tapeworm acquired by the consumption of raw fish in Japan. It causes few symptoms, but is long lived and may give rise to considerable emotional distress from the continued presence of its segments in the stools. *Diplogonoporus* (a related genus characterized by two sets of reproductive organs in each proglottid) is reported from humans in Japan and Korea, probably acquired through consumption of raw anchovies.

Treatment. Praziquantel is the drug of choice for treatment of all three species of *Diphyllobothrium*, in a single oral dose of 5 to 10 mg/kg body weight. Cure rate is over 95%.

For persons unable to take praziquantel, niclosamide (Niclocide) is effective and well tolerated, but may cause abdominal cramps, diarrhea, and nausea and vomiting in a small percentage of patients. The drug acts by inhibiting oxidative phosphorylation in the mitochondria of the worm. Niclosamide is administered by mouth, after a light breakfast. The chewable tablets are given in a single dose, 2 g for adults, 1.5 g for children weighing over 34 kg, and 1.0 g for those weighing between 11 and 34 kg.

As the worms are seldom passed spontaneously after administration of either drug, a saline purge may be given 1 to 2 hours later to expel them in a more or less intact condition.

Control. In most areas, humans are the primary hosts of *D. latum*, and proper disposal of human feces will do much to break the infection chain. Fish that has been thoroughly cooked, brine cured, or frozen at −10°C for 24 to 48 hours is safe to consume. It must be remembered that fish roe may be infected as well as the flesh.

Sparganosis

Infection of humans by plerocercoid larvae of various diphyllobothroid tapeworms belonging to the genus *Spirometra* is known as sparganosis. The larvae are often referred to by the generic name *Sparganum*, a relic of the days in which this stage was thought to represent a separate genus. Man is an acceptable second intermediate host for certain species that normally develop to the adult stage in other mammals. Sparganosis in humans is cosmopolitan, though it is rarely seen in most parts of the world. The infection may be acquired by drinking water containing copepods infected with the procercoid larval stage of the parasite, in which the larva penetrates the gut wall and works its way into the muscles or subcutaneous tissues, where it grows into the *Sparganum* larva. These larvae may migrate actively in the subcutaneous tissues. The authors have seen several such cases, apparently acquired in the southern United States.

In various areas snakes or tadpoles are consumed raw for medicinal reasons. If they happen to be infected with plerocercoids, these parasites may be capable of penetrating the intestinal wall to infect humans, causing sparganosis. Another manner in which human infections have been known to take place is through the practice of placing poultices of frog or snake flesh on open wounds or other lesions, especially of the eyes. If the flesh is infected with plerocercoid larvae, these may actively penetrate into the poulticed lesion. Ocular sparganosis acquired in this manner is not uncommon in parts of the Orient, especially in China and Vietnam. It will be appreciated that under such circumstances humans serve as a transport or paratenic host, in all ways analogous to the fish that ingests the minnow originally infected with *D. latum*, except that the full life cycle is unlikely to be completed.

The sparganum is a wrinkled, whitish, ribbon-shaped organism, a few millimeters wide and up to several centimeters long. The anterior end is capable of invagination and bears suggestions of the sucking grooves of the mature scolex. In a few instances in Japan and in single case reports from Florida, Taiwan, Paraguay, and Venezuela, human infections with a peculiar budding type of larva known as *Sparganum proliferum* have been reported. These larvae may occur almost anywhere in the body, and the branched proliferating larvae may break up into segments capable of further independent development. Infection with this form of parasite is extremely serious.

The early migratory stages in the development of the sparganum are asymptomatic, but when it has reached its final site and begins to grow, its presence elicits a painful inflammatory reaction in the surrounding tissues. The larvae apparently do not become encysted. Ocular sparganosis produces an especially intense reaction, with periorbital edema. If the larvae are retrobulbar in position, the orbit may be forced out so that the lids do not close, and corneal ulcers develop. Cerebral sparganosis is characterized by seizures, paresthesias, hemiparesis, and similar CNS symptoms. Most reported cases have been cured by surgical resection after localization (though not identification) of the lesion by computed tomography (CT) or magnetic resonance imaging (MRI) (Holodniy et al., 1991).

Diagnosis is made following surgical removal of the worms, which on section are seen to possess a rather homogeneous parenchyma in which are scattered the laminated, intensely basophilic calcareous corpuscles characteristic of cestode tissue (Fig. 7-5). A presumptive preoperative diagnosis might be made on demonstration of a painful migratory subcutaneous nodule.

Treatment. Surgical removal of one or a few sparganum larvae is usually possible. Praziquantel is apparently effective when administered at a total dose of 120 to 150 mg/kg body weight, over a 2-day period.

Prevention. In areas of endemic infection, people should be advised of the dangers of drinking water from ponds and ditches, which may contain infected copepods. The use of potentially infected animals for medicinal purposes must be discouraged.

Taenia solium

The pork tapeworm occurs wherever people eat cured or undercooked pork. Infection with *T. solium* is rarely encountered in the United States except in immigrants from areas where it is prevalent such as Mexico, Latin America, the Iberian peninsula, the Slavic countries, Africa, India, Southeast Asia, and China. The life cycle of this tapeworm (Fig. 7-6) requires one intermediate host, the pig. Embryonated eggs ingested by a pig develop into the infective larval

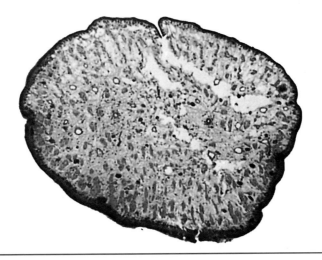

FIGURE 7-5   ■   Cross section of sparganum removed at surgery.

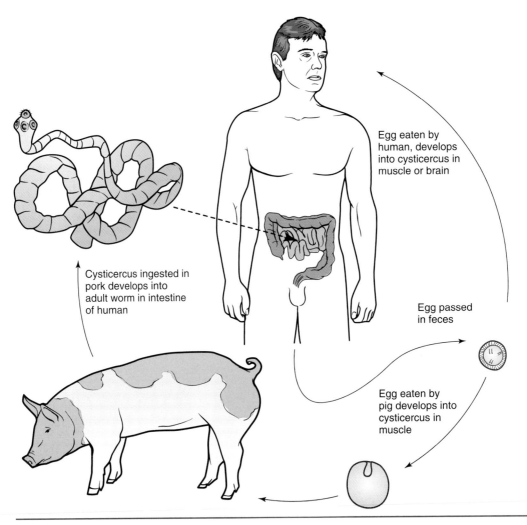

Egg eaten by human, develops into cysticercus in muscle or brain

Cysticercus ingested in pork develops into adult worm in intestine of human

Egg passed in feces

Egg eaten by pig develops into cysticercus in muscle

FIGURE 7-6   ■   Life cycle of *Taenia solium*.

stages or cysticerci in the muscles. A cysticercus is essentially a thin-walled bladder within which a single scolex develops. The larvae are 0.5 cm or more in diameter. People become infected by eating pork containing these larvae. When humans eat insufficiently cooked cysticercus-infected meat, all but the scolex portion is digested, and the scolex attaches to the intestinal wall to begin growing a chain of proglottids.

Although the adult tapeworm develops in humans after the ingestion of infected meat, infection with the larval stage or cysticercus occurs after the ingestion of eggs, either from exogenous sources or from their own stools. Although not proved, it is thought that reverse peristalsis may carry intestinal contents with eggs to the upper portions of the duodenum, where after hatching the oncospheres penetrate directly into the intestinal wall. For these reasons, infection with adults of *T. solium* is dangerous both to the patients and to those with whom they come in contact.

While pigs and humans are the usual intermediate hosts of *T. solium*, dogs can also become infected by ingestion of the eggs of this tapeworm. The European brown bear (*Ursus arctos*) has long been suspected of being another intermediate host, and recent DNA testing has confirmed that the American black bear (*Ursus americanus*) may become infected. Humans are the only known definitive hosts.

Adult *T. solium* worms may attain a length of several meters. The scolex (Fig. 7-7) is muscular and bears in addition to the four suckers a double crown of prominent hooks, which function in attachment to the intestinal mucosa. Mature segments (Fig. 7-8) are wider than they are long and contain one set of male and female reproductive organs. Gravid segments

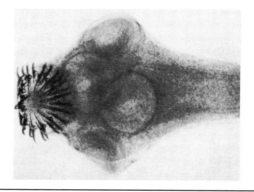

FIGURE 7-7 ■ *Taenia solium*, scolex. (Photomicrograph by Zane Price.)

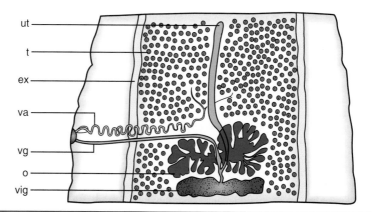

FIGURE 7-8 ■ Mature proglottid of *Taenia:* (*ex*) excretory canal; (*o*) ovary; (*t*) testis; (*ut*) uterus; (*va*) vas deferens; (*vg*) vagina; (*vig*) vitelline gland.

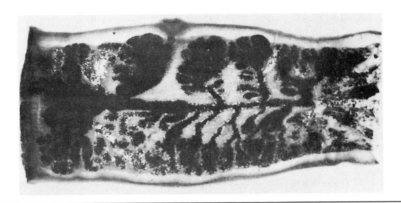

FIGURE 7-9 ▪ *Taenia solium,* gravid proglottid. (Photomicrograph by Zane Price.)

(Fig. 7-9) are usually longer than they are wide and contain a branched uterus filled with eggs. A central uterine stem extends through the length of the gravid segment. From this stem arise side branches, which project laterally and extend toward the lateral margin of the proglottid. These main side branches may have a variable number of smaller secondary branches. In *T. solium,* the number of main branches on one side of the central stem varies from 7 to 13. Specific diagnosis of *T. solium* is made by counting the number of uterine side branches, which may be done in living or in stained preparations.

While gravid segments and eggs may be found in stool specimens, specific identification cannot be made on the basis of eggs alone but only on examination of gravid proglottids. Eggs and mature proglottids of *T. solium* and of *T. saginata* are very much alike and do not provide a means of specific differentiation. *Taenia* eggs (Fig. 7-10, *C, D*; see also Plate X) may be found free in the feces. They may also be recovered by means of a cellophane tape swab (refer to *Enterobius*). The oncosphere is enclosed in a thick, radially striated coat called the embryophore, usually dark brown in color. The six-hooked embryo can be easily seen in living eggs but frequently become shriveled and opaque in preserved material. The radially striated coat is, however, sufficiently characteristic so that *Taenia* eggs cannot be confused with any of the other eggs of human helminths.

Symptoms. The adult worms probably cause no symptoms in the majority of patients. Vague abdominal discomfort, hunger pangs, and chronic indigestion have been reported but are undoubtedly seen more often in patients who are aware of their parasitic infection than in those who are not. Moderate eosinophilia frequently occurs.

Treatment. Praziquantel, administered in a single dose of 5 to 10 mg/kg body weight, is the drug of choice, with cure rates approximating 100%. Niclosamide, given as for diphyllobothriasis, is also effective.

Cysticercosis

The common larval stage of typeworms of the genus *Taenia* is known as a cysticercus, or bladder worm. When these stages were first discovered, their relationship to the adult worm was not known, and they were therefore given generic and specific names of their own. Thus, the bladder worm of *T. solium* was known as *Cysticercus cellulosae*; it is still sometimes referred to by this old name, which no longer has any taxonomic validity.

The life cycle of *T. solium* (see Fig. 7-6) commonly involves swine as the intermediate host. Eggs may remain viable for many weeks in the soil after they are passed in the feces. Upon ingestion by hogs or by humans, the outer shell disintegrates in the small intestine, and the contained embryo or oncosphere is able to invade the intestinal wall and enter a blood vessel by means of the six hooklets that it bears. It may be carried in the bloodstream

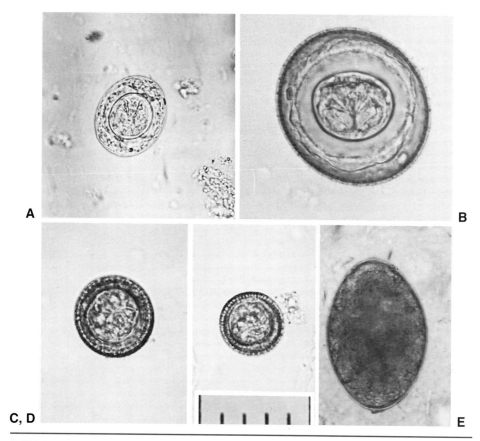

FIGURE 7-10 ■ Cestode eggs. **A,** *Hymenolepis nana.* **B,** *Hymenolepis diminuta.* **C, D,** *Taenia* sp. **E,** *Diphyllobothrium latum.* All eggs photographed at same magnification; scale equals 50 μm.

to any part of the body and may lodge in any tissue, but it most frequently develops in voluntary muscle. The cysticercus larva completes development in about 2 months. It is semitransparent, opalescent white, and elongate oval in shape and may reach a length of 0.6 to 1.8 cm (Fig. 7-11). The bladder is fluid filled, and on one side is a denser area containing the scolex.

Symptoms and Pathogenesis. In humans, cysticerci most commonly come to our attention when they occur in the central nervous system; in swine they are usually found in the muscles. This may well represent a true difference between the activities of the parasite in the two species, but muscle infections in human are often overlooked. While light infections with the bladder worm are often asymptomatic, in heavier infections the chance of cysts lodging in the brain (Fig. 7-12) or eye, where they are most likely to cause symptoms, is increased. Some 60% of patients with cysticerci are found to have them in the brain, and 3% in the eye; however, a large percentage of persons with known cerebral infections are asymptomatic. Autopsy data from Mexico City indicate a prevalence rate of 1.4% to 3.6% for neurocysticercosis among the general population of the city, most of which infections are unsuspected during life.

Cysticerci can develop in any voluntary muscle. Though the majority of such infections are asymptomatic, invasion of muscle by the larvae may give rise to myositis, with accompanying fever and eosinophilia, and in rare cases to a condition known as muscular pseudohypertrophy, with the initial muscle swelling then leading to atrophy and fibrosis. Frequently the cysticerci die and become calcified without giving rise to any symptoms (Fig. 7-13).

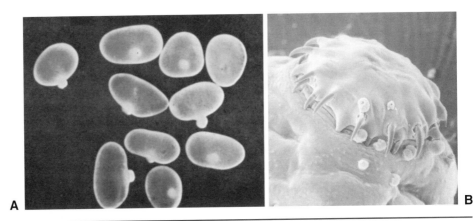

FIGURE 7-11 ■ **A,** Cysticercus larvae of *Taenia solium*. **B,** Scanning electron micrograph of scolex from cysticercus, showing hooklets. (Courtesy of the U.S. Department of Agriculture.)

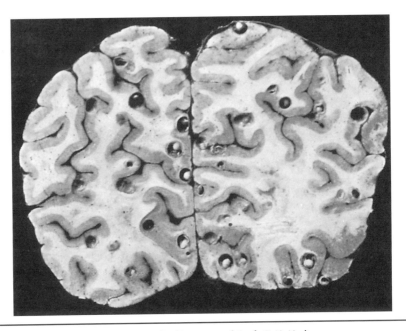

FIGURE 7-12 ■ Cerebral cysticercosis. (Courtesy of Prof. C. H. Hu.)

Their unsuspected presence in the muscles may have diagnostic importance, and soft tissue films of the thighs are often useful in the workup of a patient with unexplained seizures.

Subcutaneous cysts are easily palpated and may resemble small lipomas. Surgical removal (usually for purposes of diagnosis) is readily performed.

Cysticerci may be found within the orbit, in either the anterior or the posterior chamber or in the retinal tissues. They are often readily seen with an ophthalmoscope. Depending on their location, they may give rise to visual difficulties that fluctuate with eye position, or to a generalized decrease in visual acuity, retinal edema, hemorrhage or vasculitis, or detachment. Cysts developing along the optic tracts may give rise to visual field defects.

Worldwide, neurocysticercosis (NCC) is the most common parasitic disease of the CNS. It may present itself in many forms, depending on localization of the cysts and disease activity. As infection may take place over a period of many years, it is possible for one host to exhibit multiple forms of the disease. In a large series of cases (Sotelo et al., 1985) in

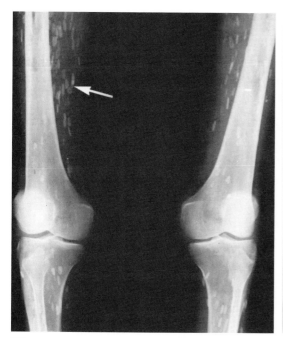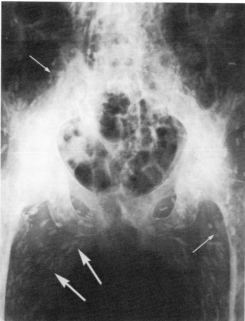

FIGURE 7-13 ■ Extensive calcified cysticercosis of muscle. Numerous elliptical calcifications having variable sizes are evident in the muscle planes of the pelvis and lower extremities and are aligned along the long axis parallel to the muscle planes *(large arrows)*. Nearly all the calcifications have a small lucent center *(small arrows)*. When viewed from the side, they resemble a ring calcification. (From Keats T. *Missouri Med* 1961; 58:457.)

Mexico City, over 90% of individuals were found to have some form of active disease, whereas more than 60% had symptoms related to dead cysts, the so-called inactive disease. About half exhibited two or more forms of NCC.

The most common form of active NCC, characterized by the presence of living cysts (see, Diagnosis, which follows), occurring in about half the patients in the series cited above, was arachnoiditis, with spinal fluid pleocytosis, increased cerebrospinal fluid protein, and a positive CSF serologic test for cysticercosis. In about a quarter of the patients, the intense inflammatory reaction provoked by this meningeal localization resulted in obstructive hydrocephalus; other sequelae may be cranial nerve involvement, intracranial hypertension, arterial thrombosis, and stroke. Parenchymally located active (noncalcified) cysts (seen in about 13% of cases) may cause no symptoms while alive and often do not result in CSF changes, but they may also give rise to cerebral edema, epileptic seizures, focal deficits, and intracranial hypertension. Other forms of active NCC include vasculitis with resultant brain infarction, mass effect produced by large cysts or clumps of cysts, intraventricular cysts, and spinal cysts. Intraventricular cysts may be asymptomatic, or if they block the flow of CSF they may cause intermittent or continuously increased intracranial pressure. Cysts developing within the spinal cord may produce an arachnoiditis, or symptoms similar to those resulting from any mass lesion.

Classified as inactive NCC are calcified parenchymal cysts, seen in about 60% of cases, and hydrocephalus secondary to meningeal fibrosis, found in about 4%.

In the series just cited, epilepsy was seen in just over half of the patients, headache occurred in 43%, papilledema in 28%, vomiting in 27%, pyramidal tract signs in 21.5%, intellectual deterioration in 16%, ataxic gait in 10%, diminished visual acuity in 10%, and optic atrophy in 6.5%. A number of other signs or symptoms, such as psychotic episodes, diplopia, vertigo, cranial nerve palsies, and behavioral disturbances, were seen in fewer than

5% of patients. Some 26% of patients had normal neurologic findings. This constellation of signs and symptoms depends on the localization of the cysts and on whether they are alive, dying, or dead and calcified. Meningeal cysts cause intense arachnoiditis, which may lead to obstructive hydrocephalus, cranial nerve involvement, intracranial hypertension, arterial thrombosis, and stroke. Parenchymal cysts may give rise to cerebral edema, epileptic seizures of various types, focal deficits, and intracranial hypertension. Intraventricular cysts, rare in the patients from Mexico City but found in up to 15% of patients in some series, may be asymptomatic, or if they block the flow of CSF may cause intermittent or continuously increased intracranial pressure, with its attendant severe persistent headache, papilledema, and progressive loss of vision. Nausea and vomiting may also result from increased intracranial pressure.

Parenchymal cysticerci that do not come in contact with the subarachnoid space and cysticerci in the ventricles that do not obstruct the flow of CSF may cause no symptoms while alive, but an intense inflammatory reaction may develop around the dead or dying parasites, with an exacerbation of symptoms. It has been suggested that this may be secondary not only to the release of antigenic substances by the dead or dying worms but also to cessation of their active immunosuppression, considered to deplete complement, suppress lymphocyte activity, reduce eosinophil activity, and have an active cytotoxic effect.

Diagnosis. Surgical removal of subcutaneous or intracranial cysts, with demonstration of the organism (Fig. 7-14), radiographic demonstration of calcified cysts in the muscle, or visualization of the cysticercus within the orbit, is diagnostic. Signs and symptoms of a space-occupying lesion of the central nervous system may be highly suggestive of cysticercosis in the presence of demonstrable cysticerci elsewhere in the body or of a positive serologic test for cysticercosis (the more important of these tests are mentioned in Chapter 16). However, serologic test results are often negative in cysticercosis of the central nervous system.

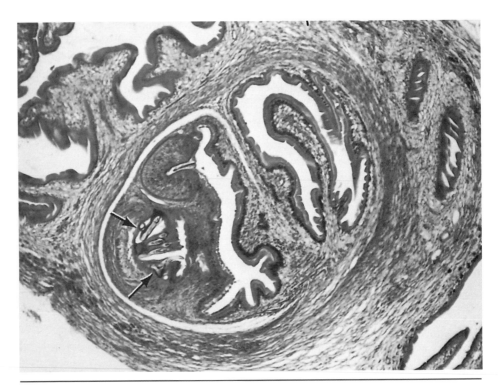

FIGURE 7-14 ■ Section through scolex of cysticercus showing hooklets *(arrows)*. (Photograph by Zane Price.)

Plain skull films may reveal calcified cysts within the brain, but computed tomography (CT) shows both calcified and uncalcified cysts, and with the use of contrast medium may show enhancement indicative of inflammatory changes, which may be used to distinguish active cysts from inactive ones. It is not useful for the demonstration of intraventricular cysts. Figure 7-15, *A, B* contrasts CT and magnetic resonance imaging (MRI) of the same parenchymal cyst. MRI is inferior for detecting parenchymal calcifications but demonstrates intraventricular cysts (Fig. 7-15, *C*) not seen on CT.

Racemose cysts (Fig. 7-16) are aberrant cysticerci, which at times are found developing in the ventricles or subarachnoid space. Such larvae form no scolex, and the cyst wall grows in an irregular branching and budding fashion to a diameter of several centimeters. Figure 7-15, *D, E*, is an MR image of such a cyst, which is noted to have the same density as the spinal fluid but is seen to produce unphysiologic enlargements within the ventricular system. The cysts may resemble *Sparganum proliferum* larvae but in section can be distinguished by the presence of a cavity within the parenchyma as well as by the demonstration of specific immune complexes.

Epidemiology. Humans acquire cysticercosis through ingestion of eggs passed in human feces. Proper disposal of feces, to avoid contamination of food, soil, and water, is essential. Cysticercosis is seen principally in areas where pork is consumed raw or undercooked, so that the prevalence of *T. solium* infection is high, and where poor hygiene allows contamination of foodstuffs by human feces.

Immigrants from Mexico, Central and South America, and Southeast Asia account for most cases in the United States. Infection rates, as determined by serologic testing of rural villagers, are reported as ranging from over 22% in Bolivia to about 11% in Mexico and 8% in Peru, and neurologic symptoms among those infected from 9.3% in a Beijing hospital to 21% in Rwanda and 47% in Bombay (Tsang and Wilson, 1995). Neurocysticercosis accounts for up to 2% of the neurology/neurosurgery admissions in southern California (Evans et al., 1997). The number of cases in Los Angeles County averages more than 100 per month, with 90% occurring in the Hispanic population (Potera, 2000). A survey involving a network of 11 U.S. university-affiliated emergency departments identified 38 (2.1%) of 1801 seizure patients as having neurocysticercosis (Ong et al., 2002). The disease was associated with Hispanic ethnicity, immigrant status, and exposure to areas of endemicity. A small percentage of infections are acquired within this country, usually by persons in close contact with such individuals. Four cases of neurocysticercosis in an orthodox Jewish community in New York City prompted serologic testing of a representative sample of the 7000 households in that community and indicated a prevalence rate of about 1.3%. Household seropositivity was linked to employment of housekeepers from Central America (Moore et al., 1995).

Treatment. As evidenced by the autopsy rate of neurocysticercosis in Mexico City, many cases are asymptomatic and require no treatment. Until recent years, all that could be offered symptomatic patients was anticonvulsants to relieve seizures, corticosteroids if necessary to control symptoms secondary to meningitis or cerebral edema, and surgery in selected cases. Surgical treatment includes direct excision of ventricular cysts, shunting procedures to relieve hydrocephalus, and removal of cysts by means of stereotaxic endoscopy. With the introduction of CT, we have not only found that the prevalence of neurocysticercosis is much greater than was thought but had to alter our ideas about the natural history of the disease. Spontaneous disappearance of parenchymal cysticerci is well documented, especially in children, suggesting to some the advisability of symptomatic treatment in those for whom it is effective and following the evolution of the lesions with CT or MRI. Such treatment, including the administration of dexamethasone (24 to 32 mg/day during the acute stage), is advised by various authorities for those few patients who develop an acute cysticercotic encephalitis, whose condition would probably be exacerbated by anticysticercal treatment. A study involving children with neurocysticercosis in New Delhi, India, determined that

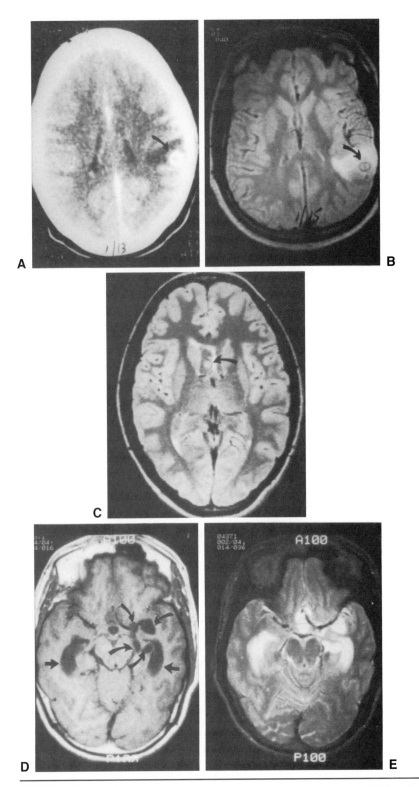

FIGURE 7-15 ■ Neurocysticercosis as seen by computed tomography (CT) and magnetic resonance imaging (MRI). **A, B,** The same parenchymal cyst (**A,** CT with contrast; **B,** proton density-weighted MRI). **C,** Proton density-weighted MRI of intraventricular cyst. **D, E,** The same racemose intraventricular cyst (**D,** T1-weighted MRI; **E,** T2-weighted MRI; *curved arrows,* cysts; *straight arrows,* lateral ventricles). (Courtesy of Prof. T. Hans Newton, University of California San Francisco, CA.)

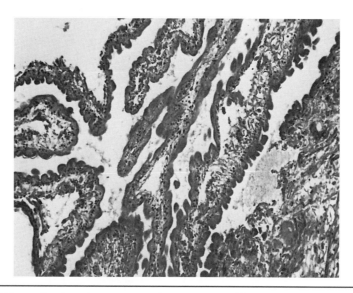

FIGURE 7-16 ■ Section of racemose cysticercus removed from ventricle of human brain. Note scalloped surface of bladder wall. (Photomicrograph by Zane Price.)

albendazole (discussed later) was not beneficial in treatment. The frequency of healing between the albendazole-treated group and the placebo group was not statistically significant (Gogia et al., 2003).

Excellent discussions of the therapy of all forms of neurocysticercosis are given by Del Brutto et al. (1992, 1993). For active parenchymal brain cysts and subarachnoid (racemose) cysts they recommend albendazole, 15 mg/kg body weight daily (maximum 800 mg per day) for 8 days. Others suggest treating for as long as 30 days. Garcia et al. (2004) conclude from a study carried out in Lima, Peru, that treatment of adult patients having neurocysticercosis with 800 mg of albendazole per day and 6 mg of dexamethasone per day for 10 days was safe and effective in decreasing the parasite burden and in reducing the number of seizures. Serum levels are increased if taken with a fatty meal. Albendazole, a member of the benzimidazole group of drugs that includes thiabendazole and mebendazole, is generally well tolerated; side effects include dizziness or headache, abdominal pain, diarrhea, nausea, and vomiting. It should not be taken during pregnancy.

The alternative drug, praziquantel, seems slightly less effective than albendazole. Praziquantel is usually administered at the rate of 50 mg/kg body weight in three divided doses daily for 15 days. The simultaneous administration of steroids (e.g., dexamethasone 24 to 32 mg/day) is considered essential in the treatment of subarachnoid cysts, but not for parenchymal cysts. Dexamethasone administration may result in decreased plasma levels of praziquantel (for which some upward adjustment of dosage may be indicated) but actually increases those of albendazole. For treatment of other forms of NCC, Del Brutto's papers and those of Badres and coworkers (1992) should be consulted. Chemotherapy should *not* be used for intraocular cysticercosis. Surgical removal is often possible.

Results of treatment may be monitored by contrast-enhanced CT, generally done after an interval of 3 months. Remission or marked improvement in seizure activity is usually seen after therapy (Vasquez and Sotelo, 1992).

Control. Thorough cooking of pork or freezing to −5°C for 4 days, −15°C for 3 days, or −24°C for 1 day kills the larvae and if universally practiced would eliminate the infection from both humans and pigs.

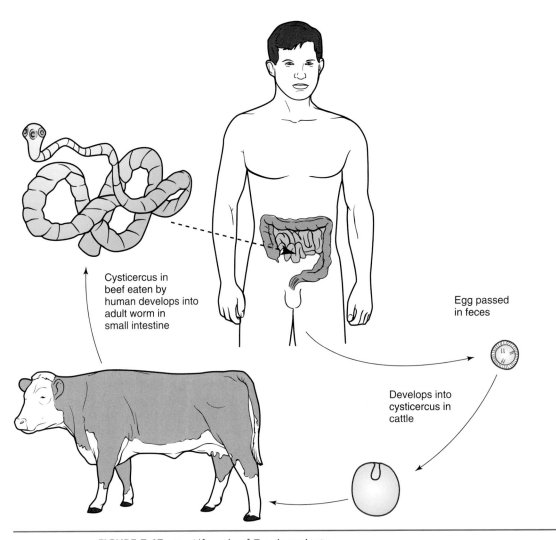

Cysticercus in
beef eaten by
human develops into
adult worm in
small intestine

Egg passed
in feces

Develops into
cysticercus in
cattle

FIGURE 7-17   ■   Life cycle of *Taenia saginata*.

Taenia saginata

The beef tapeworm, *T. saginata*, has worldwide distribution. Unlike *T. solium*, infection with *T. saginata* is frequently encountered in the United States. The life cycle is somewhat similar to that of *T. solium*, but cattle are the intermediate host, while humans are hosts only to the adult worms (Fig. 7-17). Embryonated eggs are passed with the feces and must be ingested by cattle. The larva grows in the flesh of cattle and eventually develops into an infective cysticercus. It is acquired by humans through the ingestion of raw or insufficiently cooked beef. The prevalent (and from a parasitologist's, if not a gourmet's, point of view, deplorable) liking for rare steak is one means of successful survival of this species in the United States. An important difference between *T. solium* and *T. saginata* is that cysticercosis of humans due to *T. saginata* apparently does not occur.

Adults of *T. saginata* exceptionally attain a length of 25 m, but they are usually less than half this size. The scolex (Fig. 7-18) bears four muscular suckers and a small rostellum without hooks. Presence or absence of hooks may thus serve to differentiate the two species of *Taenia*. Mature proglottids are either wider than long or nearly square, whereas gravid proglottids, which are eventually passed in the stool, are considerably longer than they are wide. Usually the gravid proglottids of *T. saginata* (Fig. 7-19) are longer than those of *T. solium*. The structure

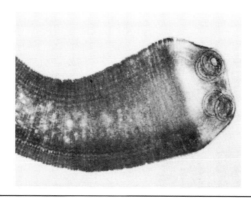

FIGURE 7-18 ■ *Taenia saginata*, scolex. (Photomicrograph by Zane Price.)

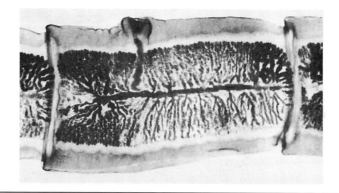

FIGURE 7-19 ■ *Taenia saginata*, gravid proglottid. (Photomicrograph by Zane Price.)

of the uterus is very much like that of *T. solium*, but the number of main side branches on each side of the central stem is 15 to 20. Eggs are similar to those of *T. solium*; specific identification may be made by examining the gravid segments as outlined for *T. solium*.

The symptoms and treatment are as outlined for taeniasis solium.

Taenia saginata asiatica (Asian Taenia)

First reported from Taiwan, this *Taenia* species has now been found also in Korea, China, the Philippines, Thailand, Malaysia, and Indonesia. In the latter country, particularly in North Sumatra and Bali, raw or rare roasted pork is consumed, and the adult worms found in humans are the Asian *Taenia*. In Irian Jaya neurocysticercosis is pandemic, but there the adult worm is *T. solium*. Apparently, the Asian taeniid does not produce cysticercosis in humans (Flisser et al., 2004). DNA testing suggests that this worm, morphologically similar to *T. saginata* but with a scolex suggestive of *T. solium*, is genetically distinct and should be considered a subspecies of *T. saginata* (Fan et al., 1995; González et al., 2004) though some would consider it a separate species, *T. asiatica* (Eom et al., 2002). It infects a range of intermediate hosts (cattle, goats, monkeys, and wild boar) in addition to swine, with cysticerci being found primarily in the liver.

Multiceps multiceps (Coenurus Disease)

The adult of *M. multiceps*, a taeniid worm of moderate size, is found in dogs and other Canidae. The larval stage, known as a coenurus, occurs in a variety of herbivorous mammals and has been reported occasionally from humans in various parts of the world, including the United States. It is possible that more than one species of *Multiceps* can produce human disease, but it is very difficult to distinguish species in this genus.

Following ingestion of the egg of *Multiceps*, the oncosphere hatches in the small intestine and makes its way into a blood vessel in the intestinal wall in the same manner as larvae of *Taenia*. The embryo is carried in the bloodstream to various parts of the body but most frequently develops in the central nervous system. Multiple scolices bud from the inner surface of the cyst wall, instead of the single one that characterizes the bladder worm. The coenurus larva is larger than a cysticercus (up to 2 cm diameter); it is semitransparent, glistening white, and filled with fluid. Numerous denser white spots on the wall indicate the position of the attached scolices. The coenurus may form a single vesicle, or it may be branched to a greater or lesser degree. It may be impossible to distinguish a sterile coenurus from a racemose cysticercus.

In sheep, the most common intermediate host, the parasite produces a disease known as gid, from the unstable gait, or giddiness, that marks the infected animals. In humans, most reported patients have had coenuri in the brain or spinal cord and symptoms suggestive of space-occupying lesions of the central nervous system. In tropical Africa, coenurus larvae, which may be those of a species other than *M. multiceps*, have been found in the muscles or subcutaneous tissues. A preoperative diagnosis of coenurus infection is unlikely, as there are no specific serologic tests for it.

Treatment is surgical. There are no reports of the use of praziquantel or albendazole, but mebendazole has been found not to be effective.

Echinococcus granulosus, E. multilocularis, and *E. vogeli (Hydatid Disease)*

The genus *Echinococcus* contains three species for which humans are host to the larval stage, or hydatid. These three species are all found as adult worms in Canidae. A fourth, *E. oligarthrus*, whose status as a human parasite is disputed, occurs as an adult in felids. The life cycle of all these worms is similar to that of *E. granulosus* (Fig. 7-20).

The adult worm (Fig. 7-21) is 0.6 cm or less in length and possesses a scolex, neck, and usually three proglottids. One proglottid is immature, one is mature, and one is gravid. The eggs cannot be distinguished from those of *Taenia*. Eggs of *Echinococcus* contain an embryo, called an onchosphere or hexacanth because of the six hooklets it bears. Upon ingestion by the intermediate host, the embryos, released from their surrounding membranes by action of the digestive juices, bore actively into the intestinal wall and enter a blood vessel. They may lodge in any organ or tissue but most frequently are found in the liver and lungs. In humans, 80% to 95% of hydatids develop in these two organs, the majority in the liver. The embryo develops slowly into the hydatid cyst, reaching a diameter of 1 cm in 5 months or so and thereafter enlarging steadily so that at the end of 10 or more years' growth it may contain some liters of fluid. Ultimate growth depends on location; in some areas of the body they are unable to expand freely, whereas in others modest growth results in serious impairment to the function of vital structures or even in death.

By the time the cyst of *E. granulosus* has reached the diameter of 1 cm, its wall is differentiated into a thick outer laminated, noncellular layer, or limiting membrane, which covers the thin germinal epithelium. From the germinal epithelium, masses of cells grow into the cavity of the cyst. They become vacuolated and are known as the brood capsules. Protoscolices bud from the inner wall of the brood capsule. Occasionally, daughter cysts appear within the hydatid (Fig. 7-22); these in turn produce brood capsules, which may contain protoscolices. The daughter cysts are replicas in miniature of the complete hydatid, possessing even the laminated outer layer; their mode of development is obscure. Gradually, the brood capsules and daughter cysts break down, liberating the developed scolices. A granular material, consisting of free protoscolices, daughter cysts, and amorphous material, is found in older cysts. This is the "hydatid sand" (Fig. 7-23) that is sometimes aspirated for diagnostic purposes. Some cysts may never produce brood capsules, or the brood capsules

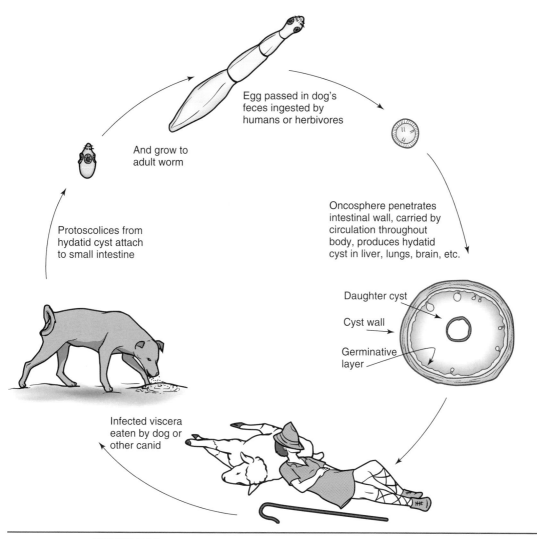

FIGURE 7-20 ■ Life cycle of *Echinococcus granulosus.* (Adapted from Brown WJ, Voge M. *Neuropathology of parasitic infections,* Oxford, 1982. Oxford University Press.)

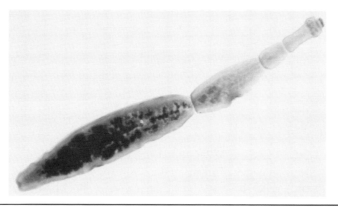

FIGURE 7-21 ■ *Echinococcus granulosus,* adult worm.

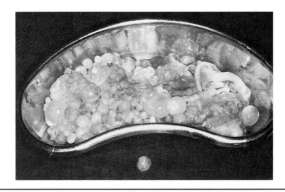

FIGURE 7-22 ■ Numerous small and medium-sized daughter cysts, recovered from a single hydatid cyst of the liver. (From Saidi F. *Surgery of hydatid disease*, Philadelphia, 1976, WB Saunders.)

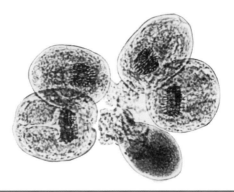

FIGURE 7-23 ■ *Echinococcus granulosus,* hydatid sand. (Photomicrograph by Zane Price.)

may fail to produce protoscolices. In other cases, hydatids may become sterile because of secondary bacterial infection or they may die and become calcified.

When the hydatid cyst is formed in bone (Fig. 7-24), development is markedly abnormal, and the limiting membrane is not formed. The hydatid develops first in the marrow cavity, from which it expands and frequently erodes large areas of bone.

The minute tapeworm *E. granulosus* lives as an adult in the intestines of dogs and other Canidae. Two different cycles—pastoral and sylvatic—and a number of different strains have been recognized. Intermediate hosts in the pastoral cycle are chiefly herbivores, in whose organs and tissues the hydatid cyst develops. The most important of these intermediate hosts is sheep, but in some areas *E. granulosus* is a common parasite of goats, swine, cattle, and horses. In North Africa, Iraq, and Iran, hydatid cysts occur with high frequency in the lungs of camels. Human infection is seen principally in the sheep-raising areas of the world, including southern Brazil, Argentina, Uruguay, Chile, and Peru; in Yugoslavia, Bulgaria, Sardinia, Cyprus, Turkey, and Lebanon; in scattered parts of Africa; in central Asia and northern China; and in New Zealand and southern Australia. While not widespread in North America, a number of cases have been reported from California, Arizona, Utah, New Mexico, and the lower Mississippi valley. Prevalence rates vary with local customs, the highest in the world being among the Turkana in the northwest corner of Kenya, bordering Ethiopia, the Sudan, and Uganda, because of the uniquely close association between the Turkana and their dogs.

In some areas, more than a single strain of *E. granulosus* may be distinguished. In Great Britain sheep-and-dog and horse-and-dog strains are recognized, with physiologic and enough morphologic differences between the two so that the subspecific name *E. granulosus*

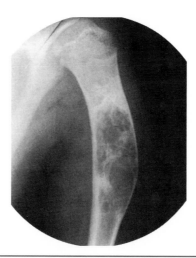

FIGURE 7-24   ■   Hydatid cyst involving the upper humerus of child. (From Saidi F. *Surgery of hydatid disease,* Philadelphia, 1976, WB Saunders.)

equines has been proposed for the horse strain, which seems not to infect humans. The Swiss cattle-and-dog strain also shows morphologic differences from strains originating from domestic animals elsewhere, and unlike those of most bovine strains, the cysts are fertile.

The sylvatic cycle occurs in wolves, the hydatids developing in wild ungulates (moose and reindeer) in Alaska, Canada, Scandinavia, and northern Eurasia. In Australia, the wallaby-and-dingo strain is more important than the sheep-and-dog strain. Humans are less likely to become infected as accidental hosts in the sylvatic cycle.

E. multilocularis was for many years thought to represent an abnormal variant of *E. granulosus* but is now recognized as a distinct species with its own life cycle. Foxes are the primary definitive hosts, while various rodents (voles, lemmings, shrews, mice) serve as intermediate hosts. Within rural communities domestic cycles may become established, with domestic dogs (and occasionally cats) as definitive hosts; rodents are again the usual intermediate hosts, but it is in this setting that humans may also become infected. *E. multilocularis* is enzootic throughout much of the subarctic area of the world—in Alaska, Canada and the North Central states bordering on Canada, the former Soviet republics including Siberia, northern China, and the northern islands of Japan—as well as Central Europe into Germany and in India.

Minor morphologic differences are seen between adults of *E. granulosus* and *E. multilocularis,* and the hydatid cysts of the two species are quite distinct. The limiting membrane is thin in *E. multilocularis,* and the germinal epithelium may bud externally, to proliferate in any direction or even to metastasize. It is because of their appearance that they are called alveolar or multilocular cysts. These cysts usually occur in the liver in humans and grow very slowly, so that they may be present for many years before causing symptoms, which are generally related to pressure from the expanding tissue. Unlike the unilocular hydatid cysts of *E. granulosus,* there is little fluid in alveolar hydatids, which consist of many small vesicles embedded in a dense connective tissue stroma (Fig. 7-25). Growth into the vena cava or portal vein may lead to metastases, usually to the lungs or brain.

E. vogeli occurs in Central and South America as a parasite of the bush dog, with its polycystic larval stage in rodents (pacas and spiny rats). Human cases have been reported from Panama, Colombia, Brazil, Peru, and Ecuador. The germinal membrane of the hydatid proliferates both inward, in the original cyst, forming septa that divide it into many sections (Fig. 7-26), and outward, to form new cysts. The vesicles forming a polycystic hydatid are relatively large and fluid filled.

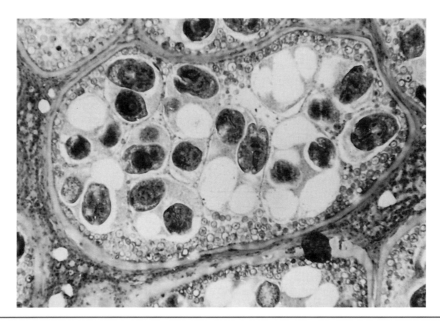

FIGURE 7-25   ■   Section through cyst of *Echinococcus multilocularis* in liver. (Photomicrograph by Zane Price.)

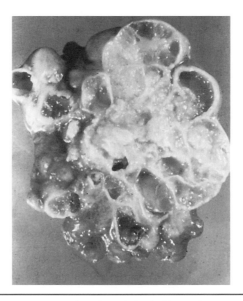

FIGURE 7-26   ■   *Echinococcus vogeli:* Polycystic hydatid cyst, human pericardium. (From D'Alessandro A et al. *Am J Trop Med Hyg* 1979; *28*:303.)

In humans, hydatids of *E. vogeli* are found in the liver, but also the lungs, pleura, pericardium, and heart; the intercostal muscles and diaphragm; and in the stomach, omentum, and mesenteries.

The fourth species, *E. oligarthrus*, is found in Central and South America. Having its adult stage in wild felids, it is likewise characterized by the formation of polycystic hydatid cysts in its rodent intermediate hosts. It has been reported on rare occasions to cause hydatid disease in humans, but some believe that these human cases were in fact misidentified *E. vogeli*.

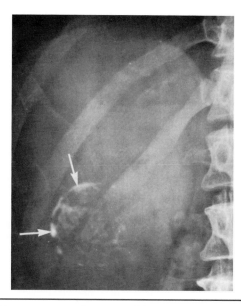

FIGURE 7-27 ■ *Echinococcus granulosus* cyst of liver. There is a single, round, partially calcified hydatid cyst in the inferior portion of the right lobe (*white arrows*). (From Teplick JG et al. *Roentgenologic diagnosis,* vol. 1, ed 3, Philadelphia, 1976, WB Saunders.)

Human infections with *E. oligarthrus* and *E. vogeli* have been reported from Suriname (Basset et al., 1998).

There is no unanimity as regards classification of the genus *Echinococcus*. Some authorities recognize as many as nine "strains" of *E. granulosus*, on the basis of differing intermediate hosts (and definitive hosts—there is a strain in Africa in which the adult worm is found only in lions), DNA sequencing, geographic location, and so forth. Four of these "strains" are considered to be sufficiently different as to warrant being called separate species (Lymbery and Thompson, 1996). Similarly, four strains of *E. multilocularis* are recognized. The diagnostic and therapeutic significance of these findings, if they are confirmed, remains to be determined.

Diagnosis. Many asymptomatic hydatid cysts are first discovered on radiographic examination (Fig. 7-27). The cyst shows a sharp outline, and fluid levels can sometimes be detected within it. Photoscans may indicate the presence of space-occupying lesions of the liver or spleen. Ultrasound and CT are also of value (Fig. 7-28). If the cyst is abdominal and large, a characteristic thrill can sometimes be elicited. After surgical exposure of a presumed hydatid cyst, aspiration of a portion of its contents can be performed, and examination of fluid removed in this manner may reveal hydatid sand. It should be remembered that some hydatid cysts are sterile and contain no sand. A number of serologic tests available for the diagnosis of hydatid disease are outlined in Chapter 16. The indirect hemagglutination test (IHA) and enzyme-linked immunosorbent assay (ELISA) seem most satisfactory. Serologic cross reactions have been noted between cysticercosis and hydatid disease and also between cysticercosis and sparganosis (personal observation).

Symptoms. Symptoms of hydatid disease vary according to the location of the cyst. If, as is most commonly the case, the cyst is in the liver, it may cause no symptoms and will be noted only when its increasing size calls attention to its presence. Hepatic cysts may cause early symptoms if the location in the liver is such that their expansion produces pressure on a major bile duct or blood vessel or if intrabiliary rupture occurs. Cysts in the lungs ordinarily are asymptomatic until they become large enough to give rise to cough, shotness of breath,

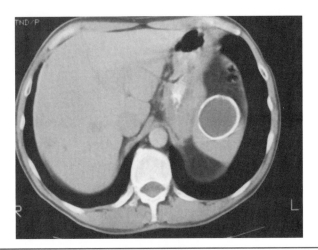

FIGURE 7-28 ■ CT shows hydatid cyst of spleen. (Courtesy of Dr. J. F. Catchpool, Sausalito, CA.)

or pain in the chest. Cysts in the central nervous system produce serious damage, symptoms very similar to those seen in ocular sparganosis.

Pathogenesis. The expanding hydatid cyst causes pressure necrosis of surrounding tissues, although as growth is slow a good deal of accommodation may take place before any vital structures are compromised. This obviously depends on the location of the cyst. Slow leakage of hydatid fluid from the cyst sensitizes the patient and elicits eosinophilia. Rupture of an abdominal hydatid cyst, either through trauma or in the course of surgery, carries with it both the grave risk of anaphylactic shock and the possibility of spread of the infection through seeding the peritoneal cavity with hydatid sand or bits of germinal epithelium, which are capable of producing new cysts. Rupture of a pulmonary cyst into a bronchus may be marked by severe allergic symptoms and coughing with the production of blood-flecked fluid, which may contain recognizable hydatid tissue. At times this results in spontaneous cure, but secondary infection may lead to chronic lung abscess.

Circulating immune complexes have been detected and membranous nephropathy demonstrated in patients with hydatid disease.

Epidemiology. Although hydatid disease caused by *E. granulosus* is most prevalent in sheep-raising areas such as Australia and New Zealand, other domestic and wild animals serve as intermediate hosts of the parasite elsewhere. Where sheep-and-dog strains are chiefly responsible for continuation of the cycle, the most successful control programs to date have consisted of routine 6-weekly deworming of the dogs with praziquantel. The adult worms are acquired by sheep dogs or stray dogs feeding on infected entrails that lie about abattoirs or that are discarded after slaughtering animals at home. Feral dogs and other canidas acquire the infection by scavenging or by preying on sheep or wild herbivores. Transmission to humans may occur whenever infected dogs live in close proximity to them.

Hydatid disease is widely distributed throughout the South American continent. In North America, *E. granulosus* occurs in Alaska, Canada, and the contiguous United States. Animal reservoirs are dogs, coyotes, and wolves; the hydatid cysts occur in sheep, pigs, deer, and other wild herbivores.

E. multilocularis is somewhat more restricted in distribution than is *E. granulosus* (see Figs. 2-7 and 2-8). Reservoir hosts of *E. multilocularis* in nature are dogs, wolves, foxes, and cats; the larval stages occur in wild rodents, particularly voles, which are an important food item of wild carnivores as well as of dogs and cats in rural areas; there is also a domestic life cycle involving adult worms in house cats, hydatids in mice. Thus, transmission to humans can occur by means of the accidental ingestion of eggs passed by dogs or cats. In addition, hunters and trappers could be infected while handling foxes or wolves.

There is growing concern in Europe about alveolar hydatid disease as the number of foxes increases in both rural and urban setting. A study in southwestern Germany reported that 75% of the foxes were infected with *E. multilocularis* (Romig et al., 1999). In Zürich, Switzerland, praziquantel-containing bait was distributed in an urban study area in an attempt to reduce the prevalence of *E. multilocularis* in the wild fox population (Hegglin et al., 2003). Examination of fox fecal samples in the baited area demonstrated a 92% reduction in infection when compared to the nonbaited control area. A concomitant reduction in infected rodents also was noted in the baited area.

The zoonotic cycle of *E. vogeli*, involving bush dogs (*Speothus venaticus*), pacas, and spiny rats, would not seem to impinge very directly upon humans. Yet pacas are large rodents, highly prized for food and hunted with dogs. Domestic dogs have been found infected naturally, and infection may be readily accomplished experimentally. It seems probable that domestic dogs, perhaps infected by being given the viscera of the paca, are the source of human infections.

Treatment. The first drug found to have any effect against the hydatid stage of *Echinococcus* was mebendazole. Albendazole is better absorbed and penetrates well into hydatid cysts, and therefore is now generally preferred over mebendazole (Gil-Grande et al., 1993), although neither drug gives impressive cure rates in most studies (Todorov et al., 1992). Albendazole is generally administered at the rate of 10 mg/kg body weight, or 400 mg twice daily for 4 weeks, repeated as necessary for up to 12 cycles each separated by an intrval of 2 weeks (Cook, 1990). The results of therapy are best judged by ultrasonography or MRI, repeated at intervals of approximately 3 months. It is generally agreed that chemotherapy should be instituted a day or so before surgery or aspiration, and continued for a month after such procedures.

Until recently the surgical removal of hydatid cysts, discussed in detail by Saidi (1976), was the only form of therapy possible. Recently many reports favor the use of percutaneous aspiration for pulmonary, hepatic, and other cysts accessible to this type of procedure. The most commonly used form of therapy is described by the acronym PAIR (*Percutaneous Aspiration, Injection*—of hypertonic saline or other scolicidal fluid—and *Reaspiration*), as detailed by Akhan et al. (1994, 1996), Bastid et al. (1994), Salama et al. (1995), Khuroo et al. (1997), and Smego et al. (2003) all of whom find it a safe and effective form of therapy in selected cases.

Praziquantel has some protoscolicidal effect. Yasawi et al. (1993) report excellent results when it is given in conjunction with albendazole; ivermectin injected directly into cysts has been found to kill all protoscolices in experimental animals (Ochieng-Mitula and Burt, 1996).

E. multilocularis is said to respond to albendazole, given in the same dosage as recommended for *e. granulosus*, in a similar fashion (Liu et al., 1993); a single report (Meneghelli et al., 1986) suggests that the same is true of *E. vogeli*.

Dipylidium caninum

D. caninum is common in cats and dogs all over the world. Occasionally it is found in humans, particularly small children. The larvae of this species are known as cysticercoids. The cysticercoid develops when the egg is ingested by a cat or dog flea larva and is retained within the adult flea. Infection takes place through the accidental ingestion of these fleas (Fig. 7-29). The cysticercoids grow into adult worms in the small intestine. The gravid proglottids possess a remarkable degree of motility and may migrate actively from the anus. They contract and expand vigorously upon reaching the exterior of the host and may remain attached to the fur surrounding the anal area for some time. It is probable that these contractions function in the release of the eggs, which are then ingested by the flea larvae.

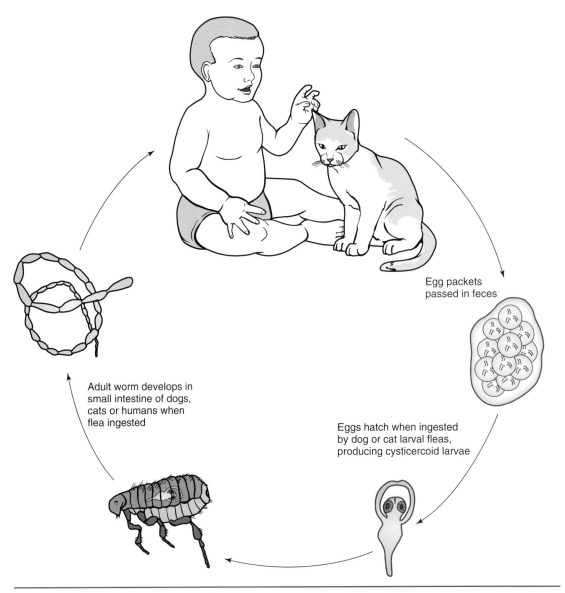

FIGURE 7-29 ■ Life cycle of *Dipylidium caninum.*

Adults of *D. caninum* are relatively small, averaging about 15 cm in length. They may reach a length of 80 cm. Many specimens may be present in one individual host. The scolex bears four suckers and a conical, retractile rostellum with several circles of small hooks. Mature proglottids (Fig. 7-30, *A*) are longer than they are wide and contain two sets each of male and female reproductive organs. The developing uterus appears in the form of a network, which, as the segment becomes gravid (Fig. 7-30, *B*), eventually breaks up into discrete units called egg packets (Fig. 7-31; see also Plate X). Each egg packet may contain 5 to 30 eggs. Gravid segments are considerably longer than they are wide and are barrel-like in outline as they appear in the stool or perineal area.

Diagnosis of this species is made on finding in the stool the characteristic proglottids or, more rarely, egg packets.

Symptoms. Light infections are often asymptomatic, but abdominal pain, diarrhea, and anal pruritus may occur in some individuals.

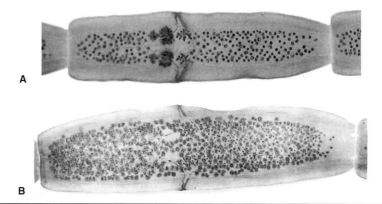

FIGURE 7-30 ■ *Dipylidium caninum.* **A,** Mature proglottid. **B,** Gravid proglottid. (Photomicrographs by Zane Price.)

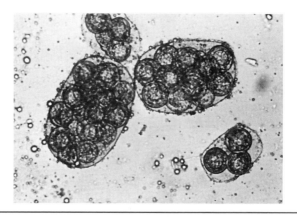

FIGURE 7-31 ■ Egg packets of *Dipylidium caninum.* (Photograph by H. J. Griffiths. From Zaiman H [ed.]. *A pictorial presentation of parasites.*)

Epidemiology. Human infection requires ingestion of infected dog or cat fleas and is thus most likely to occur in small children who kiss or are licked by their infected pets.

Treatment. Praziquantel is very effective, given in a single oral dose of 5 to 10 mg/kg body weight. Niclosamide, administered as outlined for *D. latum* infections, is an alternative.

Control. Periodic deworming of infected dogs and cats and control of fleas so that the animals do not become reinfected are essential. Niclosamide is now available in injectable form for veterinary use.

Hymenolepis nana

H. nana, the dwarf tapeworm of humans, is a common parasite of the house mouse and is found all over the world. Infection with *H. nana* is seen most frequently in children but occurs in adults as well. A relatively high prevalence of this tapeworm has been reported in surveys conducted in central Europe and in Latin America.

H. nana is unique in that the adult worm develops following ingestion of the egg by humans. Swallowed eggs hatch in the small intestine. The six-hooked oncosphere burrows into a villus of the intestinal mucosa, where, within a few days, it develops into a cysticercoid larva. The cysticercoid is a small larva (see Fig. 7-29), containing a single scolex but without the bladder characteristic of a cysticercus. When fully grown, the larva breaks out of the villus into the lumen of the small intestine, where it grows into an adult worm. Experimental evidence obtained from studies on mice suggests that in these animals a certain degree of immunity to reinfection results from the occurrence in them of the tissue phase.

Eggs of *H. nana* may also develop into infective cysticercoids in various intermediate hosts, particularly grain beetles. When ingested accidentally with contaminated grain products, the larvae grow into adult worms in mice, and probably in humans also. Adults of *H. nana* are relatively small worms, only a few centimeters long. The scolex has four suckers and a rostellum armed with one circle of hooks. All segments are wider than they are long. Mature proglottids contain one set of male and one set of female reproductive organs. Gravid segments contain a saclike uterus filled with eggs. Eggs are usually liberated from the gravid segments before they become detached. The eggs of *H. nana* (see Fig. 7-10, *A*; Plate XI, 1-3) are broadly ovoid, have a thin and smooth outer shell, and measure 30 to 47 μm. They contain the six-hooked (hexacanth) oncosphere within a rigid membrane. This membrane has two polar thickenings or knobs from which project four to eight long, thin filaments called polar filaments. The presence of these polar filaments is diagnostic and serves to differentiate the eggs of *H. nana* from those of *Hymenolepis diminuta* described subsequently.

Symptoms. Light infections are asymptomatic. When large numbers of worms are present, they may give rise to abdominal pain, diarrhea, headache, dizziness, anorexia, and various nonspecific symptoms.

Epidemiology. The estimate of 20 million *H. nana* infections worldwide made a good many years ago is no doubt a conservative figure now. Most infected persons are small children, and as these infections are usually transmitted through the ingestion of eggs, nursery schools are an important source of infection. Humans infected through ingestion of grain products contaminated by infected insects do not possess the relative tissue immunity conferred by harboring cysticercoids. Eggs produced by these worms, hatching in the intestine, encounter less tissue immunity and may give rise to the syndrome of hyperinfection.

Treatment. Praziquantel, given in a single oral dose of 25 mg/kg body weight, is the drug of choice. Niclosamide (see treatment of *D. latum*) must be given daily for 5 days because of the tissue phase of the infection. The daily dose is 2 g for adults, 1.5 g for children weighing over 34 kg, and 1 g for children weighing between 11 and 34 kg.

Nitazoxanide (Alinia), FDA-approved for *Cryptosporidium* and *Giardia*, but considered investigational for *H. nana*, may be used as an alternative treatment (Ortiz et al., 2002). Administered orally, the adult dosage is 500 mg a day for 3 days. The pediatric dosage is 100 mg twice a day for 3 days for children 1 to 3 years of age and 200 mg twice daily for 3 days for children 4 to 11 years old.

Hymenolepis diminuta

H. diminuta, despite its specific name, is much larger than *H. nana*. While *H. diminuta* commonly parasitizes rats, it may occasionally be encountered in human beings, cases having been reported from many parts of the world, including several areas of the United States. Completion of the life cycle requires an arthropod intermediate host. More than 20 different species of insects have been shown to serve as suitable hosts for the development of the cysticercoid larvae. The most important are flour moths and flour beetles. Upon ingestion of infected insects from flour contaminated by the droppings of infected rats, larvae grow into adults in the small intestine of humans or rats. The size of adult worms varies considerably and, as in other tapeworm species, depends in part on the number of worms in the intestine. The greatest length reported for an adult specimen of *H. diminuta* from a person is 1 m. Usually, adults are 20 to 50 cm long and as much as 4 mm wide (see Fig. 7-1). The scolex bears four suckers and a small rostellum without hooks. Diagnosis of this species is

TABLE 7-1 ▪ Key to the Gravid Proglottids of the Major Human Tapeworms

a. Uterus forms rosette in center of proglottid	*D. latum*
Uterus otherwise disposed	b
b. Uterus with central stem running length of proglottid	c
Uterus without central stem	d
c. Central stem with 7 to 13 main lateral branches	*T. solium*
Central stem with 15 to 20 main lateral branches	*T. saginata*
d. Proglottid wider than long	*Hymenolepis* spp.
Proglottid longer than wide	*Dipylidium caninum*

made on finding the characteristic eggs (Fig. 7-10, *B*) in the stool. Eggs are slightly ovoid and brown; the shell is relatively thick. In some specimens, fine concentric striations may be observed in the outer shell. The onchosphere is enclosed in a membrane that has two polar thickenings but no polar filaments. The absence of polar filaments readily differentiates this species from *H. nana*.

Symptoms. Most infections are in all probability asymptomatic, but occasional patients may present with mild gastrointestinal complaints such as nausea, anorexia, abdominal pains, and diarrhea.

Epidemiology. Primarily a zoonosis, hymenolepiasis diminuta may be prevented in humans by rodent control measures and by protection from rodents and their droppings and from insects of cereals, grains, and other foodstuffs that may be consumed without cooking.

Treatment. Praziquantel is very effective, given in a single oral dose of 25 mg/kg body weight. Niclosamide, administered as outlined for *D. latum* infections, is an alternative. Presumably, nitazoxanide, as outlined for *H. nana*, would be an effective alternative treatment.
Table 7-1 gives a key to the gravid proglottids of the major human tapeworms.

Uncommon Cestode Parasites of Humans

As is the case with the trematodes, humans are incidental hosts to various tapeworms. Here are a few examples; many more exist.

Bertiella

Bertiella studeri in Africa, India, Southeast Asia, and the Philippines and *B. mucronata* from South America are adult parasites of monkeys, with a cysticercoid stage in mites. Human infections involve ingestion of infected mites.

Diplogonoporus grandis

This tapeworm, related to *Diphyllobothrium*, is a parasite of whales, and has been reported a number of times from Japanese patients, who probably acquired the infection through the consumption of raw anchovies or sardines containing the plerocercoid larva.

Hymenolepis microstoma

The rodent tapeworm, *H. microstoma*, has been reported as an intestinal parasite of humans in Western Australia (Macnish et al., 2003). Various insects serve as intermediate hosts for the tapeworm, and rodent and human infections follow the ingestion of insects containing cysticercoid larvae. Molecular probes were used to identify the worms in human mixed infections with *H. nana*.

TABLE 7-2 ■ Review of Cestode Infections of Humans

Disease	Parasite	Means of Human Infection	Location of Larvae in Humans	Location of Adults in Humans	Clinical Features	Laboratory Diagnosis
Diphyllobothriasis	*Diphyllobothrium latum* (fish tapeworm)	Ingestion of larvae in fish	(Present as sparganosis)	Small intestine (attached)	Majority asymptomatic; can cause vitamin B$_{12}$ deficiency, anemia	Undeveloped operculate eggs or proglottids in stool
Taeniasis	*Taenia saginata* (beef tapeworm) *T. solium* (pork tapeworm)	Ingestion of larvae in beef or pork	Not present (for *T. solium* see cysticercosis below)	Small intestine (attached)	Vague digestive disturbances, anorexia; majority asymptomatic	Embryonated eggs or proglottids in stool
Cysticercosis	*Cysticercus cellulosae* (larva of *T. solium*)	Ingestion of eggs	Subcutaneous tissues, muscle, eye, brain	As for *T. solium*	Asymptomatic to Jacksonian seizures, hydrocephalus, visual problems	X-ray, CT, MRI, serologic tests
Echinococcosis (hydatid disease)	*Echinococcus granulosus* *E. multilocularis* *E. vogeli*	Ingestion of eggs	Liver, lungs, other organs	Not present (in canines)	Chronic space-occupying lesions of involved organs	X-ray, ultrasound, CT, aspirate of "hydatid sand," serologic tests
Hymenolepiasis	*Hymenolepis nana* (dwarf tapeworm) *H. diminuta* (rat tapeworm)	Ingestion of eggs (of larvae in insects for *H. diminuta*)	Villi of small intestine (not present in *H. diminuta*)	Small intestine (attached)	Enteritis, diarrhea, abdominal pain, anorexia; majority asymptomatic	Embryonated eggs in stool

Mathevotaenia

This intestinal tapeworm was described from a patient living in Bangkok, Thailand, following treatment with niclosamide (Lamom and Greer, 1986). The worms closely resembled *Mathevotaenia symmetrica*, a cosmopolitan intestinal tapeworm of rodents for which various insects serve as intermediate hosts. The diarrhea associated with the infection resolved after anthelminthic treatment.

Mesocestoides

Twenty-seven cases of human *Mesocestoides* infection have been reported from Africa, Asia, and the United States. The cases in the United States were in California, Louisiana, Mississipi, Missouri, New Jersey, Ohio, and Texas (Fuentes et al., 2003). Adult worms are intestinal parasites of various primates, carnivores, and birds of prey. The infective metacestode stage (tetrathyridium) is found in the body cavity and tissues of reptiles, birds, and small mammals. Human infection is acquired from eating insufficiently cooked meat of some animal that serves as an intermediate host for the larval metacestode stage. The species of *Mesocestoides* identified with human infection are *M. variabilis* and *M. lineatus*.

Praziquantel, a single oral dose of 10 mg/kg body weight, is effective in treatment.

Raillietina celebensis

A parasite of rats, this tapeworm has been reported in humans from Japan, Taiwan, the Philippines, Australia, and French Polynesia. As the entire life cycle of this parasite is not known, the method by which humans become infected is still a matter of speculation.

Table 7-2 summarizes some important features of the more common cestode infections of humans.

References

Akhan O et al. Percutaneous treatment of pulmonary hydatid cysts. *Cardiovasc Intervent Radiol* 1994; *17*:271–275.

Akhan O et al. Liver hydatid disease: Long-term results of percutaneous treatment. *Radiology* 1996; *198*:259–264.

Badres JC et al. Extraparenchymal neurocysticercosis: Report of five cases and review of management. *Clin Infect Dis* 1992; *15*:799–811.

Basset D et al. Neotropical echinococcosis in Suriname: *Echinococcus oligarthrus* in the orbit and *Echinococcus vogeli* in the abdomen. *Am J Trop Med Hyg* 1998; *59*:787–790.

Bastid C et al. Percutaneous treatment of hydatid cysts under sonographic guidance. *Digestive Dis. Sci.* 1994; *39*:1576–1580.

Cook GC. Use of benzimidazole chemotherapy in human helminthiases: Indications and efficacy. *Parasitol Today* 1990; *6*:133–136.

Del Brutto OH et al. Albendazole therapy for giant subarachnoid cysticerci. *Arch Neurol* 1992; *49*:335–338.

Del Brutto OH et al. Therapy for neurocysticercosis: A reappraisal. *Clin Infect Dis* 1993; *17*:730–735.

Eom KS et al. Identification of *Taenia asiatica* in China: Molecular, morphological, and epidemiological analysis of a Luzhai isolate. *J Parasitol* 2002; *88*:758–764.

Evans C et al. Controversies in the management of cysticercosis. *Emerg Infect Dis* 1997; *3*:403–405.

Fan PC et al. Morphological description of *Taenia saginata asiatica* (Cyclophyllidea: Taeniidae from man in Asia. *J Helminthol* 1995; *69*:299–303.

Flisser A et al. Portrait of human tapeworms. *J Parasitol* 2004; *90*:914–916.

Fuentes MV et al. A new case report of human *Mesocestoides* infection in the United States. *Am J Trop Med Hyg* 2003; *68*:566–567.

Garcia HH et al. A trial of antiparasitic treatment to reduce the rate of seizures due to cerebral cysticercosis. *N Engl J Med* 2004; *350*:249–258.

Gil-Grande LA et al. Randomized controlled trial of efficacy of albendazole in intra-abdominal hydatid disease. *Lancet* 1993; *342*:1269–1272.

Gogia S et al. Neurocysticercosis in children: Clinical findings and response to albendazole therapy in a randomized double-blind, placebo-controlled trial in newly diagnosed cases. *Trans R Soc Trop Med Hyg* 2003; *97*:416–421.

González LM et al. Differential diagnosis of *Taenia saginata* and *Taenia saginata asiatica* taeniasis through PCR. *Diag Microbiol Infect Dis* 2004; *49*:183–188.

Hegglin D et al. Anthelmintic baiting of foxes against urban contamination with *Echinococcus multilocularis*. *Emerg Infect Dis* 2003; *9*:1266–1272.

Holodniy M et al. Cerebral sparganosis: Case report and review. *Rev Infect Dis* 1991; *13*:155–159.

Khuroo MS et al. Percutaneous drainage compared with surgery for hepatic hydatid cysts. *N Engl J Med* 1997; *337*:681–687.

Lamon C, Greer GJ. Human infection with an anoplocephalid tapeworm of the genus *Mathevotaenia*. *Am J Trop Med Hyg* 1986; *35*:824–826.

Liu Y-H et al. Cerebral alveolar echinococcosis treated with albendazole. *Trans R Soc Trop Med Hyg* 1993; *87*:481.

Lymbery AL, Thompson RCA. Species of *Echinococcus*: Pattern and process. *Parasitol Today* 1996; *12*:486–491.

Macnish MG et al. Detection of the rodent tapeworm *Rodentolepis* (=*Hymenolepis*) *microstoma* in humans. A new zoonosis? *Int J Parasitol* 2003; *33*:1079–1085.

Meneghelli UG et al. Polycystic hydatid disease (*Echinococcus vogeli*): Clinical and radiological manifestations and treatment with albendazole of a patient from the Brazilian Amazon region. *Arg Gastroenterol* 1986; *23*:177–183.

Moore AC et al. Seroprevalence of cysticercosis in an orthodox Jewish community. *Am J Trop Med Hyg* 1995; *53*:439–442.

Ochieng-Mitula PJ, Burt MDB. The efficacy of ivermectin on the hydatid cyst of *Echinococcus granulosus* after direct injection at laparotomy. *J Parasitol* 1996; *82*:155–157.

Ong S et al. Neurocysticercosis in radiographically imaged seizure patients in U.S. emergency departments. *Emerg Infect Dis* 2002; *8*:608–613.

Ortiz JJ et al. Comparative clinical studies of nitazoxanide, albendazole and praziquantel in the treatment of ascariasis, trichuriasis and hymenolepiasis in children from Peru. *Trans R Soc Trop Med Hyg* 2002; *96*:193–196.

Potera C. Parasitic brain disease crosses the border. *ASM News* 2000; *66*:6–7.

Romig T et al. An epidemiologic survey of human alveolar echinococcosis in southwestern Germany. *Am J Trop Med Hyg* 1999; *61*:566–573.

Saidi F. Surgery of *hydatid disease*, Philadelphia, 1976, WB Saunders.

Salama H et al. Diagnosis and treatment of hepatic hydatid cysts with the aid of echo-guided percutaneous cyst puncture. *Clin Infect Dis* 1995; *21*:1372–1376.

Smego RA et al. Percutaneous aspiration-injection-reaspiration drainage plus albendazole or mebendazole for hepatic cystic echinococcosis: A meta-analysis. *Clin Infect Dis* 2003; *37*:1073–1083.

Sotelo J et al. Neurocysticercosis. A new classification based on active and inactive forms. A study of 753 cases. *Arch Intern Med* 1985; *145*:442–445.

Todorov T et al. Chemotherapy of human cystic echinococcosis: Comparative efficacy of mebendazole and albendazole. *Ann Trop Med Parasitol* 1992; *86*:59–66.

Tsang VCW, Wilson M. *Taenia solium* cysticercosis. An underrecognized but serious health problem. *Parasitol Today* 1995; *11*:124–126.

Vasquez V, Sotelo J. The course of seizures after treatment for cerebral cysticercosis. *N Engl J Med* 1992; *327*:696–701.

Yasawi MI et al. Combination of praziquantel and albendazole in the treatment of hydatid disease. *Trop Med Parasitol* 1993; *44*:192–194.

The Intestinal Nematodes

The nematodes have been said to be the most wormlike of the various groups of parasitic animals lumped under the loose title of worms. This is perhaps a reflection of the fact that they are shaped like the common earthworm, which seems the prototype for all worms. Actually, the earthworm is not a nematode, being a representative of the segmented worms, or annelids. Nematodes, belonging to the phylum Nematoda, are nonsegmented, generally cylindrical, tapered at both ends, and covered by a tough protective covering or cuticle. They have a complete digestive tract with both oral and anal openings. The sexes are separate; generally males are such smaller than female worms. Reproductive organs are tubular and lie coiled in the body cavity. In the male there is a single tubule, which at its smaller end consists of testicular cells; it extends into a vas deferens and seminal vesicle and terminates in an ejaculatory duct opening into the cloaca. The female worm has two cylindrical ovaries, which expand into uteri. The uteri may open to the exterior through a single vulva, or there may be a common vagina between the vulva and uteri. The vulva is frequently located near the middle of the body but varies in position in different species.

In contrast to the trematodes and cestodes, all of which are parasitic, the majority of nematodes are free living. There are an estimated 500,000 species of nematodes. Many have considerable economic importance as plant parasites, others as causes of disease in animals, and a dozen or more are commonly encountered in humans.

Parasitic nematodes are generally a light cream-white color, but the females of the smaller forms may appear darker when filled with dark-colored eggs. Certain structural modifications are important in the identification of various species. The mouth in primitive forms is surrounded by three lips, but in hookworms it has become modified into a buccal capsule furnished with cutting plates or teeth. The anterior portion of the digestive tract, the esophagus, is muscular in most forms. In one group, of which *Trichuris* and *Trichinella* are examples, the esophagus is much reduced and has the appearance of a fine tubule running lengthwise through a column of large cuboidal cells. The muscular esophagus of certain nematodes is of uniform caliber throughout; this type is called filariform. If the esophagus is expanded posteriorly into a bulb that contains a valve mechanism, it is referred to as rhab-ditiform. Male nematodes usually have a pair of copulatory spicules, while lie in pouches near the ejaculatory duct and may be inserted into the vagina of the female. In some forms the posterior end of the male is expanded into a thin-walled copulatory bursa, supported by thickened rays. The arrangement of these rays may be of importance in identification of the worms.

Stages in the life cycle of nematodes include the egg; larvae, which undergo several molts; and adults. The filariform type of esophagus generally characterizes infective-stage larvae, which in their free-living stages (or those passed in intermediate hosts) may have had an esophagus of the rhabditiform type.

As has been mentioned, the majority of nematodes are free living. The parasitic forms include representatives of several groups, which may be assumed to have independently evolved a parasitic mode of existence. The nematodes exemplify, as does no other group, many of the stages that may be considered to lead from a wholly free-living to an obligate parasitic existence. If one desires to set up such a series, at one end might be placed the vinegar eel, *Turbatrix aceti*. *Turbatrix* is a free-living nematode that frequently was found multiplying to enormous numbers in vinegar in the era when that commodity was dispensed from wooden casks and not sterilized when bottled at the factory. The vinegar eel has been found on occasion in the vagina, where it apparently is able to survive for some time if introduced in a douche. This organism exhibits some potentialities for becoming a parasite but cannot establish itself permanently in the vagina. *Strongyloides stercoralis* is a small nematode that, if conditions are suitable, may pass several free-living generations in the soil but sooner or later produces larvae of a type that must complete their development as parasites. The hookworms are invariably parasitic in the adult stage, but their larvae must undergo a free-living developmental period in the soil. *Ascaris* eggs must develop for a period outside the body before they mature and become infective, but then they are ingested and no stages of the life cycle are free living. Finally, the filarial worms, such as *Wuchereria*, might be considered perfect examples of obligate parasitism, having larval stages that develop in an insect and adults that live in humans or other mammals. At no time can the worm exist outside the body of one or the other host.

The nematode parasites of humans are moderately long-lived worms. *Ascaris* usually die out in about a year in the absence of reinfection, whereas *Trichuris* live several times that long, and hookworm infections may persist as long as 8 to 16 years. Autoinfection with *Strongyloides* (and perhaps *Enterobius*) enables these parasites to persist for indefinite periods in the absence of reinfection.

Diagnosis of intestinal nematode infection is generally made by demonstration of the characteristic eggs in the feces. These eggs, and the larvae of *Strongyloides*, are shown in Figure 8-3 and Plate XI. Occasionally adult worms are found in the stools, but except for *Ascaris* they are so small that they are frequently overlooked unless a special search is made.

Ascaris lumbricoides

The specific name of the large intestinal roundworm, *A. lumbricoides* (Fig. 8-1), is a tribute to its superficial resemblance to the common earthworm, *Lumbricus*. Female worms range from 20 to 35 cm in length, while males are seldom more than 30 cm long. The female worms may be as thick as a lead pencil; the males are definitely more slender and may be

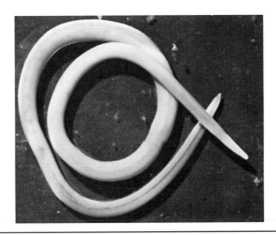

FIGURE 8-1 ■ *Ascaris lumbricoides,* female worm passed spontaneously. (Photograph by Zane Price.)

distinguished by an incurved tail. Both sexes are creamy white, sometimes with a pinkish cast, and the cuticle has fine circular striations.

Ascaris infections are found throughout the temperate and tropical areas of the globe, and under conditions of poor sanitation virtually 100% of the population harbor the parasite. The per capita worm burden may reach staggering levels, with hundreds or even a thousand or more worms in a single individual. A graphic illustration of Ascaris density was given by Stoll in 1947, who calculated a total of 18,000 tons of Ascaris eggs produced annually by those worms affecting the people of China alone, and by a 1989 Lancet editorial that stated the Ascaris burden worldwide to be so enormous that if placed head to tail the worms would encircle the world 50 times!

The life cycle of A. lumbricoides is illustrated in Figure 8-2. Ascaris eggs are unsegmented when passed; under favorable conditions they require a period of about 2 or 3 weeks outside the host to develop to the infective stage. Excessive heat and dryness soon kill them, but they

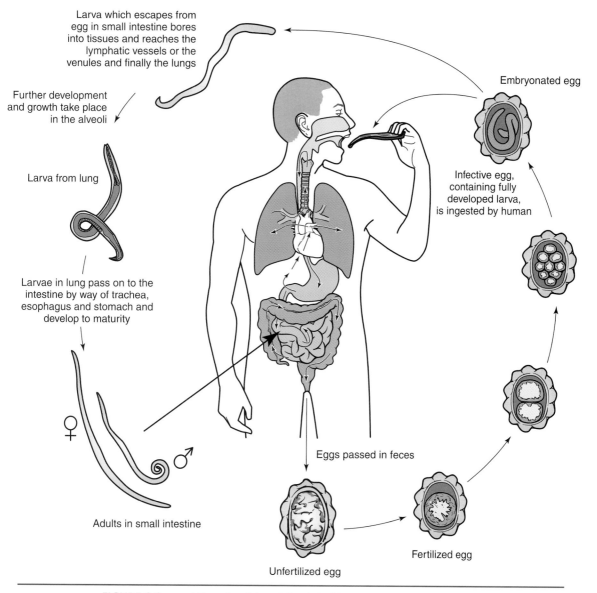

Larva which escapes from egg in small intestine bores into tissues and reaches the lymphatic vessels or the venules and finally the lungs

Further development and growth take place in the alveoli

Larva from lung

Larvae in lung pass on to the intestine by way of trachea, esophagus and stomach and develop to maturity

Adults in small intestine

Embryonated egg

Infective egg, containing fully developed larva, is ingested by human

Eggs passed in feces

Fertilized egg

Unfertilized egg

FIGURE 8-2 ■ Life cycle of *Ascaris lumbricoides*.

remain viable in moist soil for long periods. When fully embryonated eggs are swallowed, they hatch in the duodenum and then undergo an extraordinary migration through the body before returning to settle down in the intestine and grow to adulthood. The larvae first penetrate the wall of the duodenum and enter blood or lymphatic vessels to be carried to the liver, to the heart, and thence into the pulmonary circulation. They are filtered out by the capillaries of the lungs and break from them into the alveoli. There they grow and molt, and after about 20 days migrate through the respiratory passages to reach the esophagus and eventually once again the small intestine. Two or 3 months after ingestion of the eggs, the mature worms commence egg laying in the intestine. There is suggestive evidence that while infection may take place constantly and the larvae undergo a migratory cycle, they are not able to grow to adulthood in the intestine as long as any considerable number of worms remain from a previous infection. Batches of adult worms may succeed each other in hyperendemic areas at periods dependent on the longevity of the adult worms in the intestine.

Mature female worms have been estimated to produce daily an average of 200,000 eggs. In all but the rare infections in which only male worms are present, diagnosis can usually be made with ease on examination of even unconcentrated stool. The fertilized egg of *Ascaris* (Fig. 8-3, *A*) is readily recognized. It is broadly oval, measuring 45 to 75 μm by 35 to 50 μm. The outer covering is an albuminoid coat, usually stained a golden brown by bile as seen in the fresh stool. The outer coast is coarsely mammillated and lies directly on top of a thick, smooth shell, which is usually not easily distinguished. Some eggs will be seen to have lost the outer albuminoid coat (see Fig. 8-3, *A*; Plate XI), and in these the thick yellowish inner shell is obvious. It is thicker than the shell of a hookworm egg, which these decorticated *Ascaris* eggs otherwise resemble. Infertile eggs (Fig. 8-3, *B*) are longer and narrower than the fertile ones. They may measure about 90 by 40 μm. Both the inner shell and outer albuminoid coat may be thin, and if the latter is absent and the inner shell very thin, they may resemble *Trichostrongylus* eggs (Fig. 8-3, *C*).

Ascaris infections are sometimes diagnosed on radiography, either as worm-shaped radiolucent areas in a barium-filled intestine, sometimes with their own intestinal tracts outlined as well by barium they have ingested (Fig. 8-4), or in cholangiograms (Fig. 8-5).

Symptoms.   The ingestion of small numbers of infective eggs at any one time probably gives rise to no recognizable symptoms, but larger numbers may provoke pneumonitis during larval migration through the lungs. This may occur from 4 days to 2 weeks after infection. During this period sensitive persons may develop asthma attacks, which can continue until the eventual elimination of the adult worms; the sudden development of asthma in a previously nonasthmatic person who has traveled to an area with poor sanitation should raise suspicion of ascariasis. A few adult worms in the bowel are unlikely to cause symptoms unless they migrate through the ampulla of Vater into the pancreas, bile ducts, gallbladder, or liver, or up the esophagus (from whence they may enter the respiratory passages or bronchial tree); perforate the intestine; or occlude the appendix. Such migration is fortunately uncommon but may be provoked by fever, certain drugs, and anesthetic agents. However, moderate *Ascaris* infections can produce symptomatic lactose maldigestion or intolerance in preschool children. A heavy infection is likely to cause bowel obstruction, especially in children. In one series, three fourths of children with bowel obstruction presented with fever and generalized malaise. Abdominal distention and tenderness, vomiting, and rebound tenderness were also commonly seen. X-ray evidence of obstruction occurred in about two thirds of cases, but a significant eosinophilia was noted in only about 10%. A review of case reports of intestinal obstruction due to *Ascaris* infection (de Silva et al., 1997) indicates that obstruction accounts for nearly three quarters of all complications of this infection, that the incidence is in the range of 0 to 0.25 cases per 1000 population in endemic areas, related in a nonlinear fashion to the prevalence of infection, and is seen largely in children under the age of 10 years (mean age 5 years or younger), with a mean fatality rate of 5.7%.

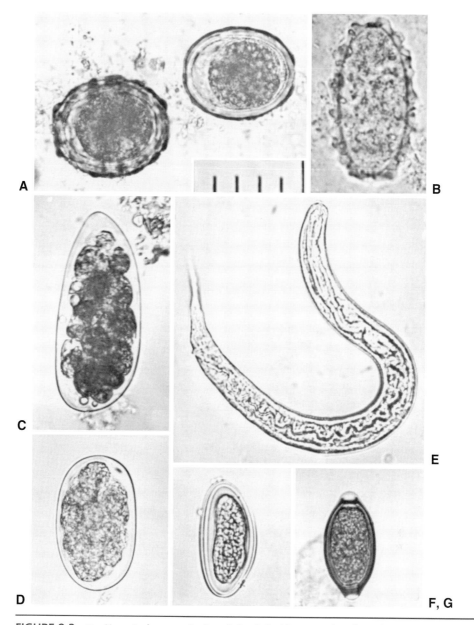

FIGURE 8-3 ■ Nematode eggs. **A,** *Ascaris lumbricoides* normal and nearly decorticated. **B,** *Ascaris lumbricoides* unfertilized. **C,** *Trichostrongylus* sp. **D,** Hookworm. **E,** *Strongyloides stercoralis* rhabditiform larva. **F,** *Enterobius vermicularis.* **G,** *Trichuris trichiura.* All photographs at same magnification; scale equals 50 μm.

Pathogenesis. An impressive eosinophilia is not characteristic of ascariasis, but it usually peaks during the period of tissue migration, declining after the worms reenter the gut. Increased levels of IgG, and especially of IgE, are seen in infected persons. Aside from the immune responses, the damage caused by ascarids seems largely related to their size. The larvae, 20 μm in diameter, and trapped in the 10-μm alveolar capillaries, break out with consequent (usually minor) hemorrhage. The large and muscular adult worms do not attach to the intestinal wall but maintain their position by constant movement. It is not surprising that they occasionally force their way into extraintestinal sites or, if present, in large numbers form tangled masses that occlude the bowel. Young children are at greatest risk of infection

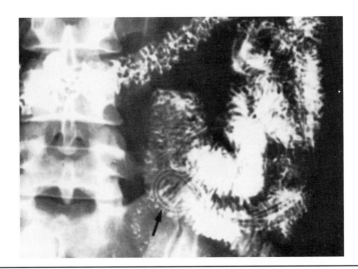

FIGURE 8-4 ▪ *Ascaris lumbricoides* in small intestine *(arrow)*. (Courtesy of Dr. Herman Zaiman, Mercy Hospital, Valley City, ND.)

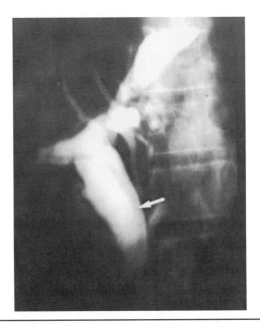

FIGURE 8-5 ▪ *Ascaris lumbricoides* in common bile duct, visualized by transduodenal cholangiography. (Courtesy of Dr. Ralph Bernstein, Highland-Alameda County Hospital, Oakland, CA.)

and ectopic migration of the parasites. A number of studies suggest that ascariasis adversely affects the nutritional status of its host, but critical review indicates these studies either to have been faulty in design or to have failed to demonstrate such an effect.

A study by Cooper et al. (2003) in Ecuador suggests that infection with intestinal helminths, particularly *Ascaris*, protects against the development of severe inflammatory diarrhea in children. The possible protective mechanism may be the production of antimicrobial substances by the worms or the increase in mucosal resistance through modulation of the mucosal immune response. Infection with intestinal helminths has also been used as an experimental remedy for inflammatory bowel disease (Wickelgren, 2004).

Epidemiology. Ascariasis affects more of the world's population than any other parasitic disease—perhaps as many as 1.3 billion persons. In China alone, 500 million people are infected (Zhou et al., 1999). While cosmopolitan in distribution, it is more prevalent in areas of poor sanitation and where human feces are used for fertilizer. The swine ascarid, *Ascaris suum*, is distinct from *A. lumbricoides* but can infect humans and even cause intestinal obstruction. It is suggested that pig manure, popular with organic gardeners, carries a risk of such infection. *Ascaris* eggs are able to survive for some months in fecal matter, sewage, or even in the 10% formalin solution used for stool preservation!

Treatment. In mixed infections with *Ascaris* and other intetinal parasites, it is good practice to treat initially with a drug effective against *Ascaris* to obviate the change of stimulating that worm to untoward activity. Albendazole (Albenza, Zentel), a nitroimidazole that binds irreversibly to tubulin, blocking microtubule assembly and inhibiting glucose uptake by the worm, is now considered the drug of choice in treatment of ascariasis and of all other intestinal roundworms with the exception of *Strongyloides*. A single oral dose of 400 mg (200 mg for children under 2 years of age) is highly effective. Side effects are minimal, consisting of diarrhea and abdominal pain. Hypersensitivity to albendazole has been reported, but is rare. Stimulation of migratory activity by the worms may occur during treatment.

Mebendazole (Vermox) has the same side effects and much the same spectrum of activity against intestinal roundworms as does albendazole, but it must be administered at the rate of 100 mg orally twice daily for 3 days.

Alternatively, pyrantel pamoate (Antiminth), a pyrimidine, may be administered in a single oral dose of 11 mg/kg body weight (maximum dose 1 g). It depolarizes the myoneural junction in the worms, paralyzing them in a spastic condition. Occasional side effects of headache, dizziness, fever, nausea, and vomiting occur; abdominal cramps and diarrhea may also be seen. The drug is ineffective in strongyloidiasis and trichuriasis.

When *Ascaris* worms obstruct the sphincter of Oddi or migrate up the biliary tree, producing acute abdominal pain suggestive of the passage of a gallstone, pancreatitis or cholangitis may result, and surgical or endoscopic removal of the worm has often been necessary. Biliary ascariasis is a regularly encountered complication in China, where traditional Chinese medicine, using nonoperative procedures involving herbal prescriptions, is used in treatment. Ninety-five percent of 9192 diagnosed cases of biliary ascariasis were successfully treated by such noninvasive procedures (Zhou et al., 1999).

Intestinal obstruction due to ascarids is treated by nasogastric suction until vomiting is controlled. One or 2 hours after suction is discontinued, an anthelmintic may be administered through the nasogastric tube, which is allowed to remain in place. Although albendazole, also available as an oral suspension, would seem the logical choice for treatment of this complication, we have seen no published reports of its use, and its proclivity to stimulate migratory activity on the part of the worms might be a reason not to use it in a patient who is obstructed. The present recommendation is to treat with an initial dose of piperazine, 150 mg/kg body weight (maximum dose 3.5 g). If vomiting recurs and suction must be resumed, additional doses may be given at the rate of 65 mg/kg (maximum 1 g) every 12 hours for six doses. If there is no vomiting, the second dose is given orally, 24 hours after the first, and is repeated at 12-hour intervals for a total of six doses. The amount given is again 65 mg/kg. If this treatment is not successful or if the obstruction is complete, surgical intervention will probably be necessary.

Control. The control of ascariasis, as of other helminthic diseases, depends on education as well as chemotherapy. The latter may involve, depending on circumstances, either mass treatment of populations in which the infection is very heavy, targeted treatment aimed at that segment of the population in which infection is heaviest, or identification and treatment of infected persons. The last of these alternatives is obviously the most expensive under virtually all circumstances. Mass treatment with ivermectin was an effective means of reducing the

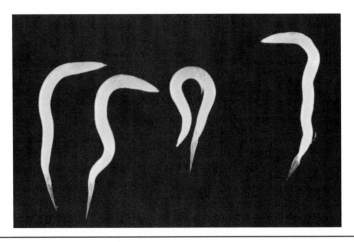

FIGURE 8-6 ■ *Enterobius vermicularis* adult female worms. Note shapes and the clear, attenuated and pointed posterior end. (Courtesy of The Louisiana State University School of Medicine.)

prevalence of intestinal helminthic diseases in a poor community in northeast Brazil (Heukelbach et al., 2004).

Enterobius vermicularis

The pinworm *E. vermicularis* (Fig. 8-6) is by all odds the most common helminth parasite of those temperate regions where sanitation measures are relatively rigorous. It has been estimated that as much as 10% of the pediatric population may be infected in these areas. Spread of pinworm infection is no doubt facilitated by crowded indoor living in temperate climates, but it is also common in the tropics. Less attention is paid to pinworm in tropical areas, probably because of the relative prevalence of more important parasites. Conversely, the importance of *Enterobius* is frequently overrated in the United States.

The life cycle of *E. vermicularis* is illustrated in Figure 8-7. The male pinworm is inconspicuous, about 2 to 5 mm long and no more than 0.2 mm wide. The female reaches a length of 8 to 13 mm and a width of up to 0.5 mm. They are a light yellowish white; the female is distinguished by a long, thin, sharply pointed tail, which characteristic gave rise to the common name. The adult worms inhabit the cecum and adjacent portions of the large and small intestines. The female worms, when fully gravid, migrate down the intestinal tract to pass out the anus and deposit their eggs (Fig. 8-8). The worms may migrate several inches out of the anus, depositing eggs as they crawl or liberating masses of them as the worms dry and literally explode. The eggs are fully embryonated and are infective within a few hours of the time they are deposited; if climatic conditions are suitable they survive for some weeks outside the body. The eggs live longest under conditions of fairly high humidity and moderate temperature. Reinfection of the patient by contamination of the hands is common and makes control of the parasite very difficult. Development of the adult worms is said to require about 6 weeks; shorter periods have, however, been reported. Infection of others through contaminated clothing, bedding, and so forth is frequently the cause of familial outbreaks. The eggs may survive for some days in dry dust, and airborne eggs may infect persons at some distance. A type of autoinfection described as "retrofection" involves hatching of the embryonated eggs after their deposition in the perianal area and subsequent migration back into the rectum and large intestine.

Diagnosis of pinworm infection is made on recovery of the characteristic eggs, although it may be suspected in children who have pruritus ani. Occasionally, the adult female worms are seen crawling in the perianal region or in the feces. Eggs may be found

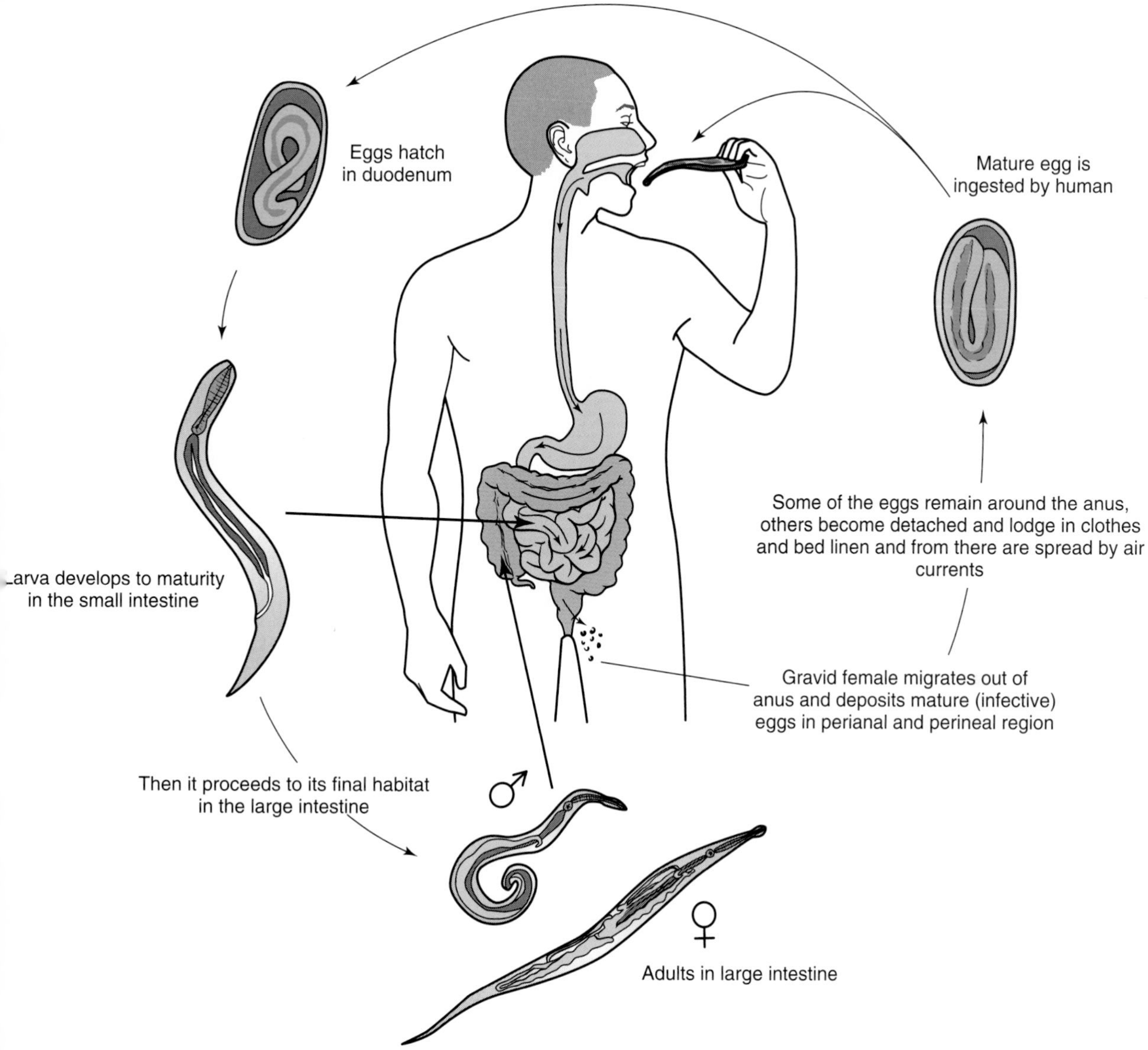

Eggs hatch in duodenum

Mature egg is ingested by human

Larva develops to maturity in the small intestine

Some of the eggs remain around the anus, others become detached and lodge in clothes and bed linen and from there are spread by air currents

Gravid female migrates out of anus and deposits mature (infective) eggs in perianal and perineal region

Then it proceeds to its final habitat in the large intestine

♂

Adults in large intestine

♀

FIGURE 8-7 ■ Life cycle of *Enterobius vermicularis*.

in the stools, but this is exceptional, as the females ordinarily do not oviposit until they leave the intestinal tract. Various methods of recovery of eggs from the perianal region (see Chapter 14) provide the most efficient means of diagnosis. The eggs (Fig. 8-3, *F*) are 50 to 60 μm in length, 20 to 32 μm in breadth, and have a translucent shell of moderate thickness. They are usually conspicuously flattened on one side, and this flattening and consequent reduction in diameter, plus the thicker shell, differentiates them from hookworm eggs.

Symptoms. The symptoms associated in the popular mind with *Enterobius* infections are many and exaggerated. Migration of the female worms from the anus in some persons produces pruritus, which may at times be severe. In small children, the worms may invade the vagina after leaving the rectum, thereby producing a local irritation. The local itching undoubtedly may interfere with the sleep of children or adults who are infected, as the

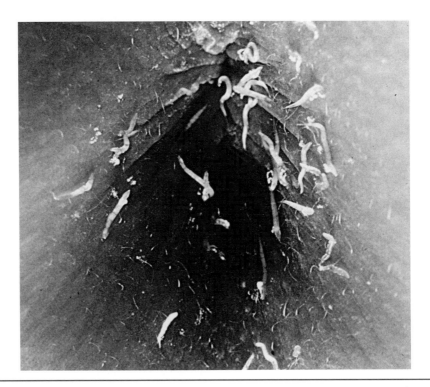

FIGURE 8-8 ■ Pinworms crawling from anus. (Courtesy Weber M. Pinworms. *N Engl J Med* 1993; *328*:927. Copyright 1993, Massachusetts Medical Society. All rights reserved.)

worms migrate from the anus during the resting hours. It is probable that *Enterobius* causes no symptoms in the majority of infected adults and children.

Pathogenesis. *Enterobius* may, for all practical purposes, be considered a commensal in all persons save those whose hypersensitivity to the secretions and excretions of the worms leads to rectal pruritus. Attachment of the adult worms to the intestinal wall may produce some inflammation. Invasion of the appendix might be expected to be the common occurrence that it is (Fig. 8-9), but any relationship between this invasion and appendicitis remains unproven. Entrance into the peritoneal cavity via the female reproductive system may result in the formation of granulomas around eggs or worms; these are rarely of clinical significance but have been thought to be responsible for a chronic pelvic peritonitis. Pinworms or their eggs have occasionally been reported from other ectopic sites, such as liver and lung.

Treatment. The worms may be eliminated by a variety of drugs and by means as simple as warm tap water enemas, yet their eggs are so resistant and widespread that their reintroduction into a household containing small children is generally only a matter of time. In a family situation in which reintroduction of the parasite seems probable, one may treat only those persons who are symptomatic or empirically treat the entire family. Tap water enemas, repeated as necessary, control symptoms. If drug therapy is desired, a single oral dose of albendazole, 400 mg (200 mg in children under 2 years of age), is the drug of choice. It should be repeated in 2 weeks in order to kill any worms that might have hatched from eggs present at the time of initial treatment. Pyrantel pamoate, in a single oral dose of 11 mg/kg body weight (maximum dose 1 g) and repeated in 2 weeks, may also be used.

Ancylostoma duodenale

The Old World hookworm, *Ancylostoma duodenale*, is the only hookworm of Europe and the areas bordering the Mediterranean, of the west coast of South America, and of parts of India

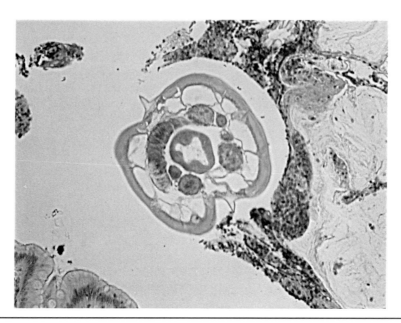

FIGURE 8-9 ■ Cross section of *Enterobius vermicularis* in appendix.

and China. It is found together with *Necator americanus* in certain areas in Brazil, a part of India, most of China, and throughout southeast Aisa, Indonesia, and the islands of the South and the Southwest Pacific. Within these areas, it is generally confined to those parts of the Northern Hemisphere south of the 36th parallel and of the Southern Hemisphere north of the 30th parallel, except where local conditions may be especially favorable, as in mines.

Ancylostoma adults are grayish white or pinkish. The head has a slight bend in relation to the rest of the body. The male worm measures nearly 1 cm by 0.5 mm; the female is somewhat longer and stouter. The mouth is well developed (Fig. 8-10), with a pair of teeth on either side of the median line and a smaller pair in the depths of the buccal capsule. The male worm is provided with a prominent copulatory bursa posteriorly (Fig. 8-14, *2*).

Hookworm eggs (see Fig. 8-3, *D*; Plate XI), when passed in the feces, are unsegmented or in the early cleavage states. Under optimal conditions, when deposited on moist sandy soil, the larvae develop and hatch within 24 to 48 hours (Fig. 8-11). Growth and development take place in the soil as the larvae feed on bacteria and organic material and undergo a first molt. After about 7 days the worms stop feeding and molt a second time, transforming from rhabditiform to filariform or infective larvae. The infective larvae do not eat and probably can live for only about 2 weeks if they do not find a host. Infective larvae usually live in the upper layers of the soil, and when the soil is cool and moist they climb to the highest point covered by a film of moisture. They extend their bodies into the air and remain waving about in this position until driven down by drying of their surroundings or by heat, or until they come in contact with the skin of a suitable host. It is probable that humans are the only normal host of *A. duodenale*; although larval penetration can take place in other mammals, development to the adult stage does not occur.

Diagnosis of hookworm infection depends on recovery of the eggs from the stools. The hookworm egg is unsegmented or in an early segmentation stage when passed. In specimens that have been allowed to stand at room temperature for a period of hours, especially if the weather is warm, a larva may be seen within the egg shell. Rarely, eggs may hatch and liberate larvae, which are then found free in the stool and must be differentiated from those of *Strongyloides*. If a stained smear is made of the stool, it is easy to differentiate between the rhabditiform larvae of hookworm and *Strongyloides* larvae (Fig. 8-12), as the former have a distinct long buccal capsule between the oral opening and the esophagus while in *Strongyloides* this

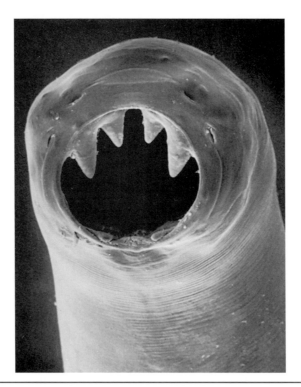

FIGURE 8-10 ■ Scanning electron micrograph of *Ancylostoma duodenale*, mouth parts showing teeth.

structure is very short. The eggs are regularly oval and 56 to 60 μm long by 36 to 40 μm in breadth. The shell is thin and colorless. Although *Ancylostoma* eggs are on average somewhat smaller than those of *Necator*, no attempt at differentiation of the two genera is ordinarily made on stool examination. Rough estimates of the numbers of worms present may be made on the basis of egg counts, as described in Chapter 14.

In humans, larvae of *Necator* must penetrate through the skin, whereas *Ancylostoma* infections may be percutaneous, oral, transmammary, and probably transplacental. Having once penetrated into the body, the larvae enter adjacent venules and are carried passively to the lungs, where they break out into alveoli. From the lungs, the larvae migrate up the trachea to be swallowed and reach the small intestine, where they mature. They attach by means of their stout mouth parts to the intestinal mucosa (Fig. 8-13) and suck blood and tissue juices of the host. The average prepatent period is 7 or 8 weeks; however, there is a strain in India that has a prepatent period of approximately 30 weeks.

Ancylostoma caninum, a hookworm of dogs, is known not only to produce an abortive infection in humans, in which the larvae, unable to complete their life cycle, migrate through the subcutaneous tissues (see Cutaneous Larva Migrans, later in this chapter), but also rarely to complete that cycle and establish an intestinal infection. A recent epidemic of eosinophilic enteritis (characterized by abdominal cramping pain, diarrhea, weight loss, melena, elevated levels of serum IgE, and in some cases a peripheral eosinophilia; also, surgery may reveal an intense segmental inflammation with eosinophilic infiltration) has been reported since the 1990s from northeastern Australia. The area is heavily populated by dogs infected with *Ancylostoma caninum*, and immature worms of this species have been recovered from a number of patients. Subclinical infections have also been noted on colonoscopy for other indications, and in that part of Australia the syndrome of obscure abdominal pain when associated with a peripheral eosinophilia is commonly responsive to treatment with mebendazole (Croese et al., 1994).

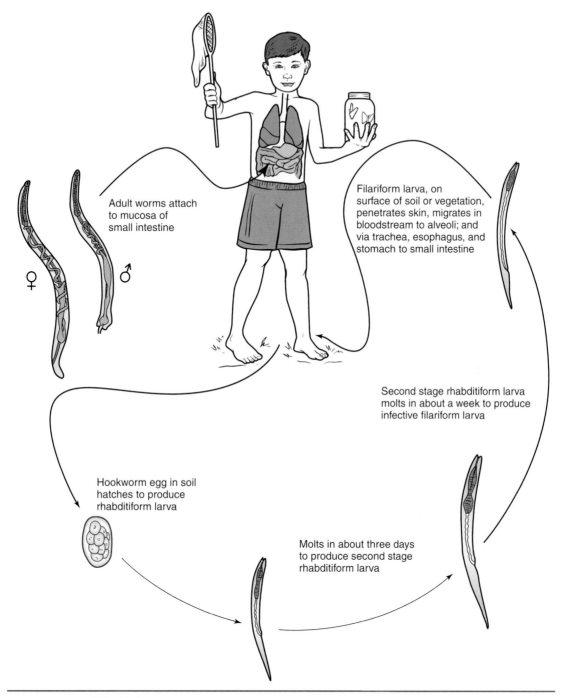

FIGURE 8-11 ■ Hookworm life cycle.

Adult worms attach to mucosa of small intestine

Filariform larva, on surface of soil or vegetation, penetrates skin, migrates in bloodstream to alveoli; and via trachea, esophagus, and stomach to small intestine

Second stage rhabditiform larva molts in about a week to produce infective filariform larva

Hookworm egg in soil hatches to produce rhabditiform larva

Molts in about three days to produce second stage rhabditiform larva

Necator americanus

The New World hookworm, *Necator americanus*, while prevalent over large portions of the Western Hemisphere, was probably introduced from Africa with the slave trade. In addition to being the only hookworm found in North America and large areas of South America, it is the native hookworm of Africa south of the Sahara and the only one found in parts of India. *Ancylostoma* and *Necator* occur together elsewhere in India, in much of China, in

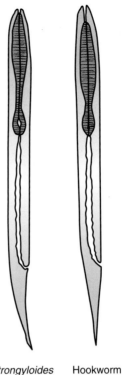

Strongyloides   Hookworm

FIGURE 8-12 ■ Diagram of hookworm and *Strongyloides* rhabditiform larvae from stool, showing differentiation on basis of buccal cavities. Hookworm larvae have a long buccal cavity, the space between the oral opening and the esophagus, whereas *Strongyloides* has a short buccal cavity.

southeast Asia, in Indonesia, in the islands of the South and Southwest Pacific, and in parts of Australia. With increasing rapidity of communications and with the exposure of large numbers of persons to the hazards of infection in various parts of the world, it is probable that the geographic boundaries between the two genera of human hookworms will disappear.

Hookworm infection is still prevalent in some parts of the United States. As recently as 1972, 12% of rural school children on the coastal plain of Georgia were infected. At about the same time, infection rates of nearly 15% were reported from upper grade elementary school students in rural Kentucky. More recent studies suggest that in Kentucky the prevalence has declined dramatically in recent years.

Adults of *N. americanus* resemble those of *Ancylostoma* but are slightly smaller. The males range from 5 to 9 mm in length, while females are usually about 1 cm long. The head is sharply bent in relation to the rest of the body (Fig. 8-14, *3*), forming a definite hook shape at the anterior end, from which the worms derive their common name. The buccal capsule of *Necator* is armed with a pair of cutting plates, while *Ancylostoma* (see Fig. 8-10) has teeth. There are also decided differences in the structure of the rays supporting the copulatory bursa in the two genera. However, with a little practice one may be able to distinguish with the eye between adults of *Necator* and *Ancylostoma*, as the anterior hook is very much more pronounced in the former genus.

The life cycles of the two genera of hookworms are very similar. The adult *Ancylostoma* being larger than *Necator*, worm for worm it is more likely to bring about iron deficiency. Eggs of *Necator* closely resemble those of *Ancylostoma* but are slightly larger, averaging 64 to 76 μm by 36 to 40 μm.

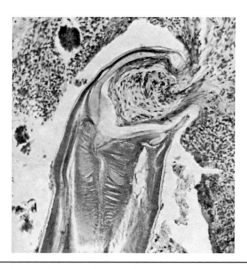

FIGURE 8-13 ■ Longitudinal section through hookworm attached to intestinal mucosa. (From U.S. Army Museum collection.)

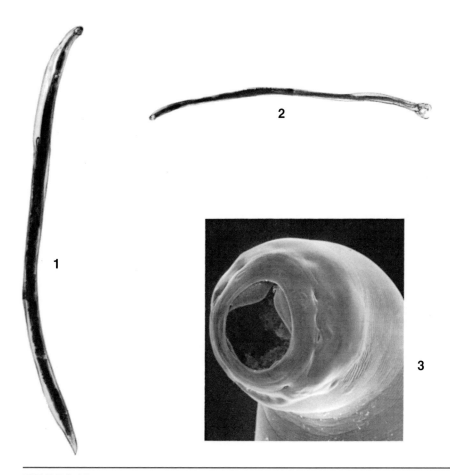

FIGURE 8-14 ■ *Necator americanus* adults, *1*, female worm; *2*, male worm showing copulatory bursa (right end) (magnification approximately 10×); *3*, frontal view of head showing pronounced anterior bend or "hook" and cutting plates (scanning electron micrograph, magnification approximately 400×). (Photomicrographs by Zane Price.)

Symptoms. In penetrating the skin, the larvae may cause an allergic reaction known as ground itch. This is less common with *Ancylostoma* than with the New World hookworm, *N. americanus*. Hookworm larvae are smaller than those of *Ascaris* and do not usually cause as severe pulmonary symptoms. If the infecting dose is large, pneumonitis may be produced by numbers of larvae breaking into the alveoli in a short space of time. Maturation of the worms may be marked by gastrointestinal discomfort or diarrhea, particularly when a previously uninfected person first acquires a heavy infection.

Even small numbers of hookworm larvae may be sufficient to produce symptoms in immunologically naive persons. Volunteers exposed to percutaneous infection with approximately 50 actively motile *N. americanus* larvae each had an initial pruritic rash during the first 6 days after infection but were then asymptomatic until approximately day 30. All reported increased flatulence and abdominal or epigastric pain or discomfort between the 30th and 45th days. Nausea, vomiting, and diarrhea were noted by some. In one patient the symptoms were sufficiently severe to warrant treatment on day 40. Eggs were found in the stools of the untreated volunteers between days 48 and 58. Eosinophilia increased progressively after 2 to 3 weeks, peaking between days 38 and 64 at levels ranging from 1350 to 3828 cells per microliter.

In chronic infections, if the number of worms is considerable, blood loss will be serious. Acute gastrointestinal hemorrhage is rare and appears to occur principally in children and young adults. If the diet is adequate in protein and if sufficient iron is taken to replace that lost through the activity of the hookworms, there may still be no evident symptoms. If iron intake is insufficient, symptoms of iron deficiency anemia gradually develop. In some tropical areas, children may be seen whose anemia has developed over a long period and who remain asymptomatic with hemoglobin levels in the range of 4 g/dl blood. Yet such children are on the verge of cardiac decompensation, which can be brought on by intercurrent infection or injury. Hypoproteinemia, another consequence of such long-term blood loss, evidences itself in facial and peripheral edema. Eosinophilia is variable, ranging up to 70%.

Pica, the habitual ingestion of nonfood substances, is thought to have diverse causes, one of which is iron deficiency anemia. Certainly, pica, with ingestion of various substances, including soil, may be observed in persons with hookworm disease and ironically may expose them to further infection with hookworm or other worm infections such as toxocariasis or to toxoplasmosis.

Pathogenesis. A significant negative correlation between worm burden and hemoglobin level can be demonstrated in any representative series of patients infected with hookworm. When anemia is present, it is of the microcytic hypochromic type. The bone marrow is generally markedly hyperplastic, and there may be erythroid and myeloid hyperplasia of the spleen. Radioisotope measurements indicate a host blood loss per day per *A. duodenale* considerably greater than that calculated for *N. americanus*. Histologic changes in the mucosa of the affected intestine appear to be minimal. Flattening or atrophy of the intestinal villi has been noted on occasion, but more frequently examination of a biopsy specimen demonstrates a completely normal mucosal pattern. Malabsorption is apparently uncommon, and malnutrition does not seem to be characteristic of pure hookworm disease in areas where a good diet is available. Emaciation and mental and physical retardation frequently associated with this disease are more properly ascribed to a combination of other nutritional and disease factors that are common in many endemic areas. *A. duodenale* lives 1 to 5 years; *N. americanus* may survive as long as 18 years.

Epidemiology. Because initial infection occurs through the skin, prerequisite to widespread hookworm infection is a population significant parts of which defecate directly onto the soil and do not customarily wear shoes, at least during part of the year. Additional factors include appropriate ambient temperature, sufficient rainfall, and a loose sandy loam soil. These conditions limit areas of endemicity primarily to the tropics and subtropics, although they

extend into some more temperate zones. The observation that in the laboratory certain animals (rabbits, lambs, calves, pigs) can act as paratenic hosts when fed infective larvae of
A. duodenale and are then infective when fed to puppies is interesting, but its epidemiologic
significance remains unknown.

Treatment. Albendazole, in a single oral dose of 400 mg (200 mg in children under 2 years
of age), is the drug of choice for treatment of both *Ancylostoma* and *Necator*. Equally effective
is mebendazole, 100 mg twice daily for 3 days, to adults and children over 2 years of age.
Pyrantel pamoate, in the dose employed for ascariasis, is also effective.

Hookworm infections, if symptomatic, are so generally because of the concomitant
anemia, and unless this is corrected eradication of the worms will be of little avail. In severe
infections, ferrous sulfate, 200 mg, should be administered three times daily, at the time
anthelmintic treatment is begun, and continued for about 3 months after the hemoglobin
value returns to normal in order to replenish depleted iron stores.

Cutaneous Larva Migrans

If humans come in contact with infective larvae of the dog or cat hookworms *Ancylostoma*
braziliense or *A. caninum*, penetration of the skin may take place, but the larvae are then usually
unable to complete their migratory cycle. Trapped larvae of *A. braziliense* may survive for
some weeks or even months, migrating through the subcutaneous tissues, whereas those of
A. caninum encyst and remain dormant in skeletal muscle after a shorter cutaneous migratory
period. They may evoke a fairly severe reaction (Fig. 8-15), forming serpiginous tunnels
through the tissues, erythematous and sometimes vesicular at the advancing end, fading out
and becoming dry and encrusted in the older portions. There is often intense pruritus, and
scratching may lead to secondary bacterial invasion. This syndrome is referred to as creeping
eruption or as cutaneous larva migrans to distinguish it from the visceral type of larva
migrans discussed in Chapter 9.

Epidemiology. *A. braziliense* infects both dogs and cats, whereas *A. caninum* is found only
in dogs. Both are most common in the same tropical and subtropical regions in which

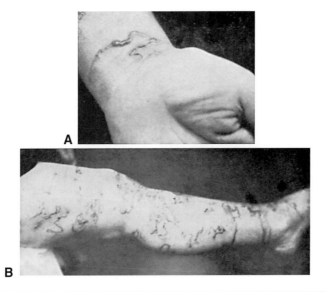

FIGURE 8-15 ■ Creeping eruption. **A,** lesions on wrist. **B,** Extensive lesions on leg of
3 weeks' duration. (**A,** Courtesy of Drs. J. B. and Bedford Shelmire. **B,** Courtesy of Dr. J. Lee
Kirby-Smith.)

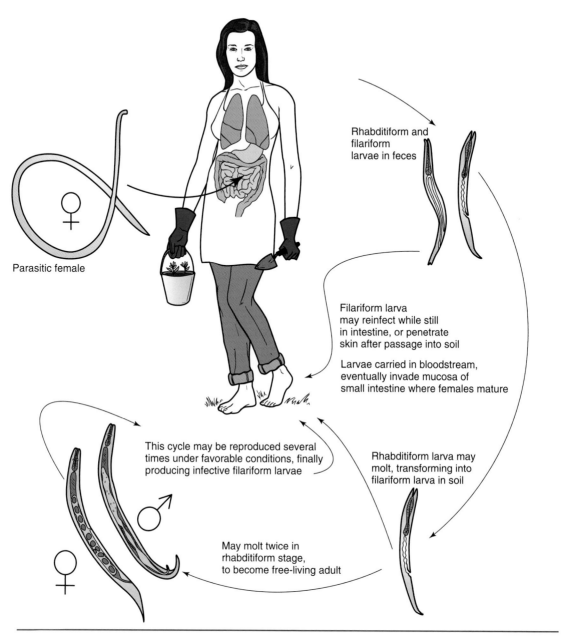

Rhabditiform and filariform larvae in feces

Filariform larva may reinfect while still in intestine, or penetrate skin after passage into soil

Larvae carried in bloodstream, eventually invade mucosa of small intestine where females mature

Parasitic female

This cycle may be reproduced several times under favorable conditions, finally producing infective filariform larvae

Rhabditiform larva may molt, transforming into filariform larva in soil

May molt twice in rhabditiform stage, to become free-living adult

FIGURE 8-16 ▪ Life cycle of *Strongyloides stercoralis.*

human hookworms can best complete their life cycles. Human infection usually occurs in areas where recreational exposure to contaminated soil may take place, such as sandy beaches on which dogs are allowed to roam free or children's sandboxes that are not protected from feline visitation. In the United States, creeping eruption is most frequent in the southeastern and Gulf states. An excellent account of cutaneous larva migrans in travelers is given by Jelinek et al. (1994).

Treatment. Albendazole, 400 mg by mouth daily for 3 days, is the treatment of choice (Albanese et al., 2001). Oral ivermectin, 200 mcg/kg body weight daily for 1 to 2 days, may also be used. Where lesions are few, thiabendazole ointment, applied several times daily for

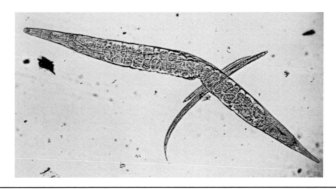

FIGURE 8-17 ▪ *Strongyloides stercoralis,* free-living female and larvae. (Photomicrograph by Zane Price.)

10 days or longer, gives good results but is unavailable in the United States or Canada. The oral suspension of this drug, applied to the area surrounding the advancing end of the larval burrow, may be used in its place.

Strongyloides stercoralis

Although the temperature and moisture requirements of *S. stercoralis* during the free-living phase of its life cycle are similar to those of hookworm, and their geographical distribution is likewise similar, the prevalence of strongyloidiasis is generally lower than that of hookworm disease. A number of species of *Strongyloides* are known, and generally they are quite host specific. Cats and dogs may both be infected with *S. stercoralis,* and human infection from a canine source has been reported.

When environmental conditions are optimal, *Strongyloides* may exist for some time as a free-living nematode, completing two or more generations in this manner (Fig. 8-16). The adults of the free-living generations, like other soil nematodes, are very small, being only about 1 mm long (Fig. 8-17). More frequently, perhaps, there is but a single free-living generation, producing rhabditiform larvae, which transform into infective filariform larvae. The filariform larvae are incapable of further development in the soil and must penetrate the skin of their host to continue the life cycle. Rhabditiform larvae that pass out of the host in the stools may also transform into filariform larvae directly, without developing into free-living adults. Penetration through the skin and the subsequent migration through the lungs and eventually to the small intestine is similar to that seen with hookworms. However, it has been demonstrated that migratory routes involving organs other than the lungs not only are possible but may predominate.

The parasitic males, if indeed they exist, are eliminated from the body early in the infection. It seems likely that the larvae, produced over a period of months, develop parthenogenetically. The females (Fig. 8-18), which may attain a length of slightly over 2 mm, burrow into the mucosa of the intestinal tract (Fig. 8-19), where they lay their eggs. The eggs, similar in appearance to those of hookworms, hatch in the mucosa and liberate rhabditiform larvae (see Fig. 8-3, *E*; Plate XI), which make their way to the lumen of the intestine. The larvae may feed and molt once before being passed in the feces. When they molt within the intestinal tract, they usually retain their rhabditiform characteristics but may transform into infective filariform larvae. If filariform larvae are formed, they may penetrate immediately into the wall of the gut and enter the bloodstream, where they begin the same types of migratory cycles as the larvae that penetrate the skin from the soil.

Diagnosis is by demonstration of the characteristic larvae in the stools (Fig. 8-20). Larvae resemble those of hookworms but can be distinguished by their very short buccal cavity (see Fig. 8-12). With severe diarrhea, the embryonated eggs may be present in the stools and can be differentiated from hookworm eggs by the fact that they always contain

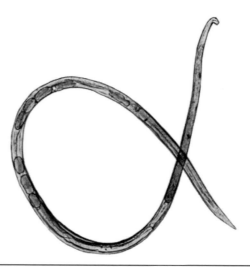

FIGURE 8-18 ■ *Strongyloides stercoralis,* parasitic female. (Photomicrograph by Zane Price.)

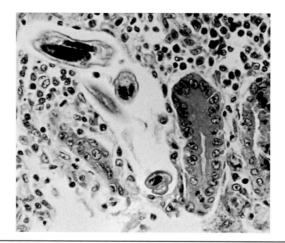

FIGURE 8-19 ■ Section through intestinal mucosa containing *Strongyloides stercoralis.*

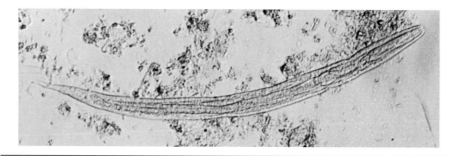

FIGURE 8-20 ■ *Strongyloides stercoralis.* Larva in stool specimen preserved in formalin. (Photomicrograph by Zane Price from material furnished by Dr. Lawrence Ash.)

well-developed larvae. If larvae are scarce, it may be necessary to concentrate the stool. The larvae may be concentrated with zinc sulfate, but more efficient means of recovery are described in Chapter 14. Duodenal aspiration occasionally reveals larvae when the stools consistently do not, and the string-capsule method (Entero Test) gives good results. In disseminated strongyloidiasis, larvae may at times be found in the sputum. A number of serologic tests have been described (see Chapter 16).

A characteristic x-ray picture is reported in severe strongyloidiasis with loss of mucosal pattern, rigidity, and tubular narrowing (Fig. 8-21).

Symptoms. Lesions resembling the ground itch of hookworm infection are sometimes seen following penetration of the skin by *Strongyloides* larvae. Pneumonitis may be produced by the larvae, but as in hookworm infection it is generally less severe than in ascariasis. The adult worms in the intestine may give rise to no demonstrable symptoms or to moderate to severe diarrhea. A malabsorption syndrome with steatorrhea has been described. It has been considered to be characteristic only of those cases in which there is severe protein malnutrition, to be reversible if the malnutrition is corrected even without elimination of the parasites, and to persist after treatment of the infection if the malnutrition remains uncorrected. Heavy infection may involve the large as well as the small bowel, and ulceration of the intestinal mucosa may give rise to symptoms suggestive of duodenal ulcer or of ulcerative colitis. Melena may be seen, or there may be massive lower gastrointestinal bleeding, with passage of bright red blood per rectum.

At times the normal life cycle of the parasite is altered, primarily because of an increase in the proportion of rhabditiform larvae that transform into filariform larvae while still within the gut. The mechanisms that promote this change are unknown, but it results in a large increase in the worm burden. If only the gastrointestinal tract and lungs are involved, the condition is referred to as the hyperinfection syndrome. Hyperinfection may lead to

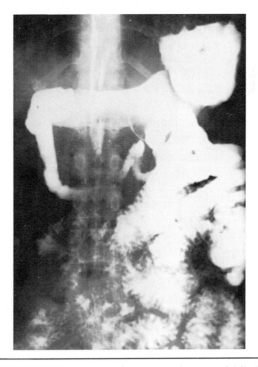

FIGURE 8-21 ■ Small bowel radiograph of patient with strongyloidiasis shows pipestem deformity of duodenum and thickening of mucosal folds in jejunum. (Courtesy of Dr. Herman Zaiman.)

severe debilitation or death. Patients who have the hyperinfection syndrome usually present with fever, gastrointestinal symptoms, dyspnea, wheezing, hemoptysis, cough, and weakness. Eosinophilia may not be present. When the numbers of migrating larvae are so great as to injure other organs such as the liver, heart, adrenals, pancreas, kidneys, or central nervous system, a multiplicity of other symptoms may be present, and we refer to the condition as disseminated strongyloidiasis, seen primarily in patients whose normal defenses have become compromised through malnutrition, intercurrent illness, especially with human lymphotropic virus type I (HTLV-I), or various forms of immunosuppression including acquired immunodeficiency syndrome (AIDS), chemotherapy for malignancies, and corticosteroids in high doses. Defective T-lymphocyte function is seen in many such patients. Other risk factors are hematologic malignancies and prior gastric surgery. Disseminated strongyloidiasis has been reported in both of the recipients of kidney allografts from a single cadaver donor and could presumably be transmitted through other organ transplants.

Because under ordinary circumstances some rhabditiform larvae transform to the filariform stage within the gut, strongyloidiasis may persist for many years in nonendemic areas. In a series of some 500 British former prisoners of war interned in the Far East during World War II, all of whom were repatriated by 1949, 78 (15.6%) were still infected with *Strongyloides* some 35 years after leaving the endemic area. Comparable levels of infection have been reported among American prisoners of war who were confined in the same area. The infection rate among Vietnam War veterans seems to have been considerably lower. Gastrointestinal symptoms were noted in only 5% of those infected in World War II, but 84% exhibited a characteristic dermal lesion similar to cutaneous larva migrans caused by dog hookworms. The strongyloid track advances at a much faster rate (5 to 10 cm/hour) than that of the dog hookworm larva in humans, and for this reason the lesion has been referred to as *larva currens*. Larva currens does not seem characteristic of strongyloidiasis acquired in the United States.

Pathogenesis. Although local lesions occur on penetration of the larvae into the skin, these are generally minor; chronic cutaneous larval migration (larva currens) is perhaps more common than was appreciated in the past. More severe skin lesions, including giant hives, are rare. The pulmonary response to larval migration is generally not severe; in heavy infections there may be a patchy pneumonitis, and larvae may be found in the sputum. The adult female worms may be found in all parts of the intestinal tract, although they are most common in the jejunum. Heavy infections, such as are seen with the hyperinfection syndrome or in disseminated strongyloidiasis as discussed earlier, can produce extensive ulceration and sloughing of the mucosa, and fibrosis and inflammatory infiltration of the submucosal layers and granulomas surrounding the larvae may be found in other affected organs. Microhemorrhages may occur around such larvae in the central nervous system.

Eosinophilia of 10% to 40% is common; in occasional patients it is higher. Lack of eosinophilic response is occasionally seen, generally in overwhelming infections. Early in the infection there may be polymorphonuclear leukocytosis. Total serum IgE is usually elevated.

Epidemiology. As mentioned previously, strongyloidiasis occurs in much the same tropical and subtropical areas of relatively heavy rainfall as does hookworm infection, though prevalence rates for the former disease seem generally lower. It differs importantly from hookworm infection in that, while the infection dies out over a period of some years in persons with hookworm infection who have moved from an endemic area, strongyloidiasis may persist by virtue of autoinfection, and prolonged absence from an endemic area is no guarantee of freedom from infection.

Treatment. Both albendazole and ivermectin are effective in the treatment of strongyloidiasis. Recommended dosage of albendazole is 400 mg (for children under 2 years of age, 200 mg) twice daily for 2 days; treatment may be repeated if necessary in 3 weeks. For the hyperinfection syndrome, 400 mg daily for 15 days is suggested. In chronic strongyloidiasis doses of 400 mg twice daily for 3 days resulted in a 75% cure rate; re-treatment of initial treatment failures was successful in only about one third of cases.

Ivermectin (see Chapter 9, treatment of *Wuchereria bancrofti*) has been found to produce cure rates approaching 100% when administered at the rate of 200 mcg/kg body weight daily for 2 days; in a small number of AIDS patients, 200 mcg/kg body weight daily for 2 days, repeated in 2 weeks, had similar results. A patient with *Strongyloides* hyperinfection and paralytic ileus, who was unable to tolerate oral therapy, was successfully treated with ivermectin administered as a rectal enema (Tarr et al., 2003).

Strongyloides fulleborni

Two other types of human strongyloidiasis have been found, one in Central Africa and the other in Papua New Guinea. In Ethiopia, the Central African Republic, Cameroon, Congo, Zimbabwe, and Zambia, *S. fulleborni*, a parasite of monkeys, also infects humans, and is common in infants under 6 months of age. In Zambia some 30% of *Strongyloides* infections have been ascribed to this species. *S. fulleborni* differs morphologically from *S. stercoralis* in some minor respects, but its eggs and not larvae are found in the feces, while larvae have been found in the milk of nursing mothers. Whether this is the usual mode of transmission is not known.

In Papua New Guinea and at least one area of Irian Jaya a subspecies, *S. fulleborni kellyi*, not only differs from the African worm in minor details of morphology, but produces in some infants a syndrome not known in other types of strongyloidiasis. Eggs, not larvae, are found in the stools, and *S. fkellyi* infects very young infants, with prevalence rates up to 80% to 100% in those 3 weeks to 1 year of age, and decreasing with age to about 5% to 20% of adults. Infections in infants are universally heavy, while those in adults are light. Most infants and adults are asymptomatic, but some infants suffer from what is locally referred to as "swollen belly sickness," characterized by abdominal distention, respiratory distress, generalized edema, and hypoproteinemia. This affliction was almost uniformly fatal until vast numbers of *Strongyloides* eggs were found in their stools. Therapy as recommended for *S. stercoralis* is curative if begun early.

Several interesting questions are posed by Papua New Guinea strongyloidiasis. While *S. fulleborni* in Africa has a primate reservoir, there are no nonhuman primates in Papua New Guinea, and no areas of *S. fulleborni* infection between the two localities. How did the infection get to Papua New Guinea? And while larvae of *S. fulleborni* are found in the milk of at least some African mothers with this infection, extensive efforts have failed to reveal evidence of transmammary transmission in Papua New Guinea. How, then, does the initial infection take place in a very young infant? Prenatal infection seems unlikely, as the prepatent period is under 2 weeks, while the youngest known infected infant was 18 days old. Infants are carried in bags lined with banana leaves, infrequently changed, so very high infection rates in the first few months of life are most likely the result of autoinfection (Ashford et al., 1992).

Zoonotic Strongyloidiasis/Creeping Eruption

Bearing an interesting relationship to "swimmer's itch" caused by penetration of the skin by avian schistosome cercariae, the "swamp itch" seen in hunters, trappers, and oil workers exposed to the swampy waters of the Mississippi River delta in southern Louisiana is considered to be a zoonotic infection.

Raccoons (*Procyon lotor*) and nutria (*Myocastor coypu*) are common in these swamps; each is infected with its own species of *Strongyloides*—*S. myopotami* of nutria and *S. procyonis* of raccoons, and larvae of both are abundant in swamp waters. Application of larvae of either species to the skin of a human volunteer produces creeping eruptions (Fig. 8-22) essentially identical to those accompanying *S. stercoralis* infection. In the laboratory, sensitization by means of successive exposures to the animal *Strongyloides* larvae seems necessary before the eruptive condition appears. The same preconditioning would easily be met by those frequenting the swampy areas.

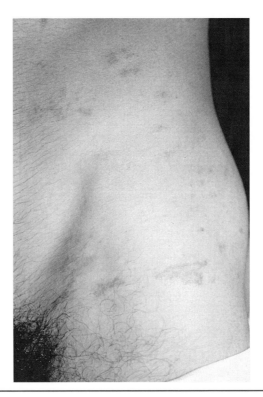

FIGURE 8-22   ▨   Zoonotic strongyloidiasis ("swamp itch") in a Louisiana frog trapper.

Capillaria philippinensis

Intestinal capillariasis was first observed in 1962, in the province of Ilocos Sur, on the island of Luzon in the Philippines. It reached epidemic proportions (1400 cases and 95 deaths) from 1967 to 1970. While its prevalence has declined since 1970, in all, 1877 cases with 115 deaths were reported through 1988. It also occurs elsewhere in the Philippines and in Thailand, and there have been scattered reports from Taiwan, Japan, Korea, Egypt, Iran, and Colombia.

Adult worms are slender, approximately 4 to 5 mm long. They live in the intestinal mucosa, primarily in the jejunum (Fig. 8-23), where they may be present in enormous numbers. The finding of larval stages, and of oviparous as well as larviparous females in the bowel, suggests that the parasite multiplies in the intestine and that overwhelming infections are the result of autoinfection. Eggs voided by infected persons, measuring about 45 by 21 μm, develop outside the host and are ingested by fresh-water and brackish-water fish, in which larval stages have been found. The complete life cycle is not known. Laboratory diagnosis is made by finding the characteristic eggs (Fig. 8-24) in the stool.

Symptoms. Although asymptomatic or mildly symptomatic cases occur, many infected persons exhibit a rather characteristic clinical picture. Abdominal pain, borborygmus (gurgling), and diarrhea appear early. The diarrhea may be protracted and may be accompanied by anorexia, nausea and vomiting, and hypotension. The patient may become cachectic, with generalized anasarca. Visible peristaltic waves may be seen over the distended abdomen.

Pathogenesis. Pronounced eosinophilia, surprisingly, does not seem to be a consistent feature of this disease. Hypoproteinemia; low blood calcium, potassium, and cholesterol levels; and other features of a protein-wasting enteropathy are encountered and are reflected in the pathologic picture. The villi are blunted, flattened, or completely obliterated, with

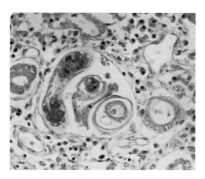

FIGURE 8-23 ■ Section through intestinal mucosa containing *Capillaria philippinensis.*

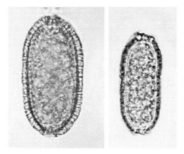

FIGURE 8-24 ■ Eggs of *Capillaria hepatica (left)* and *Capillaria philippinensis (right),* taken at the same magnification.

deepening of the crypts of Lieberkühn and an inflammatory submucosal infiltrate. Total thickness of the mucosa is generally reduced. These nonspecific changes are seen in various malabsorption stages and have been mentioned in relation to giardiasis and coccidiosis.

Epidemiology. Presumably a zoonotic infection, the natural cycle of *C. philippinensis,* recently redescribed as *Paracapillaria philippinensis* (Moravec, 2001), is not known. Experimentally, eggs hatch and develop into larvae if fed to various fresh- and brackish-water fish, and to the adult stage if the infected fish are fed to monkeys. Various fresh-water fish are eaten raw in the endemic area of Luzon, and human infection is presumably acquired by this means. Since 1973 there has been a considerable decline in incidence of the infection, perhaps because of successful treatment and, with fewer eggs contaminating the surrounding waters, a decrease in the number of infected fish. Two other capillarias cause rare human infections: *C. hepatica,* causing hepatic capillariasis, and *C. aerophila,* causing pulmonary capillariasis.

Treatment. Mebendazole has been the drug of choice for treatment of Philippine capillariasis. The recommended dosage is 200 mg twice daily for 20 days. This dosage may need to be repeated in some chronic cases. Although there has been little experience with its use, an alternative suggested treatment is albendazole, 400 mg daily for 10 days. In management of the acute illness, fluid and electrolyte replacement and a high-protein diet are important.

Trichuris trichiura

The whipworm, *T. trichiura,* has a worldwide distribution but is more common in tropical areas and in regions where sanitation is poor. The common name of whipworm is most descriptive, the thick posterior part of the body forming the stock, and the long thin anterior portion the

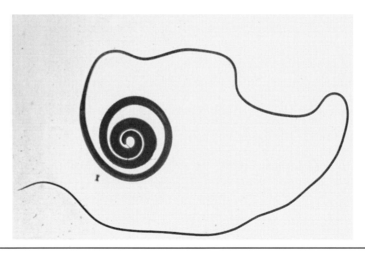

FIGURE 8-25   ■   *Trichuris trichiura,* adult male. (Photomicrograph by Zane Price.)

lash (Fig. 8-25). The generic name (*Trichuris,* hair tail) is less fortunate, having been applied under the impression that the attenuated portion of the worm was its posterior end. Subsequently the name *Trichocephalus* was given to the genus and has been adopted by some workers. It is much more apt but unfortunately should not be used, as the name *Trichuris* has priority.

The adult worms are from 3 to 5 cm long. As is usual among the nematodes, the females are larger than the males. The thin, almost colorless anterior three fifths of the body consists of the much reduced esophagus. The expanded posterior part of the worm is pinkish gray and contains the intestine and reproductive organs.

The life cycle of *T. trichiura* is illustrated in Figure 8-26. Infection is acquired by ingestion of the fully embryonated eggs. These are passed in the unsegmented condition and require a period of 10 days or more outside the body to reach the infective stage. The shell is digested in the small intestine, where the larvae lodge temporarily. After a period of growth, larvae pass to the cecal area, where they attach themselves permanently with their attenuated anterior ends embedded in the mucosa (Fig. 8-27). In heavy infections, worms may be found as far down as the rectum.

Diagnosis is by demonstration of the characteristic barrel- or football-shaped eggs in the feces (see Fig. 8-3, G; Plate XI). Each female worm produces 3000 to 7000 eggs daily. The eggs measure 50 to 54 μm in length, with refractile prominences (usually referred to as polar plugs) at either end. The zinc sulfate flotation method is extremely efficient in demonstrating them.

Symptoms. Light whipworm infections are usually asymptomatic. Heavier infections may be characterized by abdominal pain and distention, bloody or mucoid diarrhea, tenesmus, weight loss, and weakness. Prolapse of the rectum is occasionally seen, usually in children with heavy infections. Worms may be visible on the prolapsed, edematous rectum. Anemia and moderate eosinophilia may be seen in heavy infections. Nutritional deficiencies may occur in children with heavy whipworm infections.

Pathogenesis. The anterior ends of the worms, interlaced in the colonic mucosa, apparently produce little damage to the host unless present in large numbers. Some authorities believe that bacterial invasion of the mucosa is facilitated by the penetration of the worms. Appendicitis, brought about by blockage of the lumen of that organ by worms, has been frequently reported. Edema of the rectum, produced by numbers of worms embedded in that area, is responsible for rectal prolapse. The blood loss per worm is apparently slight; with

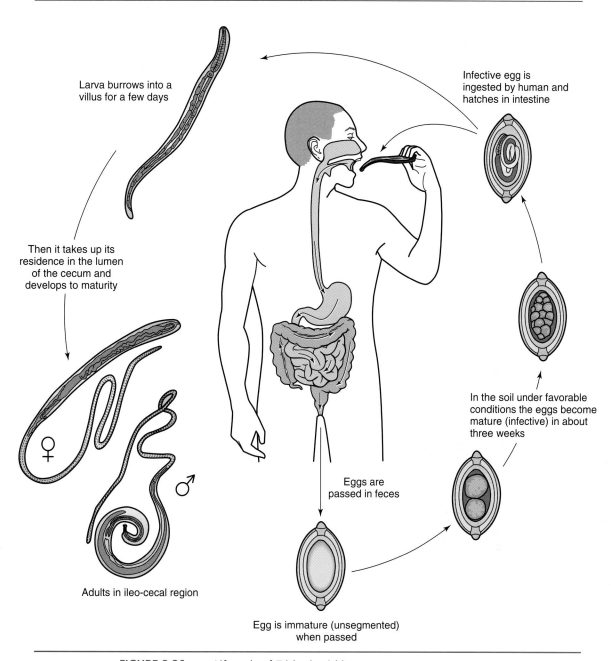

Larva burrows into a villus for a few days

Infective egg is ingested by human and hatches in intestine

Then it takes up its residence in the lumen of the cecum and develops to maturity

In the soil under favorable conditions the eggs become mature (infective) in about three weeks

Eggs are passed in feces

♀

♂

Adults in ileo-cecal region

Egg is immature (unsegmented) when passed

FIGURE 8-26 ▓ Life cycle of *Trichuris trichiura*.

radioisotope techniques it has been calculated to be approximately 0.005 ml per worm per day. Infections of 200 worms or more in children may cause chronic dysentery, profound anemia, and growth retardation, though catch-up growth is the rule in treated children. In many ways trichuriasis mimics inflammatory bowel disease, but unlike that condition it is readily curable.

Epidemiology. Prevalence and intensity of whipworm infection vary greatly with the level of sanitation. Where defecation onto the soil takes place or where human feces are used for fertilizer, prevalence rates are high—as high as 50% to 80% in some parts of Asia. In North America, whipworm infection is seen primarily in rural areas of the southeastern states and

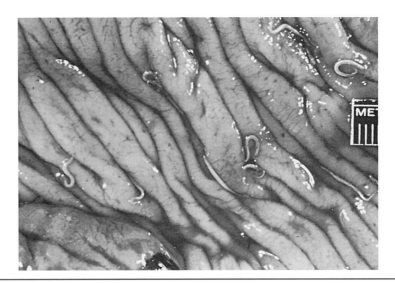

FIGURE 8-27 ■ *Trichuris trichiura* attached to intestinal mucosa. (Photograph by B. Guett. From Zaiman H [ed.]. *A pictorial presentation of parasites.*)

in immigrants from tropical areas. The life span of the worms if the infection is untreated may be from 4 to 8 years.

Treatment. While not as effective as it is in treatment of most intestinal nematodes, albendazole is the drug of choice in trichuriasis. An oral dose of 400 mg per day for 3 days is recommended for adults (200 mg for children under 2 years of age). Alternatively, oral mebendazole may be used at a dose of 100 mg twice a day for 3 days, or 500 mg once. In diarrheic patients, loperamide hydrochloride (Imodium) may help by increasing contact time between drug and parasites.

Trichostrongylus spp.

The genus *Trichostrongylus* contains a number of species that are primarily parasites of herbivores and are found throughout the world. Human infections have been reported on occasion from many regions and are accidental. *Trichostrongylus orientalis* is fairly common in Japan, Korea, China including Taiwan, and Armenia; a number of other species infecting humans have also been reported from the former Soviet Union.

Trichostrongyles are related to the hookworms, and the adults are rather similar in appearance. The various species reported from humans are smaller than the hookworms, but their eggs are larger. Identification of the various species of *Trichostrongylus* from the eggs is difficult, but differentiation of the eggs from those of hookworm can be readily accomplished. Trichostrongyle eggs (see Fig. 8-3, *C*; Plate XI) are symmetrical and thin shelled and differ from hookworm eggs in their size (73 to 95 μm by 40 to 50 μm) and their more pointed ends.

Symptoms and Pathogenesis. Eggs hatch in the soil, and if the hatched larvae contaminate foodstuffs, they may be ingested. The larvae do not undergo a pulmonary migration but when swallowed attach themselves to the intestinal mucosa and grow to adulthood in 3 to 4 weeks. They ingest blood; only in rather heavy infections is the blood loss clinically significant. Heavily infected patients may become emaciated.

Epidemiology. Trichostrongyle eggs passed in the feces of infected herbivores of humans hatch and develop in the soil in much the same manner as hookworm eggs do. Although *Trichostrongylus* worms are principally zoonotic, the use of human feces for fertilizer, an almost universal practice in the Orient, no doubt facilitates human-to-human spread of the infection in those areas.

Treatment. Mebendazole, 100 mg twice daily for 3 days, has been considered the treatment of choice for both adults and children. Although there are no published reports on the use of albendazole, it seems probable that a single dose of 400 mg (200 mg in children under 2 years of age) would be equally effective.

Anisakiasis

Marine fish in many parts of the world are infected with larval stages of nematodes of the family Anisakidae. Adult anisakids are parasites of the gastrointestinal tract of a wide variety of animals, but those of medical importance are parasites of marine mammals (seals, sea lions, whales, and dolphins). Eggs, passed in the feces of the mammalian host, hatch to liberate larvae, which may then be ingested by marine crustaceans. In these animals the larvae grow and molt, and if the crustacean is then eaten by fish or squid, the contained third-stage larvae are liberated to penetrate into the body cavity or muscles of that host. The fish or squid acts as a transport, or paratenic, host, in which the larvae may grow but do not molt to become adults. If, as is often the case, the first transport host is in turn ingested by a larger fish or squid, the larva continues to infect the new host. In this manner, fish at the top of the food chain may become very heavily infected. When these fish are eaten by marine mammals, the larvae develop into adult worms. If infected fish are consumed, either raw or improperly prepared, by humans, the larvae are unable to complete their development and attempt once again to adapt to a paratenic host (Fig. 8-28).

Human infections are principally the result of ingestion of third-stage larvae belonging to the genera *Anisakis* or *Pseudoterranova* (also called *Terranova* and *Phocanema*). Such larvae may reach a length of 50 mm and a diameter of 1 to 2 mm, though many are smaller. Classification of the larvae of anisakids is difficult; they are generally identified by "type" on the basis of the structure of the digestive tract (see Fig. 8-29). *Anisakis* larvae are usually found in herring and mackerel, and salmon in North America. The larvae of *Pseudoterranova* usually parasitize cod, halibut, rockfish (Pacific red snapper), sardine, and squid.

Most human infections have been reported from Japan and the Netherlands; in Japan primarily from the consumption of sushi and sashimi and in the Netherlands from pickled herring. The majority of infections from Japan have involved gastric invasion, and those from the Netherlands and adjacent areas invasion of the intesinal tract. In North America, while invasive gastrointestinal anisakiasis is sometimes seen, a more benign form of infection, known as transient anisakiasis, is more common, and seems to involve infection by *Pseudoterranova* rather than *Anisakis*.

Symptoms. Invasion of the intestinal wall may be characterized by the abrupt onset, 1 to 5 days after the ingestion of raw fish, of abdominal pain, nausea, and sometimes vomiting or diarrhea, with signs of peritoneal irritation and incomplete ileus of the small intestine. Perforation of the bowel has been reported, with the finding of an anisakid larva in an inflammatory omental mass. Segmental inflammation and thickening of the intestinal wall may be noted at surgery, and the resected tissue is found to have an eosinophilic infiltrate surrounding the larva, usually of the *Anisakis* type. Gastric anisakiasis frequently presents with severe epigastric pain, nausea, and vomiting, sometimes coming on within a few hours after raw fish has been consumed; it is also reported to produce chronic illness. Gastroscopic removal of the worm is usually readily accomplished, at least in patients who experience onset of illness shortly after eating raw fish. A threadlike filling defect is seen in the stomach of about half of such patients examined with an upper gastrointestinal tract film series.

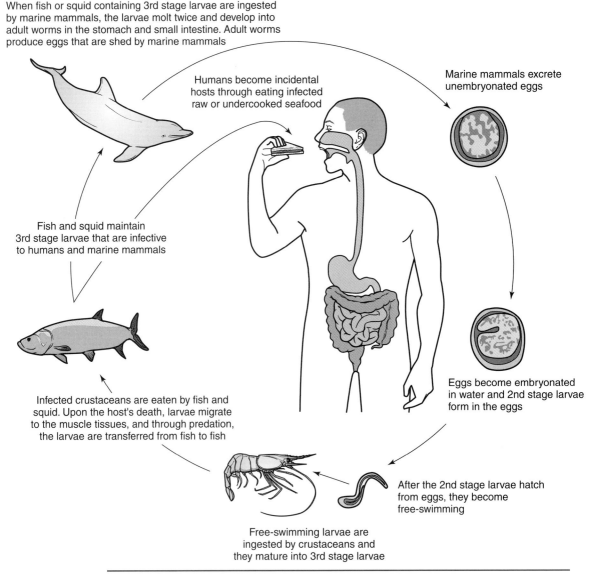

When fish or squid containing 3rd stage larvae are ingested by marine mammals, the larvae molt twice and develop into adult worms in the stomach and small intestine. Adult worms produce eggs that are shed by marine mammals

Humans become incidental hosts through eating infected raw or undercooked seafood

Marine mammals excrete unembryonated eggs

Fish and squid maintain 3rd stage larvae that are infective to humans and marine mammals

Infected crustaceans are eaten by fish and squid. Upon the host's death, larvae migrate to the muscle tissues, and through predation, the larvae are transferred from fish to fish

Eggs become embryonated in water and 2nd stage larvae form in the eggs

After the 2nd stage larvae hatch from eggs, they become free-swimming

Free-swimming larvae are ingested by crustaceans and they mature into 3rd stage larvae

FIGURE 8-28 ■ Life cycle of *Anisakis*.

Transient anisakiasis has been reported primarily from North America. There may be some nausea and gastric distress within a few hours after ingestion of the fish, but frequently there are no such symptoms or only a mild throat irritation, and a larva is coughed up some days later. It seems probable that many such transient infections are never diagnosed. While most infections have been reported from the Pacific coast, and a few from the Atlantic, they might occur in any part of the country. Fresh salmon shipped from the Pacific Northwest and purchased from supermarkets in Michigan were all found to be infected with living larvae of *Anisakis*.

A presumptive diagnosis can be made on the basis of the patient's food habits. Definitive diagnosis rests upon the demonstration of worms obtained by gastroscopy, at surgery (Fig. 8-30), or vomited by the patient. If vomited larvae are well preserved, they may be cleared in glycerin (see Chapter 14) and identified by the structure of the digestive tract (Fig. 8-29), which differs in the three types of anisakid larvae.

Esophagus

Ventriculus

Intestine

Anisakis

Esophagus

Intestinal cecum

Ventriculus

Intestine

Pseudoterranova

Esophagus

Intestinal cecum

Ventriculus

Ventricular appendix

Intestine

Contracaecum

Type	Ventriculus	Anteriorly projecting intestinal cecum	Ventricular appendix
Anisakis	Present	Absent	Absent
Pseudoterranova	Present	Present	Absent
Contracaecum	Present	Present	Present

FIGURE 8-29 ▨ Comparative morphology of the digestive tracts of the three types of anisakid larvae. (Modified from *Pathology of tropical and extraordinary disease.* Armed Forces Institute of Pathology, 76-6005.)

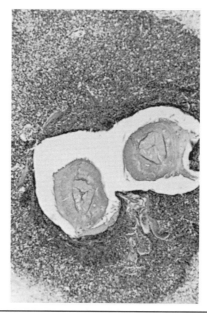

FIGURE 8-30 ▨ Cross section of larval *Anisakis* in eosinophilic abscess in submucosa of stomach. (Courtesy of Dr. Muneo Yokogawa, Chiba University, Japan.)

Epidemiology and Prevention. Human infection results from the consumption of raw or insufficiently smoked or salted or marinated fish. The prevalence of larval anisakids in fish depends in turn on the prevalence of marine mammals, which is high in the North Sea, in Japanese and Alaskan coastal waters, and is increasing along the Pacific cost of North America. In fish frequently consumed raw on the Pacific coast, the prevalence of anisakid worms may be higher than 80%, and individual fish may be heavily infected. Fish kept frozen at −20°C for at least 5 days are considered safe for consumption in dishes such as sashimi, sushi, ceviche, and poisson cru. Smoking fish kills the parasites only if the temperature of the flesh reaches 65°C during the process (a temperature not achieved by all types of smoking). Salting or marinating fish cannot be depended on to kill the parasites. Larvae may be found in the gut, the visceral cavity, and the flesh of fish. In some species, such as herring, few or none are found in the flesh during life and if the fish are cleaned promptly the flesh will be free of larvae. When fish are iced (but not frozen) for transportation to harbor processing plants, larvae tend to migrate from the gut into the muscles. Human anisakiasis has virtually disappeared from the Netherlands since it became mandatory to freeze herring.

Treatment. Other than reassurance, no treatment is needed for transient anisakiasis. In the gastrointestinal form of infection, where worms are embedded in the stomach or bowel wall, a diagnosis can be made only by gastroscopy or surgery, which should also be curative. A history of consuming raw fish shortly before the onset of symptoms should suggest the possibility of anisakiasis (or, as we shall see, eustrongyloidiasis), and depending on the symptoms gastroscopy or surgery may be in order. Albendazole, 400 mg twice daily for 21 days, has been reported to successfully treat a patient with anisakiasis (Moore et al., 2002).

Uncommon Intestinal Nematodes of Humans

A few examples of the numerous species of nematodes, normally parasites of domestic or wild animals, that are sporadically encountered in humans are given next. Many are seen so infrequently that drug therapy has never been attempted.

Eustrongylides spp.

Parasitic as an adult in various wading birds, the larvae of various species of *Eustrongylides* are found in fish. Four instances of human infection have involved fishermen (in Maryland and New Jersey) who consumed live bait minnows. In three of these cases, and another related to the consumption of sushi (Wittner et al., 1989), the human paratenic hosts of *Eustrongylides* required surgery because worms were invading the abdominal cavity. *Eustrongylides* is closely related to *Dioctophyma renale* (see Chapter 9), the giant kidney worm of carnivores and mustelids.

Gongylonema spp.

Cosmopolitan parasites of ruminants, these threadlike nematodes are also found in swine, bears, hedgehogs, monkeys, and occasionally humans. The adult worm migrates within the wall of the duodenum, stomach, esophagus, and (in humans) the buccal cavity. Adult females may reach of length of 145 mm in some hosts, but are smaller in humans; male worms are smaller than females. Intermediate hosts are cockroaches and other insects, and human infection must be the result of ingestion of these insects or of water containing the larval stages derived from disintegrating insects. Nine human cases have been described from the United States (Eberhard and Busillo, 1999).

Oesophagostomum spp.

These worms are parasitic in ruminants, pigs, and monkeys in China, the Philippines, Indonesia, and Africa. Individual human cases have been found in Ethiopia, Java, and Brazil, while the

TABLE 8-1 ■ Review of Intestinal Nematode Infections of Humans

Disease	Parasite	Means of Human Infection	Location of Larvae in Humans	Location of Adults in Humans	Clinical Features	Laboratory Diagnosis
Ascariasis	*Ascaris lumbricoides*	Ingestion of eggs	Lungs	Small intestine (lumen)	Cough, pneumonitis, vague GI symptoms	Undeveloped eggs in stool
Enterobiasis	*Enterobius vermicularis* (pinworm)	Ingestion of eggs	Lumen of small intestine	Cecum, adjacent large and small bowel (superficial attachment)	Anal pruritus, restless sleep	Embryonated eggs on cellophane tape preparation
Ancylostomiasis (necatoriasis)	*Ancylostoma duodenale, Necator americanus* (hookworms)	Larvae penetrate the skin	Skin, lungs	Small intestine (attached)	Dermatitis, cough, diarrhea, abdominal pain, anemia, eosinophilia	Undeveloped eggs in stool
Cutaneous larva migrans (creeping eruption)	*Ancylostoma braziliense, A. caninum* (cat and dog hookworms)	Larvae penetrate the skin	Skin, in serpiginous tunnels	Not present (in cats and dogs)	Dermatitis, pruritus, secondary infection	Larval tracks in skin
Strongyloidiasis	*Strongyloides stercoralis* (threadworm)	Larvae penetrate the skin (also by autoinfection)	Skin, lungs, duodenal mucosa	Deep in duodenal mucosa (females)	Cough, epigastric pain, diarrhea, eosinophilia	Rhabditiform larvae in stool
Trichuriasis	*Trichuris trichiura* (whipworm)	Ingestion of eggs	Mucosa of small intestine	Cecum to rectum (attached)	Abdominal pain, mucous diarrhea, eosinophilia	Undeveloped eggs in stool
Anisakiasis	*Anisakis* spp. and related genera	Ingestion of larvae in marine fish	Mucosa of stomach and intestine	Not present (in marine mammals)	Epigastric pain, nausea, vomiting, diarrhea, variable eosinophilia	None (identification of larvae)

infection is common in a small area of northern Togo and Ghana, bordering in Burkina Faso, where an estimated 250,000 people are infected with the human parasite *O. bifurcum* (Storeg et al., 2000). The worms resemble hookworms; their eggs are indistinguishable. Larvae develop in the soil, and when ingested, by both their human and animal hosts, penetrate the intestinal wall, where some develop rapidly into adults and reenter the intestine. Other remain in an immature state for long periods, forming nodules in the intestinal wall, the omentum, or even the abdominal wall. Two clinical conditions have been described in human esophagostomiasis (de Gruijter et al., 2004). The unilocular disease, referred to as "Dapaong tumor" or as "turtle in the belly" by indigenous healers, is a painful abdominal mass that frequently adhers to the abdominal wall. The multilocular disease involves hundreds of pea-sized nodules in the submucosa and subserosa of the large intestine. DNA studies have demonstrated that *O. bifurcum* of humans is generally distinct from *O. bifurcum* of monkeys and baboons of the same geographic area (de Gruijter et al., 2004). Surgery is the only treatment for worms in these extraintestinal foci (Polderman and Blotkamp, 1995), while albendazole in a single dose of 400 mg is quite effective in eliminating the intestinal worms (Krepel et al., 1993; Ziem et al., 2004).

These and other unusual infections occur when two normally separate ecologic systems come to overlap. Sometimes, as in the case of *Eustrongylides*, these may indeed be sporadic events, while in other instances (such as in Philippine capillariasis) human involvement in what was originally a strict zoonosis may become quite common.

Acanthocephala

The acanthocephala, or thorny-headed worms, while superficially resembling nematodes, belong to their own phylum. Although they are only of minor importance as human intestinal parasites, they will be briefly discussed here.

Acanthocephalans are cylindrical worms with a spiny proboscis. The adult worms possess no digestive tract, and all are parasitic in the intestinal tract of vertebrates. Larvae require an arthropod as intermediate host, and some go through a juvenile stage in a second intermediate host; the vertebrate becomes infected by ingesting the first or second intermediate host.

Moniliformis moniliformis is a rodent parasite of cosmopolitan distribution. Male worms are 4 to 5 cm long, and females 10 to 27 cm. Beetles and cockroaches are intermediate hosts. Isolated and scattered reports of human infections attest to humankind's omnivorous nature. *Macracanthorhynchus hirudinaceus* is a parasite of pigs, both domestic and wild. Adult worms are about twice the size of *Moniliformis*, and beetles serve as intermediate hosts of this parasite. Human infection is rare but was at one time said to be common in the Volga valley, where raw *Melolontha* beetles were consumed. *Macracanthorhynchus ingens*, a common intestinal parasite of raccoons, has been reported from an infant who presumably acquired it by ingesting an infected beetle.

Acanthocephalans, in addition to anisakid and eustrongylid nematodes, may be acquired by eating sashimi. *Bulbosoma* has a life cycle involving crustaceans as first intermediate hosts, fish as a second intermediate host; the adult worms are found in sea mammals such as whales. Rare reports of infection with this or similar acanthocephalans are known from Japan and among fish-eating Inuit (Eskimos).

Table 8-1 summarizes some important features of the more common intestinal nematode infections of humans.

References

Albanese G et al. Treatment of larva migrans cutanea (creeping eruption): A comparison between albendazole and traditional therapy. *Int J Dermatol* 2001; *40*:67–71.

Ashford RW et al. *Strongyloides fuelleborni kellyi*: Infection and disease in Papua New Guinea. *Parasitol Today* 1992; *8*:314–318.

Cooper PJ et al. Geohelminth infections protect against severe inflammatory diarrhea in children. *Trans R Soc Trop Med Hyg* 2003; *97*:519–521.

Croese J et al. Human enteric infection with canine hookworms. *Ann Intern Med* 1994; *120*:369–373.

de Gruijter JM et al. Genetic substructuring within *Oesophagostomum bifurcum* (nematode) from human and non-human primates from Ghana based on random amplified polymorphic DNA analysis. *Am J Trop Med Hyg* 2004; *71*:227–233.

de Silva NR et al. Morbidity and mortality due to *Ascaris*-induced intestinal obstruction. *Trans R Soc Trop Med Hyg* 1997; *91*:31–36.

Eberhard ML, Busillo C. Human *Gongylonema* infection in a resident of New York City. *Am J Trop Med Hyg* 1999; *61*:51–52.

Heukelbach J et al. Selective mass treatment with ivermectin to control intestinal helminthiases and parasitic skin diseases in a severely affected population. *Bull WHO* 2004; *82*:563–571.

Jelinek T et al. Cutaneous larva migrans in travelers: Synopsis of histories, symptoms and treatment of 98 patients. *Clin Infect Dis* 1994; *19*:1062–1066.

Krepel HP et al. Treatment of mixed *Oesophagostomum* and hookworm infection: Effect of albendazole, pyrantel pamoate, levamisole and thiabendazole. *Trans R Soc Trop Med Hyg* 1993; *87*:87–89.

Moore DAJ et al. Treatment of anisakiasis with albendazole. *Lancet* 2002; *360*:54.

Moravec F. Redescription and systematic status of *Capillaria philippinensis*, an intestinal parasite of human beings. *J Parasitol* 2001; *87*:161–164.

Polderman AM, Blotkamp J. *Oesophagostomum* infections in humans. *Parasitol Today* 1995; *11*:451–456.

Storey PA et al. Clinical epidemiology and classification of human oesophagostomiasis. *Trans R Soc Trop Med Hyg* 2000; *94*:177–182.

Tarr PE et al. Case report: Rectal administration of ivermectin to a patient with *Strongyloides* hyperinfection syndrome. *Am J Trop Med Hyg* 2003; *68*:453–455.

Wickelgren I. Can worms tame the immune system? *Science* 2004; *305*:170–171.

Wittner M et al. Eustrongyliasis—a parasitic infection acquired by eating sushi. *N Engl J Med* 1989; *320*:1124–1126.

Zhou X et al. Treatment of biliary ascariasis in China. *Trans R Soc Trop Med Hyg* 1999; *93*:561–564.

Ziem JB et al. The short-term impact of albendazole treatment on *Oesophagostomum bifurcum* and hookworm infections in northern Ghana. *Ann Trop Med Parasitol* 2004; *98*:385–390.

The Blood- and Tissue-Dwelling Nematodes

A diverse group of nematodes parasitize the blood vascular system and other organs and tissues of humans. For a few of these, humans are the only known definitive host, some are shared with other species of vertebrates, and for a large number humans are a relatively uncommon accidental host.

The Filariae

The filariae are long, threadlike nematodes, various species of which inhabit portions of the human lymphatic system, and others the subcutaneous and deep connective tissues. In addition to the eight species that commonly infect humans, a number of filariae that are primarily parasites of other animals are reported occasionally from humans. The adults of all species of filariae are parasites of vertebrate hosts. The female worms produce eggs that during their development become elongate and wormlike in appearance, a modification that adapts them for life within the vascular system or for migration through the tissues. These highly modified eggs, referred to as microfilariae, are generally capable of living for a long period within the vertebrate host but not of developing further until ingested by their intermediate host and vector, an insect. In the insect, the microfilariae molt and grow, transforming into infective larvae, which are deposited on the skin when the insect next takes blood from a suitable host.

The most important of the filarial diseases of humans are the lymphatic filariases, so called because the adult worms are found in the lymphatic system. Agents of lymphatic filariasis are *Wuchereria bancrofti, Brugia malayi,* and *B. timori.*

Wuchereria bancrofti

Bancroftian filariasis is widely distributed throughout the tropics and subtropics. It is found through much of central Africa, in Madagascar, and in the Nile delta. Scattered cases have been reported from Turkey. In Asia, the disease may be found along the Arabian seacoast, in India, Pakistan, Sri Lanka, Myanmar (Burma), Thailand, Southeast Asia, Malaysia, and the Philippines, as well as in the southern part of China. It occurs extensively throughout the Pacific islands. In the New World, it is found in Haiti, the Dominican Republic, Guyana, Surinam, French Guiana, and coastal Brazil. An endemic focus formerly occurred in the region of Charleston, South Carolina. The World Health Organization (WHO) estimated in 1994 the number of persons world-wide suffering from overt bancroftian filariasis to approximate 106.2 million. Of these, some 45.5 million are to be found in India, and 40 million in Sub-Saharan Africa.

It has been speculated that *Wuchereria bancrofti* originated in Southeast Asia, where its closest known relative, *W. kalimantani,* parasitizes the Indonesian leaf monkey. From there it was presumably carried by the earliest migrants to the islands of the South Pacific, perhaps as long ago as the second millennium BC. Another migration from the same area of Southeast Asia, known to have settled in Madagascar sometime before 500 AD, may have brought filariasis to that island and subsequently to the mainland of Africa. Filariasis is known to have spread throughout Central Africa and into Arabia by the 14th or 15th century (with no evidence of its presence in Egypt in Pharaonic times), and to have been imported to the New World via the slave trade of the 17th and 18th centuries. It was introduced into northeastern Australia during the 19th century, but has since been eradicated.

The life cycle of *W. bancrofti* (Fig. 9-1) is of more than usual interest, as Manson's discovery, in 1878, of the transmission of this parasite by mosquitoes was the first demonstration of an arthropod as vector of a parasitic organism. The mosquito Manson found infected in China was *Culex fatigans*; since then it has been found that various species of *Aedes* and *Anopheles* are the important vectors in some other parts of the world. The mosquito is more than a simple agent of transmission of the parasite; an essential developmental cycle takes place within the body of the insect. Upon taking blood from an infected person, the mosquito may ingest microfilariae with its blood meal. The microfilariae bore through the stomach wall to enter the body cavity of the insect, where they migrate to the thoracic musculature

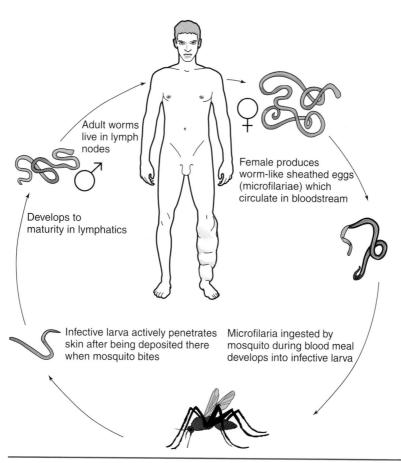

Adult worms live in lymph nodes

Female produces worm-like sheathed eggs (microfilariae) which circulate in bloodstream

Develops to maturity in lymphatics

Infective larva actively penetrates skin after being deposited there when mosquito bites

Microfilaria ingested by mosquito during blood meal develops into infective larva

FIGURE 9-1 ■ Life cycle of *Wuchereria* and *Brugia.*

for a period of growth. During the next 10 days or so, the larvae grow and molt to become infective-stage larvae. During this period they have increased in length from about 300 μm to 1.5 to 2 mm. The infective larvae enter the proboscis of the mosquito and when the next blood meal is taken escape from the proboscis onto the skin. They enter through the puncture hole left by the mosquito, to infect their new host. The subsequent development in humans is not as completely known. Infective larvae gain access to the peripheral lymphatics and thence to the regional lymph nodes and larger lymph vessels. They molt twice before they mature in the lymph nodes or vessels; if male and female worms are present in the same area they mate and microfilariae are produced. The time necessary for the worms to grow to sexual maturity is probably several months; adult worms are known to live for some years. Adults are threadlike white worms. The males measure 2.5 to 4 cm and the females 5 to 10 cm.

Microfilariae of *W. bancrofti* (Fig. 9-2) are said to be sheathed. The sheath is actually the egg shell, which is very thin and delicate and surrounds the embryo as it circulates in the blood; it is not lost until it is digested away in the stomach of the mosquito. In thick blood films, microfilariae range in length from about 245 to nearly 300 μm. A large number of distinct nuclei can be seen in the body of a well-stained specimen, as well as the rudiments of some organs of the adult worm. There is no alimentary canal. The cylindrical body is bluntly rounded anteriorly; posteriorly it tapers to a point. Nuclei are not seen in the terminal portion of the tail, and this characteristic serves to differentiate microfilariae of this species from other sheathed microfilariae. A key to the microfilariae found in the blood is given at the end of this section (Table 9-1).

In most parts of the world where filariasis is endemic, the infection is seen in its so-called periodic form. Microfilariae, present in very small numbers in the circulating blood during the daytime hours and often virtually undetectable then, appear at their greatest density at night, generally between the hours of 10 PM and 2 to 4 AM. The subperiodic form of filariasis occurs throughout the Pacific islands. Persons infected with this strain exhibit microfilaremia at all times, but the organisms are present in greatest numbers between noon and 8 PM. The subperiodic form has also been found in some areas of Vietnam. The suggestion has been made that the subperiodic form be recognized as a separate variety, *Wuchereria*

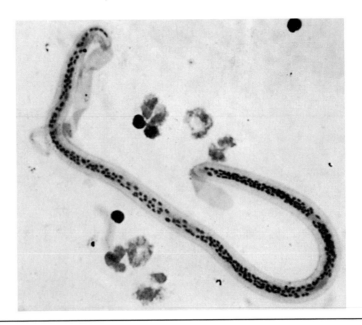

FIGURE 9-2 ■ Microfilaria of *Wuchereria bancrofti* in thick blood film (hematoxylin stain). (Photomicrograph by Zane Price.)

bancrofti var. *pacifica*, or that it should form a distinct species, *Wuchereria pacifica*. Neither proposal has been widely accepted, as the morphologic differences reported between adult worms of the periodic and nonperiodic forms are extremely minor, and microfilariae of the two sorts appear to be identical.

The basis of filarial periodicity remains largely unknown; it may be altered by a change in the habits of the host, as when waking and sleeping hours are transposed. It takes about a week for such reversal to be effected, suggesting that sleeping and waking as such do not affect the periodicity but that the entire 24-hour rhythm of the host is in some way responsible for this phenomenon. When absent from the peripheral circulation, the microfilariae are found primarily in the capillaries and small vessels of the lungs. Some of the factors that influence migration of microfilariae of the periodic strain of *W. bancrofti* to the lungs are increased pulmonary pO_2 and increased exertion. Obviously, while normal daily activity can in this manner influence migration of the nocturnally periodic or common strain of *W. bancrofti*, it must affect the Pacific or diurnally subperiodic strain differently. Presumably other factors are also important in influencing the microfilarial migration, which determines periodicity. In general, it has been noted that where the nonperiodic disease occurs the vectors take blood during the day and that in areas of the periodic disease the mosquitoes do so at night.

Diagnosis of filarial infection is frequently made on strict clinical grounds, particularly in endemic areas, but demonstration of microfilariae in the circulating blood is the only means by which one may make a certain diagnosis. The microfilariae may be found by examination of a fresh blood film, where their movements make them conspicuous. If they are present in small numbers, it may be necessary to prepare a thick blood film or concentrate of a larger volume of venous blood to detect them. The "provocative" administration of diethylcarbamazine may enable an examiner to detect the presence of nocturnally periodic microfilariae in blood samples taken during the day. Microfilariae can be demonstrated, at about one third of nocturnal number, three quarters of an hour to 2 or more hours after the administration of an oral dose of 100 mg of diethylcarbamazine (a slow-acting microfilaricidal drug).

This phenomenon does not apply to the subperiodic or Pacific variant strain of *W. bancrofti*. A *fall* in circulating microfilariae to about 8% of pretreatment levels has been found 1 hour after the oral administration of diethylcarbamazine, 5 mg/kg body weight (the usual treatment dose). This also occurs in the Pacific strain following the administration of very small (5 to 10 mg total) doses of the same drug (Markell, unpublished data).

Details of two concentration techniques, nucleopore filtration and Knott concentration, are given in Chapter 15. In areas where more than one kind of filarial disease exists, well-stained slides are essential, as the different filarial infections are distinguished by differences in structure of the microfilariae (Fig. 9-3). A skin test using an extract of the dog heartworm,

TABLE 9-1 ■ Key to Microfilariae Commonly Found in the Blood

a. Larvae possess sheath	b
Larvae unsheathed	e
b. Nuclei found in tip of tail	c
Nuclei do not extend to tip	*Wuchereria bancrofti*
c. Nuclei form continuous row in tail	*Loa loa*
Nuclei not continuous, two at end of tail	d
d. Cephalic space ratio 2:1	*Brugia malayi**
Cephalic space ratio 3:1	*Brugia timori*
e. Nuclei found in tip of tail	f
Nuclei do not extend to tip	*Mansonella ozzardi*
f. Nuclei often form double row, terminal nucleus or nuclei separate	*Mansonella perstans*
Nuclei in single row, tail curved	*Mansonella streptocerca*

*Sheath, which may be cast in thick film, stains heavily with Giemsa.

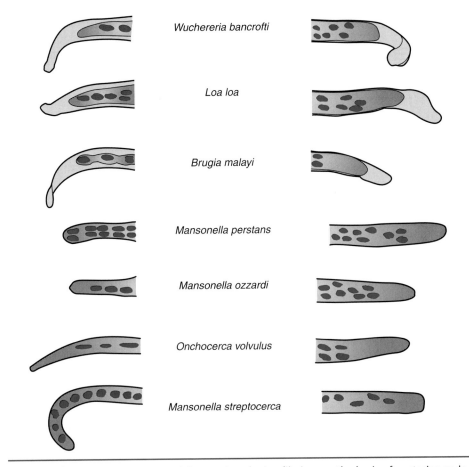

Wuchereria bancrofti

Loa loa

Brugia malayi

Mansonella perstans

Mansonella ozzardi

Onchocerca volvulus

Mansonella streptocerca

FIGURE 9-3 ■ Differentiation of the species of microfilariae, on the basis of posterior ends *(left)* and anterior ends *(right)* of the microfilariae. Note the distribution of nuclei, their presence or absence in the extreme caudal portion, and the presence or absence of a sheath.

Dirofilaria immitis (not available in the United States), is group specific for filarial infections, as are various serologic tests (Chapter 16).

Radiographs can at times give evidence of infection (Fig. 9-4), as the worms die and become calcified. Lymphangiography may demonstrate characteristic changes in filarial elephantiasis (Fig. 9-5), and ultrasonography may show the movements of adult worms in the lymphatics (see under Symptoms).

While the presence of the signs and symptoms of filarial infection, described below, may provide a presumptive diagnosis in persons from endemic areas, demonstration of microfilariae in the blood has long been the diagnostic goal. However, filarial infection may occur without demonstrable microfilaremia. This is commonly seen in immunologically naive persons, coming from nonendemic areas, and in such cases represents hyperreactivity to the microfilariae, resulting in their rapid destruction by immune mechanisms of the host. Tropical pulmonary eosinophilia (discussed later in this chapter), Meyers and Kouwenaar's syndrome (lymphadenopathy with splenomegaly, transient pulmonary infiltrates, and hypereosinophilia), and sowda (discussed under onchocerciasis) are other examples of such generally amicrofilaremic states.

In some instances microfilariae, while present, may simply be too few for detection by the usual techniques, which involve the examination of thick films made from 20 to 60 μl of blood. Dreyer and others (1996), rechecking 100 male long-time residents of an endemic area in Brazil found negative on the examination of 60 μl nocturnal blood samples,

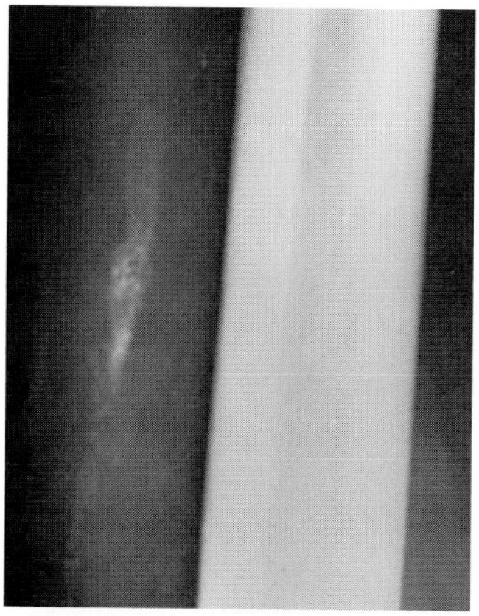

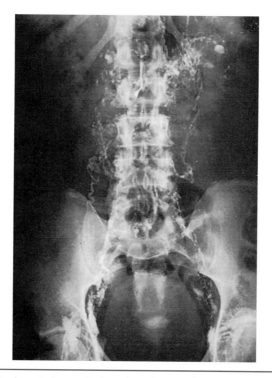

FIGURE 9-4 ■ Calcified *Wuchereria bancrofti* in tissue.

FIGURE 9-5 ■ *Wuchereria bancrofti*. Lymphangiogram shows enlarged nodes and dilated, tortuous lymph channels. (Courtesy Dr. Herman Zaiman.)

were able, by membrane filtration (see Chapter 15) of incremental increases of blood samples to 1, 5, and 10 ml, to demonstrate microfilariae in 27 of these men. By ultrasonography they could see the "filarial dance sign" (see under Symptoms) in another 10 individuals. In how many more were adult filariae situated in sites where they could not be visualized?

In one endemic area in which microfilaremia was found in 29% of individuals, filarial antigens were detected in the blood of an additional 17% of apparently asymptomatic amicrofilaremics (Weil et al., 1996). Diagnosis of filarial infection by detection of circulating filarial antigens would obviate the problems seen in persons with low level microfilaremia, but such tests are available in the United States only through the Centers for Disease Control and Prevention (CDC) and certain reference laboratories (see Chapter 16). An ELISA kit test employing monoclonal antibodies to detect the circulating antigens of *W. bancrofti* is commercially available from Tropical Biotechnology Pty Ltd, Queensland, Australia (Nicolas, 1997). A commercially available (AMRAD, Australia) whole-blood antigen card test (ICT) for filariasis was used to detect infection in Sri Lanka following a mass treatment program using single dose diethylcarbamazine (Chandrasena et al., 2002). ICT appeared to be more sensitive and specific than standard parasitological methods of diagnosing lymphatic filariasis (thick blood films and membrane filtration). However, the unit cost of ICT was considerably more, approximately 10 times greater.

Of all those infected with lymphatic filariasis worldwide, a WHO review indicates that nearly two-thirds are microfilaremic without overt symptoms but with subclinical renal and lymphatic damage; nearly one quarter of male have hydrocele, and a little over one eighth of infected persons have elephantiasis and/or lymphedema with accompanying attacks of acute lymphangitis of lymphadenitis (Ottesen and Ramachandran, 1995).

Symptoms. Clinical manifestations of infection are variable and probably depend on constitutional factors in the host, numbers of infecting organisms, and possibly strain differences in the parasite itself. Some persons become heavily infected without showing any signs of disease other than large numbers of microfilariae in the circulating blood. It has long been considered that because such persons have an infection that has not resulted in disease, they need not be treated. Recent studies have shown that this assumption is incorrect. In a Brazilian investigation (Dreyer et al., 1992), 9 of 20 randomly selected asymptomatic microfilaremic soldiers, with no recognized medical causes for renal disease, were found to have microscopic hematuria (7 of 20) and/or proteinuria (4 of 20). Standard treatment was found to exacerbate the hematuria and proteinuria transiently in the affected patients, and to induce these findings temporarily in most of those who had been initially negative. Following therapy, all patients had normal urinary findings. Lymphangioscintigraphy has allowed the visualization of the peripheral lymphatics in patients with filarial infection (Witte et al., 1993), with the finding of significant abnormalities in lymphatic structure and function in asymptomatic microfilaremics (Freedman et al., 1994, 1995). Renal and lymphatic disease in these "asymptomatic" individuals strongly suggests the advisability of treatment.

In some, the presence of even a few worms provokes severe reactions. Such hyperreactivity is characteristic of immunologically naive persons rather than those who are native to the endemic area, whose maternally acquired antibodies have been augmented by early infection and who frequently show no signs of disease.

Early manifestations of filariasis are fever, lymphangitis, and lymphadenitis. Febrile attacks may be seen with or without associated lymphangitis, although the latter are less common. These attacks are sometimes referred to as "filarial" or "elephantoid" fever. The attack usually begins with a chill, and the fever remains high for 1 or 2 days and gradually subsides over the following 2- to 5-day period. Lymphangitis commonly affects the limbs but may occur in the breast, scrotum, or elsewhere. When seen on the limbs it usually develops centrifugally, starting in the region of a lymph node and progressing distally along the lymphatic channel. The affected lymphatic vessel is distended and acutely tender, and the overlying skin is tense, erythematous, and hot. The surrounding area is frequently edematous. Attacks of lymphangitis recur periodically. Occasionally they are accompanied by abscess formation, either along the course of the lymphatic or at a lymph node. When such abscesses are opened or drain spontaneously, remnants of adult worms are sometimes found in the drainage. Lymphadenitis, either alone or in combination with periodic lymphangitic attacks, most commonly affects the femoral and epitrochlear nodes which, once enlarged, tend to remain so. They are firm, discrete, and somewhat tender. Enlargement of the epitrochlear lymph nodes occurs early in the subperiodic form of filariasis, while it is relatively less common in the periodic form.

The scrotal lymphatics appear to be a preferential site for localization of the adult worms. Ultrasonographic examination of the scrotal lymphatics of 14 asymptomatic microfilaremic males resulted in the demonstration of random movements—the "filarial dance sign" (FDS)—of adult filariae in the dilated lymphatics of 7 individuals (Amaral et al., 1994). Subsequently, 10 persons exhibiting the FDS were examined several times weekly for 12 consecutive weeks, during which time no worm was observed to have changed its location. Weekly ultrasonographic examination of the scrotal lymphatics of 100 microfilaremic men, none of whom had been treated for filariasis, carried out for 6 weeks, revealed the FDS in 80. Its presence was strongly correlated with higher microfilarial blood levels (Norões et al., 1996), but it has also been noted in amicrofilaremic individuals. Administration of diethyl-carbamazine has been associated with disappearance of the FDS in some worms.

Orchitis and inflammation of the spermatic cord are common, and some permanent thickening of the cord is seen in a large percentage of the cases that are symptomatic. A lymph varix of the cord may appear and rupture into the scrotal sac, leading to a condition known as lymphocele. Lymphocele is one type of hydrocele, a condition that may also develop gradually as a result of recurrent attacks of orchitis. Microfilariae may be found in the hydrocele fluid if it is wholly or partially made up of lymph. Rupture of lymph varices into any part of the urinary tract leads to the passage of lymph in the urine (chyluria). Chyluria usually comes on suddenly and lasts for a few days. There may be repeated episodes, separated by long intervals. Microfilariae may be found in the chylous urine.

Intraocular filariasis is an extremely rare condition, with only 42 such cases reported in the world literature. A recent report from Vellore, India (Mathai and David, 2000), describes a case in which a 2 cm adult male *W. bancrofti* was surgically removed from the anterior chamber of the eye of a patient who, for a week prior, had experienced redness, irritation, and diminished vision. Since the eye has no lymphatics, entry to the eye was presumed to be hematogenous.

Elephantiasis, the enlargement of one or more limbs, the scrotum, breasts, or vulva with dermal hypertrophy and verrucous changes, is a relatively uncommon and late complication of filariasis (Figs. 9-6 and 9-7). It must be emphasized that elephantiasis is by no means the inevitable result of filarial infection. Even in endemic areas where the population is exposed to infection during their entire lives, many persons who become infected never develop overt symptoms or signs other than a microfilaremia. Others develop lymphadenopathy or may have recurrent attacks of fever and lymphangitis, but the disease does not progress to elephantiasis.

Pathogenesis. Adult worms are found in lymph vessels throughout the body but principally in or around the axillary, epitrochlear, inguinal, and pelvic nodes, and the lymphatics distal to them, as well as those of the testis, epididymis, and cord. Inflammatory changes in and around the lymphatic vessels comprise the basic reaction to infection, though the expression of this reaction may be variable. Attacks of lymphangitis and lymphadenitis may begin before the worms mature. These attacks are marked by retrograde lymphangitis if a limb is involved; funiculitis, epididymitis, or orchitis may be seen if the worms are located in the scrotal lymphatics; fever and other constitutional symptoms without localizing signs are seen if the pelvic or abdominal lymphatics are the site of inflammation. It is now recognized that bacterial or fungal superinfection of the already compromised lymphatics may play an important role in the recurrent attacks of adenolymphangitis.

Repeated attacks of inflammation lead to dilation and thickening of the affected lymphatic vessels, which may become incompetent and lead to lymphedema. Lymphedema may be intermittent early in the course of the disease, but lymphatic vessels tend to become fibrosed after repeated attacks of lymphangitis. With chronic lymphedema, there is hyperplasia of the connective tissue, and infiltration of plasma cells, macrophages, and eosinophils.

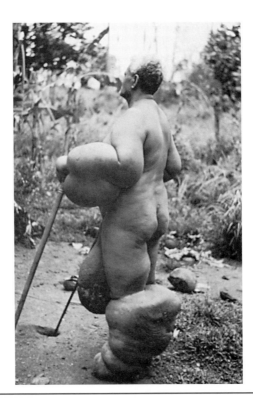

FIGURE 9-6 ■ Extreme elephantiasis of all four limbs and scrotum. (Courtesy Dr. John F. Kessel.)

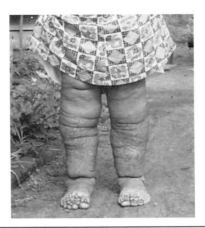

FIGURE 9-7 ■ Moderately advanced elephantiasis involving both legs. Note verrucous hyperplasia of skin over toes.

Finally, woody induration of the tissues may take place, with thickening and verrucous changes of the skin, producing the condition known as elephantiasis (Figs. 9-6 and 9-7).

Elephantiasis may develop in any limb; scrotal elephantiasis is common, and in women elephantiasis of the breasts and vulva is sometimes seen. Elephantiasis is a disfiguring and frequently disabling condition, and because circulation is badly impaired an elephantoid limb or organ is in constant danger of secondary bacterial or fungal infection.

Involvement of the scrotal lymphatics may lead to hydrocele far earlier, and more commonly, than to scrotal elephantiasis. Lymph varices may form in any affected vessels. If in the urinary tract rupture of such varices may bring on attacks of chyluria, and if near the surface of the scrotum they may be readily seen and palpated through the skin and may rupture. This rare condition is known as lymph scrotum.

Death of an adult worm generally leads to severe localized inflammation. Often the worms are absorbed, sometimes they calcify and can be identified on radiographs (see Fig. 9-4), and at other times an abscess forms around them.

Much of what has been learned of the immunology of lymphatic filariasis comes from experiments with *Brugia malayi* and *B. pahangi*, as these parasites, unlike *W. bancrofti*, infect laboratory animals. The two genera are closely related, and their effects on the human host are similar, so that we can assume that what is learned from *Brugia* applies also to *Wuchereria*.

Lymphangitis and its sequelae occur as a result of reactions to the products of developing, adult, or dying worms or from bacterial or fungal infection. Microfilariae seem not be directly responsible for any of the major manifestations of lymphatic filariasis. Antifilarial antibodies of three classes—IgG, IgM, and IgE—have been identified in patients with bancroftian filariasis. The lowest antibody levels were seen in patients with asymptomatic microfilaremia and the highest in amicrofilaremic persons, while levels in those with filarial fever and chronic lymphatic disease were intermediate. The lymphocytic proliferative response was also greater in amicrofilaremic persons than in those with clinical disease. Antisheath antibodies (reacting with surface antigens of microfilariae) have been detected almost exclusively in amicrofilaremic persons, and opsonizing antibodies, promoting in vitro adherence of normal leukocytes to microfilariae, were found in amicrofilaremic persons who had high titers of antisheath antibodies.

Epidemiology. While *W. bancrofti* is capable of larval development in a large number of species of mosquitoes, a rather small number of anthropophilic species are important as vectors. Night-biting *Anopheles* and *Culex* mosquitoes are vectors of the nocturnally periodic *W. bancrofti*, whereas the subperiodic Pacific strain is carried by the daytime-biting *Aedes polynesiensis*. As there are no reservoir hosts for this species, endemicity of the infection demands both an adequate human reservoir and sufficient numbers of circulating microfilariae in the blood of those infected. The importance of these two criteria lies in the fact that transmission of the disease may be interrupted when either the number of persons infected in a given area or the microfilariae level in those infected falls below a critical level. Of course, measures directed against the adult mosquitoes or their larvae are also important in control of the disease. The incidence of demonstrable infection is low in young children, but in endemic areas it probably remains constant after the first few years of life. In many areas, clinical infection appears to be more common in males than in females; this may have a physiologic basis, as has been found to be the case in experimental infections with the filaria *B. pahangi*.

Bancroftian filariasis is widely distributed in the tropics and subtropics between 40°N and 30°S latitude. Transmission is restricted to the more humid areas, and it is thought that this restriction may be a result of the way in which invasion of the definitive host takes place. When infective larvae escape onto the skin from the proboscis sheath of the biting mosquito, they carry with them minute drops of mosquito hemolymph, which protects the larvae from desiccation while they are finding and penetrating the puncture wound left by the mosquito bite. In less humid areas, this protection would be quickly lost.

The possibility of reintroduction of filariasis into the United States is raised by the observation that 6.7% of some 600 Haitian refugees in South Florida were found to have microfilaremia. Laboratory strains of the only mosquito considered to be a likely vector, *Culex quinquefasciatus*, did not become infected, but infection of wild strains was not attempted.

Treatment. Attacks of filarial lymphangitis often respond to the administration of antihistamines and analgesics; in more advanced cases in which secondary infection may be involved, antibiotic therapy is appropriate. In such cases, careful hygienic measures may help prevent recurrent infection and lymphangitis.

Diethylcarbamazine (DEC) (Hetrazan, Notezine)* is an effective microfilaricidal drug, but it eliminates the adult worms more slowly. Its mechanism of action is unclear. In vitro, DEC possesses no microfilaricidal activity; in vivo, its effect is dependent on integrity of the cellular and humoral immune mechanisms of the host. Most of the microfilariae are destroyed by the reticuloendothelial cells of the liver.

DEC is generally administered at the rate of 6 mg/kg of body weight. In the past it was usually given either daily for 12 days, or once a month for a year. Comparable results are obtained by use of a single annual dose, more practical for mass treatment programs. With all such treatment programs microfilariae disappear from the blood of most patients within 2 weeks, to reappear in smaller numbers within 3 to 6 months. On the basis of parasite antigen levels before and following treatment, it is suggested that DEC administered at 6 mg/kg body weight daily for 12 days has approximately a 50% *macro*filaricidal effect; the once-yearly administration has a lesser impact on the adult worms.

The long-term effect of three different treatment strategies for mass DEC administration was assessed in Tanzania 10 years following treatment (Meyrowitsch et al., 2004). The strategies included (1) the standard 12-day treatment, (2) a semiannual single-dose treatment, and (3) a monthly low-dose treatment. All treatments were for 1 year. Ten years after the treatment of infected individuals, microfilarial intensities were 11%, 13%, and 2% of the pretreatment levels for the three treatment strategies, 1, 2, and 3, respectively.

A practical method of administration of DEC in mass treatment programs is by addition to table salt. This has been utilized in several very successful Chinese programs (Fan et al., 1995; Liu et al., 1992), and in Tanzania (Meyrowitsch et al., 1996). Addition of 0.2 to 0.4 per cent by weight of DEC to either plain or iodized salt is effective and safe, and this concentration, when used steadily for 6 months to a year, will virtually eradicate the infection.

Better long-term suppression of microfilaremia is obtained by the concurrent administration of DEC plus ivermectin (Mectizan), on the same, once-yearly dosage schedule. Ivermectin, a macrocyclic lactone antibiotic belonging to the group of avermectins derived from *Streptomyces avermitilis*, was first used in veterinary medicine for the treatment of various nematode and cutaneous arthropod infections. Its efficacy in the treatment of filarial infections in animals led to a trial of ivermectin in human onchocerciasis and other filarial diseases. Ivermectin is thought to act by modifying release of the neurotransmitter gamma-aminobutyric acid (GABA), resulting in paralysis of the microfilariae.

Given once, a single dose of ivermectin of 400 mcg/kg body weight seems as effective as a 12-day course of DEC of 6 mg/kg daily, while repetition at 6-month intervals is even more effective in suppressing microfilaremia (Nguyen et al., 1996), comparable in that respect to the results achieved with once-yearly administration of ivermectin, 400 mcg/kg plus DEC 6 mg/kg (Moulia-Pelat et al., 1996). However, the combination of DEC and ivermectin seems preferable because of the macrofilaricidal properties of DEC. For mass treatment programs, it seems that such yearly drug treatment should be continued for at least 4 years.

Periodic checks of microfilarial load (either by microfilaria counts on thick blood smear, by membrane filtration technique, or by one of the newer antigenic assays) may be used as a guide to re-treatment, both of mass treatment programs and for the individual patient.

Also recommended in areas where intestinal roundworms are a problem is the yearly administration of either DEC or ivermectin, in the doses mentioned earlier, along with a single dose of albendazole, 400 mg for adults or 200 mg for children. Either of these combinations is said to produce suppression of microfilariae comparable to that seen with DEC

*May be obtained from the CDC Drug Service, Centers for Disease Control and Prevention, Atlanta, GA 30333; (404) 639-3670.

plus ivermectin, with the added advantage of the elimination of *Ascaris*. The benefit of the therapy is obvious to the patient and an added incentive to compliance with therapy.

Allergic reactions to death of the microfilariae may occur early in treatment; these reactions consist of fever, urticaria, and lymphangitis, and are usually well controlled with antihistamines. Later, bullous reactions may occur, requiring the use of corticosteroids. These uncommon reactions are also thought to be allergic in nature. Filarial abscesses, which may occur at any point along a lymphatic chain, denote death of the adult worm and a hypersensitivity reaction to its remains. Portions of the dead worm can at times be observed when the abscess is drained. Generalized malaise, vertigo, headache, nausea, and vomiting are occasional side effects of administration of these drugs.

Surgical procedures for treatment of scrotal elephantiasis are generally satisfactory; hydrocele may also be treated by the accepted surgical means. Newer surgical techniques produce fair results in treatment of elephantiasis of the extremities. The use of elastic bandages or Unna's paste boots may gradually reduce the size of affected limbs. Corticosteroids, administered with cautious supervision and never in the presence of bacterial or fungal infection, may be used for a short time in conjunction with bandaging at the onset of treatment of elephantoid extremities to soften the woody induration.

Control. Transmission of the filarial diseases depends on two factors: the availability of a suitable intermediate host (the vector) and the presence in the population of persons who can infect that vector. It is never necessary to achieve total eradication of an infection to prevent its transmission, as defense mechanisms in both vector and human host serve to ensure that small numbers of microfilariae will not infect the vector and that relatively large numbers of bites by infected vectors are necessary to establish infection in the human host. In bancroftian filariasis, larvicides, residual spraying, and at times other means can be used to reduce the mosquito population, depending on the habits of the particular mosquito vector. The biological control of mosquito larvae using the bacterium *Bacillus sphaericus* has been somewhat successful in an urban area of Recife, Brazil (Regis et al., 2000). Mass treatment of the infected population may serve to lower microfilaremia to the point where either mosquitoes do not become infected or infections are so infrequent and light that transmission does not take place. These strategies have proved successful in smaller, isolated areas such as Tahiti but become more and more difficult to apply as the size of the infected area increases. Control of some of the filarial diseases is complicated by the presence of reservoir hosts. Fortunately, this is not true of bancroftian filariasis. Protection of the individual visiting or residing in infected areas may be increased by the use of insect repellents, screening, bed nets, and so forth.

In 1993 the International Task Force for Disease Eradication identified lymphatic filariasis as one of six diseases as being eradicable or potentially eradicable. The World Health Assembly, in 1997, passed a resolution proposing the global elimination of lymphatic filariasis in the 80 nations where it was endemic. Since that time, progress has been steady toward the goal. The international campaign to eliminate filariasis is now overseen by the Global Program to Eliminate Lymphatic Filariasis, which is coordinated by the World Health Organization. By the year 2002, national programs were active in 38 of the 80 countries, reaching almost 90 million people. The target was to reach 350 million people by 2005 and 1.1 billion by 2020 (Ottesen, 2002).

Brugia malayi

Some 30% of cases of the Malayan form of lymphatic filariasis occur in South China and 20% occur in India, while the rest are found in Indonesia, Thailand, Vietnam, Malaysia, the Philippines, and South Korea. The distribution of this species obviously overlaps that of *W. bancrofti*.

The life cycle of *B. malayi* is similar to that of *W. bancrofti*, except that in most areas the principal mosquito vectors belong to the genus *Mansonia*. In some areas, *Anopheles* may be an important vector or the only one. Macaques (*Macaca* spp.) and leaf monkeys (*Presbytis* spp.) are important reservoirs of at least certain strains of *B. malayi*, which can also be transmitted to cats and civet cats. In Indonesia, zoophilic and anthropophilic strains are recognized. The zoophilic strain, transmitted by *Mansonia* mosquitoes, may be aperiodic, nocturnally subperiodic, or nocturnally periodic in humans, while in experimental animals (jirds) it is usually nocturnally subperiodic. It is found in Kalimantan (Borneo), Malaya, Sumatra, and Buru (one of the Maluku Islands of Indonesia), usually in swampy areas. The anthropophilic strain, found primarily in rice-growing areas of Sulawesi (Indonesia), is transmitted by *Anopheles* mosquitoes, always exhibits nocturnal periodicity, and experimental animals may be infected only with difficulty and do not retain the infection. Thus, at least in the Indonesian areas investigated, humans may be infected with both anthropophilic and zoophilic strains, the latter making more difficult any control measures.

The microfilariae are sheathed and average 200 to 275 μm in length; body nuclei extend almost to the tip of the tail, whereas the tail of *W. bancrofti* microfilariae contains no nuclei. Two terminal nuclei are distinctly separate from the others in the tail, and this characteristic serves further to differentiate the microfilariae from those of *Loa loa*, discussed later. Adults of *B. malayi* seem to be somewhat smaller than those of *W. bancrofti*, although few as yet have been recovered. Laboratory diagnosis is accomplished by examining blood films stained to demonstrate the differential morphologic features of the microfilariae (see Fig. 9-3).

Symptoms and Pathogenesis. Clinical features of Malayan filariasis are generally similar to those seen in bancroftian infections. Lymphadenitis occurs most frequently in the inguinal area, and may be followed by a retrograde lymphangitis, often accompanied by lymphedema of the foot and ankle. Occasionally (and more commonly than in bancroftian filariasis) there is ulceration of the affected node. Involvement of the genitalia (funiculitis, orchitis, epididymitis, hydrocele) and chyluria are not characteristic of brugian filariasis. When elephantiasis occurs in Malayan filariasis, it involves the leg below the knee (Fig. 9-8) or, less commonly, the arm below the elbow.

Pulmonary nodules, seen on radiographs and surgically explored, have not infrequently been found to contain filarial worms. Most of these represent zoonotic infections and are

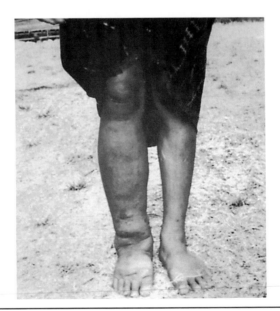

FIGURE 9-8   ■   Malayan elephantiasis. Note involvement of leg below knee only. (Courtesy Dr. Felix Partono, University of Indonesia, Jakarta.)

discussed elsewhere, but some have been found that contain human *Brugia* or *Wuchereria* parasites.

Treatment. Treatment is the same as for filariasis bancrofti. Allergic reactions tend to be severe in filariasis malayi; treatment with DEC may be initiated with smaller doses, or antihistamines may be administered as a routine measure.

DEC has been demonstrated to kill both adult worms and microfilariae of *B. malayi*, though the microfilariae are destroyed more rapidly. In Malaysia, where *Mansonia* is the vector, cumulative doses of 36 mg/kg body weight of DEC, whether given at the rate of 6 mg/kg weekly for 6 weeks or at the same daily dose over a period of 9 days (with an interval of 3 days between the first and subsequent doses), were found to produce a reduction of about 80% in the number of microfilaremic individuals and of more than 90% in the mean density of circulating microfilariae. These decreases were sustained, in the absence of any mosquito control measures, for at least 18 to 24 months after treatment. DEC-medicated salt has been found to give excellent results in mass treatment programs (Liu et al., 1992).

Invermectin, given as a single dose of 20, 50, 100, or 20 mcg/kg body weight, and repeated in 6 months, gave results comparable to those seen in *W. bancrofti* infections. While results favored 200 mcg/kg, they were not strikingly different from those obtained with 20 mcg. Side effects were milder than those following administration of DEC (Sheuoy et al., 1992).

Brugia timori

Microfilariae of a new type were first reported from the island of Timor in 1964. Subsequently they were found in persons from surrounding islands of the Lesser Sunda group in Indonesia, where prevalence rates for this parasite are quite high. The disease closely resembles bancroftian filariasis in its clinical expression, though the rate of abscess formation (Fig. 9-9) seems higher; however, there is a preponderance of elephantiasis of the legs, as in *B. malayi* infection. Microfilariae of *B. timori* can be readily distinguished from those of *B. malayi*. They are somewhat longer than those of *B. malayi* (Fig. 9-10), averaging 310 μm. The cephalic space (that part of the microfilariae anterior to the body nuclei) has a length-width ratio of approximately 2:1 in *B. malayi* (Fig. 9-11), but 3:1 in *B. timori*. The sheath of *B. malayi* stains deeply with Giemsa stain, whereas that of *B. timori* does not. In microfilariae of *Brugia*, unlike those of *Wuchereria*, nuclei extend to the tip of the tail.

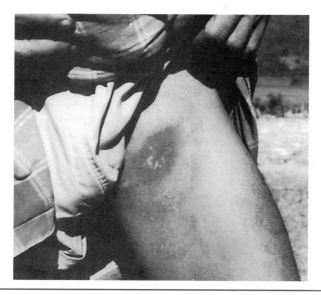

FIGURE 9-9 ■ Timoran filariasis. Typical scar following rupture of infected inguinal node. (Courtesy Dr. Felix Partono, University of Indonesia, Jakarta.)

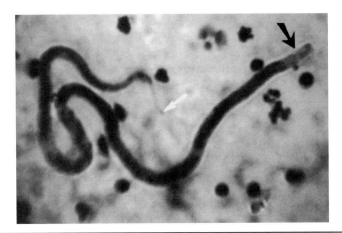

FIGURE 9-10 ■ Microfilaria of *Brugia timori* (Giemsa stain). Note long cephalic space *(black arrow)*, nuclei at tip of tail *(white arrow)*. (Courtesy Dr. Felix Partono, University of Indonesia, Jakarta.)

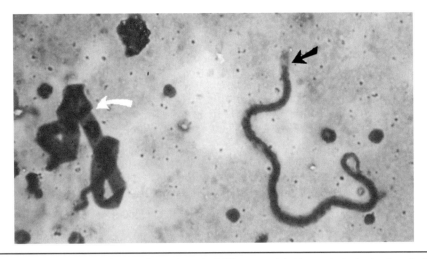

FIGURE 9-11 ■ Microfilaria of *Brugia malayi* (Giemsa stain). Note relatively short cephalic space *(black arrow)*, deeply stained cast sheath *(white arrow)*. (Courtesy Dr. Felix Partono, University of Indonesia, Jakarta.)

The microfilariae exhibit a nocturnal periodicity. The vector is *Anopheles barbirostris*, and as far as is known, humans are the only definitive host.

Treatment. DEC has been used for mass treatment, and it seems probable that Timoran filariasis responds better to drug therapy than the other lymphatic filariases, though the long-term aspects of their reported programs may also be a factor.

In one village on the island of Flores, DEC was administered to all the inhabitants at the rate of 5 mg/kg body weight daily for 10 days. This was repeated for all the inhabitants 3 years later. Yearly, for the first 5 years of the program, all new residents, all of whom were initially microfilaremic, and all of whom had an attack of adenolymphangitis during the preceding year, received the same course of treatment. Additionally, at the time of an attack of adenolymphangitis, each adult received a course of DEC, 300 mg daily for 10 days (150 mg daily for children under 10 years old). Eleven years after the program started, a complete clearance of microfilaremia was noted, with resolution of elephantiasis in approximately three-quarters of those initially infected, principally in those with less advanced disease. Filarial antigen levels dropped dramatically (Partono et al., 1989).

Administration of DEC at low dosage over an extended period has also been found effective. Weekly dosage of the drug for 18 months (25 mg to children under 10 years of age, 50 mg to all others) resulted in a drop in microfilarial levels to those detectable only by membrane filtration (see Chapter 15) at 1 year, a decline in adenolymphangitis and a slower but dramatic effect on elephantiasis. Side effects of this low-dosage treatment were mild and confined to the first few weeks of therapy. A single oral dose of 6 mg/kg body weight of DEC combined with 400 mg albendazole has been shown to have a long-term suppressive effect on *B. timori* microfilariae for at least 1 year (Fischer et al., 2003).

No studies of the use of ivermectin in the brugian filariases have been published, but Partono (personal communication) has not found it to be more effective than DEC.

Loa loa

The African eye worm, *L. loa* (Fig. 9-12), is found throughout the rain forest areas of the Sudan, the basin of the Congo, and West Africa. The adult *Loa* migrates actively throughout the subcutaneous tissues of the body and derives its popular name from the fact that it is most conspicuous and irritating when crossing the conjunctiva. The scientific name comes from a native term for the worm. In hyperendemic areas, estimates of infection rates in adults range from 9% to 70% of the population.

Adult males of *L. loa* are 2 to 3.5 cm long, and females generally 5 to 7 cm (Fig. 9-13); neither is more than 0.5 mm wide. The microfilariae, which are 250 to 300 μm long and sheathed, differ from the microfilariae of *Wuchereria* and *Brugia* in having body nuclei that are continuous to the tip of the tail. While adult worms migrate through the subcutaneous and deeper connective tissues, the microfilariae make their way into the bloodstream, where they circulate, having a diurnal periodicity, and may be ingested by any of several species of mango fly. The mango fly, *Chrysops*, is large, with mouth parts that can produce a painful bite. The microfilariae undergo a developmental cycle in the thoracic musculature of the fly similar to that of *Wuchereria* in the mosquito, and after 10 to 12 days reach the infective stage. When the fly bites, the infective larvae migrate out onto the surface of the skin and then enter through the bite wound.

Diagnosis of loiasis is most frequently made on the basis of a history of Calabar swellings (also known as fugitive swellings) or the appearance of the worm in the conjunctivae, since microfilariae frequently do not appear in the blood until years after the worms or the results of their activities become apparent. It is estimated that only one third of those infected in Gabon have microfilaremia. At times, circulating microfilariae (see Fig. 9-3) are found quite early in the disease.

Symptoms. Migration of the adult worms through the tissues is not painful and seldom is noticed unless they happen to pass over the bridge of the nose or through the conjunctival tissue across the eyeball. While they migrate rapidly, they can often be immobilized with a few drops of 10% cocaine instilled into the eye and excised while passing through the conjunctiva. There may be some edema of conjunctiva and lids when the worms are in that area. At other times, patches of localized subcutaneous edema (Calabar swellings) may appear anywhere on the body. The swellings, named for the coastal Nigerian town where they were first recorded, may be several inches in diameter and are often preceded by localized pain and pruritus. They last several days to some weeks and subside slowly. It is thought that Calabar swellings are a type of allergic reaction to the metabolic products of the worms or to dead worms. A worm is not necessarily present in the area of a Calabar swelling when it appears. The subcutaneous injection of a small amount of the extract of *Dirofilaria immitis*, formerly used as a skin test antigen in the diagnosis of filariasis, results in formation of a Calabar swelling in that area.

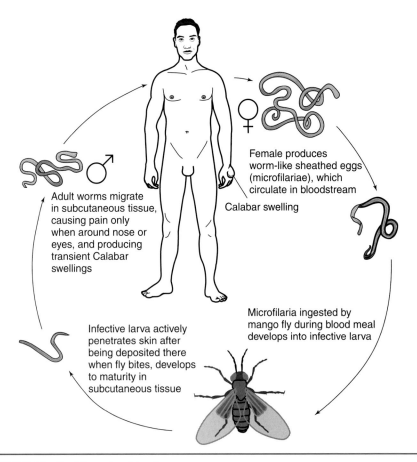

Female produces
worm-like sheathed eggs
(microfilariae), which
circulate in bloodstream

Calabar swelling

Adult worms migrate
in subcutaneous tissue,
causing pain only
when around nose or
eyes, and producing
transient Calabar
swellings

Microfilaria ingested by
mango fly during blood meal
develops into infective larva

Infective larva actively
penetrates skin after
being deposited there
when fly bites, develops
to maturity in
subcutaneous tissue

FIGURE 9-12 ■ Life cycle of *Loa loa*.

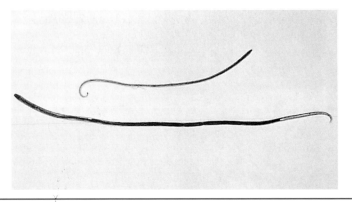

FIGURE 9-13 ■ *Loa loa* adult male (top) and adult female. (Photograph by Zane Price from material supplied by Dr. Tom Orihel.)

Loa in ectopic sites may provoke unusual reactions. Clinical features that have been described are hydrocele and orchitis in patients with adult *Loa* in the tunica vaginalis or spermatic cord, a colonic lesion causing obstruction in a patient with an adult *Loa* in the bowel wall, and membranous glomerulonephritis in a patient who, probably following therapy with DEC, developed loal encephalitis and diffuse vascular obstruction of the small vessels of all organs with fibrin thrombi surrounding degenerating microfilariae.

Fibroblastic endocarditis, retinopathy, arthritis, and peripheral neuropathy have also been described in loiasis, but are rare in persons native to the endemic areas.

As has been seen to be the case in bancroftian filariasis, loiasis may present a different picture in persons not native to endemic areas. In one report 20 persons who had acquired loiasis after temporary residence in West Africa were investigated. Only 5 were asymptomatic (but were diagnosed after a persistent or high eosinophilia was noted); 15 had pruritus, 14 had Calabar swellings, and urticaria was noted by 11 patients. All patients had markedly elevated levels of antifilarial antibody; all had eosinophilia, with levels greater than 3000 per μl in 18 of the 20. All but two had elevated levels of serum IgE. Only 3 of the 20 patients had microfilaremia. One patient was found to have endomyocardial fibrosis; six had renal abnormalities (five with hematuria and one with proteinuria) without evidence of urinary infection.

Pathogenesis. There is little to suggest that the adult *Loa* produces any lasting damage to its host during life. Its quite rapid migration through subcutaneous tissue (about 1 cm per minute) may be completely painless in areas other than the face. Eosinophilia of 50% to 70% is frequently noted, especially when Calabar swellings are present. IgE levels are increased, markedly so in a majority of patients.

Hypersensitivity reactions to worms and microfilariae have already been mentioned. Lymphadenitis of a type considered characteristic of loiasis, marked by distention of the subcapsular and medullary sinuses by histiocytes and eosinophils and by atrophy of lymphoid follicles, may also represent a local reaction to dead microfilariae. Amicrofilaremic persons may have high filarial antibody titers.

Epidemiology. Several species of African monkeys harbor a *Loa* that is morphologically indistinguishable from the *L. loa* of humans; the monkey strain exhibits nocturnal periodicity and is carried by a species of *Chrysops* that is arboreal and bites at night. The human infection has been experimentally transmitted to monkeys, but the possibility that the reverse occurs in nature remains unproven. The two strains of *Loa* probably represent a relatively early stage in a "radiative evolution," which might ultimately result in morphologically distinguishable species. Of possible public health concern is the report that *L. loa* can develop in the American deerfly, *Chrysops atlanticus*, and is infective for monkeys after development in this insect.

The infection is long lived, and the prepatent period in some cases may be as long as 10 years, although generally it is perhaps closer to 1 year.

Treatment. Surgical removal of the migrating adult worms, most readily affected when they are found crossing the bridge of the nose, or in the conjunctiva, is a relatively simple matter.

DEC treatment is effective, but not without risk, as it readily penetrates the blood-brain barrier and in heavily infected persons may cause a fatal encephalitis (Carme et al., 1991). Its administration has also been associated with retinal hemorrhage and possibly with exacerbation of renal lesions. Use of DEC is contraindicated in persons with blood microfilaria counts of 500 or more per 20 μl, as determined by samples taken on two or more occasions at the appropriate time of day. The usual dosage of DEC is 2 mg/kg body weight, three times daily for 21 days.

DEC has also been found to be of value in prophylaxis of loiasis in uninfected persons entering endemic areas for an extended stay. For this purpose, the suggested adult dosage is 300 mg once a week.

Ivermectin is also an effective microfilaricide in loiasis. Its onset of action is slower than that of DEC, and the severe reactions resulting from a massive destruction of these organisms generally are not seen with its use. Side effects of treatment are mild; pruritus is the most common one. However, Boussinesq et al. (1998) report several cases with severe neurologic complications, including coma, in patients being treated for onchocerciasis who had concomitant infections (50,000 or more microfilariae per ml of blood) with *Loa loa*. Following treatment with a single dose of 400 mcg/kg body weight, microfilaremia has been noted to decrease to about one fifth of the pretreatment level by day 2, to reach a low point of approximately 9% of that level by days 8 to 10, and to remain constant thereafter for over 3 months (Martin-Prevel et al., 1993). Treatment of nearly 900 persons (in a village with initial microfilaremia of 30%) with ivermectin, 200 mcg/kg every 3 months for 2 years, resulted in a reduction of microfilaremia to approximately 6% and of mean microfilarial density to 8% of its initial value (Ranque et al., 1996).

As is true for the other filarial diseases, no satisfactory *macro*filaricidal drug is presently available.

Mansonella ozzardi

The only filaria parasitizing humans that is confined to the New World, *M. ozzardi* is found in northern Argentina, Bolivia, the Amazon basin of Brazil and Peru, Venezuela, Colombia, Guyana, French Guiana, Panama, Guatemala, the Yucatan peninsula, and the West Indies islands of Trinidad, St. Vincent, St. Lucia, Martinique, Guadeloupe, Antigua, Nevis, Vieques (Puerto Rico), and Hispaniola (both Haiti and the Dominican Republic). Prevalence rates vary from a few per cent in Nevis, St. Lucia, and St. Vincent to 50% to 90% in endemic areas of Trinidad, Guyana, and Colombia.

The adult stage of *M. ozzardi* has been redescribed with the result that two species previously classified in the genus *Acanthocheilonema* or *Dipetalonema* (*Mansonella streptocerca* and *M. perstans*) have been recognized as also belonging to the genus *Mansonella*. Adults of *M. ozzardi* inhabit the mesenteries and visceral fat; the unsheathed nonperiodic microfilariae are found in the blood, and also may be obtained by means of skin biopsy. When found in the skin, they are primarily confined to capillaries, and even in the intravascular spaces do not seem to cause inflammatory changes. Nuclei of the body of the microfilariae (see Fig. 9-3) do not extend to the tip of the tail as in *M. streptocerca*, and the tail is shorter and less tapered than that of *Onchocerca volvulus*, the other microfilariae that may be found in skin biopsies. Throughout most of its range, *M. ozzardi* is transmitted by *Culicoides* flies (Fig. 9-14) but in the Amazon basin by the blackfly, *Simulium*, or by both vectors.

Mansonellosis ozzardi is generally an asymptomatic infection, although inguinal adenopathy has been reported, as have pruritic and maculopapular skin lesions, arthritis, fever, and marked eosinophilia. A careful clinical evaluation of 150 patients with mansonelliasis in Haiti failed to find any morbidity that could be related directly to that infection. However, as in other filarial infections, symptoms may be more severe in infected persons not native to the endemic areas.

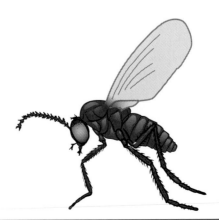

FIGURE 9-14 ■ *Culicoides,* vector of the mansonellas.

Treatment. Asymptomatic cases do not require treatment. DEC apparently has no effect. Ivermectin may be used in a single oral dose of 200 mcg/kg of body weight.

Mansonella streptocerca

M. streptocerca (formerly *Dipetalonema streptocerca*) is found in both monkeys and humans in the Congo basin. Unsheathed microfilariae are found primarily in the skin but also in the blood. Nuclei extend to the tip of the tail, which is characteristically bent in the form of a shepherd's crook. Differential morphologic features of the microfilariae are shown in Figure 9-3.

Small midges belonging to the genus *Culicoides* transmit this filaria. Infection in humans is characterized by a pruritic dermatitis, with hypopigmented macules and inguinal adenopathy.

Treatment. Drugs of choice are either DEC, 6 mg/kg body weight per day orally for 14 days, or ivermectin, a single oral dose of 15 mcg/kg of body weight. DEC is active against both the adult worms and microfilariae, whereas ivermectin is active against only the microfilariae. Mild to severe pruritus is a common side effect of administration of both drugs; the appearance of cutaneous papules containing worms (dead when biopsies were taken toward the end of treatment) is described following DEC therapy.

Mansonella perstans

M. perstans (formerly *Dipetalonema perstans*) is a common parasite of humans and apes in large areas of Africa. On the West Coast it ranges from Senegal to Angola, and throughout Central Africa north to southwest Sudan, east to Uganda, Kenya, and Tanzania, and south to Zimbabwe. It also is found on the Yucatan peninsula, in Panama, Colombia, Venezuela, Guyana, Surinam, French Guiana, and the Amazon basin of Brazil, and on the islands of Trinidad, St. Vincent, St. Lucia, Guadeloupe, Nevis, and Hispaniola (Dominican Republic). Prevalence figures are highly variable; from 2% in western Nigeria to 86% in parts of Zaire, and 12% to 70% in Guyana. A number of years ago it was estimated to affect 19 million persons in Africa and 8 million in tropical America. The adult worms, similar in size to the other filariae that have been discussed, live in the deep connective tissues. Their unsheathed microfilariae are found in the peripheral blood, where they exhibit no periodicity, and in the skin. These microfilariae (see Fig. 9-3) are characterized by nuclei that extend to the tip of the tail. The terminal nucleus or pair of nuclei is separated slightly from the other caudal nuclei. This filaria is also transmitted by *Culicoides*.

Symptoms. The majority of infections are benign, although symptomatic cases occur throughout the endemic areas. It is difficult to evaluate reported symptoms, but Calabar-like swellings, pruritus, hives, fever and headache are reported from both Africa and South America. In Uganda, a condition known as Kampala or Ugandan eye worm has been found to be the result of invasion of the conjunctiva or periorbital connective tissues by adult *M. perstans*. Edema and inflammatory changes surround these worms, and granulomas form around dead filariae. Similar findings have been reported from the Sudan, Nigeria, and possibly Zaire. In Zimbabwe, infection with what is considered to be this species is frequently associated with arthralgias and fever.

In South America, numerous investigators find bone and joint pains, lymphadenitis, and hydrocele to characterize mansonelliasis perstans. An eosinophilia is usually present, and may be quite intense.

Treatment. Treatment is probably unnecessary in most cases. DEC seems ineffective, as does ivermectin. Mebendazole, 100 mg twice daily for 30 days, reportedly has a high cure rate. Albendazole, 400 mg twice daily for 10 days, also is recommended.

Control of the Mansonelliases. No vector control program has been instituted for any of the mansonelliases. Protection of visitors to endemic areas is best afforded by the use of insect repellents. Both *Culicoides* and *Simulium* are small enough to pass readily through screening or mosquito nets.

Onchocerca volvulus

O. volvulus (Fig. 9-15) is widely distributed throughout Central Africa. It is also present in Saudi Arabia, Yemen, and in the Western Hemisphere in limited areas in Mexico, Guatemala, Venezuela, Colombia, Ecuador, and Brazil. It is generally considered to have been introduced into the Americas by the slave trade. In all of these areas its distribution is restricted by the breeding habits of its vector, larvae and pupae of which develop in rivers or streams.

The intermediate host and vector of *O. volvulus* may be one of a number of species of *Simulium*, the blackfly or buffalo gnat. These minute insects are widespread in their distribution, but only certain species are suitable vectors, possibly because of their feeding habits or perhaps for other reasons. Upon biting an infected person the simuliid ingests microfilariae, which have a developmental cycle in the insect similar to that of other filarial larvae, transforming into infective forms that may enter a new host when the simuliid again takes a blood meal. After introduction into the new host, the developing worms wander through the subcutaneous tissues but settle down, usually in groups of two or more; most worms finally become encapsulated. Nodules, produced by encapsulation of the adult worms in a fibrous tissue tumor-like mass, usually form within a year after infection. They are most frequently subcutaneous but may occur in connective tissues deeper in the body. The nodules

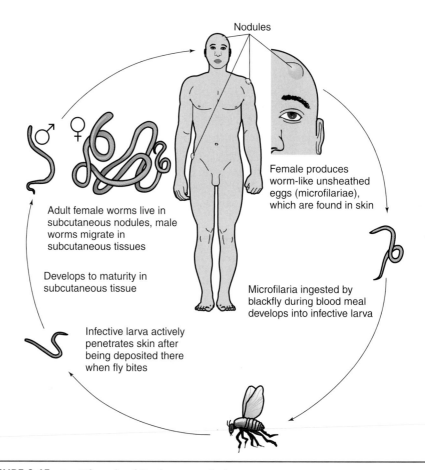

Nodules

Female produces worm-like unsheathed eggs (microfilariae), which are found in skin

Microfilaria ingested by blackfly during blood meal develops into infective larva

Infective larva actively penetrates skin after being deposited there when fly bites

Develops to maturity in subcutaneous tissue

Adult female worms live in subcutaneous nodules, male worms migrate in subcutaneous tissues

FIGURE 9-15   ■   Life cycle of *Onchocerca volvulus*.

range from a few millimeters to several centimeters in diameter and may be numerous. In Venezuela and in Africa the majority of nodules are located on the patient's trunk or limbs, and few form on the head, whereas in Mexico and Guatemala they are frequently seen in the patient's scalp (Fig. 9-16) and less often on other parts of the body. The reason for this difference in distribution of lesions is by no means apparent, but it may be related to the biting habits of the several vectors. Studies have suggested that the African and American strains are distinct; it is possible that there are several distinct strains in Africa.

The wirelike, whitish adult worms lie coiled within fibrous tissue capsules (Fig. 9-17). The female may be as long as 50 cm, though it is less than 0.5 mm in diameter. Males are considerably shorter, not more than 5 cm. Microfilariae make their way out of the nodules and migrate actively through the dermis and in the connective tissues, not only in the vicinity

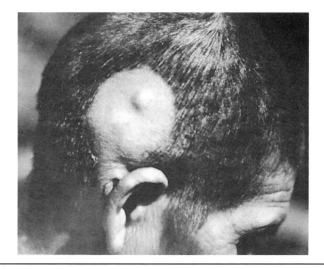

FIGURE 9-16 ■ *Onchocerca volvulus* nodules on scalp. Note also thickened, wrinkled skin in front of ear. (Armed Forces Institute of Pathology, #79, 133D.)

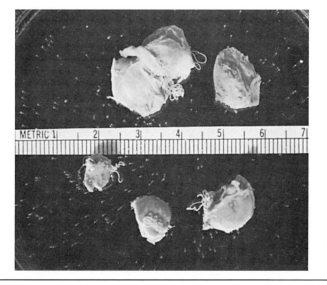

FIGURE 9-17 ■ *Onchocerca volvulus* nodules. Portions of contained adult worms protruding. (Photograph by Zane Price.)

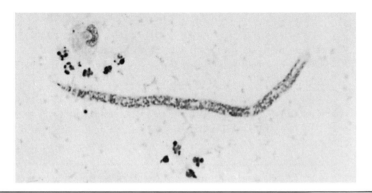

FIGURE 9-18 ■ *Onchocerca volvulus,* microfilaria from scarification preparation. (Photomicrograph by Zane Price.)

of the nodules but at some distance from them. Rarely, microfilariae may be found in urine, blood, or sputum. As seen in skin biopsies, the larvae are unsheathed and are 150 to over 350 μm long.

Diagnosis is by identification of the microfilariae in "skin snips" (Fig. 9-18). The bits of tissue needed for diagnosis may be secured by two different techniques. After preparing the skin with a volatile antiseptic agent, a fold of skin may be squeezed between the thumb and forefinger of one hand while a thin slice of skin is removed with a razor blade held in the other, or a needle may be used to catch and raise a small cone of skin, which is then removed with scissors or a razor blade. The tissue is then placed in saline and may be teased to facilitate liberation of the microfilariae, or incubated for 4 hours in a culture medium such as NCTC 135 in Hanks' balanced salt solution. It may be necessary to take multiple skin snips from patients with light infections. In Africa, skin snips are customarily taken from the buttock region, and in Mexico and Guatemala from the shoulders. In Liberia, the overall sensitivity of examining six skin snips (one from each shoulder, hip, and calf) was estimated to be 91.6%. When the number of microfilariae was 3.5 or more per milligram of skin, there were no false negative results (Taylor et al., 1989). Obviously, an adequate skin snip specimen is essential.

Although microfilariae are more often found in the skin than elsewhere, microfilaruria is not uncommon. In an area in Guatemala where infection is seen in virtually 100% of the population, 80% had microfilariae in skin snips, and 17% to 30% of those aged 10 years or older had microfilaruria. The numbers of microfilariae in the urine may be increased following the administration of an oral dose of 50 mg DEC, at which time they may also be found in the blood and sputum.

In the tropical rain forest of Africa, microfilariae of *M. streptocerca* may also be found in skin snip specimens. They are generally smaller than those of *O. volvulus,* but for differentiation the microfilariae should be stained. In stained smears, nuclei are seen to extend to the tip of the tail of *M. streptocerca* whereas the tail of *O. volvulus* is free of nuclei.

If skin snips reveal no microfilariae, a presumptive diagnosis may be made by means of the Mazzotti test. This consists of the oral administration of a single dose of 50 mg DEC, which generally provokes intense pruritus within a few hours. Itching can then be controlled by short-term administration of corticosteroids and subsides without such treatment in 2 to 3 days. Severe systemic or ocular complications (see Treatment) are uncommon but may occur. A patch test—local application of 10% DEC anhydrous lanolin covered with an occlusive dressing—is reported to provoke in infected person local dermatitis without systemic reaction.

Biopsy of the onchocercomas may be undertaken not only for therapeutic but for diagnostic purposes, and sections of these nodules reveal a characteristic picture (Fig. 9-19). Ultrasonography has also been suggested (Leichsenring et al., 1990) for detection of

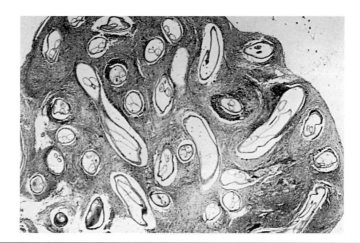

FIGURE 9-19 ■ Section of onchocercoma removed from forehead.

onchocercal nodules in the deeper tissues. A very characteristic pattern is produced by the onchocercomas.

Symptoms. The nodules, though sometimes disfiguring, are not painful, and the importance of the infection lies not in the adult worms but in the effects their microfilariae may produce. In persons living in Mexico and Guatemala, an acute inflammatory reaction, involving usually the face, eyes, ears, neck, or shoulders but sometimes found elsewhere on the body, may occur spontaneously. The skin is hot, edematous, and often painful. There may be associated pruritus. The inflammation subsides slowly and may recur many times, eventually resulting in permanent thickening of the skin, which may also assume a violaceous color. This reaction is thought to be caused by death of microfilariae in the skin and liberation of antigenic materials from them. It may be provoked by the administration of drugs known to kill the microfilariae and prevented by administration of corticosteroids. It has been estimated that in heavily infected persons approximately 100,000 microfilariae die every day (Mawson and WaKabongo, 2002).

Onchodermatitis seems to assume somewhat distinct forms in different areas. In the Western Hemisphere, the patchy purplish or reddish eruption that characterizes acute attacks (Fig. 9-20) is known as *mal morado* or *erisipela de la costa*. Chronically infected skin is atrophic and wrinkled, with subcutaneous thickening. In African patients, atrophy of the skin and subcutaneous lymphedema are also seen, along with depigmentation producing a "leopard skin" appearance, and the presence of papular to pustular nodules up to 1 cm in diameter, caused by inflammatory reactions to localized collections of microfilariae in the skin. These lesions are locally referred to as *craw-craw*.

In Yemen, dermal manifestations of onchocerciasis are usually confined to a single extremity. Typically, one leg is involved, occasionally an arm; rarely is the trunk affected. There is a pruritic papular eruption; the skin is swollen and dark; regional lymph nodes are enlarged and soft. Microfilariae are scarce in the skin, but more likely to be seen if biopsies are taken around the ankles (which may, because of the type of clothing worn in the region, be the area most frequently bitten). The disease is referred to locally as sowda, in reference to the darkened skin. Ocular involvement seems not to be a feature of sowda, perhaps because of the small numbers of microfilariae usually present.

The infected skin loses its elasticity and becomes deeply wrinkled and atrophic. In Mexico and Guatemala, this is seen mainly in the head and neck region, producing an appearance of premature senility, and sometimes rather leonine facies. In Africa, the same process occurring around the hip region is responsible for the spectacular complication

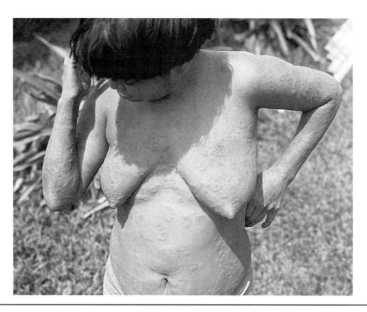

FIGURE 9-20   ■   Acute onchodermatitis.

known as "hanging groin" (Fig. 9-21), a condition in which a sac of tissue forms in the inguinal region. It may contain inguinal or femoral lymph nodes and may hang down as far as the knees. Lymphedema of the external genitalia and scrotal elephantiasis are seen as complications of onchocerciasis in some areas of Africa.

As a measure of the severity of the eye lesions in onchocerciasis, it has been estimated that while blindness is two to four times more prevalent in an area where trachoma is endemic than in a control area such as Europe, it is at least six times more common in areas of high *Onchocerca* endemicity. Different degrees of eye involvement are noted in different parts of the Cameroon. In the rainforest, some 80% to 90% of children 5 to 9 years old are infected, and of these about 2% are blind; in the savannah areas only 60% to 70% of a comparable age group are infected, but 5% are blind. Among persons older than 40 years, the figures for blindness in the two areas are 4.2% and 14.4%, respectively. Onchocercal blindness in Guatemala is found only in areas of high prevalence (more than 80% of the population) and intensity of infection (more than 22 microfilariae per milligram of skin). A similar situation occurs in Ecuador, where blindness and other chronic changes (elephantiasis, hanging groin, hydrocele) are seen only in the inhabitants of hyperendemic areas.

Intrauterine transmission of *Onchocerca* microfilariae is known to take place—they have been found in the umbilical cords and in skin snips taken from newborn infants. Comparison of two otherwise similar areas in Ecuador, one hyperendemic and the other nonendemic for onchocerciasis, indicated a marked drop in the incidence of spontaneous abortion in the hyperendemic area after the onset of treatment with ivermectin, whereas there was no significant change in rate in the nonendemic area (Guderian et al., 1997).

Pathogenesis. Encapsulation in the characteristic onchocercomas is by no means the universal fate of adult *O. volvulus*. Some worms, especially during the early stages of the disease in young children and in lightly infected persons, produce no apparent tissue reaction; these worms are found free in the tissues. The dermal lesions are without doubt an allergic reaction, and they can be exactly duplicated by the administration of small doses of DEC, resulting in the death of large numbers of microfilariae in the skin. Such acute reactions, occurring either spontaneously or as the result of therapy, can be suppressed by the administration of corticosteroids. The loss of elasticity of the skin of the pelvic region, seen in chronic African

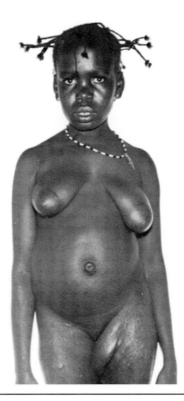

FIGURE 9-21 ■ Patient with hanging groin caused by underlying obstructive onchocercal lymphadenitis and loss of dermal elasticity. Note also onchodermatitis. (Photograph by Dr. Daniel H. Connor, Armed Forces Institute of Pathology, #68-10066-1)

onchocerciasis, results not only in the hanging groin mentioned earlier but in a high prevalence of inguinal and femoral hernias. It is possible that the deposition of immune complexes in tissues, as a result of the constant antigenic stimulation provided by the microfilariae, is basic to the inflammation, fibrosis, and eventual obstructive lymphadenitis seen in some of these patients.

Differences in frequency of the various ophthalmic lesions between the African and American strains of *Onchocerca* have been noted but are not well explained. The earliest lesions noted consist of punctate keratitis; at this time microfilariae may be found in the cornea and the anterior chamber. These opacities may coalesce, usually in the lower portions of the cornea; there may be inflammation of the limbus of the cornea and of the adjacent scleral tissue, as well as formation of pterygia, which grow out over the cornea. Iridocyclitis appears somewhat later than the corneal changes; posterior synechiae frequently displace the pupil, which becomes fixed and sometimes distorted. An exudate may form and cover the pupillary area, finally leading to blindness. These lesions of the cornea, anterior chamber, and iris are seen in both African and American onchocerciasis, but they tend to be more severe in the latter. Lesions of the posterior chamber are less common in both areas. Microfilariae are not seen adherent to or within the lens substance or in the posterior chamber. Onchocercal retinochoroiditis and optic atrophy are seen, but they cannot readily be distinguished from those resulting from toxoplasmosis or other causes.

Wolbachia bacteria have been known to be endosymbionts of filarial parasites, including *W. bancrofti, B. malayi, and O. volvulus*, since the 1970s. However, only recently has the role of these bacteria in inflammation and possible blindness been investigated in a mouse model of river blindness (Saint André et al., 2002). *Wolbachia* are essential symbionts, which occur in all stages of *O. volvulus*, with embryogenesis being dependent on their presence. Using the mouse model just discussed, researchers injected soluble extracts of *O. volvulus* into the corneal stroma and observed that the predominant inflammatory response in the cornea was due to the endosymbiotic *Wolbachia*. Further research is needed to determine the precise role of the microfilarial proteins versus the microfilarial symbiotic bacteria in the inflammatory response and subsequent blindness.

The localized onchocercal infection seen in sowda contrasts with the generalized infection seen elsewhere and is not readily explained. Some suggest that Yemenites may be hyperreactors or conversely, that those infected with onchocerciasis in other areas exhibit a degree of immune tolerance. Such tolerance might be lacking in Yemenites if onchocerciasis has recently been introduced to that area. It has been noted that the disease in Europeans who contract onchocerciasis in Africa often resembles sowda.

Epidemiology. African and American forms of onchocerciasis exhibit certain differences, some of which may be related to vector biting habits (localization of the onchocercomas) and some to strain or other differences as yet unexplained (rainforest versus savannah). Onchocerciasis was presumably introduced to the Americas by the slave trade, and observations in Colombia of the present-day distribution of the disease in that country are of some interest. The simuliid vectors in Colombia are zoophilic, and where domestic livestock is found the human infection has died out, to persist only in areas where no large domestic animals are kept. Onchocerciasis has been sporadically reported from many nonendemic areas such as Great Britain, and at least some of these cases represent zoonotic infections with onchocercas from horses or other domestic animals.

Simuliid gnats have larval stages that are aquatic, most of them requiring swiftly flowing streams in which the larvae and pupae attach to submerged rocks or vegetation. Some species develop in more quiet waters and certain African species attach themselves to freshwater crabs. It follows that endemic areas generally coincide with the course of rivers or streams, hence the common name for the disease: river blindness.

Treatment. DEC is very effective in killing the microfilariae of *Onchocerca*, but the rapidity of onset of its action (basis of the Mazzotti test mentioned earlier) can lead to severe side effects. The sudden death of enormous numbers of microfilariae in the skin may give rise to intense pruritus and localized edema, while in the eye it may lead to chorioretinal damage and keratitis. Other side effects of the use of DEC include myalgias and arthralgias, headache, dizziness, and rarely, hypotensive episodes.

Fortunately, ivermectin exerts its microfilaricidal effect more slowly; pruritic reactions are less severe, and ocular reactions minimal. All the side effects mentioned for DEC may occur with the use of ivermectin, but are usually quite mild. However, it is prudent to check for the presence of microfilariae in the anterior chamber or cornea and, if they are found, to pretreat with steroids (such as prednisone 1 mg/kg body weight daily) for 2 to 3 days before the administration of ivermectin. The usual dose of ivermectin is 150 mcg/kg body weight, given once. Numbers of skin microfilariae drop sharply after a single dose of ivermectin, but small numbers remain after a year. Treatment is repeated every 6 to 12 months until microfilariae are eliminated. It has been found that the drug has little initial effect on the adult worms, and the sustained reduction in microfilariae is due to interference with embryogenesis to the microfilaria stage. However, when ivermectin at a dosage of 150 mcg/kg was repeated every 3 months, Duke et al. (1992) found progressive reduction in the numbers of microfilariae being produced (none after 24 months) and in percentages of live female worms as compared with those in nodules from control subjects. In a very large study in Malawi, involving administration of 150 to 200 mcg/kg of ivermectin yearly for 3 years, no serious side effects were noted (Burnham, 1993).

Since 1988, Merck & Co., Inc., has donated ivermectin for mass drug treatment programs in Yemen, sub-Saharan Africa, and the Americas, with the goal of eliminating onchocerciasis as a public health problem. Ten countries in West Africa have subsequently eliminated onchocerciasis as a disease of public health importance (Molyneux et al., 2003).

Ivermectin has been distributed on an annual basis to individuals at risk of exposure to infection. In areas of west and central Africa, where *O. volvulus* and *L. loa* coexist, encephalopathy may result from ivermectin treatment of individuals with high *Loa* microfilaremias, further complicating mass distribution programs. Doxycycline treatment of individuals with 100 mg per day for 6 weeks, which acts against the *Wolbachia* endosymbionts, will produce permanent sterility in adult female *O. volvulus* (Hoerauf et al., 2000). Elimination of the worm's endosymbiotic bacteria by antibiotics may become an adjunct to control in the overall management of onchocerciasis.

Suramin* (see Chapter 5) is a *macro*filaricide when used for the treatment of onchocerciasis. It is quite toxic, and its use for this purpose is now seldom warranted.

Nodulectomy—the surgical removal of palpable nodules—has long been practiced in Mexico and Guatemala, and is credited with markedly decreasing the ocular complications of the disease. Special teams of paramedics make periodic visits to the remote coffee plantations where the disease is most prevalent to perform this procedure.

OTHER FILARIAL INFECTIONS IN HUMANS

Zoonotic filarial infections are reported sporadically from humans in various parts of the world, and it is interesting that about half of them have originated in the United States. Probably the most common type are those found in nodules in the subcutaneous tissues; these worms are usually immature. Some mature microfilaria-containing worms found in this location have been identified as *Dirofilaria tenuis*, which is commonly found in the subcutaneous tissues of raccoons and is transmitted by mosquitoes; *Dirofilaria ursi*–like parasites (*D. ursi* is found in bears and transmitted by blackflies) have been reported from humans in the United States and Canada. In Europe, Africa, and Asia, similar infections may be caused by *D. repens*, a parasite of dogs and cats, also transmitted by mosquitoes. *D. immitis*, the heartworm of dogs, has been found in the heart and lungs in humans. Some have been found at autopsy; more often they are first noted as solitary pulmonary nodules (coin lesions) on x-ray examination, and their true nature discovered only after surgery. Pulmonary infarction has been described secondary to the presence of *Dirofilaria* in the pulmonary artery or elsewhere in the lungs. *D. immitis* or closely related species have also been found causing arterial obstruction in the fingers; they might well lodge in other areas without producing symptomatic circulatory compromise. Transmission of these infections to humans is without doubt by the agency of the same insects that infect their usual hosts. Some 60 cases of human pulmonary dirofilariasis have been reported from the United States. Its distribution roughly parallels that of the infection in dogs, which is common in the Gulf Coast and Atlantic states, but has been reported from virtually all parts of the country. A case from California is discussed by Roy et al. (1993). Another case of *D. immitis* infection in California involved the spermatic cord, produced significant symptoms, and required orchiectomy (Theis et al., 2001).

A number of cases of lymphatic infection with filarial worms belonging to the genus *Brugia* have been reported from the United States, principally from northeastern and north central states but a few from other parts of the country (Eberhard et al., 1993). Identification has been made after surgical removal of enlarged nodes, most of which were nontender. Two species of *Brugia* are known from the United States, *B. beaveri*, from raccoons in Louisiana and bobcats in Florida, and *B. lepori,* found in rabbits in Louisiana. An unidentified *Brugia* has been found in domestic cats in California, and it is probable that other species exist in mammalian hosts in this country. Zoonotic *Brugia* infections have also been reported from Colombia, Ecuador, Brazil, Peru, and Ethiopia. The vectors of these brugias are not known.

Among the various parasites that invade the anterior chamber or vitreous of the eye, a number have been considered to be filariae, but positive identifications have been few.

---

*May be obtained from the CDC Drug Service Centers for Disease Control and Prevention, CDC, Atanta, Ga 30333; (404) 639-3670.

Tropical Pulmonary Eosinophilia

Eosinophilic lung disease, or tropical pulmonary eosinophilia, is a syndrome characterized by persistent hypereosinophilia, cough and wheezing with scanty production of sputum, and a variable x-ray appearance. There may also be low-grade fever, weight loss, and adenopathy. Characteristically, eosinophil counts are more than 3000 per μl blood, IgE levels are 1000 units per ml or greater, and high titers of antifilarial antibodies are present both in the blood and in fluid obtained by bronchoalveolar lavage. Microfilariae are not found in the peripheral blood, even by membrane filtration techniques, but they may be found in biopsy specimens from the lung and elsewhere; those of *W. bancrofti, B. malayi,* and unidentified species have been recovered in this way.

The *sine qua non* of diagnosis is response to DEC, which is generally prompt. The suggested dose is 2 mg/kg three times daily for 7 to 10 days. Repeated courses are occasionally necessary.

Nonfilarial Elephantiasis

An elephantiasis of nonfilarial origin is not uncommon in northern and central East Africa (Ethiopia, Uganda, Kenya, Tanzania, Rwanda, Burundi, and the Sudan), where its range overlaps that of bancroftian filariasis. It seems to be confined to areas where the soil contains large quantities of iron and aluminum salts and the clay kaolinite. Persons affected go barefoot all or much of the time and are thought to absorb these materials through abrasions on the feet. Crystals of silicates, with iron and aluminum salts, are found in the hypertrophied lymphatics of these individuals. Some 100,000 persons are said to be victims of this disease in Ethiopia, where the average age at onset is 18 years. Onset is generally distal, and it proceeds upward on the leg, rarely extending above the knee.

The Guinea Worm

Dracunculus medinensis

The guinea worm, *D. medinensis,* is of imposing antiquity among known agents of human disease. It is thought that the "fiery serpents" that plagued the Israelites by the Red Sea were *Dracunculus*; the disease they cause was recognized and named by Galen.

The guinea worm has been an important parasite in the Middle East (Saudi Arabia, Iran, Yemen), in central India and Pakistan, and in Africa in the Sudan, scattered through central equatorial Africa, and on its west coast. It was once found in the West Indies, Guyuna, Surinam, French Guiana, and Brazil but apparently no longer occurs in the Western Hemisphere except in reservoir hosts. It is a parasite of dogs and other carnivores in North America and of a number of different mammalian hosts in the areas from which human infections are reported.

Though it is sometimes classed with the filarial worms, *Dracunculus* is not a true filaria. The worms are elongate (Fig. 9-22), females measuring up to a meter or slightly more in length but averaging less, and with a diameter of less than 2 mm. The little-known male worm is inconspicuous and 2 cm long.

Dracunculiasis is acquired through ingestion of water contaminated by the presence of infected copepods, the intermediate host. These minute crustaceans (commonly known as water fleas) themselves become infected by the consumption of dracunculid larvae liberated into the same water source by infected persons (or other mammalian hosts of the adult worm).

Larvae of *Dracunculus,* unlike microfilariae, have a well-developed digestive tract and are never found in the blood or tissues of the host, being discharged directly into water. If ingested (Fig. 9-23) by suitable copepods (belonging to several different genera), the larvae

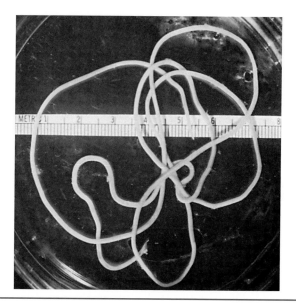

FIGURE 9-22 ▪ *Dracunculus medinensis,* female worm removed surgically. (Photograph by Zane Price.)

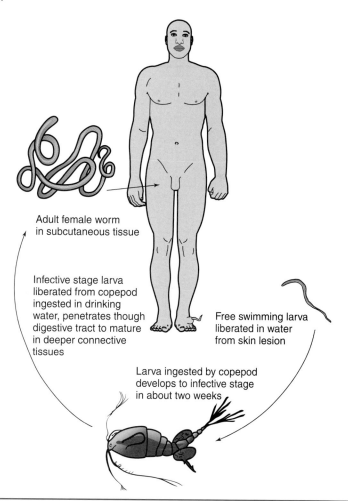

Adult female worm
in subcutaneous tissue

Infective stage larva
liberated from copepod
ingested in drinking
water, penetrates though
digestive tract to mature
in deeper connective
tissues

Free swimming larva
liberated in water
from skin lesion

Larva ingested by copepod
develops to infective stage
in about two weeks

FIGURE 9-23 ▪ Life cycle of *Dracunculus medinensis.*

mature in their host into infective forms in about 2 weeks. Frequently, wells, streams, or other sources of drinking water contain large numbers of copepods; whenever the ulcer of an infected person is immersed in water, larvae are liberated, so that in endemic areas a large proportion of copepods may be infected. If such copepods are swallowed, the contained larvae are liberated to penetrate through the digestive tract, entering the deep connective tissues where they mature. Maturation apparently takes about 1 year.

Females migrate to the subcutaneous tissues when they become gravid. The body of the fully gravid female worm is almost completely filled by a uterus distended with larvae. A papule is produced in the skin where the head of the female lies just under the dermis, and this becomes vesicular and finally ulcerates, exposing the worm. A loop of uterus prolapses through the body wall of the worm, to lie in the ulcer opening (Fig. 9-24); when the ulcer is immersed in water, larvae are discharged in large numbers.

Diagnosis usually presents no problems in endemic areas, as the development of the local lesion is quite characteristic. Once the ulcer is formed, larvae may be obtained for diagnostic purposes by flooding the area with water.

Symptoms and Pathogenesis.   One or many worms may be seen at one time, in any part of the body but usually on the legs or feet. The majority of infections consist of a single worm, but in endemic areas repeated reinfection is the rule. The presence of maturing worms may give rise to mild allergic symptoms such as urticaria. When the gravid female seeks a position close to the skin, there may be some localized erythema and tenderness in the area where the ulcer will form. The patient frequently exhibits some generalized symptoms at this time, with pruritus, sometimes nausea, vomiting, or diarrhea, or asthma attacks. These symptoms usually disappear with the appearance of the ulcer, the drainage of fluid that has formed around the female worm, and the initial discharge of larvae. A localized reaction, often quite painful, persists around the site of the ulcer during the entire period while the worm continues to discharge its larvae. Forty percent of patients experience severe disability, lasting an average of 6 weeks; about 1% suffer permanent damage from ankylosis of a joint. Discharge is intermittent, whenever the affected part comes in contact with water, and may take as long as 3 weeks to be completed. After the uterus has been emptied, the worm may withdraw into the tissues and become resorbed or it may be expelled. If the lesion does not become secondarily infected, healing is rapid after all larvae have been discharged. It has been estimated that approximately 50% of the lesions become infected, causing problems

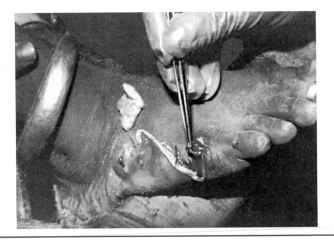

FIGURE 9-24   ■   Extraction of *Dracunculus medinensis* from ulcerated lesion on foot. Near ankle is a vesicle produced by another worm about to break through the skin. (Courtesy Dr. Michael Kliks, University of Hawaii Medical School.)

lasting for up to a year after the worms emerge (Ogunniyi et al., 2000). If the worms are removed surgically, the wound heals promptly. A rare complication of infection is invasion of the extradural space by the guinea worm, leading in some cases to abscess formation and paraplegia.

The calcified remains of worms that have died in the subcutaneous tissues may be found on x-ray examination. They may appear as linear calcific densities up to 25 cm in length, as tightly coiled bodies, or as rather dense, usually somewhat elongate, nodules.

Epidemiology and Control. Transmission of *Dracunculus* depends almost entirely on water sources that can become breeding grounds for copepods, with which infected persons come in direct contact and from which drinking water is obtained directly. The step wells of India, into which persons desiring water must descend, are almost ideal for transmission of the parasite. *Cyclops* breeds in standing water, as in wells, ponds, or open cisterns; it is not usually seen in flowing streams or rivers.

Control of dracunculiasis is perhaps simpler than that of any other infectious disease, as provision of safe drinking water, requiring only minimal filtration, is all that is needed. In 1985 the World Health Organization decided to attempt eradication of dracunculiasis during the next decade. In 1986 there were an estimated 3,600,000 cases worldwide, and by the end of 1996 that figure had dropped to approximately 100,000. The disease has been almost completely wiped out in Asia, and great progress made in Africa, where the Sudan remains the only country in which eradication efforts have made little progress. Currently there remain an estimated 75,000 cases of dracunculiasis in 12 sub-Saharan African countries, with most of them, 63%, occurring in the Sudan. It seems safe to predict that within a very few years this infection will be regarded as a sporadic zoonosis.

Treatment. Surgical removal of the worms by methods as primitive as twisting them around a stick has been practiced for centuries and may be quite successful if the worm is removed whole. If in the process of its removal the worm is broken, secondary infection almost always develops.

Metronidazole is the drug of choice, the dose for adults being 250 mg three times daily for 10 days, and for children 25 mg/kg body weight in three divided doses, not to exceed the daily adult dose. Thiabendazole, 50 mg/kg daily for 2 days, also gives good results, but side effects are more common than with metronidazole. Neither drug kills the worm, but drug treatment facilitates its removal. Mebendazole, 400 to 800 mg per day for 6 days, apparently kills the worms.

Other Tissue Nematodes

Trichinella spiralis and other *Trichinella* spp.

Discussed here because of the importance of the tissue phase of its life cycle, *T. spiralis* could as readily be considered with the intestinal helminths. The intestinal infection, in which adult worms are found in the mucosa, is transitory and usually asymptomatic or nearly so, whereas the phase of migration and encystment of larvae in the muscles is prolonged and frequently accompanied by serious symptoms.

Since 1835, controversy has surrounded the discovery and description of *Trichinella*. In that year the organism was initially seen by a first-year medical student, James Paget, later famous for other medical achievements, but it was named and described by his professor, Richard Owen. It was *T. spiralis* that Paget discovered and Owen named, and until recently that species was the only one known. However, five distinct species of *Trichinella* are now recognized (Pozio et al., 1992), all of which parasitize humans and a wide variety of carnivorous mammals. While *T. spiralis* is the most important of these parasites in most parts of the world, being cosmopolitan in distribution and of high pathogenicity, three of the other four species are of more regional importance. They may be distinguished as follows:

T. nativa—occurs in arctic and subarctic zones; of high pathogenicity, high resistance to freezing.

T. nelsoni—occurs in tropical Africa; intermediate in pathogenicity.

T. britovi—occurs in temperate Paleoarctic region; very low pathogenicity.

T. pseudospiralis—cosmopolitan; does not encyst, infectious to birds, pathogenicity in humans not well characterized.

Three additional species of *Trichinella* have been described: *T murrelli,* a parasite of wild carnivores in North America, having moderate to severe pathogenicity for humans and no resistance to freezing (Pozio and La Rosa, 2000); *T. zimbabwensis*, a parasite of crocodiles in Zimbabwe, experimentally infective in mammals, including primates (Pozio et al., 2002); and *T. papuae*, a parasite of wild and domestic pigs in Papua New Guinea, experimentally infective in reptiles (Pozio et al., 1999, 2004). *T. zimbabwensis* was the first species of *Trichinella* to be described from a cold-blooded animal. Like *T. pseudospiralis*, it does not encyst.

T. spiralis, a parasite of carnivorous mammals, is especially common in rats and in swine fed uncooked garbage and slaughterhouse scraps. It may occur in humans who consume uncooked pork and is most common in groups who make a practice of consuming raw pork products such as various types of salami and wurst. Bears are heavily infected, as numerous hunters have learned, to their sorrow. *Trichinella* is cosmopolitan in its distribution but occurs much more frequently in areas where raw garbage containing pork scraps is fed to hogs. It was once prevalent in many European countries, but enlightened sanitation practices have markedly lowered the rate in many areas, so that a few years ago the United States was said to enjoy the doubtful distinction of having three times as much trichinellosis as the rest of the world combined. Prevalence of trichina infection in this country, estimated on the basis of autopsy findings covering the years 1931 to 1942, was in the vicinity of 16% of the population; it has been stated that approximately 4% of these infections were sufficiently heavy to cause symptoms. Many states have adopted or are adopting laws requiring cooking of garbage fed to hogs; a lower incidence of infection has resulted. The highest incidence of trichinellosis is now reported from China (10,000 cases annually). It is also still common in Spain, France, Italy, and Yugoslavia. Six European outbreaks have been traced to infected horsemeat, and infected cattle are reported from China.

Infection is initiated by the consumption of raw or undercooked pork or other meat containing the encysted larvae (Fig. 9-25). The larvae excyst after the cysts are digested and penetrate into the intestinal mucosa, developing to adult worms within the short space of 30 to 40 hours. Male worms are generally less than 2 mm long, while females may reach a length of almost 5 mm. Mating may take place as soon as the worms are mature, and larvae may be produced within 3 days after fertilization. Thus, within about 5 days the larvae grow to maturity and begin the stage of larval deposition, which continues for as long as the female worms remain in the intestine. The duration of the intestinal infection probably depends on a number of factors, including the number of worms present in the intestine and the immune status of the host as determined by previous infections. The intestinal phase persists in congenitally athymic (nude) mice much longer than in those heterozygous for the athymic gene, indicating that T cell-dependent antigen is necessary for protection against the intestinal phase of the infection. Human intestinal infections have been known to persist for as long as 54 days; the average duration is probably shorter.

On being deposited in the mucosa, the larvae enter lymphatic vessels and from them gain access to the general circulation. They are 80 to 120 μm long and 5 or 6 μm in diameter and, so, are readily transported throughout the body. They leave the capillaries in striated muscle to penetrate through the sheaths of the muscle fibers. Degenerative and inflammatory changes are seen in infected fibers, and within about a month the larvae have reached their full size (Fig. 9-26). They are, except for *T. pseudospiralis*, coiled in a spiral and gradually

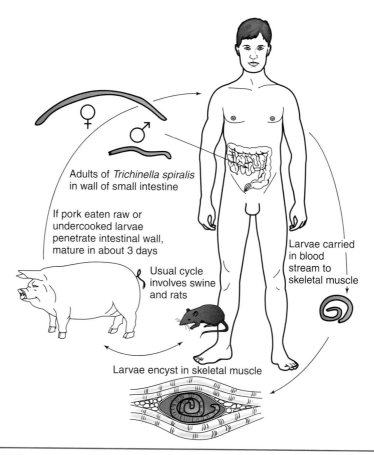

FIGURE 9-25 ■ Life cycle of *Trichinella spiralis*.

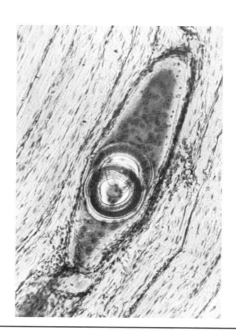

FIGURE 9-26 ■ *Trichinella spiralis* larva in muscle. (Photomicrograph by Zane Price.)

become surrounded by a sheath derived from the muscle fiber. The fully developed larva measures about 1 mm long. Encysted trichinae may remain viable for many years, even after the capsule has calcified.

The diagnosis may be fairly obvious on the basis of clinical symptoms and history but should be confirmed by laboratory examination or serologic tests. Several serologic tests are now available (see Chapter 16). Biopsy of skeletal muscle, usually gastrocnemius, may reveal the encysting larvae at any time after the first week of infection. Knott or membrane filtration concentrates of venous blood taken during the period of larval migration may demonstrate these organisms (see Chapter 15).

Symptoms. Symptoms during the intestinal phase may be so minor as to go unnoticed or they may be moderately severe. If present, they usually appear suddenly and are those of a nonspecific gastroenteritis. Diagnosis of the disease is seldom made at this stage, but an epidemic outbreak of gastroenteritis, from 2 to 7 days after ingestion of uncooked pork products by a group, should suggest trichinosis. Diarrhea, with or without abdominal pain, may last for several weeks.

During the stage of muscle invasion, symptoms vary, again according to the intensity of infection. Fever and eosinophilia are rather consistently seen when the infection is sufficiently severe to produce any symptoms, and eosinophilia probably accompanies even asymptomatic cases. It usually reaches its height in the third or fourth week, and at that time may range from 10% or less to 90%. In some overwhelming infections, eosinophilia may not appear. Characteristically, the eosinophilia increases rapidly during the early stages of the disease and gradually declines thereafter over a period of some months. Leukocytosis is common but not always present. Hyperimmunoglobulinemia E is characteristic. Myositis appears early, and with it, almost invariably, occurs the classic sign of trichinosis, circumorbital edema. This sign is rarely absent in patients who develop clinical symptoms of infection; it is thought to be related to the vasculitis responsible for the production of splinter hemorrhages. Edema of the eyelids appears as early as the seventh day of infection but may come on much later. In some patients, photophobia, diplopia, or other visual disturbances may occur. Muscle pain may be severe and usually reaches its height from the 12th to 20th day of infection. Muscles are often sensitive to pressure. While radiographs will not demonstrate the calcified cysts in muscle, they may be seen by xeroradiography. Splinter hemorrhages beneath the nails are seen in a large percentage of patients. Central nervous system involvement, with symptoms suggestive of acute psychosis, meningoencephalitis, cerebrovascular accident, or brain tumor, is seen in a small percentage of patients with clinical trichinosis. In moderate infections, symptoms usually begin to abate during the fifth or sixth week. In severe cases, death may occur 4 to 6 weeks after infection.

Analysis of an outbreak of trichinellosis acquired from walrus meat in an Inuit (Eskimo) village in northern Quebec provides strong evidence for two clinical syndromes associated with *T. nativa* infection. A primary infection was seen to produce symptoms similar to those described for *T. spiralis*, while with a secondary or subsequent infection the intestinal phase is prolonged, characterized by 5 to 15 nonbloody, nonmucoid stools daily, lasting for several weeks, with little edema or myalgia (MacLean et al., 1992). A similar syndrome has been reported from Greenland.

Pathogenesis. The intestinal phase of a *Trichinella* infection ends when the adult worms are rejected because of the development of local tissue immunity. The development of immunity can be suppressed and the intestinal phase prolonged by the administration of corticosteroids, facts that must be borne in mind if steroids are used in therapy. The primary pathogenic effect of *Trichinella* comes from destruction of the striated muscle fibers in which it encysts. Vasculitis may accompany the migration of the larvae, accounting for the splinter hemorrhages and perhaps the periorbital edema. Certain of the neurologic manifestations of trichinellosis may also be due to vasculitis; granulomas that sometimes contain *Trichinella* larvae have also been found in the brains of patients who succumb to this infection. Clinically apparent trichinal myocarditis is rare. Death from trichinellosis may generally be ascribed to myocarditis, encephalitis, or pneumonitis.

A possible connection between trichinellosis and polyarteritis nodosa has been frequently noted and may involve deposition of circulating immune complexes in vessel walls, cross-reactivity between parasitic antigens and human vessel walls, high levels of circulating IgE reacting in several different ways to initiate or sustain inflammatory vascular disease, and hypereosinophilia-induced tissue damage.

Epidemiology and Control. In the 1930s it was estimated (on the basis of autopsy findings) that one out of every six persons in the United States became infected with *T. spiralis* during their lifetime; more recent studies indicate that the infection rate had declined to approximately one in 25 by 1970, and at that time was less than one in 50 for those younger than 45 years. Although trichinellosis is a reportable disease in the United States, the number of clinical cases reported annually in the decade from 1980 to 1989 ranged from a high of 206 to a low of 30. In contrast to the overall decline in clinical cases, the incidence among refugees from Southeast Asia (principally those from Cambodia and Laos) remains high (more than 25 times the national average in the years 1974 to 1984) and represents a challenge for health education.

Among the factors responsible for the general decrease in the disease are legislative measures requiring heat treatment of garbage used as hog food, low temperature storage of pork (refrigeration at −15°C for 20 days or more or quick freezing at −37° C), public awareness of the danger involved in eating undercooked pork, and perhaps a decline in the consumption of pork and pork products. Sporadic outbreaks are still seen, generally associated with the consumption of homemade sausage (Centers for Disease Control, 1991). Current recommendations for safe cooking of pork products were established from studies in which meat was cooked in conventional ovens, and United States Department of Agriculture regulations state that "*all parts* of pork muscle tissue must be heated to a temperature not lower than 137° F (58.3° C)." Pork roasts, cooked in microwave ovens following the procedures recommended by the oven manufacturer and the national Pork Council, have been found to contain *Trichinella* larvae that were still viable and infective to rats. Additionally, it must be remembered that freezing may not kill the larvae of *T. nativa*, which have been found in horsemeat—a testimony to the fact that equines are not necessarily strict vegetarians. Indeed, freezing–of whatever duration—cannot be relied on to destroy all larvae of any *Trichinella* species.

Of the many flesh-eating mammals that may become infected with *T. spiralis*, only two are of epidemiologic importance in addition to swine. Rats may become infected by feeding on scraps of infected pork or through cannibalism, and they are sometimes an important source of infection for hogs. Bears are frequently infected and are a source of occasional outbreaks of the disease. A recent outbreak of trichinellosis nativa in northern Saskatchewan, involving 78 individuals, resulted from the consumption of black bear meat (Schellenberg et al., 2003). Species identification was made by polymerase chain reaction (PCR). Treatment with antiparasitic drugs (mebendazole and albendazole) and prednisone was effective in limiting the severity and duration of the illness. Wild pigs may be as heavily infected as their domesticated brethren. An outbreak in southern Spain, involving 38 people, 15 of whom were hospitalized, was caused by *T. britovi*, acquired by consuming sausage made from a mixture of uninspected wild boar meat and inspected pork (Gomez-Garcia et al., 2003). Larvae were identified by indirect immunofluorescence and Western blot assay.

Treatment. In severely symptomatic infections, corticosteroids are beneficial and may at times be lifesaving. Recognition that, as mentioned previously, the intestinal phase of the infection may be prolonged by their use suggests that they should be reserved for cases in which there is considerable toxicity. The initial dose may be 20 to 60 mg prednisone, or its equivalent, reduced after the first few days to the lowest dose that alleviates symptoms and then gradually discontinued.

Mebendazole is the drug of choice for treatment of trichinellosis. The dosage for adults and children over the age of 2 years is 200 to 400 mg three times daily for 3 days, followed by 400 to 500 mg three times daily for 10 days. An alternative drug is albendazole at a dosage of 400 mg twice a day for 8 to 14 days.

An outbreak of trichinellosis caused by *T. pseudospiralis* and affecting 59 persons, with one fatality, occurred in southern Thailand in 1994–1995. The source of the epidemic was consumption of raw pork from a wild pig. The most striking clinical features were the persistence of the muscular swelling, myalgia, and weakness, with these symptoms lasting in some patients longer than 4 months. Muscle biopsies showed unencapsulated, actively migrating larvae, positively identified as *T. pseudospiralis* by DNA analysis. Treatment with thiabendazole and mebendazole was ineffective, although administration of albendazole (dosage unreported) for 2 weeks seemed effective (Jongwutiwes et al., 1998).

Visceral Larva Migrans

Larvae of nonhuman ascarids such as *Toxocara canis* or *T. cati* are capable of limited development in human hosts. The adult worms, similar to *Ascaris lumbricoides* in appearance but only a quarter to half its size, live in the small intestine of dogs and cats. Their eggs, which require a period of maturation outside the host, are infective for dogs, cats, and humans. In all of these hosts, infective eggs hatch in the intestine and liberate larvae that burrow into the wall of the intestine. In puppies younger than 5 weeks, the larvae complete a migratory and developmental cycle similar to that of A. *lumbricoides* in man and become mature *Toxocara* in the intestinal tract. In older puppies or adult dogs, or in humans, the larvae are unable to complete their development. They may wander for some time in the tissues (Fig. 9-27), finally encysting as second-stage larvae. By some mechanism not yet understood, these larvae may excyst in a pregnant bitch and cross the placenta, to grow to adult worms in the pups. Eggs of *T. cati*, ingested by cats, apparently complete their developmental cycle and become adult worms in the intestine.

If humans or any of a variety of other animals ingest infective eggs of *T. canis* or *T. cati*, development proceeds only as far as second-stage larvae, which after a period of migration encyst in the tissues. When rats or mice so infected are eaten by dogs or cats, the larvae complete their development in the new host, becoming adult worms in the intestine.

Various studies have assessed the prevalence of *Toxocara* eggs in places where they might be ingested by children. In two parks in the St. Joseph–Benton Harbor area of Michigan, these eggs were found in approximately one-third of all soil specimens examined; they were present in 11% of soil samples collected from backyards and gardens of 146 private homes in Baltimore, Maryland. Seroprevalence rates in children are in the range of 5% in the

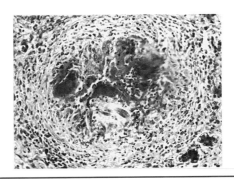

FIGURE 9-27 ■ Visceral larva migrans. Section through larva surrounded by granuloma. (Photomicrograph by Zane Price.)

United States; similar or higher rates are reported from England and France. In Trinidad, the seroprevalence rates were 62% for schoolchildren aged 5 to 12 years (Baboolal and Rawlins, 2002).

Eggs of *Toxocara* resemble those of *Ascaris,* but are larger, less elongate, and have a thinner shell and albuminoid outer covering. Those of *T.* canis measure about 85 by 75 μm; *T. cati* eggs have a diameter of 65 to 70 μm, while fertile *Ascaris* eggs have extreme measurements of 75 by 50 μm.

An additional mode of infection in humans has recently been reported from various parts of the world. This involves the ingestion of various raw meats such as chicken and rabbit giblets and lamb liver. Although the evidence is circumstantial, based largely on serologic findings, ingestion of infected meats from these paratenic hosts would seem a logical explanation for the acquisition of visceral larva migrans by adults.

Diagnosis of visceral larva migrans in humans is generally made on clinical grounds. Chronic eosinophilia, especially in a young child who has been exposed to ascarid-infected pets, accompanied by hepatomegaly or chronic nonspecific pulmonary disease, is suggestive of this condition. Various serologic tests using cultured second-stage *Toxocara* larvae as the antigen give excellent results, especially if the patient's serum is first adsorbed with *Ascaris* antigens. Needle biopsy is not an effective method of diagnosing hepatic infection; more productive is laparoscopy and biopsy of suspicious-looking liver nodules under direct visualization.

Symptoms. Visceral larva migrans affects primarily children, probably because they are more likely to come in contact with dog and cat ascarid eggs in the soil. Hypereosinophilia is very common; hepatomegaly may be seen, and some patients have symptoms of chronic pulmonary inflammation, with cough and fever. In rare cases, pulmonary involvement has been sufficiently severe to lead to considerable respiratory embarrassment, and deaths have been reported from this condition. Visual difficulties may indicate a toxocaral retinochoroiditis or peripheral retinitis; such involvement would be expected to be unilateral. Epilepsy and myocarditis have also been associated with *Toxocara* infections in humans.

An expanded spectrum of symptoms in toxocaral disease is suggested by observation that in a series of 84 patients, seropositive for this infection by ELISA, the most common clinical features were abdominal pain, hepatomegaly, anorexia, nausea, vomiting, lethargy, sleep and behavioral disturbances, pneumonia, cough, wheezing, cervical adenitis, headache, myositis, and fever. Twenty-three of these patients had normal eosinophil counts.

Pathogenesis. Wandering of the second-stage larvae through the tissues produces tracks marked by hemorrhage, necrosis, and infiltration of lymphocytes and eosinophils. Granulomatous foci are produced around dead larvae. Epileptic children have been found to have significantly higher *Toxocara* antibody titers than nonepileptic controls; however, no difference has been noted between children with idiopathic epilepsy and epilepsy with known cause. Epilepsy-associated mental retardation, hyperactivity, and pica were thought to predispose these children to *Toxocara* infection.

Ocular larva migrans is rare, but its consequences may be severe. It is usually unilateral, and may be the result of penetration of the orbit by a single larva. It is thought usually to be seen in light infections, where larval migration is relatively unimpeded by tissue reaction and symptoms of visceral involvement are lacking. Diminished vision, strabismus, leukokoria, a fixed pupil, and on funduscopic examination a posterior retinochoroiditis are frequent findings. Occasionally an infection may be subclinical, and toxocaral granulomas misdiagnosed as retinoblastomas may lead to unnecessary enucleation of the eye. The results of serologic testing are often helpful in making what is frequently a difficult diagnosis.

Prevention. Dogs are the chief culprits in spreading this disease because of their indiscriminate defecatory habits. Some 50% of puppies and 20% of older dogs are infected with *Toxocara*. If they cannot be kept away from small children, they should be dewormed on a regular basis. The more fastidious feline is usually a problem only if it shares a sandbox with children.

Treatment. The disease is self-limited, frequently first coming to the attention of the physician at a time when the symptoms are at their worst. Watchful waiting is advised, and corticosteroids (employed as in trichinellosis) are reserved for patients who are severely symptomatic except in the ocular form of infection, where their early use may be of great benefit. Drugs of choice are albendazole, 400 mg twice a day for 5 days, or mebendazole, 100 to 200 mg twice a day for 5 days.

ANGIOSTRONGYLUS CANTONENSIS

The rat lungworm, *A. cantonensis*, is widespread, and the infection seems to be increasing in rats and bandicoots in the tropics and subtropics, very probably through the agency of infected rats traveling as stowaways on ships. It has been found in rats in New Orleans and in Egypt, where human cases are not known to occur. First reported in the United States in 1987, *A. cantonensis* is now endemic in Louisiana wildlife and has been responsible for the deaths of zoo animals in Lafayette and New Orleans (Kim et al., 2002). Human infections that cause eosinophilic meningitis have been reported from Hawaii, Tahiti, Japan, mainland China, Taiwan, Thailand, Vietnam, Malaysia, Indonesia, Vanuatu, American Samoa, the Ivory Coast, and Jamaica. An outbreak of *A. cantonensis*–caused eosinophilic meningitis was described in a group of 12 U.S. travelers returning from Jamaica (Slom et al., 2002). Unconfirmed cases have been noted from other Pacific islands, Hong Kong, the Philippines, Papua New Guinea, Australia, New Caledonia, Réunion, Mauritius, Cuba, and Puerto Rico. Two other species are possible agents of human eosinophilic meningitis, *A. mackerrasse* in Australia, and *A. malaysiensis* in Sarawak (Malaysia), in Thailand, and in Indonesia. Ocular infection with *A. cantonensis* has been reported from Thailand, Taiwan, Indonesia, Japan, South Vietnam, and Sri Lanka but is rare (Wariyapola et al., 1998).

A. cantonensis is a slender worm, up to 25 mm long. Larval stages develop in slugs and land snails. When eaten by rats, the larvae migrate to the meninges and develop in the brain for about a month. Young adults then migrate to the pulmonary artery, where they attain maturity. The incidence of this infection in rats and snails may be quite high in endemic areas.

In human hosts, *Angiostrongylus* does not complete its developmental cycle. When third-stage larvae are ingested, they penetrate into blood vessels in the intestinal tract and are carried to the meninges but are unable to migrate to the lungs, as they do in rats. Rarely, worms develop to the young adult stage in the meninges, but they soon die, and it is the death of the larvae or young adults and the inflammatory reaction provoked by the dead worms that cause the characteristic signs and symptoms of human infection.

A presumptive diagnosis may be made in patients from areas where the disease is endemic on the basis of meningitis with blood and spinal fluid eosinophilia. Lesions may be seen in the meninges by computed tomography (CT), with serologic confirmation of the infection by ELISA.

Sources of human infection are slugs, land snails, or fresh-water prawns and other paratenic (transport) hosts (Fig. 9-28), which are often consumed raw in islands of the Pacific, in Thailand, and in Vietnam. In Thailand and Malaysia, snails of the genus *Pila* are eaten raw, either mixed with vegetables or as a form of medication. The giant African land snail, *Achatina fulica*, has spread throughout the Pacific islands and is apparently a common vector. Raw prawns are a frequent article of diet in Tahiti, and larvae found in them are infective to laboratory rats. The contamination of fresh vegetables by carnivorous land planarians that have fed on infected snails appears to be another important means of infection in New Caledonia and perhaps elsewhere.

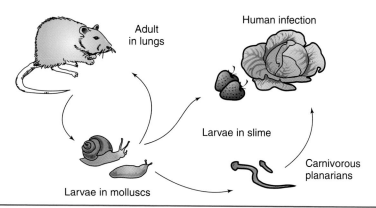

FIGURE 9-28 ▪ Life cycle of *Angiostrongylus cantonensis*. (From Brown WJ, Voge M. *Neuropathology of Parasitic Infections,* Oxford, 1982, Oxford University Press.)

Symptoms. The incubation period of the disease varies and apparently can be as long as 47 days. Infection in man is usually benign and self-limited, although fatalities have occurred. The first fatality in the Western Hemisphere was reported from Jamaica and occurred in a 14-month-old Jamaican boy (Lindo et al., 2004). Sections of multiple worms were observed in the brain and lungs at autopsy. Symptoms of meningitis or meningoencephalitis—headache and stiff neck, often with sensorial changes—are of abrupt onset. A radiculomyeloencephalitis, with pains and paresthesias of the lower trunk and legs, bowel and bladder dysfunction, and one death, was seen in 16 of 21 Korean fishermen who ate giant African land snails in Samoa and in none of five who ate cooked snails. A CSF pleocytosis of more than 500 per μl occurred in 80% of infected persons, and on autopsy worms were found in the subarachnoid space of the lumbar cord, with invasion of the white and gray matter. The spinal fluid usually contains 100 to 2000 white blood cells per μl generally accompanied by a marked eosinophilia. Other common symptoms include nausea and vomiting, fever, and, early in the infection, abdominal pain, malaise, and constipation. A blood eosinophilia is also common; total leukocyte counts are moderately elevated.

Eye invasion is marked by visual impairment, ocular pain, blepharospasm, circumcorneal injection, keratitis, cells and flares in the anterior chamber and vitreous, iritis, and retinal edema. Living worms have been noted and on occasion removed surgically.

Pathogenesis. Little is known about the effects of this parasite on the central nervous system, since most patients recover uneventfully. On autopsy, sections of immature *Angiostrongylus* have been seen in the cerebrum and cerebellum, as well as the spinal cord, associated with infiltrates of eosinophils, monocytes, and foreign-body giant cells. Marked tissue necrosis has been seen in some areas in connection with dead worms. Immature worms have been found in spinal fluid obtained by lumbar puncture; adult worms have been found in the eye and the pulmonary artery.

Treatment. Trials of specific therapy are still inconclusive. Thiabendazole and mebendazole have some effect in animal infections, but thiabendazole was found to be ineffective in reported human cases. Symptomatic treatment is all that is needed in the majority of these infections, but where specific anthelmintic treatment seems necessary, mebendazole, 100 mg twice daily for 5 days, is a recommended investigational regimen for adults.

Angiostrongylus costaricensis

The adult of *A. costaricensis* ordinarily inhabits the mesenteric arteries of the cotton rat (*Sigmodon hispidus*) and several other species of wild rodents. It has been encountered as a human parasite principally in Costa Rica, though additional cases have been reported from most other parts of Central America, from Mexico (Yucatan), and from Brazil (São Paulo). Most such infections have been found in children.

Egg laying takes place in arterioles of the intestinal wall of the rodent host; the eggs hatch to produce larvae, which migrate through the intestinal wall to appear in the feces. First stage larvae, ingested by the slug *Vaginulus plebeius*, grow and undergo two molts, after which they are infectious to rats or humans. Children are likely to become infected while playing in the grassy areas infested by these slugs; infection has also been traced to contaminated salad vegetables. Physid snails may also serve as intermediate hosts.

In humans, the larvae penetrate the wall of the intestine and first enter lymphatic vessels, migrating usually to the ileocecocolic branches of the anterior mesenteric artery; they may be found in ectopic locations such as the spermatic arteries. Ectopic migration may in other instances place the worms where their eggs reach the liver. The presence of the adult worms (Fig. 9-29) provokes an inflammatory reaction that damages the endothelium of the occupied vessels, causing localized thrombosis and necrosis of the tissues perfused by the thrombosed vessel. An eosinophilic infiltrate and granuloma formation occur around the eggs and larvae. In the most common form, with localization of the worms in the region of the cecum, there is usually pain in the right flank and iliac fossa and tenderness to palpation. A tumorlike mass is often palpable, and the x-ray picture on barium enema may mimic that of a malignancy. The intestinal wall may become thickened even to the point of obstruction. If the worms become lodged in the spermatic arteries they may cause obstruction and necrosis, with acute testicular pain. If the eggs and larvae reach the liver, the clinical picture may resemble the hepatic involvement seen in visceral larva migrans. In most cases there is a leukocytosis of 15,000 to 40,000 cells per µl, and 20% to 50% eosinophilia.

A skin test antigen has been prepared and is reported to give good results. A precipitin test has also been developed. Neither of these tests is generally available. Diagnosis is usually made by surgery, which is the only available form of treatment, although thiabendazole and mebendazole have also been recommended. Eggs and larvae do not appear in the stools of humans.

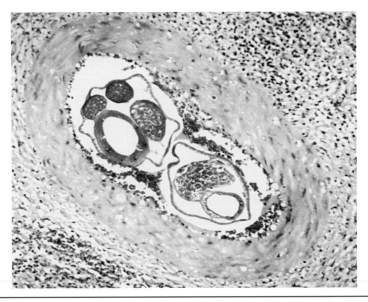

FIGURE 9-29 ■ *Angiostrongylus costaricensis* in section of human appendix. (Photomicrograph by Zane Price from material furnished by Dr. Pedro Morera.)

Gnathostoma spinigerum

Larval stages of roundworms belonging to the genus *Gnathostoma* are acquired by man through ingestion of raw, insufficiently cooked, or fermented fresh-water fish or amphibians, or paratenic hosts such as birds and snakes. While many species of *Gnathostoma* have been described, *G. spinigerum* is of primary medical importance. Human infections with this parasite are fairly common in Japan and have also been reported from China, Thailand, Malaysia, Indonesia, the Philippines, Israel, Tanzania, and other areas where raw or pickled fish are part of the diet. Gnathostomiasis was first reported in Mexico in 1970, and human cases seem to be increasing, with more than 1000 reported between 1980 and 1996, primarily along the Gulf and Pacific coasts (Ogata et al., 1998). During the 4-year period, 1993 to 1997, 98 cases of gnathostomiasis were identified in Acapulco, Mexico, the major Mexican city where cases have been reported (Rojas-Molina et al., 1999). The epidemiology of the infection in these areas is unclear, but it very likely includes the eating of raw or insufficiently cooked fresh-water fish, especially in the form of sushimi or ceviche, a lime-marinated fish salad originally from South America and now popular in Mexico.

The life cycle of *G. spinigerum* involves two intermediate hosts; the first is a copepod, the second any of a number of fresh-water food fish, frogs, snakes, or birds. The larval worms, about 4 mm long with numerous spines on the head and body (Fig. 9-30), encyst in the second intermediate host. Adult worms are normally found in dogs and cats, where they live coiled in the wall of the alimentary tract. When ingested by humans, the larvae do not mature but migrate throughout the body.

Other species of *Gnathostoma* have occasionally been reported as human parasites (Sato et al., 1992).

Symptoms and Pathogenesis. A few days after they are ingested, migration of the larvae through the intestinal wall and into the abdominal cavity may produce epigastric pain, fever, vomiting, and anorexia, which may persist for several weeks. These symptoms clear when the characteristic cutaneous manifestations begin. Circumscribed patches of edema, usually on the abdomen, may last a few days and recur at different sites, depending on the path of the migrating worm. The edematous areas may be the size of a fist, slightly erythematous, and accompanied by pruritus, rash, and stabbing pain. They may also produce lesions similar to those of cutaneous larva migrans. An eosinophilia between 35% and 80% is reported in patients with cutaneous involvement.

An eosinophilic myeloencephalitis may result from invasion of the central nervous system by migration of the worms along nerve tracts. Characteristically this is initiated by sudden severe nerve root pain, followed by paralysis of extremities and sensory impairment. Eosinophilic pleocytosis with bloody or xanthochromic spinal fluid is suggestive of eosinophilic

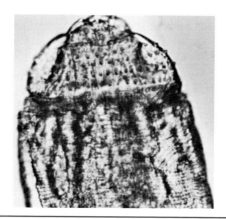

FIGURE 9-30 ▪ Head portion of larva of *Gnathostoma spinigerum.*

meningitis caused by *A. cantonensis*, but the clinical presentations of the two infections differ. Subarachnoid hemorrhage may be detected by CT scan. Ocular involvement may be marked by palpebral edema, exophthalmos, or subconjunctival hemorrhage; if the vitreous, retina, or corneal or lenticular structures are involved, blindness may result.

Presumptive diagnosis may be made on the basis of clinical symptoms and the patient's history in relation to food habits and residence. The differential diagnosis may also include sparganosis, cutaneous paragonimiasis, cutaneous larva migrans, and myiasis. Definitive diagnosis rests on the recovery and identification of the worm. While gnathostomiasis is principally a disease of the Far East, the case in which subarachnoid hemorrhage was diagnosed by CT mentioned earlier and another involving a Laotian, residing in the United States for 3 years, who developed costovertebral pain, hematuria, and fever and passed a gnathostome in his urine, suggest that more such infections may be seen in Western countries.

Treatment. Worms may be surgically removed from subcutaneous and other accessible loci. Albendazole, 400 mg twice a day for 21 days, is reported to produce cure rates of over 90%. Ivermectin, 200 mcg/kg daily for 2 days, may also be used. The infection is prevented by thorough cooking of all meats and fish.

Uncommon Tissue Nematodes

Baylisascaris procyonis

An ascarid found in raccoons, this worm produces a visceral larva migrans syndrome in humans and a variety of mammals and birds, with an apparent predilection for the central nervous system. Raccoons develop an intestinal infection after ingesting either the eggs or the tissues of other animals in which the larval stage is found. A 13-month-old child with neurologic symptoms was diagnosed as infected with *B. procyonis* on the basis of serologic testing and was treated with thiabendazole, prednisone, and a single dose of ivermectin. He survived with persistent severe neurologic deficit (Cunningham et al., 1994). At least two other children who ingested the eggs are known to have contracted a fatal eosinophilic meningoencephalitis. It is thought also to cause a unilateral neuroretinitis in adults, who presumably ingest smaller quantities of eggs. Larvae may be apparent to patients as "floaters" and may be seen through the ophthalmoscope or revealed by their random tracks in the retina. Immunofluorescence and ELISA have been used in diagnosis but are not readily available. Laser photocoagulation has been employed to destroy larvae in the retina; there is no known effective systemic treatment. *Baylisascaris* seems widespread in raccoons, its eggs remain infective in the soil for long periods, and it may represent a largely unrecognized public health problem.

The prevalence of *B. procyonis* infection in raccoons is often high as evidenced by a study in southern California in which 24 of 26 roadkill raccoons were found to be infected (Moore et al, 2004). In northern California, approximately 50% of raccoon defecation sites (latrines) were found to contain *B. procyonis* eggs (Roussere et al., 2003). In the Atlanta area, 22% of live-trapped raccoons were found to be infected (Eberhard et al., 2003).

Dioctophyma renale

This large nematode is found in the kidneys of dogs, mink, and other fish-eating mammals. Females may reach 100 cm in length, the males as much as 40 cm; they may invade and destroy the kidney and are also found in the abdominal cavity. Eggs, passed in the urine, are ingested by annelids, and if these are eaten by fish, the larvae develop to a stage infectious for the mammalian host. Only a handful of human infections, presumably acquired through eating raw fish, have been reported. Diagnosis is made by finding the barrel-shaped eggs, with thick pitted brownish shells, measuring about 66 by 42 µm, in the urine. The only known treatment is surgical.

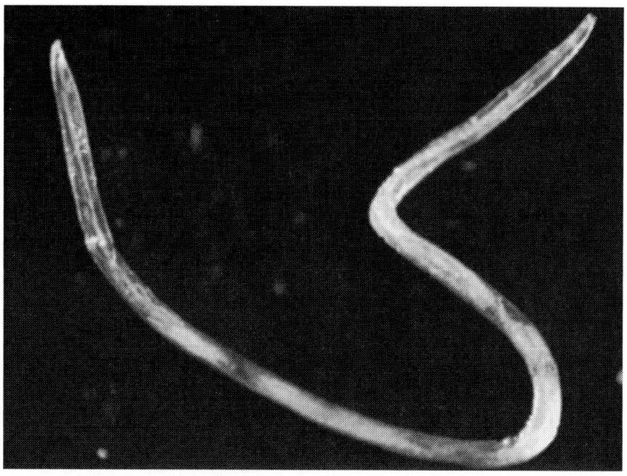

FIGURE 9-31 ■ *Thelazia californiensis* from human eye. (Photograph by Zane Price.)

Lagochilascaris minor

A parasite of the cloudy leopard, *Felis nebulosa*, this worm has been reported from humans in Trinidad, Tobago, Surinam, and Brazil. An intestinal parasite in its normal host, it occurs in such aberrant loci as the tissues of the neck, mastoid, eye, and lungs in humans. The worms are small, males reaching up to 9 mm in length, females to 15 mm. The eggs resemble those of *Toxocara cati*. Treatment has been primarily surgical. Levamisole (approved in the United States and Canada only for treatment of colorectal carcinoma and melanoma) is reported to have some value in treatment of this infection (De Aguilar-Nascimento et al., 1993).

Micronema deletrix

Ordinarily not parasitic, but living a saprophytic existence on decaying organic matter, this worm has been known to cause nasal, maxillary, and renal granulomas and meningoencephalitis in horses. Two cases of fatal human meningoencephalitis caused by *Micronema* have been reported; in both, the mode of infection seems obscure.

Syngamus laryngeus

A parasite of the upper respiratory tract of ruminants, *Syngamus* has been reported as an accidental parasite of humans in the United States, Canada, Australia, the Caribbean, Guyana, Brazil, and the Philippines. It causes respiratory distress and coughing, and at times a transient pulmonary infiltrate. The worms may be expelled during paroxysms of coughing or removed by laryngoscopy. Eggs, occasionally found in the feces, measuring 78 to 85 by 42 to 45 μm, have a shell resembling that of *Capillaria* but without polar plugs. The life cycle and mode of infection are unknown. A single report suggests the efficacy of thiabendazole in treatment.

Thelazia californiensis

Not really a tissue nematode, *Thelazia*, commonly known as the eyeworm of deer, jack rabbits, and coyotes in California, is occasionally found in the conjunctival sac of humans (and of dogs and cats). The worms are 1 to 15 cm long, grayish white, and threadlike (Fig. 9-31). They cause a severe conjunctivitis but are readily removed without any lasting ill effects. They are transmitted by a fly of the genus *Fannia*. An eyeworm of dogs, *T. calipaeda*, is reported to infect humans in China, Korea, Japan, Thailand, and the former Soviet Union. In China this worm is transmitted by the housefly, *Musca domestica*. Table 9-2 summarizes important features of the more common tissue nematode infections in humans.

TABLE 9-2   ■   Review of Tissue Nematode Infections of Humans

Disease	Parasite	Means of Human Infection	Location of Larvae in Humans	Location of Adults in Humans	Clinical Features	Laboratory Diagnosis
Lymphatic filariasis	*Wuchereria bancrofti, Brugia malayi, B. timori*	"Bite" of infected mosquito (*Anopheles, Aedes, Culex, Mansonia*)	Skin, lymphatics (while developing to adults)	Lymphatic system	Lymphangitis, lymphadenitis, edema, fever, eosinophilia (hydrocele, elephantiasis)	Microfilariae in blood (periodicity nocturnal in most areas), serologic tests
Loiasis	*Loa loa* (eye worm)	"Bite" of infected deerfly (*Chrysops*)	Subcutaneous tissue (while developing to adults)	Migrating in subcutaneous tissue	Calabar (fugative) swellings, pruritus, eosinophilia, worm migrates across eye	Microfilaria in blood (diurnal periodicity)
Onchocerciasis (river blindness)	*Onchocerca volvulus* (blinding worm)	"Bite" of infected blackfly (*Simulium*)	Skin and subcutaneous tissue (while developing to adults)	Subcutaneous or deeper connective tissues	Subcutaneous nodules, pruritic dermatitis, hyperpigmentation, visual disturbances, blindness	Microfilaria in skin biopsy, biopsy of onchocercal nodules
Dracunculiasis	*Dracunculus medinensis* (Guinea worm)	Ingestion of larvae in infected copepods (*Cyclops* and others)	Intestinal tract, deep connective tissues	Deep connective tissues, subcutaneous tissue, dermis	Pruritus, blister, ulcer, eosinophilia, secondary infection	Adult worm in lesion, larvae from worm in ulcer
Trichinellosis	*Trichinella spiralis*	Ingestion of larvae in pork and other meats	Striated muscle (encysted)	Mucosa of small intestine (embedded)	Fever, eosinophilia, muscle pain, orbital edema	Larvae in muscle biopsy, serologic tests
Visceral larva migrans	*Toxocara canis, T. cati*	Ingestion of eggs	Liver (also lungs, eyes, brain)	Not present (in dogs and cats)	Hepatomegaly, hypereosinophilia, hyperglobulinemia	Serologic tests

References

Amaral F et al. Live adult worms detected by ultrasonography in human bancroftian filariasis. *Am J Trop Med Hyg* 1994; *50*:753–757.

Baboolal S, Rawlins SC. Seroprevalence of toxocariasis in schoolchildren in Trinidad. *Trans R Soc Trop Med Hyg* 2002; *96*:139–143.

Boussinesq M et al. Three probable cases of *Loa loa* encephalopathy following ivermectin treatment for onchocerciasis. *Am J Trop Med Hyg* 1998; *58*:461–469.

Burnham GM. Adverse reactions to ivermectin treatment for onchocerciasis. Results of a placebo-controlled double-blind trial in Malawi. *Trans R Soc Trop Med Hyg* 1993; *87*:313–317.

Carme B et al. Five cases of encephalitis during treatment of loiasis with diethylcarbamazine. *Am J Trop Med Hyg* 1991; *44*:684–690.

Centers for Disease Control. *Trichincella spiralis* infection–United States, 1990. *MMWR* 1991; *40*:57–60.

Chandrasena TGAN et al. Evaluation of the ICT whole-blood antigen card test to detect infection due to *Wuchereria bancrofti* in Sri Lanka. *Trans R Soc Trop Med Hyg* 2002; *96*:60–63.

Cunningham CK et al. Diagnosis and management of *Baylisascaris procyonis* infection in an infant with nonfatal meningoencephalitis. *Clin Infect Dis* 1994; *18*:868–872.

De Aguilar-Nascimento JE et al. Infection of the soft tissues of the neck due to *Logochilascaris minor*. *Trans R Soc Trop Med Hyg* 1993; *87*:198.

Dreyer G et al. Renal abnormalities in microfilaremic patients with Bancroftian filariasis. *Am J Trop Med Hyg* 1992; *46*:745–751.

Dreyer G et al. Amicrofilaremic carriers of adult *Wuchereria bancrofti*. *Trans R Soc Trop Med Hyg* 1996; *90*:288–289.

Duke BOL et al. Effects of three-month doses of ivermectin on adult *Onchocera volvulus*. *Am J Trop Med Hyg* 1992; *46*:189–194.

Eberhard ML et al. Zoonotic *Brugia* infection in Western Michigan. *Am J Surg Pathol* 1993; *17*:1058–1061.

Eberhard, ML et al. *Baylisascaris procyonis* in the metropolitan Atlanta area. *Emerg Infect Dis* 2003; *9*:1636–1637.

Fan PC et al. Follow-up investigations on clinical manifestations after filariasis eradication by diethyl-carbamazine medicated common salt on Kinmen (Quemoy) islands, Republic of China. *J Trop Med Hyg* 1995; *98*:461–464.

Fischer P et al. Long-lasting reduction of *Brugia timori* microfilariae following a single dose of diethyl-carbamazine combined with albendazole. *Trans R Soc Trop Med Hyg* 2003; *97*:446–448.

Freedman DO et al. Lymphoscintigraphic analysis of lymphatic abnormalities in symptomatic and asymptomatic human filariasis. *J Infect Dis* 1994; *170*:927–933.

Freedman DO et al. Abnormal lymphatic function in presymptomatic Bancroftian filariasis. *J Infect Dis* 1995; *171*:997–1001.

Gomez-Garcia V et al. Short report: Human infection with *Trichinella britovi* in Granada, Spain. *Am J Trop Med Hyg* 2003; *68*:463–464.

Guderian RH et al. Onchocerciasis and reproductive health in Ecuador. *Trans R Soc Trop Med Hyg* 1997; *91*:513–317.

Hoerauf A et al. Endosymbiotic bacteria in worms as targets for a novel chemotherapy in filariasis. *Lancet* 2000; *355*:1242–1243.

Jongwutiwes S et al. First outbreak of human trichinellosis caused by *Trichinella pseudospiralis*. *Clin Infect Dis* 1998; *26*:111–115.

Kim DY et al. *Parastrongylus (=Angiostrongylus) cantonensis* now endemic in Louisiana wildlife. *J Parasitol* 2002; *88*:1024–1026.

Leichsenring M et al. Ultrasonographic investigations of onchocerciasis in Liberia. *Am J Trop Med Hyg* 1990; *43*:380–385.

Lindo JF et al. Fatal autochthonous eosinophilic meningitis in a Jamaican child caused by *Angiostrongylus cantonensis*. *Am J Trop Med Hyg* 2004; *70*:425–428.

Liu J et al. Mass treatment of filariasis using DEC medicated salt. *J Trop Med Hyg* 1992; *95*:132–135.

MacLean JD et al. Epidemiologic and serologic definition of primary and secondary trichinosis in the arctic. *J Infect Dis* 1992; *165*:908–912.

Martin-Prevel Y et al. Tolerance and efficacy of single high-dose ivermectin for the treatment of loiasis. *Am J Trop Med Hyg* 1993; *48*:186–192.

Mathai E, David S. Intraocular filariasis due to *Wuchereria bancrofti. Trans R Soc Trop Med Hyg* 2000; *94*:317–318.

Mawson AR, WaKabongo M. Onchocerciasis-associated morbidity: Hypothesis. *Trans R Soc Trop Med Hyg* 2002; *96*:541–542.

Meyrowitsch DW et al. Mass diethylcarbamazine chemotherapy for control of bancroftian filariasis through community participation: Comparative efficacy of a low monthly dose and medicated salt. *Trans R Soc Trop Med Hyg* 1996; *99*:74–79.

Meyrowitsch DW et al. Long-term effect of three different strategies for mass diethylcarbamazine administration in bancroftian filariasis: Follow-up at 10 years after treatment. *Trans R Soc Trop Med Hyg* 2004; *98*:627–634.

Molyneux DH et al. Mass drug treatment for lymphatic filariasis and onchocerciasis. *Trends Parasitol* 2003; *19*:516–522.

Moore L et al. *Baylisascaris procyonis* in California. *Emerg Infect Dis* 2004; *10*:1693–1694.

Moulia-Pelat JP et al. Associations de l'ivermectine et de la diethylcarbamazine pour obtenir un meilleur controle de l'infection en filariose lymphatique. *Parasite* 1996; *3*:45–48.

Nguyen NL et al. Control of bancroftian filariasis in an endemic area of Polynesia by ivermectin 400 μg/kg. *Trans R Soc Trop Med Hyg* 1996; *90*:689–691.

Nicolas D. New tools for diagnosis and monitoring of Bancroftian filariasis parasitism: The Polynesian experience. *Parasitol Today* 1997; *13*:370–375.

Norões J et al. Occurrence of living adult *Wuchereria bancrofti* in the scrotal area of men with microfilaremia. *Trans R Soc Trop Med Hyg* 1996; *90*:55–56.

Ogata K et al. Short report: Gnathostomiasis in Mexico. *Am J Trop Med Hyg* 1998; *58*:316–318.

Ogunniyi TAB et al. Disinfectants/antiseptics in the management of guinea worm ulcers in the rural areas. *Acta Trop* 2000; *74*:33–38.

Ottesen EA, Ramacfhadran CP. Lymphatic filariasis infection and disease: Control strategies. *Parasitol Today* 1995; *11*:129–131.

Ottesen EA. Major progress toward eliminating lymphatic filariasis. *N Engl J Med* 2002; *347*:1885–1886.

Partono F et al. Towards a filariasis-free community: Evaluation of filariasis control over an eleven-year period in Flores, Indonesia. *Trans R Soc Trop Med Hyg* 1989; *83*:821–826.

Pozio E, La Rosa G. *Tichinella murrelli* n.sp: Etiological agent of sylvatic trichinellosis in temperate areas of North America. *J Parasitol* 2000; *86*:134–139.

Pozio E et al. Taxonomic revision of the genus *Trichinella. J Parasitol* 1992; *78*:654–659.

Pozio E et al. *Trichinella papuae* n. sp. (nematode). A new non-encapsulated species from domestic and sylvatic swine of Papua New Guinea. *Int J Parasitol* 1999; *29*:1825–1839.

Pozio E et al. *Trichinella zimbabwensis* n.sp. (nematode): A new non-encapsulated species from crocodiles (*Crocodylus niloticus*) in Zimbabwe also infecting mammals. *Int J Parasitol* 2002; *32*:1787–1799.

Pozio E et al. *Trichinella papuae* and *Trichinella zimbabwensis* induce infection in experimentally infected varans, caimans, pythons and turtles. *Parasitology* 2004; *128*:333–342.

Ranque S et al. Decreased prevalence and intensity of *Loa loa* infection in a community treated with ivermectin every three months for two years. *Trans R Soc Trop Med Hyg* 1996: *90*:429–430.

Regis L et al. Efficacy of *Bacillus sphaericus* in control of the filariasis vector *Culex quinquefasciatus* in an urban area of Olinda, Brazil. *Trans R Soc Trop Med Hyg* 2000; *94*:488–492.

Rojas-Molina N et al. Gnathostomosis: An emerging foodborne zoonotic disease in Acapulco, Mexico. *Emerg Infect Dis* 1999; *5*:264–266.

Rouseere GP et al. Raccoon roundworm eggs near homes and risk for larva migrans disease, California communities. *Emerg Infect Dis* 2003; *9*:1516–1522.

Roy BT et al. Pulmonary dirofilariasis in California. *West J Med* 1993; *158*:74–76.

Saint André Av et al. The role of endosymbiotic *Wolbachia* bacteria in the pathogenesis of river blindness. *Science* 2002; *295*:1892–1895.

Sato H et al. Five confirmed human cases of gnathostomiasis nipponica recently found in northern Japan. *J Parasitol* 1992; *78*:1006–1010.

Schellenberg RS et al. An outbreak of trichinellosis due to consumption of bear meat infected with *Trichinella native*, in 2 northern Saskatchewan communities. *J Infect Dis* 2003; *188*:835–843.

Sheuoy RK et al. Ivermectin for the treatment of periodic malayan filariasis. A study of efficacy and side effects following a single oral dose and retreatment at six months. *Ann Trop Med Parasitol* 1992; *86*:271–278.

Slom TJ et al. An outbreak of eosinophilic meningitis caused by *Angiostrongylus cantonensis* in travelers returning from the Caribbean. *N Engl J Med* 2002; *346*:668–675.

Taylor HR et al. Reliability of detection of microfilariae in skin snips in the diagnosis of onchocerciasis. *Am J Trop Med Hyg* 1989; *41*:467–471.

Theis JH et al. Case report: Unusual location of *Dirofilaria immitis* in a 28-year-old man necessitates orchiectomy. *Am J Trop Med Hyg* 2001; *64*:317–322.

Wariyapola D et al. Second case of ocular parastrongyliasis from Sri Lanka. *Trans R Soc Trop Med Hyg* 1998; *92*:64–65.

Weil GJ et al. Parasite antigenemia without microfilaremia in bacroftian filariasis. *Am J Trop Med Hyg* 1996; *55*:333–337.

Witte MH et al. Lymphatic abnormalities in human filariasis as depicted by lymphangioscintigraphy. *Arch Intern Med* 1993; *153*:737–744.

CHAPTER

10

Arthropods and Human Disease

Arthropods are as intimately associated with humans' welfare as any other animals. The economic importance of this group to agriculture, in terms of both beneficial and destructive effects, can hardly be overemphasized. In addition, many species have a direct relationship to human health and well-being. This is not a textbook of medical entomology, and it is not our purpose to consider this subject in detail, but we will discuss a few of the more important roles assumed by arthropods in their relation to disease in humans. The majority of arthropods function indirectly in human disease, which they transmit but do not produce; some species are true parasites, whereas others may inflict direct injury by their bites, stings, or other activities. Some species are both parasites and vectors of disease. For the purposes of discussion, one may conveniently divide the arthropods of medical importance into two groups: those that are true parasites and all others that in different ways affect health or well-being.

Arthropods as Parasites

THE ITCH MITE

Sarcoptes scabiei

The itch mite, *S. scabiei* (Fig. 10-1), is cosmopolitan in distribution and thoroughly democratic in its choice of victims. The global prevalence is about 300 million cases. It parasitizes both domestic animals and humans, causing a disease known as scabies in humans and mange in animals. The female mite is larger than the male and measures a little less than 0.5 mm in length. The adult mites enter the skin, digging sinuous burrows in the upper layers of the epidermis. Eggs (Fig. 10-2) deposited in the burrows hatch after 3 or 4 days into larvae, which excavate new burrows and mature in about 4 days. Preferred sites of infestation are the interdigital (Fig. 10-3) and popliteal folds, the groin, and the inframammary folds. Many other parts of the body may also be involved. The activities and secretions of the mites cause intense itching of the affected areas. Very small vesicles may be seen on the skin surface. Scratching may result in bleeding and scab formation, frequently followed by secondary bacterial infection. The skin disease seen in scabies results from a developing delayed (type IV) hypersensitivity. Histologic studies show a dense cellular infiltrate in the perivascular areas, spreading into the epidermis near the advancing mites. Most of the infiltrating cells are mononuclear T cells; macrophages and B cells are less numerous. The incubation period, normally from 2 to 6 weeks, may be as little as 1 to 4 days in persons sensitized by prior exposure. A generalized dermatitis with extensive scaling and crusting, referred to as crusted or Norwegian scabies, may occur in immunodeficient individuals.

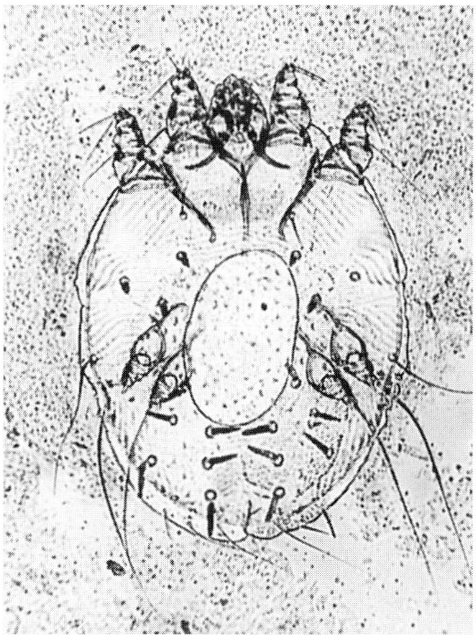

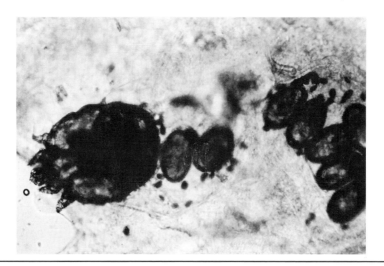

FIGURE 10-1 ■ *Sarcoptes scabiei,* adult female. (Photomicrograph by Zane Price.)

FIGURE 10-2 ■ Skin scrapings show adult and eggs of *Sarcoptes scabiei.* (From Reeves JR. *Clinical Dermatology Illustrated*, Philadelphia, 1984, MacLennan & Petty.)

Such infections have been reported in a patient with adult T-cell leukemia, in transplant patients, and in patients with AIDS and other immune deficiency states. Thousands to millions of mites may infest these patients. A hospital outbreak of scabies in Spain, involving 35 individuals, stemmed from two AIDS patients with crusted scabies. Transmission of the mites is accomplished by direct contact with infected persons or with their clothing or bedding. Spread of the infection to different parts of the body occurs through scratching and manual transfer of the mite by the afflicted individual. The infection may also be acquired from infected domestic animals, but there appear to be different strains of the mite, having distinct host preferences, so that an infection acquired from domestic animals is usually of short duration in humans.

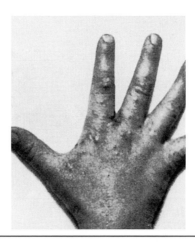

FIGURE 10-3   ■   Scabies lesions on hand. (Courtesy Dr. Hamnett A. Dixon.)

While infection with *S. scabiei* may end spontaneously after a few months, chronic cases do occur; in such cases the parasites are less numerous and consequently more difficult to find. The only way in which a definitive diagnosis of scabies can be made is by finding the parasites or their eggs. Because of their location under the surface of the skin (Fig. 10-4), scrapings must be made of the infected areas. Before scrapings are made it is best to examine the skin surface with a hand lens to find the minute burrows of the mite. While eggs may be found in any portion of a recent excavation, the adult mite is most frequently recovered from the terminal parts of a fresh burrow. It is therefore best to make scrapings in these regions. The material obtained in this fashion is placed on a microscope slide, cleared by adding one or two drops of a 20% solution of potassium hydroxide, covered with a coverslip, and examined under the low power of the microscope. However, potassium hydroxide solutions eventually will dissolve the mites and their eggs. Thus, alternatively, mineral oil may be applied to the skin before scraping. This enables organisms and eggs to adhere better to the needle or blade and the microscope slide, and mineral oil will not dissolve mites or eggs. Other methods that have been proposed for obtaining specimens, but that appear to be less useful than scraping, include the use of cellophane tape and various synthetic glues.

Treatment. For adults with noncrusted scabies, the synthetic pyrethrin, permethrin, as a 5% cream (Elimite) and gamma benzene hexachloride (lindane), 1%, are equally effective. Because of potential neurotoxicity, the use of lindane should be restricted to patients without history of neurologic disease, and is relatively contraindicated in pregnant or lactating women. The use of 10% crotamiton, N-ethyl-o-crotonotoluidide (Eurax) cream, is suggested for infants under 2 months of age, but is generally considered less effective than permethrin or lindane. Sulfur (6%) ointment is also effective, but may require more than one application, is messy, has an unpleasant odor, and stains clothing. The scabicide should be applied to all skin surfaces from the top of the head to the soles of the feet in infants, children, and the elderly. It is generally unnecessary to treat the heads of younger adults. Whichever drug is used should be applied for 8 to 12 hours and then washed off; treatment should be repeated in 1 week if live mites or eggs are still present.

For patients with crusted (Norwegian) scabies, permethrin, 5%, is usually effective, but in those who are immunocompromised, it may be necessary to combine the drug with the anthelminthic drug ivermectin, given in a single oral dose of 200 mcg per kilogram of body weight. Lindane should be used with caution because repeated applications may be necessary in these patients, who may also need crust removal with a keratolytic agent such as 3% to 6% salicylic acid in petrolatum if initial treatment is ineffective. Sulfur (6%) ointment is also effective.

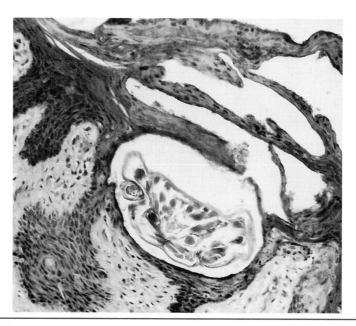

FIGURE 10-4 ▪ Section through skin containing *Sarcoptes scabiei.* (Photomicrograph by Zane Price.)

Proper treatment of all fomites is essential. They may be washed and then dried for at least 10 minutes at 50° C (122° F), dry cleaned, or stored in closed plastic containers for 7 days.

HAIR FOLLICLE MITES

Demodex spp.

The follicle mites, *D. folliculorum* (Fig. 10-5) and *D. brevis*, live in the hair follicles and sebaceous glands, especially of the face, nose, and eyelids. Both species are similar in appearance, although *D. brevis* is somewhat shorter in length. Rarely do the mites elicit a reaction in humans; nonetheless, they may be associated with acne, comedones (blackheads), or localized keratitis. Related species of *Demodex* produce demodectic mange in certain domestic animals, particularly dogs. Human *Demodex* infections rarely require treatment. Useful therapy is 1% gamma benzene hexachloride in an ointment base.

MITES OF NONHUMAN HOSTS

Chigger Mites

The larvae of several trombiculid mites are responsible for a condition known as chiggers in humans. The minute six-legged larvae are ectoparasites of various vertebrates; the eight-legged nymphs and adult mites are predators on other small arthropods or their eggs. Chiggers that are important in North America include the larvae of *Eutrombicula alfreddugesi* and *Eutrombicula splendens*. In Europe the important species is *Trombicula autumnalis*, the harvest mite.

Chiggers do not burrow into the skin, nor do they suck blood. Rather, they attach to the surface of the skin using their hooked mouth parts and feed on tissue fluids. Chiggers tend to attach to the skin where clothing is tight or restricted—ankles, legs, groin, waistline, armpits. After prolonged feeding, the engorged chiggers fall to the ground, where they undergo nymphal and adult development.

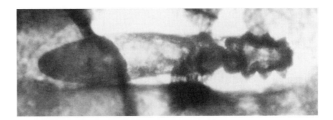

FIGURE 10-5 ▬ *Demodex folliculorum* from ulcer on forehead (acid-fast stain).

Saliva injected by the mites produces an intense pruritus and severe dermatitis, especially in persons sensitized by prior infestations. Within 24 hours red maculopapular lesions develop around the larva, which may be visible in the center of the reddened swollen area. Itching begins early in sensitized persons, but in those not previously sensitized it may not occur until a few hours after the chiggers detach. Loss of sleep and secondary bacterial infection may result from scratching. Bluish or purple ecchymoses may persist for weeks or months.

Treatment for the irritating dermatitis caused by chiggers is usually topical and palliative. Home remedies include rubbing alcohol, household ammonia, camphorated oil, and baking soda; nail polish may even offer relief from itching. Various lotions containing benzocaine in 3% to 5% strength may be somewhat more effective. The use of repellents, applied to the skin and clothing, is recommended for persons going into chigger-infested areas. The treatment of clothing with permethrin, $0.125 \ g/cm^2$, has been shown to provide protection against chigger infestation under military field conditions (Breeden et al., 1982). Permethrin acts as a toxicant rather than a repellent; apparently, chiggers are prevented from biting as a result of rapid intoxication. Permethrin retains its effectiveness for several days in treated clothing and was found to be nonirritating and odor-free (the use of clothing treated with *N*, *N*-diethyl-m-toluamide [DEET] or with M-1960, the military clothing repellent mixture, causes discomfort).

Trombiculid mites are also important as vectors of human disease. Scrub typhus, caused by *Rickettsia tsutsugamushi*, is transmitted from rodents to humans by larvae of several species of *Leptotrombidium*.

OTHER MITES THAT CAUSE DERMATITIS

A number of other mites attack the skin of humans and cause dermatitis: the rat mite, *Ornithonyssus bacoti*; mouse mite, *Liponyssoides sanguineus*; chicken mite, *Dermanyssus gallinae*; and straw itch mite, *Pyemotes ventricosus*. An outbreak of dermatitis in Austin, Texas, was traced to *Pyemotes*-infested decorative wheat being sold by an imported-goods retail store. *L. sanguineus* is the natural vector for rickettsialpox, caused by *Rickettsia akari*, in humans. Other dermatitis-producing mites are species of *Glycyphagus* (grocery mites), *Tyrophagus* (copra mites), and *Acarus* (cheese mites). These dermatitis-producing mites can be effectively eliminated by topical application of 1% gamma benzene hexachloride ointment or lotion.

MITES THAT CAUSE ALLERGY

The house dust mites, mainly *Dermatophagoides farinae* in North America and *D. pteronyssinus* in Europe, are responsible for an allergic condition known as house dust allergy. These mites have been shown to cause asthma, especially in children. Cockroach allergen also has been shown to play an important role in causing illness among inner-city children with asthma. A survey of houses for dust mites in Atlanta, Georgia, revealed that more mites were present in dust samples from furniture and bedding than from floors. Relative humidity also affected the number of mites present: the higher the humidity, the more mites. *D. pteronyssinus* was present in all houses surveyed and dominant in 11 of 20. *D. farinae* was found in 17 of 20 houses and was dominant in six. The 20 children in this study with asthma all had high titers of IgE antibody with either *D. farinae* or *D. pteronyssinus* radioallergosorbent tests (RAST). A study in Oxfordshire, England, demonstrated that wet vacuum cleaning carpets was more effective than dry vacuum cleaning in reducing house dust mite allergens.

LICE

Pediculus humanus

The human body or head louse, *P. humanus* (Fig. 10-6), is found wherever personal or general hygiene is at a low level. Lice are dorsoventrally flattened insects, sufficiently large to be detected easily with the naked eye. Males are about 2 mm, females 3 mm, long. The whole life cycle occurs on the human host. The subspecies, or biologic races, are commonly recognized.

P. humanus capitis infests the scalp. The female lice deposit their eggs on the hair, where they are firmly attached. The eggs or nits are quite small and glistening white and may be seen with the naked eye. Because nits also fluoresce under ultraviolet light, Wood's light, used in diagnosis of dermatologic conditions, is a useful tool for screening large groups of people. About 10 days after deposition they hatch into nymphs, which are structurally quite similar to the adults and mature in about 2 weeks. Both nymphs and adults feed on blood obtained by their piercing mouth parts and a pumping device located in the pharyngeal region. From 6 to 12 million individuals are infested with head lice yearly in the United States, with 72% being children who usually get the infestation from schoolmates.

The body louse, *P. h. humanus* (frequently called *P. h. corporis*), lives on the protected parts of the body. Its life history is similar to that of the head louse, which it closely resembles, although it is slightly larger. While distinct habitat preferences characterize these two varieties, the lice may be found on other parts, particularly in cases of heavy infestation. When searching for body lice it is best to examine the clothing rather than the skin surface, since the lice remain on clothing when such articles are removed or discarded.

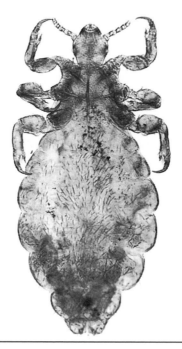

FIGURE 10-6 ▪ *Pediculus humanus.* (Photomicrograph by Zane Price.)

Head or body lice are transferred from one person to the next by direct contact or by contact with clothing, hats, or hair from "lousy" individuals. The body louse may survive for more than a week in discarded clothing. Cloth-covered seats in theaters, railway carriages, and other public places may be a source of infestation. Lice are quite sensitive to high environmental temperatures and abandon a host who has a fever. This is important in the transmission of louse-borne diseases listed in Table 10-1 on p. 349.

Phthirus pubis

The pubic, or crab, louse, *P. pubis* (Fig. 10-7), usually is found on the hairs of the genital region but may occur elsewhere on the body. *Phthirus* is somewhat shorter and broader than *Pediculus*, measuring up to 2 mm in length. It possesses powerful legs, especially adapted to attachment to the hair, on which the eggs are laid. The entire life is spent on the host, and the life cycle is completed in 30 to 40 days. Transmission is by contact with infested individuals or less commonly their clothing. While the head louse moves about rapidly, the pubic louse is much more sedentary in its habits.

Infestation with lice is generally referred to as pediculosis. Some people are very sensitive to the bites, which produce macular swellings and a great deal of pruritus. In persons who have had lice for long periods the skin may become thickened and show spots of hyperpigmentation, the maculae ceruleae. These skin changes have been referred to as vagabond's disease. Body lice are important vectors of disease, transmitting the infectious agents that cause epidemic typhus, trench fever, and the louse-borne variety of relapsing fever. The role of head lice in this regard is apparently negligible, while the pubic louse has not been incriminated in disease transmission.

Treatment. Persons infested with body lice generally require no treatment other than removal and decontamination of infested clothing. Clothing may be decontaminated by laundering at 50° C (122° F) for 30 minutes, dry-cleaning, or storage in a closed plastic container for 2 weeks.

For many years, application of 1% gamma benzene hexachloride (lindane) lotion or shampoo was the mainstay of treatment for head and crab louse infestation. However, because of its potential toxicity and increased drug resistance in lice, the current drug of choice is 1% permethrin (Nix) in a cream rinse. Permethrin is a synthetic pyrethrin. Nix is applied to the hair for 10 minutes, washed out, and followed by regular shampooing and rinse. A second application is recommended a week later to kill hatching nymphs.

An alternative treatment is use of the pyrethrin-based shampoo, RID (0.3% pyrethrins plus 3% piperonyl butoxide). A number of slightly different formulations, with different trade names, are also available. RID is applied to the hair in the same manner as Nix. A second application is recommended 7 days later. Nix and RID are the drugs of choice and alternative, respectively, for all adult and pediatric patients (Hitchcock et al., 1996; Jablon and Schneider, 1995). Treatment failures have been reported for both drugs. 5% malathion lotion (Ovide) has been used successfully to treat permethrin-resistant head lice (Yoon et al., 2003).

A study in Alexandria, Egypt, showed that a single application of ivermectin, 0.8% in liquid form, was effective in curing head lice infestation within 48 hours (Youssef et al., 1995). Ivermectin, two doses of 200 mcg/kg body weight 10 days apart, has also been used in mass treatment to control intestinal helminth infections and parasitic skin diseases including pediculosis and scabies (Heukelbach et al., 2004b).

Nits are relatively resistant to all pediculicides; thus, their removal by use of a fine-toothed comb is an important adjunct to therapy. Head and crab lice do not generally infest clothing.

FLY LARVAE THAT CAUSE MYIASIS

Myiasis, or infestation with fly larvae, is common in domestic and wild mammals all over the world. In humans, myiasis is a relatively frequent occurrence in rural regions where people are in close contact with domestic animals. Many different species of flies produce myiasis. While some of them require a host for larval development, many are opportunists only, able to develop in living animals if the occasion presents itself. Infection with fly larvae may occur when flies deposit eggs or first-stage larvae on the body or its apertures. The portions of the body affected vary with the habits and preferences of the species of fly and may depend also on other factors. An open wound or lesion, for example, may attract certain flies, which then deposit their eggs or larvae in the area of the injury. They develop and grow, establishing an infection. Larvae of certain other species invade the unbroken skin. Some gain access to the body via the nose or ears. If eggs are deposited on the lips, within the mouth, or on food, they may be swallowed and develop in the stomach or intestine, giving rise to gastric or intestinal myiasis. Genitourinary myiasis may occur when certain flies have the opportunity to oviposit on the genitourinary orifices.

In view of the large number of different myiasis-producing flies and because of the diversity in life cycle requirements, it seems best to discuss the more important species only, emphasizing their host relations and sites of predilection rather than their taxonomic affinities. One may conveniently assign the various species to three groups or categories. The first of these, the so-called specific group, includes species that require a host to complete larval development; the second or semispecific group includes species that develop in a host if entry is facilitated by the presence of wounds or sores but that can complete development without a host. The third category includes accidental invaders that usually complete larval development without a host but may in rare instances develop in one.

Specific Myiasis

Flies that require a host for the development of their larval stages belong to a large number of different species that habitually parasitize animals. Important among them are the various botflies, including the human bot, *Dermatobia hominis*, found in humid areas of Mexico and Central and South America. The female fly attaches her eggs to the abdomen of bloodsucking flies or mosquitoes. When this transport host feeds on a human or another mammal, the eggs hatch and the young larvae bore through the skin. As the larva grows, a lesion develops (Fig. 10-8), which may be quite painful. Larval development (Figs. 10-9 and 10-10) requires 6 to 12 weeks, after which the mature third-stage larva (Fig. 10-11; see Fig. 10-10) emerges from the host, falls to the ground, and pupates in the soil. Several other insects as well as ticks have been shown to carry eggs of *D. hominis* and to transport them to humans or domestic animals.

The Tumbu fly, *Cordylobia anthropophaga*, of tropical Africa is the major cause of cutaneous myiasis in residents and travelers to endemic areas. Eggs are laid in feces- or urine-contaminated soil or clothing or in damp clothing and bed linens. Larvae hatch within 2 to 3 days,

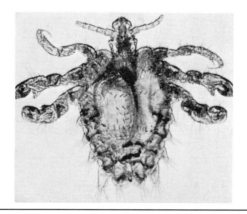

FIGURE 10-7 ▪ *Phthirus pubis.* (Courtesy Army Medical Museum.)

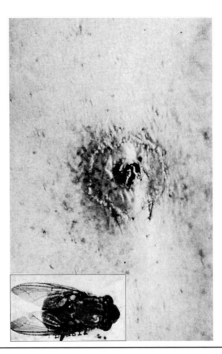

FIGURE 10-8   ■   *Dermatobia hominis* larva embedded in skin over tibia of man. The shiny spot in the center is the rear end of the larva. *Inset,* adult fly. (Courtesy Armed Forces Institute of Pathology.)

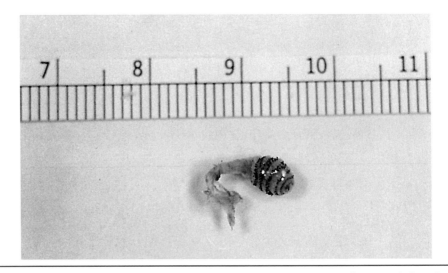

FIGURE 10-9   ■   *Dermatobia hominis,* second-stage larva, approximately 15 mm in length, removed surgically from forehead of woman after return from prolonged visit to Belize. Dark structures on bulbed end are abdominal hooklets.

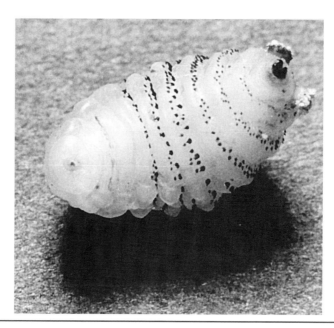

FIGURE 10-10 ■ *Dermatobia hominis,* mature third-stage larva, after emergence from furuncle on scalp of visitor to Costa Rica, approximately 9 weeks after return. Size 8 × 15 mm. (Photograph by Kevin Stephens.)

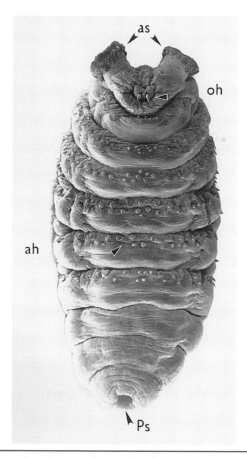

FIGURE 10-11 ■ Scanning electron micrograph of mature third-stage larva of *Dermatobia hominis* shown in Figure 10-10: ah, abdominal hooklets; as, anterior spiracles; oh, oral hooks; Ps, posterior spiracles. (SEM by Dr. David A. Henderson.)

attach to the unbroken skin of a human or animal host and penetrate, and then produce furuncular swellings. Larvae, 13 to 15 mm long, mature and leave the host in 8 to 10 days.

Another important species is the sheep botfly, *Oestrus ovis*. Worldwide in distribution, it is prevalent in sheep-raising areas. The fly deposits living larvae in the nostrils or on the eyes of sheep and goats; in humans they may develop in the conjunctival sac, producing ophthalmomyiasis. Larval development in the host takes several months.

Species of *Hypoderma*, the cattle botflies or ox warbles, are also worldwide in distribution. Eggs are deposited on the skin and hatch into larvae, which after penetrating the skin migrate throughout the body. Eventually they come to lie beneath the skin, producing local swelling. A case of ophthalmomyiasis was reported in a university farm manager in Iowa, in whom a migrating first-stage larva, most likely of *Hypoderma*, was immobilized and destroyed by laser treatment, with subsequent recovery of vision.

Horses also have botflies, which belong to the genus *Gasterophilus*. The fly deposits eggs on the hair, skin, or lips. After hatching, the larvae either penetrate the skin or are swallowed. In animals these larvae normally develop in the intestinal tract; in humans they more frequently wander beneath the skin, where they give rise to lesions similar to those produced by migration of the larvae of dog hookworms. A second-stage *Gasterophilus* larva was removed from an abdominal lesion of an infant of a rural ranching and farming area of western Washington State (Royce et al., 1999).

Some other forms producing specific myiasis are the screwworm flies. Of these, *Cochliomyia hominivorax* is prevalent in the Western Hemisphere. This fly normally parasitizes animals, depositing eggs on the unbroken skin, on the nose and ears or on wounds. The larvae are able to burrow deeply into healthy tissue and may even penetrate bone. Infection with this species is dangerous because of the vigorous activity of the larvae, which may enter the middle ear, nasal sinuses, or brain of humans. Larval development is usually completed within 10 days. Premature death of the host does not necessarily interrupt larval development, which may proceed within the dead body.

The New World screwworm fly, *C. hominivorax*, was accidentally introduced into Libya in 1988 with a shipment of infested livestock from Latin America. The infestation was restricted to an area around Tripoli, where some 14,000 livestock were reported infested and 15 human cases were confirmed. The infestation was eradicated in 1991 by using the sterile insect technique. The technique involves the mass rearing of the insect, sterilization by irradiation, and release in the infested area. When wild females mate with sterile males, no offspring are produced. Between 1990 and 1992, 1.3 billion sterile insects, produced in the Mexico–U.S. screwworm breeding plant, were transported by charter flight from Mexico to Tripoli and subsequently released in the infested zone. Although surveillance was continued until the end of 1992, the last confirmed case of New World screwworm myiasis was in April 1991. The cost of the Libyan eradication program was approximately 75 million dollars.

Other fly larvae of medical importance include the Old World screwworm, *Chrysomyia bezziana*, and several species of the sarcophagid *Wohlfahrtia*, causing human infection in Europe, the Middle East, Russia, and the United States.

One of the most interesting, although medically not nearly as important, species is *Auchmeromyia senegalensis* of tropical Africa, known as the Congo floor maggot. The adult fly lays her eggs on sand or on the floor of native huts. The larvae become active at night, crawling about in search of food. If they come upon an animal or person sleeping on the ground they will suck blood, and after the blood meal detach and hide in the soil until another meal is needed. While blood meals are necessary for the development of these larvae, their procurement seems more a predatory than a parasitic activity. It has been reported that infestation by *A. senegalensis* among the Pygmies in the Congo Republic has occurred as a consequence of their adopting a sedentary life over their former nomadic existence. A sedentary life style by the host allows the fly sufficient contact to complete its developmental cycle.

Larvae of the rodent and rabbit botfly, *Cuterebra*, have been reported to cause cutaneous myiasis in the United States. Usually, eggs are deposited on vegetation, and larvae enter their hosts through the mucous membranes of the nose, mouth, or eye. However, in human cases, larvae most likely penetrate through the skin.

Semispecific Myiasis

Among the flies that cause what is known as semispecific myiasis are some species that normally lay their eggs in decaying animal or vegetable matter. Prominent representatives of this group are species of *Lucilia*, the green-bottle flies; *Cochliomyia*, or blue-bottle flies; black bottles, belonging to the genus *Phormia*; and the blowfly, *Calliphora*. All of these are worldwide in distribution, frequenting areas of human habitation. They occasionally lay their eggs on open sores of animals or humans, especially if the sores are necrotic and malodorous. Large numbers of these flies congregate near slaughterhouses and other unclean places.

Another group that causes intestinal and other types of myiasis in humans is the flesh flies, or sarcophagids. Species of *Sarcophaga* are worldwide in distribution. They normally breed in carrion or other decomposing matter and may deposit their larvae on foods such as meat or fruit. Sarcophagid flies are larviparous, females depositing active first-stage larvae that quickly penetrate into the material on which they have been deposited. Thus, ingestion of contaminated food may be a source of infection.

Accidental Myiasis

Flies that produce accidental myiasis have no requirement or even preference for development in a host. However, eggs may be deposited accidentally on oral or genitourinary opening and the larvae gain entrance to the intestinal or genitourinary tract. *Musca domestica*, the housefly; *Fannia*, or latrine flies (Fig. 10-12); certain species of flesh flies; green- or blue-bottle flies; and many others may produce accidental myiasis.

One of the more striking species, *Eristalis tenax*, usually deposits eggs in manure, in rotting animal matter, or about privies. The larvae, known as rat-tailed maggots (Fig. 10-13), have a long, slender tail and by their peculiar appearance frequently attract attention. Human cases of intestinal and other types of myiasis due to this fly are on record; however, the presence of rat-tailed maggots in stool specimens may also be the result of contamination after the specimen has been passed.

Nosocomial Myiasis

Myiasis in hospitalized patients occurs with some frequency. Bedridden patients with open wounds or sores may become infested if flies are about. It is therefore important to keep the

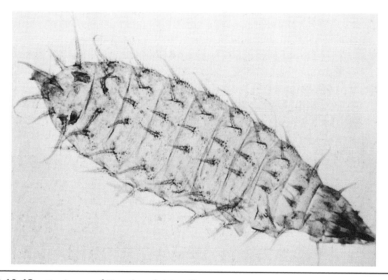

FIGURE 10-12 ■ Larva of *Fannia*, a latrine fly.

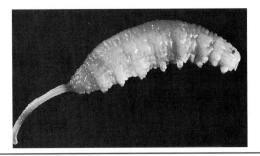

FIGURE 10-13 ■ The rat-tailed maggot, *Eristalis tenax*. (Photograph by Zane Price.)

rooms of such patients free of flies. Two cases of nosocomial infection were reported from Kuwait University Teaching Hospital. In one, *Lucilia* larvae caused nasopharyngeal myiasis, and in the other, *Megaselia* larvae produced wound myiasis (Hira et al., 2004).

Diagnosis of Myiasis

In view of the different types of myiasis caused by many diverse species of flies, it is impractical to present an adequate description of all the signs and symptoms of human infection. The clinical aspects of myiasis vary with the regions affected, with the species of fly involved, and with the numbers of maggots present. The possibility of maggot infection or infestation is frequently overlooked. The symptoms of intestinal myiasis are not specific, and neither are those of urinary myiasis. Cutaneous myiasis should be suspected in a patient with painful, indolent ulcers or furuncle-like sores of long standing. In addition, certain botfly larvae may give rise to dermal lesions similar to those of creeping eruption.

Nasal myiasis often causes obstruction of the nasal passages, severe irritation, and in some cases facial edema and fever. Death is not uncommon. Equally dangerous is aural myiasis, in which the patient may complain of crawling sensations and buzzing noises. A foul-smelling, purulent discharge may be present. If located in the middle ear, the larvae may find their way into the brain. Ophthalmomyiasis is not uncommon and is accompanied by severe irritation, edema, and pain.

A definitive diagnosis of myiasis can be made only on finding the larvae, which should be removed and kept for identification. If live maggots are obtained, they should be placed on a dish of raw meat in a glass jar containing moist sand to the height of 5 cm or more. The jar is then tightly plugged with cotton and allowed to stand at room temperature. The maggots will burrow into the meat and remain there for some time, depending on their stage of development. They will eventually leave the meat and enter the sand in order to pupate. At this time, the meat should be removed and the jar examined periodically for the presence of emergent flies. A good substitute, usually available in a hospital laboratory, is a Petri dish containing blood agar, in which maggots seem to thrive. Precise identification of the species necessitates examination of the adult fly and, as a rule, cannot be made on larvae alone. Familial, and in some cases, generic determination can be accomplished on the basis of larval morphology. Important differential characters are provided by a pair of dark-colored chitinous plates situated at the posterior end of the larva. These are the stigmal plates (Fig. 10-14), which contain the respiratory apertures or spiracles, arranged in a pattern characteristic of the particular group of flies. If stigmal plates are to be examined, they must be cut off with a sharp scalpel or razor blade and placed on a slide, and their structure is then observed under the microscope. While a good deal of information can thus be obtained by relatively inexperienced workers, it is always desirable to refer specimens of larvae or even adult flies to an experienced entomologist for identification.

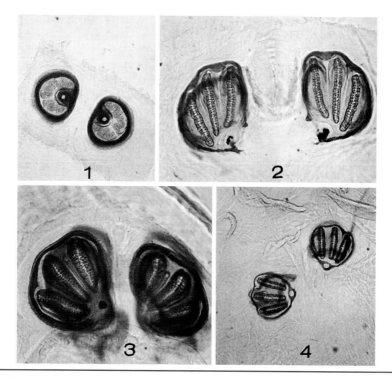

FIGURE 10-14 ■ Stigmal plates of fly larvae. *1, Musca; 2, Sarcophaga; 3, Cochliomyia; 4, Phaenicia.* (Photographs from material furnished by Dr. Ralph A. Barr.)

The Use of Maggots in Medicine

A discussion of myiasis should not fail to include mention of the medicinal use of fly maggots. Surgeons in Napoleon's armies were the first to recognize that wounded soldiers with blowfly infestation were much more likely to survive than the wounded without myiasis. During the American Civil War, army surgeons deliberately put blowfly maggots into wounds to clean away decayed tissue. The maggots consumed devitalized tissues and in doing so perhaps reduced bacterial activity and the chance of secondary infection. Blowfly maggots were used frequently for the débridement of deep wounds in soldiers, and after World War I they were used for similar purposes in civilian practice. Eventually, flies were reared under sterile conditions and used in the treatment of chronic osteomyelitis. More recently it has been shown that *Proteus mirabilis*, present in maggot salivary glands, produces substances that kill pathogenic bacteria and promote wound healing.

THE CHIGOE FLEA

Tunga penetrans

The chigoe or sand flea, *T. penetrans* (Fig. 10-15), parasitizes many different kinds of warm-blooded animals, including humans. It is found in tropical and subtropical regions of America as well as in Africa and the Far East, where it has been introduced from the New World. Chigoe fleas are relatively small, measuring no more than 1 mm. While the males and virgin females behave in the usual manner of fleas, the fertilized female has the distressing habit of burrowing into the skin, preferably under the toenails (Fig. 10-16) or between the toes, where she feeds on tissue fluids and blood. As the eggs develop, the embedded female becomes progressively larger until the abdomen assumes a nearly spherical shape. At this time,

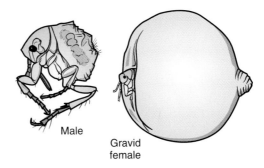

Male

Gravid
female

Tunga penetrans (chigoe)

FIGURE 10-15 ■ *Tunga penetrans,* male and female. (Modified from Hunter GW, Swartzwelder JC, Clyde DF. *Tropical Medicine,* ed 5, Philadelphia, 1976, WB Saunders.)

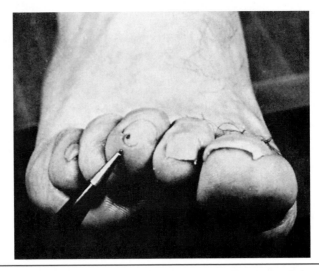

FIGURE 10-16 ■ The chigoe flea, *Tunga penetrans,* embedded in skin below nail. (Courtesy Dr. T. H. G. Aitken.)

a part of the abdomen is seen to protrude slightly beyond the skin surface. Mature eggs, sometimes as many as 100, are expelled to the outside and continue their development in the soil. The female eventually drops out of the host.

Infection with chigoe fleas is extremely irritating and usually produces inflammation and ulceration; the latter is primarily due to the development of secondary infection. Diagnosis is made by detecting the dark portion of the flea's abdomen on the skin surface. Surgical removal of the flea is indicated.

A study in an impoverished community in northeast Brazil identified 16 persons infested with a high number of sand fleas (Feldmeier et al., 2003). Each patient had greater than 50 lesions and showed signs of acute and chronic inflammation, ulceration, nail loss, and difficulty in walking. In another Brazilian study, 47 individuals entering an endemic area were examined for *T. penetrans* for a period of 6 weeks (Heukelbach et al., 2004a). Virtually 100% of the individuals were infested by the end of the third week. Studies have shown prevalences between 16% and 55% in typical endemic areas.

PENTASTOMES

Pentastomes, belonging to the phylum Pentastomida, are wormlike parasites that live mainly in the respiratory passages of carnivorous reptiles, birds, and mammals. Larval development takes place within an intermediate host, which ingests embryonated eggs that occur in the sputum or feces of an infected definitive host. Intermediate hosts may be fish, rodents, rabbits, or small ungulates. Pentastomes are related to the arthropods, although they also have some annelid-like features. Pentastomes are often referred to as tongue worms because of the generalized tonguelike shape of the genus *Linguatula*. Most pentastomid species, however, are more or less cylindrical. The head of a pentastome bears what appear to be five ventral openings (actually the mouth and four hooks), hence the parasite's name.

Human infections have been reported from Africa, Europe, Asia, and the Americas, and they are common in Malaysia and Central Africa. Infection is acquired by ingesting raw vegetables or water contaminated with pentastome eggs or by consuming uncooked infected snake meat or sheep liver or visceral lymph nodes. Ingested eggs hatch in the intestine and larvae penetrate the intestinal wall and migrate to the mesenteric lymph nodes, liver, spleen, lungs, or eye where they develop into nymphs and become encapsulated. Encapsulated nymphs, often curved into a C shape and less than 1 cm in diameter (Fig. 10-17), may calcify and be visible on radiographs of the abdomen or chest. In most cases, infection usually is asymptomatic, although described clinical manifestations include inflamed and enlarged mesenteric lymph nodes, abdominal pain, jaundice, and ocular lesions. Although rare, ocular infections have been reported from the United States, Israel, and Ecuador. The latter was a case report in which the patient, a 34-year-old woman, experienced ocular pain, conjunctivitis, and visual difficulties for a period of 2 months (Lazo et al., 1999). A *Linguatula serrata* nymph was surgically removed from the anterior chamber of the eye. A few deaths have been attributed to infection with pentastomes.

In Lebanon, a clinical condition known as halzoun is caused in part by the nymphs of pentastomes. Present in the liver and visceral lymph nodes of sheep and goats, the nymphs may attach to the nasopharyngeal mucous membranes when infected raw meat is eaten. The attached nymphs provoke a pharyngitis accompanied by pharyngeal pain, coughing, sneezing, and vomiting. A similar clinical condition in the Sudan, caused by *L. serrata*, is referred to as the marrara syndrome, named after *marrara*, a favorite Sudanese dish consisting of raw sheep or goat liver and lungs. Halzoun may also be caused by the attachment to the pharyngeal mucosa of adult *Fasciola hepatica*, ingested in raw sheep or goat liver.

Several species of *Armillifer* have been reported from humans, primarily in Africa, but also in the Far East. *L. serrata*, cosmopolitan in distribution, is the pentastome most frequently encountered in human infections, and the only species described from North America. The treatment of larval pentastomiasis is unnecessary in most instances. The halzoun syndrome is self-limited in the majority of cases, although airway protection may be necessary with severe laryngeal edema.

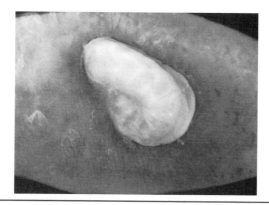

FIGURE 10-17 ■ Encysted nymph of *Armillifer armillatus* on capsular surface of liver. Specimen is from a Zairian who was a homicide victim. Note the C shape of the nymph. (Courtesy Armed Forces Institute of Pathology, #72-4561.)

Injurious Arthropods

STINGS AND BITES

A discussion of arthropods in relation to disease would not be complete without mention of their obvious and annoying activities of stinging and biting. The bloodsucking activities of fleas (Fig. 10-18), mosquitoes (see Fig. 10-34), bedbugs (Fig. 10-19), and the like, while always irritating, do not affect every person in the same manner. Some people do not suffer any appreciable harm; others react very strongly to the bites of certain arthropods, exhibiting various allergic manifestations and generalized as well as local effects. The effects of tick bites such as those of the pajaroello and related ticks (Fig. 10-20) have often been exaggerated. The pajaroello tick (*Ornithodoros coriaceus*) is found in California and Mexico. The bites may be painless but cause a mildly indurated lesion up to 20 mm in diameter, which gradually heals over a period of weeks. Rarely, the bites cause systemic reactions, with ulceration and slow healing of the lesions. It is common knowledge that some persons are not unduly affected by flea bites but may be very sensitive to the bites of mosquitoes, for example. Conversely, insects of a given kind seem to prefer certain individuals to others. In general, it may be said that the reactions to bites and stings of certain arthropods vary with the species of arthropod and with each individual person. Insects such as bees, for instance, although they inflict a painful sting, may not produce any further damage. However, in a person sensitized to bee venom, bee stings may have serious consequences and may even lead to death. In California, during a 16-year period, Hymenoptera (bees, wasps, ants) stings were responsible for 56% of the 34 deaths attributed to venomous animals. It is of interest that bee stings were once used in the treatment of arthritis; the beneficial effects ascribed to this form of therapy may possibly have been due to increased secretion of steroid hormones.

The sting of certain species of scorpions (Fig. 10-21) and the bites of centipedes and of spiders such as *Latrodectus mactans*, the black widow (Figs. 10-22 and 10-23), may be quite dangerous. The reaction to these stings and bites varies with the amount of venom injected, the site of the sting or bite, and the body size and general health of the afflicted individual. A case of black widow spider envenomation occurred through the conjunctiva when a fragment from a smashed spider lodged in the eye. The patient experienced local periorbital reaction as well as systemic effects. While healthy adults usually recover, small children or weakened persons suffer considerably and may die if proper care is not instituted immediately. It is estimated that in Mexico 1000 deaths a year are caused by scorpion strings; 75% of the victims are children younger than 5 years.

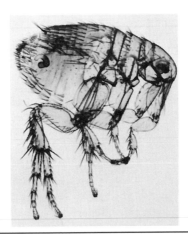

FIGURE 10-18 ■ The rat flea, *Xenopsylla cheopis,* a vector of plague. (Photomicrograph by Zane Price.)

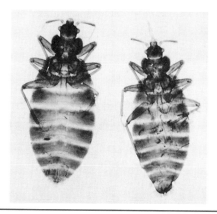

FIGURE 10-19 ■ A female and a male bedbug, *Cimex hemipterus.* (Photograph by Zane Price from material furnished by Dr. Ralph A. Barr.)

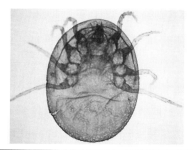

FIGURE 10-20 ■ *Ornithodoros moubata,* female, ventral view. (Photograph by Zane Price from material furnished by Dr. Ralph A. Barr.)

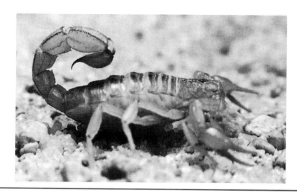

FIGURE 10-21 ■ *Centruroides sculpturatus* from Tucson, Arizona. Envenomation by this species of scorpion may be life threatening.

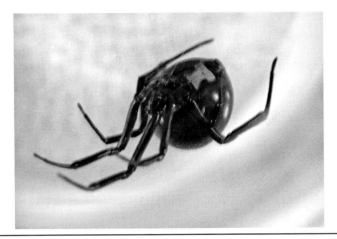

FIGURE 10-22 ■ Female black widow spider (*Latrodectus mactans*), a plump, shiny, black spider with an hourglass (red or orange) marking on the ventral surface of the abdomen, seen in its typical position of hanging upside down in the web. (Photograph by Terry Drenner of a specimen provided by Dr. Gary and Nadean Watson.)

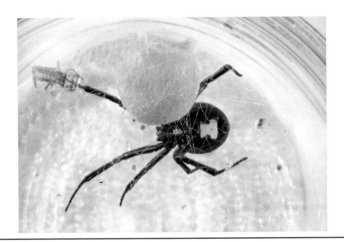

FIGURE 10-23 ■ Female black widow spider (*Latrodectus mactans*) guarding her egg sac. Object in upper left corner is a cricket nymph, food of the black widow. (Photograph by Terry Drenner of a specimen provided by Dr. Gary and Nadean Watson.)

Treatment. Hospitalization is advisable for known or suspected black widow spider bites. Muscle spasms may be severe and may require intravenous administration of calcium gluconate or other muscle relaxants. A specific antivenin is available and is valuable if given early. It is prepared from the serum of hyperimmunized horses, and patients must first be tested for horse serum sensitivity.

NECROTIC ARACHNIDISM

The bites of certain spiders may cause necrotizing skin lesions of varying extent and severity, depending on the species involved. Most important are spiders of the genus *Loxosceles*, commonly known as the brown recluse spider and the violin or fiddleback spider (Fig. 10-24). They are found in South and Central America, and several species occur in the United States. The spiders have relatively long legs and a brown body 5 to 10 mm long; some species have

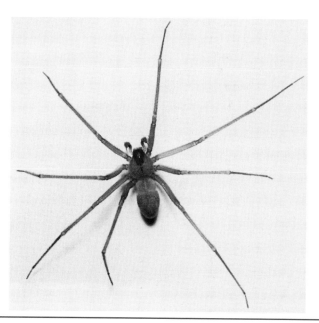

FIGURE 10-24   ■   Brown recluse spider (*Loxosceles sp.*); actual body length excluding legs is about 7 mm. (Courtesy Dr. Finley E. Russell, University of Southern California.)

an inverted fiddle-shaped marking on the dorsal cephalothorax. They are found under lumber or rocks and also near or inside human dwellings, preferring dry rather than damp habitats.

While the bite is fairly painless, mild to severe pain develops within a few hours, accompanied by erythema, vesicle formation, and itching at the site. This is frequently followed by chills, headache, and nausea. The bite of *Loxosceles laeta* may result in kidney damage and death. Viscero-cutaneous loxoscelism (VCL), in which there is systemic involvement, with intravascular hemolysis, thrombocytopenia, disseminated intravascular coagulation, and acute renal failure (ARF), has been reported in Brazil to occur in 1% to 13% of cases of *Loxosceles* bites. ARF occurs in 50% of Brazilian cases of VCL (França et al., 2002). The initial lesion ulcerates (Fig. 10-25), becomes necrotic, and unless promptly treated does not heal but continues to spread for weeks or months.

Treatment. Although most brown recluse spider bites in the United States are inconsequential and healing is uncomplicated, some persons develop a reaction that requires treatment. Nevertheless, conservative treatment is the mainstay of therapy: rest, good hydration, frequent cleansing of the bite, and tetanus prophylaxis as indicated. Analgesics are given as needed for pain. Bites should not be débrided or excised for the first 3 to 6 weeks because natural healing is excellent. Excision and skin grafting may be used for bites that have not healed in 6 to 8 weeks. Systemic steroids are not helpful in preventing or treating cutaneous necrosis but may be useful in treating hemolysis and may be administered as prednisone, 1 to 2 mg/kg per day for 3 to 5 days. Dapsone and hyperbaric oxygen, currently popular, have no proven efficacy in treatment of necrotic arachnidism. Bacterial infection accompanying brown recluse bite is uncommon, but when it does occur it should be treated specifically with antibiotics. An example is the report of a 37-year-old man who developed tularemia after being bitten by a brown recluse spider; *Francisella tularensis* presumably was introduced with the bite.

In South America, *Loxosceles* envenomation may be life threatening. In such cases, an antivenin, not available in the United States, is administered intravenously. An ELISA has been developed to confirm the diagnosis of brown recluse bite.

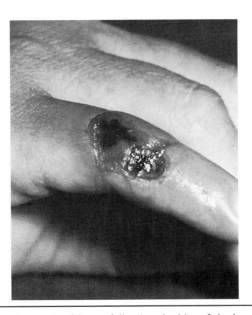

FIGURE 10-25 ■ Local necrosis of finger following the bite of the brown recluse spider, *Loxosceles reclusa*. (From Dillaha CJ, Jansen GT, Honneycutt WM, Hayden CR. North America loxoscelism: Necrotic bite of the brown recluse spider. *JAMA* 1964; *188*:33–36. Copyright 1964, American Medical Association. All rights reserved.)

Bites of the spider *Chiracanthium mildei*, commonly found in houses, also may produce necrotizing, painful lesions. However, they heal within a few weeks, are far less extensive than those caused by the brown recluse spider, and are not accompanied by systemic manifestations. Envenomation by the bite of the grass spider, *Agelenopsis aperta*, has been reported in southern California (Vetter, 1998). Clinical features included stiff neck, headache, nausea, and pain at the site of the bite, which lasted for 2 days.

It should be emphasized that the incrimination of a species of spider is not possible from the appearance of the lesion alone; the spider must be identified, and, in the absence of a specimen, a description should be obtained from the patient as soon as possible.

TICK PARALYSIS

A condition known as tick paralysis (tick toxicosis) may be induced by the bite of certain ticks. Tick paralysis has been observed in dogs, sheep, and human beings in the United States and elsewhere. Forty-three species of ticks have been found to cause tick paralysis in humans and other mammals. In North America, the occurrence of this disease coincides with the distribution of *Dermacentor* species (Fig. 10-26, *A, B*). Ixodid (Fig. 10-27) and argasid ticks cause this condition elsewhere. If the tick lodges in the occipital (or other) region of humans or animals to obtain a blood meal, an acute ascending paralysis, which can end in death, may ensue. In general, the tick must be attached for at least 4 days before symptoms begin. Prompt removal of the engorging tick usually prevents progression of the paralysis, and complete recovery takes place in a few days. An excellent review of tick paralysis may be found in the case report by Felz and colleagues (2000). As far as is known, only engorging adult female ticks cause tick paralysis. The illness is thought to be caused by a toxin in the saliva of the tick. The etiologic mechanisms of this paralysis have been studied extensively in recent years. There appear to be differences between the toxins of *Ixodes* and *Dermacentor*. Some of the effects of the toxins of *Dermacentor* and other ticks are a marked reduction in velocity of motor nerve conduction, a decrease of action potentials of nerves, and an impairment of impulse propagation of afferent fibers. In paralysis with ixodid ticks, the amplitudes of nerve action potentials apparently remain unchanged.

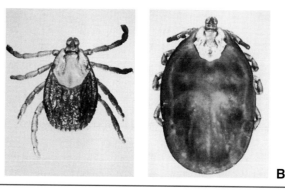

FIGURE 10-26 ■ *Dermacentor andersoni.* **A,** normal appearance. **B,** Engorged. (Photographs by Zane Price.)

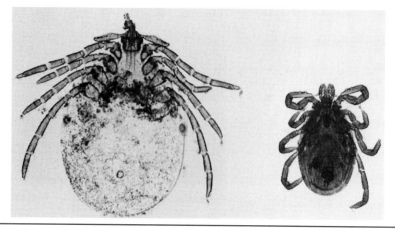

FIGURE 10-27 ■ *Ixodes scapularis,* female *(left)* and male. (Photograph by Zane Price from material furnished by Dr. Ralph A. Barr.)

A case of anaphylaxis from the bites of *Ixodes pacificus* ticks was reported in a 73-year-old man from Santa Cruz, California. An avid gardener, the man had been bitten by ticks several times a year since childhood, with reactions consisting of local erythema and induration. The last two bites, however, produced generalized urticaria, angioedema of the tongue and larynx, and hypotension. The patient responded to epinephrine, antihistamines, and corticosteroids on both occasions.

LEPIDOPTERISM AND ERUCISM

The hairs of some butterflies and moths are associated with cells or glands that secrete substances that cause severe dermatitis when the hairs are deposited on the skin. Intense itching shortly after contact is followed by papule formation, swelling, and induration. In South America, lepidopterism may occur in epidemic form during the time of year when large numbers of moths are airborne. *Hylesia alinda* moths were involved in two outbreaks of dermatitis among employees of 17 hotels in Cozumel, Mexico, during December 1989 and January 1990. An acute dermatitis characterized by erythema, pruritus, and warmth in the area of the rash occurred in 203 persons. To assess the effect of direct contact with the moths, the wings and body of a live moth were rubbed on the forearms of six volunteers. Within 5 minutes, five of the volunteers had developed intense pruritus, which was followed by an erythematous rash that lasted 3 days. During the two outbreaks, thousands of moths had appeared throughout the island.

Histamine in the urticating hairs of *Hylesia* moths has been considered to be the vasoactive mediator of the dermatitis. A case characterized by necrosis of the small vessels and nuclear fragmentation of the leukocytes in the inflammatory infiltrate suggests that antibody-mediated hypersensitivity also may be contributing to the pathogenesis of the dermatitis (Benvenuti et al., 1998).

Erucism is caused by contact with the poison hairs of different kinds of caterpillars (Figs. 10-28 to 10-30). Erythema and swelling are accompanied by burning and itching, and occasionally by nausea and fever. Usually, these symptoms disappear after 24 hours, but the lesions may persist for several days. Analysis of the nettling hair venom of *Euproctis* caterpillars has identified several serine proteases with trypsin-like and chymotrypsin-like activity and phospholipase-A activity.

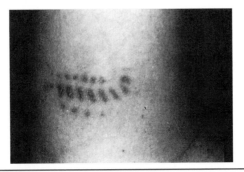

FIGURE 10-28   ■   Lesion on arm from contact with puss caterpillar, *Megalopyge opercularis*. (Courtesy Louisiana State University School of Medicine, New Orleans, Louisiana.)

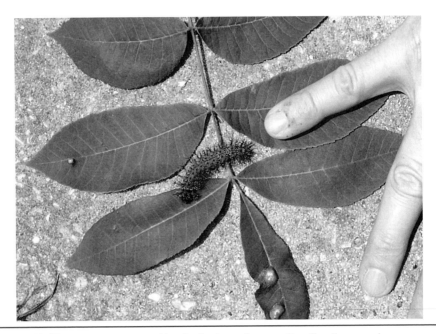

FIGURE 10-29   ■   Erucism caused by the buck moth caterpillar, *Hemileuca maia*; New Orleans, Louisiana.

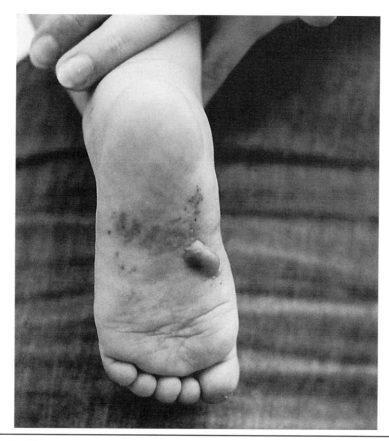

FIGURE 10-30 ■ Lesions on the foot of a child caused by the buck moth caterpillar, *Hemileuca maia*; New Orleans, Louisiana.

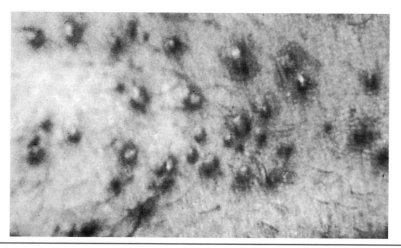

FIGURE 10-31 ■ Clusters of pustules on arm at site of fire ant stings. (From Hunter GW, Swartzwelder JC, Clyde DF. *Tropical Medicine*, ed 5, Philadelphia, 1976, WB Saunders.)

FIRE ANTS

Native fire ants are numerous in the Southeastern United States. The more aggressive imported fire ants, *Solenopsis richteri* and *S. invicta*, were introduced in the United States in 1918 and 1940, respectively, and occur in the southern states from Texas to Florida and north to the Carolinas. The fire ant attaches to a person by biting with its jaws and then it pivots around in a circle to sting in multiple sites. Their stings are painful and result in flares and wheals that may reach an inch or more in diameter, followed by the formation of fluid-filled vesicles, which often become purulent after 24 hours (Fig. 10-31). A necrotizing toxin, solenamine, has been identified as the probable active substance of fire ant venom. Whereas the venom of most Hymenoptera consists of about 50% protein, fire ant venom contains only about 1% protein. The bulk of the venom consists mainly of alkaloids, which are hemolytic and have been shown to cause histamine release and necrosis when injected into human skin. The alkaloids do not appear to be responsible for allergic reactions; rather, the proteins, of which 21 have been isolated, are the allergens. It is estimated that 16% of individuals experience systemic allergic reactions after fire ant stings. Systemic reactions to the stings may include fever, urticaria, localized edema, and necrosis. Some persons' reactions to the strings may be serious. Fatalities have been reported.

Treatment of local reactions is symptomatic. Infections, resulting from scratching the pustules, should be treated with appropriate antibiotics. Anaphylactic reactions are treated with epinephrine and antihistamines. Fire ants are controlled by the use of bait containing the insecticide tetrahydrodimethylaydrazone, which is carried into the mound by the worker ants. When ingested, the chemical will kill the queen and workers and gradually eliminate the colony over a period of several weeks. Contact insecticides sprayed onto the mounds are usually less effective because they may not kill the queen, who is hidden in a subterranean chamber.

ENTOMOPHOBIA AND DELUSIONAL PARASITOSIS

Fear of insects carried to a pathologic degree is sometimes seen and is referred to as entomophobia. Mentally disturbed patients sometimes report insect infestation to their physicians, describing the presence of minute insects on or in the skin, which give rise to biting or crawling sensations. The psychiatric syndrome is known as delusional parasitosis. The skin may be extensively excoriated by the continuous scratching of these patients, who can usually be benefited only by proper psychiatric treatment.

SPANISH FLY AND OTHER BEETLES

Among the many arthropods of interest from a medical point of view *Lytta vesicatoria*, the Spanish fly, must be mentioned. This renowned insect is actually not a fly but a beetle. It occurs in some abundance in Spain and southern France, where it is collected to be killed and ground into a power, known as cantharidin. Cantharidin is highly irritant, producing blisters when applied to the skin. Its aphrodisiac properties have long been known and exaggerated; they depend on similar irritation of the genital tract, which has sometimes produced frank hematuria.

Many other beetles may release fluids that cause mild to fairly severe skin irritation with erythema and vesicle formation. These symptoms usually disappear within a week.

Arthropods as Vectors

Arthropods are of great importance as vectors of disease-producing agents to humans and other animals. Disease transmission can be accomplished in two general ways. It may be mechanical, which means that the arthropod carries an infectious organism from one

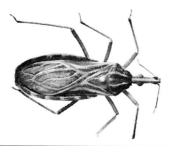

FIGURE 10-32 ■ *Rhodnius prolixus,* a vector of Chagas' disease. (Photograph by Zane Price from material furnished by Dr. Ralph A. Barr.)

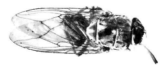

FIGURE 10-33 ■ *Glossina morsitans*, a vector of African sleeping sickness. (Photograph by Zane Price from material furnished by Dr. Ralph A. Barr.)

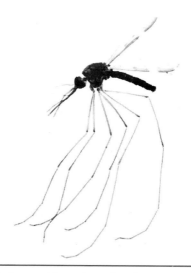

FIGURE 10-34 ■ *Anopheles quadrimaculatus,* female, a vector of malaria. (Photograph by Zane Price.)

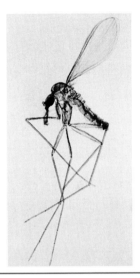

FIGURE 10-35 ■ *Phlebotomus,* a vector of leishmaniasis. (Photograph by Zane Price from material furnished by Dr. Ralph A. Barr.)

person or object to the next without serving as a host for the development or multiplication of this organism. Transmission may also be biological, in which case the infectious organism develops or multiplies within the arthropod host and is only then transmitted to the vertebrate host. Table 10-1 lists some of the arthropods of importance in disease transmission. Human granulocytic ehrlichiosis, caused by a yet-to-be described species of the rickettsia *Ehrlichia,* is the most recent addition to the list of tick-transmitted diseases. It was first reported in the United States in 1994. The organism is closely related to *E. equi,* which infects horses; *E. phagocytophila,* infecting cattle and sheep; and *E. ewingii,* the agent of granulocytic ehrlichiosis in dogs (Buller et al., 1999). Human monocytic ehrlichiosis, first reported in the United States in 1987 and now documented in 30 states, Europe, and Africa, is caused by *E. chaffeensis,* which infects mononuclear leukocytes, in contrast to the *Ehrlichia* of granulocytic ehrlichiosis, which involves predominantly neutrophils. A similar disease, caused by *E. sennetsu,* has been reported from Japan and Malaysia.

Among those diseases that may be transmitted in a mechanical manner are the bacterial enteritides. Enteric organisms may be carried by flies that feed on fecal material to foods destined for human consumption. Pathogenic bacteria may be found on the mouth parts, legs, or intestinal contents of flies feeding on excreta; some protozoan cysts may be carried in a like manner. Flies have long been thought to play a role in the mechanical transmission of those viral diseases in which the organisms are passed in the feces. Certain gnats are mechanical vectors of yaws, and it is possible that trachoma is also spread from person to person in this manner.

Some infectious organisms require an arthropod host for completion of their life cycle and also utilize this host as a vector. Some of the important biologic vectors are shown in Figures 10-32 to 10-35. Most arthropod-borne diseases are carried in this fashion, reaching the vertebrate host through the agency of the bite of the vector. Examples of such diseases are malaria and filariasis. An arthropod may serve as intermediate host for an organism that is acquired by the vertebrate host when that host ingests the infected arthropod. Direct ingestion of the invertebrate host takes place in the life cycle of *Dracunculus medinensis;* in *Diphyllobothrium* infections the arthropod host is ingested by a vertebrate second intermediate host, which in turn is eaten to pass the infection to humans or to another definitive host.

TABLE 10-1 ▪ **Some Important Diseases Transmitted by Arthropods**

Arthropod Group	Disease	Vector or Intermediate Host	Vertebrate Reservoir of Disease*	Disease Distribution
Crustacea				
Copepods	Diphyllobothriasis	*Cyclops* spp.	Dog, bear	Scandinavia, Canada, Northern United States, Finland, Russia
	Dracunculiasis (dracontiasis)	*Cyclops* spp.	Carnivores probably	Africa, India, Middle East
Crabs, crayfish	Paragonimiasis	Fresh-water crabs, crayfish	Carnivores	Asia, Africa, Philippines, Pacific Islands, South America
Arachnida				
Mites	Rickettsialpox	*Liponyssoides*	Mice	United States, Russia
	Scrub typhus (tsutsugamushi disease)	*Leptotrombidium* spp.	Rodents	Far East, Southwest Pacific, Philippines
Ticks	Babesiosis	*Ixodes* spp.	Rodents, cattle	United States, Mexico, Europe
	Boutonneuse fever (Mediterranean spotted fever)	*Rhipicephalus, Haemaphysalis, Amblyomma, Boophilus, Hyalomma*	Dog, rodents	Africa, India, Europe, Middle East
	Colorado tick fever	*Dermacentor*	Wild rodents, porcupine	Western United States
	Ehrlichiosis (human monocytic and granulocytic)	*Amblyomma, Ixodes*	Dogs, deer, rodents	United States, Europe
	Japanese spotted fever	*Dermacentor, Haemaphysalis, Ixodes*	Rodents, dogs	Japan
	Lyme disease	*Ixodes* spp.	Rodents, raccoons, deer	United States, Canada, Europe, Russia, Asia, Australia
	Q-fever	*Dermacentor, Boophilus*	Cattle, sheep, goats, bandicoot	Probably worldwide
	Relapsing fever	*Ornithodoros*	Monkeys, squirrels, rats	Africa, Asia, America, Europe
	Rocky Mountain spotted fever	*Dermacentor* spp. and other ticks	Small mammals dogs, birds	Canada, United States, Central and South America
	Sennetsu fever	*Helminths*?[†]	Helminths in fish?[†]	Japan, Malaysia
	Tick-borne viral encephalitis	*Ixodes*	Various mammals and birds	Northern Europe and Asia
	Tularemia	*Dermacentor* spp.	Rabbits	North America, Europe, Japan
Insecta				
Lice	Epidemic typhus	*Pediculus humanus*	Flying squirrels (United States)	Europe, Asia, Africa, Central America, United States
	Louse-borne relapsing fever	*Pediculus humanus*	None	Europe, Asia, Africa
	Trench fever	*Pediculus humanus*	None	Central Europe
Fleas	Cat-scratch disease	*Ctenocephalides felis*	Cats	Worldwide
	Dipylidiasis	Cat and dog fleas	Cats, dogs	Worldwide
	Plague	*Xenopsylla cheopis,* other rodent fleas	Rodents	Worldwide
	Murine typhus	*Xenopsylla cheopis,*	Rodents, opossums	Worldwide
	Murine typhus-like	*Ctenocephalides felis*	Opossums, cats	United States

Continued

TABLE 10-1 ■ **Some Important Diseases Transmitted by Arthropods—cont'd**

Arthropod Group	Disease	Vector of Intermediate Host	Vertebrate Reservoir of Disease*	Disease Distribution
Bugs	Chagas' disease (American trypanosomiasis)	*Triatoma, Panstrongylus*	Carnivores, rodents, armadillos	South America, Central America, North America
Beetles	Hymenolepiasis	Flour beetle[‡]	Mice, rats	Worldwide
Flies, gnats	African sleeping sickness (trypanosomiasis)	*Glossina* spp. (tsetse flies)	Herbivores	Africa
	Bartonellosis (Oroya fever/ verruga peruana)	*Phlebotomus* spp. (sandflies)	None	Peru, Colombia, Ecuador (1700–10,000 feet)
	Leishmaniasis (all kinds)	*Phlebotomus* spp. *Lutzomyia* spp. (sandflies)	Dogs and cats in various areas	Asia, Mediterranean, East Africa, southern Mexico, Central and South America
	Loiasis	*Chrysops* spp.	Monkeys	Tropical Africa
	Mansonelliasis	*Culicoides, Simulium* in Amazon basin	Monkeys	Africa, Central and South America, West Indies
	Onchocerciasis	*Simulium* spp. (black flies)	None	Africa, Mexico, Central and South America
	Tularemia	*Chrysops* (deer flies)	Rabbits	North America, Europe, Japan
Mosquitoes	Dengue fever	*Aedes* spp.	Monkeys	Tropics and subtropics
	Western equine	*Culex* spp.	Birds, horses	United States, Southern Canada, Argentina
	Venezuelan equine		Rodents, horses	Southern United States, Central and South America
	St. Louis } Encephalomyelitis	*Culex* spp.	Birds, horses	United States
	Eastern equine	*Aedes* and *Mansonia* spp.	Birds, horses	United States, Canada, West Indies, Central America
	Japanese B	*Culex* spp.	Birds, domestic animals	Far East
	Filariasis, bancroftian	*Culex, Aedes, Anopheles*	None	Worldwide, tropics and subtropics
	Filariasis, Malayan	*Anopheles, Mansonia*	Monkeys? cats?	India, Malaysia
	Malaria	*Anopheles* spp.	None	Worldwide
	Yellow fever	*Aedes aegypti*[‡]	Monkeys	Africa, Central and South America

*Other than humans.
[†]CDC, 2002.
[‡]Important but not only vector.

References

Benvenuti LA et al. Cutaneous leucocytoclastic vasculitis from contact with *Hylesia* moths (Lepidoptera: Saturniidae). *Trans R Soc Trop Med Hyg* 1998; *92*:428–429.

Breeden GC et al. Permethrin as a clothing treatment for personal protection against chigger mites (Acarina: Trombiculidae). *Am J Trop Med Hyg* 1982; *31*:589–592.

Buller RS et al. *Ehrlichia ewingii*, a newly recognized agent of human ehrlichiosis. *N Engl J Med* 1999; *341*:148–155.

Centers for Disease Control (CDC). Human ehrlichiosis in the United States. Centers for Disease Control and Prevention 2002; http:www.cdc.gov/ncidod/dvrd/ehrlichia/Index.htm.

Feldmeier H et al. Severe tungiasis in underprivileged communities. Case series from Brazil. *Emerg Infect Dis* 2003; *9*:949–955.

Felz MW et al. A six-year-old girl with tick paralysis. *N Engl J Med* 2000; *342*:90–94.

França FOS et al. Rhabdomyolysis in presumed viscero-cutaneous loxoscelism: Report of two cases. *Trans R Soc Trop Med Hyg* 2002; *96*: 287–290.

Heukelbach J et al. High attack rate of *Tunga penetrans* (Linnaeus 1758) infestation in an impoverished Brazilian community. *Trans R Soc Trop Med Hyg* 2004a; *98*:431–434.

Heukelbach J et al. Selective mass treatment with ivermectin to control intestinal helminthiases and parasitic skin diseases in a severely affected population. *Bull WHO* 2004b; *82*:563–571.

Hira PR et al. Myiasis in Kuwait: Nosocomial infections caused by *Lucilia sericata* and *Megaselia scalaris*. *Am J Trop Med Hyg* 2004; *70*:386–389.

Hitchcock JC et al. Head lice (*Pediculus humanus capitis*): A heady, nitpicky, and lousy problem. *California Morbidity* 1996; March:2.

Jablon L, Schneider S. Lice and scabies treatment update. *Drug Bull* 1995; Mar/Apr:5–7.

Lazo RF et al. Ocular linguatuliasis in Ecuador: Case report morphometric study of the larva of *Linguatula serrata*. *Am J Trop Med Hyg* 1999; *60*:405–409.

Meinking TL et al. The treatment of scabies with ivermectin, *N Engl J Med* 1995; *333*:26–30.

Morbidity and Mortality Weekly Report. Sexually transmitted diseases. Treatment guidelines 1985. MMWR 1985; *34*(suppl):91S–92S.

Royce LA et al. Recovery of a second instar *Gasterophilus* larva in a human infant: A case report. *Am J Trop Med Hyg* 1999; *60*:403–404.

Vetter RS. Envenomation by a spider, *Agelenopsis aperta* (Family: Agelenidae) previously considered harmless. *Ann Emerg Med* 1998; *32*:739–741.

Yoon KS et al. Permethrin-resistant human head lice, *Pediculus capitis*, and their treatment. *Arch Dermatol* 2003; *139*:994–1000.

Youssef MYM et al. Topical application of ivermectin for human ectoparasites. *Am J Trop Med Hyg* 1995; *53*:652–653.

Parasitic Infections in Immunocompromised Hosts

The most important immunodeficiency in humans is the acquired immunodeficiency syndrome (AIDS) (Reynolds et al., 2003; UNAIDS, 2004; Walker et al., 2004). Approximately 40 million people are HIV infected, with 90% of infections in sub-Saharan Africa, Asia, and South America. Co-infection with HIV and parasites is therefore common and the effects of co-infection on the outcome of both parasite and HIV infection are just now being discerned. In addition to the AIDS pandemic are other immunodeficiencies. Important among such causes are various malignancies (and, unfortunately, many of the cytotoxic drugs used to treat malignant and other diseases), the cytotoxic effects of radiation, prolonged corticosteroid therapy, and the drugs used to prevent organ transplant rejection. Patients whose immune systems are weakened for any of these reasons may more readily become infected with certain parasites.

HIV infection attacks the cells bearing the CD4 antigen and the CCR5 and CXCR4 chemokine receptors, which together allow binding and entry of HIV into T lymphocytes and macrophages, and so favor the development of infections in which cellular immunity is a major factor. Such infections are often referred to as opportunistic, to differentiate them from the usual infections that occur in immunocompetent hosts. Some innate deficiencies, such as achlorhydria and hypogammaglobulinemia, may also be important in facilitating parasitic infection. Malnutrition is an important factor in determining the severity of disease, and, as we know, malnutrition is widespread in the tropics and not unknown in temperate areas. There is evidence for suppression of helper T cells, deficient antibody responses, and decreased serum opsonic activity in protein-energy malnutrition (Keusch, 2003). A number of opportunistic parasites, which either fail to infect persons with normal immune mechanisms or cause asymptomatic to mild and self-limited infections, may cause devastating disease in persons whose cellular immunity and other protective systems are abnormal.

Looking at matters from another perspective, it has been suggested that chronic parasitic diseases (such as malaria, trypanosomiasis, schistosomiasis, and filariasis) seen in many parts of the tropics have a profound effect on the immune system and alter the host's immune response to infections such as HIV as well (Harms and Feldmeier, 2002).

If we consider only patients whose cellular immunity is weakened by HIV, we see that the opportunistic parasitic infections, such as toxoplasmosis, cryptosporidiosis, isosporiasis, and microsporidiosis, have high prevalence rates, while rates of the nonopportunistic infections, such as malaria, amebiasis, giardiasis, and schistosomiasis, are little affected. This seems to be true not only in Africa, where AIDS is prevalent and where amebic and schistosomal infections are more common, but in Europe, North America, and the

Caribbean area as well. The inclusion of other causes of immunocompromise does not greatly change the picture, although these are now of minor importance in comparison with AIDS.

Here we present an overview of the parasites that infect immunocompromised hosts. For a more extensive discussion of these parasites and of their diagnosis and treatment, the reader is referred to the appropriate sections of the text.

Organisms of Uncertain Taxonomic Status

With the DNA-based recognition of *Pneumocystis jiroveci* (formerly *P. carinii*) as a fungus—and hence its de facto transfer out of the field of parasitology—a discussion of this agent here is no longer appropriate. The reader is referred to numerous studies of pneumocystosis in the literature on AIDS, HIV, and general infectious diseases.

Blastocystis hominis, whose taxonomic position has been the subject of controversy for many decades, seems recently to have found a DNA-based home with a highly diverse protistan group, the stramenopiles (Silberman et al., 1996). The organism is widespread in the stools of a variety of populations of immunocompetent persons, with or without gastrointestinal symptoms, in at least four serologic variants. However, pathogenicity of *B. hominis* remains highly questionable, and there is no convincing evidence to suggest that it plays a more important role in immunosuppressed persons.

Protozoa

Sarcomastigophora and Ciliophora

Leishmaniasis. Overall, there is increasing evidence that visceral leishmaniasis (*L. donovani*) may be exacerbated in persons whose immunity is severely compromised by any means, including HIV/AIDS, organ transplantation, or malnutrition (Alvar et al., 1997). Leishmaniasis is exceeded only by toxoplasmosis as an opportunistic tissue parasitic infection in HIV/AIDS. It is almost always the visceral disease species of leishmania that are opportunistic infections in HIV/AIDS and not the cutaneous species. In HIV/AIDS, visceral leishmaniasis is predominantly seen in young men, reversing the usual peak of infection in children (Pratlong et al., 2003). Studies in Brazil have indicated that severely malnourished children are almost nine times as likely to develop severe visceral leishmaniasis as children in the same community who are well nourished or have only mild malnutrition. Massive infections are common in immunocompromised patients, but may occur with few or no symptoms of kala-azar, and such infections may prove refractory to treatment (Torre-Cisneros et al., 1993).

In HIV/AIDS, perhaps because of the chronicity and gradual development of the host's immunoincompetence, the effects of the viral disease on leishmaniasis are seen more in terms of greater initial susceptibility to, and hence wider prevalence of, the protozoal infection than of frank, individual virulence. Visceral leishmaniasis is becoming an important opportunistic infection in patients with AIDS, even in areas where the disease is not normally endemic (Albrecht et al., 1996). Where both cutaneous and visceral forms of leishmaniasis are endemic, the latter has even been suggested as a diagnostic criterion for AIDS. Unusual organ involvement and greater posttreatment relapse potential also may be seen (Laguna et al., 1995). In HIV-infected persons, serologic titers for leishmania are frequently low or nondiagnostic, and organisms may be difficult to demonstrate; in contrast, in some cases, peripheral blood or buffy coat examination may demonstrate amastigotes. At the same time, among 342 patients negative for HIV by Western blot analysis in Bahia, Brazil, visceral leishmaniasis was the only disease among several endemic parasitoses and other infections that gave false-positive HIV-1 results (9%) by ELISA.

Trypanosomiasis. American trypanosomiasis or Chagas' disease, the result of infection by *Trypanosoma cruzi*, is subject to modification by immunosuppression, whether due to HIV/AIDS or to other causes, both natural and iatrogenic. Infection itself with *T. cruzi* also appears to be immunosuppressive. In endemic areas, cases of cardiac transplantation (with induced immunosuppression) and of acute lymphoblastic leukemia have been complicated by either cerebral (focal), cardiac, or dermal manifestations of Chagas' disease (DiLorenzo, 1996; Gentry et al., 1994).

In HIV/AIDS, the central nervous system was involved with *T. cruzi* in 87% of one series, producing a severe, multifocal, or diffuse meningoencephalitis, clinically manifested as an expanding intracranial mass lesion; an acute, chronic, or combined myocarditis was seen in 30%. Most of these cases are interpreted as presumably due to reactivation of chronic, latent trypanosomal infection, perhaps similar to that seen in toxoplasmosis.

African trypanosomiasis has not yet been determined to be clinically affected by HIV/AIDS. Seroprevalence surveys conducted in mutually endemic areas in Africa have not indicated any epidemiologic association between the trypanosomal and retroviral diseases. However, the success of chemotherapy of both trypanosomiasis and leishmaniasis may depend on an intact immune system for clearance of the etiologic organisms.

Giardiasis. Although the flagellate *Giardia lamblia* is a common parasite in HIV-positive homosexual males due to oral-anal or penile-anal practices (odds ratio 2.9:1), it does not seem to be associated with an increase in symptoms in this group. On the other hand, prolongation of patient infection has been noted in immunosuppressed humans, and recrudescences have been demonstrated in gerbils previously infected with *G. lamblia* when injected with hydrocortisone at a time when their primary infection had waned. Moreover, persistence of cysts well beyond the 14-day fecal clearance seen in normal mice has been observed in mice infected with murine AIDS (MAIDS) virus, while *Giardia*-stimulated IL-2 and IL-4 were depressed in the MAIDS-infected group. In humans with AIDS, levels of IgG, IgM, and IgA antibodies to *Giardia* were depressed in comparison to those seen in immunocompetent controls. This was especially evident in persons in both groups who had acute symptomatic infections.

Trichomoniasis. The importance of the trichomoniasis–HIV interaction is the role of the parasite in increasing women's susceptibility to HIV infection. While the increase in susceptibility is estimated to be only two- to three-fold, the high prevalence of trichomoniasis (7 million new infections in the United States each year) results in an estimated 700 new HIV infections in the United States alone annually due to trichomoniasis (Chesson et al., 2004).

Dientamebiasis and Balantidiasis. The situation as regards the flagellate, *Dientamoeba fragilis*, or the ciliate, *Balantidium coli*, has yet to be clearly defined. In a comparison of 82 HIV-seropositive patients without diarrhea and 300 controls, one group in Argentina has reported a significantly higher prevalence of *D. fragilis* infection among the seropositive group. Although sporadic outbreaks of waterborne *Balantidium coli* infection have resulted, under favorable conditions, in relatively large numbers of cases, human infections are sufficiently rare that there have been no published observations as to any effects of immunosuppression on balantidiasis.

Amebiasis. *Entamoeba dispar* has a high prevalence rate among homosexual men, although there is no morbidity associated with this infection. It is not clear if *E. histolytica* is a substantial concern in patients with HIV/AIDS, as most studies to date have not attempted to differentiate between *E. histolytica* and *E. dispar* (Gatti et al., 1992; Haque et al., 2003; Sargeaunt et al., 1983). Nevertheless, there does not seem to be any increasing prevalence of symptomatic amebiasis in areas such as Africa, where pathogenic zymodemes are common and AIDS is widespread.

In fact, in a rural, endemic area in Tanzania, the prevalence of *E. histolytica* in HIV-positive patients was half that in HIV-negative patients (12.5% and 25.1%, respectively), although *Cryptosporidium* and *Isospora* were significantly higher in the HIV/AIDS groups. By contrast, however, a report from Argentina indicated that a group of 82 HIV-seropositive patients with diarrhea harbored a significantly higher percentage of *E. histolytica*, although no such differences were found in percentages of *Giardia lamblia, E. coli*, or *Chilomastix mesnili*. In the same study, almost equal percentages of *Dientamoeba fragilis* (25.3%) and *E. histolytica* (26.5%) were reported in the HIV-positive group (Mendez et al., 1994).

Free-Living Amebae. Opportunistic amebae of the genera *Acanthamoeba* or *Balamuthia* (a eptomyxid ameba) may produce either a granulomatous amebic encephalitis (GAE), or sinus, pulmonary, or skin infection, lacking central nervous system (CNS) involvement (Murakawa et al., 1995; Sison et al., 1995). These more indolent forms are usually seen in immunocompromised patients, although the course of acanthamoebiasis may also be acute in patients whose immune status is affected by AIDS or immunosuppressive drugs. GAE is a subacute to chronic, progressive CNS disease with an incubation period longer than 10 days, in contrast to primary amebic meningoencephalitis (PAM), a rapidly fatal CNS infection in non-immnocompromised individuals caused by *Naegleria fowleri*.

Apicocomplexa

Toxoplasmosis. From the strictly parasitologic point of view, *Toxoplasma gondii* is not a parasite of humans, but of cats, in which little disease is produced. Before the advent of the AIDS epidemic, this feline parasite had a relatively minor role in human disease in healthy individuals, although it was often far more consequential during pregnancy and in immunodeficient patients. However, owing to the high rate of asymptomatic *infection* in the adult human population, and to profound deficits in the immune system caused by HIV, *Toxoplasma* has now come into its own as a major human pathogen.

The five generally recognized classical subtypes of overt disease are congenital toxoplasmosis, with potentially severe sequelae for the infant; chronic toxoplasmic lymphadenitis, a mild and self-limited infection; retinochoroiditis; encephalomyelitis; and a local or disseminated form of the disease seen almost exclusively in (iatrogenically) immunocompromised persons. In addition, AIDS-associated toxoplasmosis (Wong et al., 1995) now encompasses multifocal involvement of the CNS, including focal abnormalities and seizures; infection of the spinal cord with transverse myelitis; a rapidly fatal panencephalitis; pulmonary disease including febrile illness with cough and dyspnea clinically indistinguishable from *P. carinii* pneumonia; ocular disease, typically a necrotizing chorioretinitis; extracerebral/disseminated toxoplasmosis; and disease caused by replication of *T. gondii* outside the CNS.

In the natural immunocompromised state in pregnancy, toxoplasmosis is potentially a serious problem for the unborn child. Maternal infection acquired in the first trimester has resulted in congenital infection in the fetus approximately 25% of the time, usually producing spontaneous abortion, stillbirth, or severe disease. If untreated, acquisition of toxoplasmosis during the third trimester increased the likelihood of congenital infection to about 65%, with many newborns having subclinical infection. However, the rates of acquired infection in pregnant women, and of congenital toxoplasmosis, appear to be decreasing, and stringent application of current diagnostic methods can markedly decrease the uncertainty of the outcome by permitting appropriate treatment of the mother. In a recent, prospective study (European Collaborative Study, 1996) of congenital toxoplasmosis in 1058 children born to women infected with HIV, only 1 child followed for a mean of 35 months developed clinical toxoplasmosis (acquired postnatally), indicating a low risk of maternal-fetal transmission of toxoplasmosis in this setting.

Toxoplasma may become encysted in the tissues without causing evident disease. Reactivation of latent infection may occur with suppression of cellular immunity. In patients requiring organ transplantation, such latent infection in transplanted tissues may be a significant problem; in most cases, transmission reportedly occurs when a seronegative recipient receives a heart from a seropositive donor. In England, among 12% to 17% of patients who became infected as a result of transplantation, 50% developed overt toxoplasmosis. In one series in the United States, 10 cases (3.4%) were reported among 290 cardiac transplants. In another cardiac transplant series, *T. gondii* infection occurred in 13% of 121 patients after transplantation, and overt clinical disease occurred in 4%. By serologic analysis, organ-transmitted infection was more frequent (61% of 18) and more often associated with acute disease than the reactivation of latent infection (7% of 69 patients). After bone marrow transplantation, on the other hand, overt toxoplasmosis appears to be due largely to reactivation in a seropositive recipient. In renal transplant patients, despite a few seroconversions, overt disease has not been a problem.

Infection with HIV leads to depletion of helper/inducer (CD4$^+$) T lymphocytes and depressed macrophage function, resulting in reactivation of latent infection. In AIDS patients, reactivation of toxoplasmosis is seen most frequently as a life-threatening encephalitis and is the most frequent cause of focal intracerebral lesions in this group: the differential diagnosis of mass or focal lesions of patients with HIV includes toxoplasmosis, 50% to 70%, with the second consideration, primary CNS lymphoma, 20% to 30%. With effective highly active antiretroviral therapy (HAART) for HIV/AIDS, CNS toxoplasmosis is much less of a problem (Samuel et al., 2002).

The median number of CD4$^+$ T lymphocytes in AIDS patients with acute toxoplasmic encephalitis was 60/μl or less, with approximately 80% of patients having a CD4$^+$ count of less than 100/μl. Nevertheless, definitive diagnosis of toxoplasmic encephalitis may be difficult, frequently resulting in empirical therapy to avoid brain biopsy. Between 20% and 47% of AIDS patients who are seropositive for *T. gondii* will ultimately develop this most serious disease, which is frequently the initial manifestation of AIDS in areas where seroprevalence rates are high (Wong et al., 1995).

In Germany and France, owing to culinary habits involving frequent consumption of raw or undercooked meats, serologic evidence of *Toxoplasma* infection may be found in 50% to 75% of the adult population; this level is equivalent to those found recently in Saudi Arabia and Ethiopia. By contrast, toxoplasmic seropositivity rates are much lower in many other parts of the world.

As in other zoonotic opportunistic infections in AIDS, the issue of pet-derived associated infections must be considered when counseling patients (Steele, 1997). Based on seroprevalence studies, approximately 30% of the cats in the United States have been infected by *T. gondii*. A summary of recommendations for the prevention of toxoplasmic encephalitis was published as a joint report by the Centers for Disease Control and Prevention (CDC) and the Infectious Disease Society of America (IDSA) in mid-1997 (Centers for Disease Control and Prevention, 1997).

Coccidiosis. Uncommon prior to the AIDS era, human disease caused by coccidian parasites of the genera *Cryptosporidium* and *Isospora* has come to be almost pathognomonic of HIV infection, and by HIV-mediated host T-cell dysfunction and T-cell–dependent B-cell dysfunction (Wittner et al., 1993). In the appropriate setting, both *C. parvum* and *I. belli* can produce profuse, watery, life-threatening diarrhea following invasion of enterocytes. The disease is most often self-limited in immunocompetent persons, exhibiting an acute illness usually lasting several days up to 2 to 5 weeks. In immunocompromised persons, by contrast, severe or chronic enteritis with profuse diarrhea is the rule. Cholangiopancreatographic changes, including biliary tract disease with common duct thickening and stenosis and acalculous cholecystitis, have also been reported in AIDS patients.

Reported prevalences of *Isospora* and *Cryptosporidium* vary geographically in both non-HIV and HIV groups, and the overall prevalence of both parasites appears to be lower in developed countries than in many developing areas of the world. Prevalences ranging from 0.2% to 3.8% among, respectively, 17,642 Australian aborigines without HIV infection and

16,953 AIDS patients in Los Angeles County, California, to double-digit levels of 20% to 30% among smaller numbers of AIDS patients in Thailand and Haiti, respectively, have been reported.

Cryptosporidiosis was first reported in humans in 1976, and even then was recognized to occur in both healthy and immunosuppressed individuals. Since that time, we have recognized that it may cause a self-limited diarrheal disease in many immunologically competent persons, and especially in children, while rarely causing severe diarrhea. In the presence of HIV, infection with *Cryptosporidium* may also, at times, be asymptomatic. However, in AIDS patients and otherwise immunocompromised hosts, the gastrointestinal symptoms are usually more severe, and cryptosporidia may be recovered from various extraintestinal sites, including the respiratory tract (Poirot et al., 1996). A hospital-acquired infection involving five of the six patients on a bone marrow transplant unit has been described, with apparent resolution of symptoms as improvement of the patients' immune functions occurred. During the 1993 outbreak of cryptosporidiosis in greater Milwaukee, Wisconsin, an estimated 403,000 residents were infected after drinking contaminated municipal water. Despite the dramatically wide spread of the parasitosis in that outbreak, illness remained significantly related to immunosuppression, and transmission ceased within 2 months of closure of the dysfunctional water plant.

Isospora belli has long been known to produce a self-limited and rather benign disease in immunocompetent persons, but with AIDS and other immunodeficiencies, it may cause severe diarrhea as is seen with *Cryptosporidium* infection. *Isospora* may also cause extraintestinal disease, having been found in mesenteric, periaortic, and mediastinal lymph nodes in a patient with AIDS. For their opportunistic pathogenicity, both parasites appear to take advantage of HIV-induced damage to the mucosal immune system, that is, the reduction of CD4$^+$ cells in the lamina propria of the gut wall. Facilitation of infection by the two agents differs according to the level of immunosuppression: *Isospora* infections are seen at a higher level of circulating CD4$^+$ lymphocytes—that is, lesser immunosuppression—than infection by *Cryptosporidium*, which appears to require a greater reduction of these cells for infection. Clinically, the two infections differ in one important aspect: *Isospora* is easily treated whereas *Cryptosporidium* is not.

Cyclosporiasis. Formerly known as a cyanobacterium-like body, *Cyclospora cayetanensis* was established as a coccidian parasite by Ortega et al. (1993, 1994). A cause of usually self-limited, watery diarrhea indistinguishable from that caused by the other coccidian enteropathies clinically, *C. cayetanensis* has been isolated from children in, and travelers to, the developing world, and from both immunocompetent adults and HIV-seropositive individuals. In immunocompromised patients with AIDS, the diarrhea may become prolonged, chronic, or recurrent (Pape et al., 1994). Since *C. cayetanensis* can be acquired through drinking water or foods washed in contaminated water, it has the potential for causing widespread outbreaks, the most dramatic of which occurred in 1996, involving 1465 cases in the U.S. linked to consumption of imported raspberries. Two more recent outbreaks involved 50 cases in Florida, associated with mesclun, a baby lettuce mixture, and 48 in Virginia, attributed to basil-pesto pasta salad; other, smaller outbreaks associated with fresh basil were also described. The potential for becoming established in the HIV-positive population under these circumstances clearly exists. A summary of recommendations for the prevention of cyclosporiasis was published as a joint report by the Centers for Disease Control and Prevention (CDC) and the Infectious Disease Society of America (IDSA) in mid-1997 (Centers for Disease Control and Prevention, 1997).

Sarcocystosis. *Sarcocystis* has not been recognized as an important enteric pathogen in HIV-infected or otherwise immunocompromised persons, but it might be expected that species for which humans are the definitive host (*S. hominis* and *S. suihominis*) would be encountered increasingly often in immunodeficient individuals. The same might be true for species of *Sarcocystis* in which humans are the intermediate host and bradyzoites are found in the tissues (Lockwood and Weber, 1989).

Malaria. There is little evidence to suggest that malaria, with the possible exception of malaria infection during pregnancy (Chai-Savaneeyakorn et al., 2002), is either more common or more severe in immunosuppressed persons. A brief report of a case of blackwater fever with 95% parasitemia due to *Plasmodium vivax* in a patient with AIDS (Katongole-Mbidde et al., 1988) stands alone in the literature, and it has been virtual dogma that HIV infection plays no role in malaria infectivity, pathogenesis, or morbidity. This perception was enhanced by a direct investigation of 484 Ugandan patients with AIDS, in whom no association could be found between HIV-1 infection and *P. falciparum* malaria in either children or adults, and no differences were found in malaria prevalence, parasite density, or response to treatment between HIV-positive and HIV-negative patients. The lack of association was further supported by a study of 3792 women at prenatal and pediatric clinics in Rwanda, in which, again, no association was found between HIV and the presence or degree of malaria parasitemia; and by the lack of an increase in splenomegaly among HIV-1 infected children in an area of Zaire holoendemic for falciparum malaria (Jackson et al., 1992).

The unknowing use of HIV-infected blood for transfusions for severe malaria has unfortunately contributed to the spread of HIV infection. As summarized most aptly by the title of one report, "Malnutrition and Malaria Gave Him Anemia, Then the Blood Transfusion Gave HIM HIV" (Addo-Yobo et al., 1992), therapeutic—frequently lifesaving—blood transfusions have had undesired and tragic side effects. In one study of 167 hospitalized children in Kinshasa, Zaire, 112 (67%) had malaria, 78 (47%) had received transfusions during the current hospitalization, and 21 (13%) were HIV-seropositive; 10 of the 11 HIV-positive malaria patients had received transfusions during the current hospitalization, and of all blood transfusions, 87% were administered to malaria patients. There are no data to support a note for malaria exacerbating HIV infection: for example, a follow-up study of 1000 emergency ward transfusions demonstrated that malaria was neither more frequent nor more severe in children with progressive HIV-1 infection and also did not appear to accelerate the rate of progression of HIV disease.

Studies on the relationship between Burkitt's lymphoma, the Epstein-Barr virus (EBV), and malaria have indicated that the lymphoma is most common in Africa and Papua New Guinea, and it is thought that this B-cell lymphoma may arise from interactions of EBV-infected B lymphocytes with immune responses to malaria (Marsh and Greenwood, 1986).

Babesiosis. Infection of humans by plasmodium-like piroplasms of the genus *Babesia* has long been recognized as associated with the modification of immunocompetence by splenectomy, at least in European cases caused by the cattle-associated species, *B. divergens*. No clear association with splenectomy or other immunocompromised state has been found for infection with *B. microti* in the United States. However, babesiosis in an asplenic, renal transplant patient and in a patient with AIDS without prior splenectomy was reported recently.

Microsporidia

Microsporidia differ sufficiently from other protozoa to be assigned their own phylum, and five genera are currently recognized as causing human infection. While remaining rare in immunocompetent persons, microsporidiosis is increasingly recognized in HIV/AIDS. There is serologic evidence of infection with one of these organisms, *Encephalitozoon cuniculi*, in a small percentage of healthy persons, and perhaps in a greater percentage of travelers returning from the tropics. However, human disease has been recognized almost entirely in those who are immunocompromised: only 10 cases of microsporidiosis had been described among persons not infected with HIV by 1994, and one cae of *E. bieneusi* microsporidiosis was reported in 1996 in an HIV-negative heart-lung transplant recipient in France. As in the case of the coccidian, the microsporidia have really "come into their own" in the context of human disease only since the beginning of the AIDS epidemic. Microsporidiosis now constitutes a major disease problem in the seriously immunocompromised population; in the HIV-infected, a spectrum of infections—from asymptomatic, to double (or multiple), to fatal—may occur. Fortunately, with effective HAART, HIV/AIDS microsporidiosis is on the decline in the developed world.

Several microsporidiosis syndromes can be constructed, to some extent depending on the infecting species (Table 11-1). As paraphrased from Atias (1995), these include (1) generalized infections with multisystem involvement; (2) enteric localization, which may cause death in AIDS patients due to intractable, large-volume diarrhea; (3) ocular infection, affecting the cornea and/or conjunctiva, and sometimes extending to the paranasal sinuses; (4) hepatic and biliary tract infection with granulomatous lesions, hepatic necrosis, or sclerosing cholangiitis: and (5) muscular infection, affecting skeletal muscle. The most frequently seen is enteric: a profuse, unremitting, watery diarrhea that tends to become chronic, and may be fatal. In the disseminated forms (Gunnarsson et al., 1995), infective microsporidial spores may be isolated from body fluids, including stool, urine, respiratory secretions, and duodenal aspirates (Visvesvara et al., 1994), suggesting that these may serve as potentially infective sources for person-to-person transmission. The extent to which infection of susceptible individuals might occur from environmental or zoonotic sources, including pets, is unclear; however, the ease of transmission or adaptation of human microsporidial strains to laboratory animals, the profound susceptibility of the immunocompromised host, and the ubiquity of the phylum do raise concerns.

It has been estimated that the coccidians *C. parvum, I. belli,* and *Cyclospora,* and the microsporidia now account for up to 50% overall of cases of persistent diarrhea in HIV/AIDS patients in the developing world, although prevalence rates vary. In one study of 250 HIV-infected individuals referred for gastrointestinal evaluation in New York in the pre-HAART era, intestinal microsporidia were found in 39% of AIDS patients with diarrhea (all with severely depressed CD4+ lymphocytes) but in only 3% of non-AIDS patients.

TABLE 11-1 ■ The Microsporidia in Human Disease

Species	Observed in		Principal Disease Site	
	Non-AIDS*	AIDS	"Local"	Disseminated
Enterocytozoon bieneusi	+	+	Small intestine (diarrhea)	Hepatobiliary tract
Encephalitozoon intestinalis (Septata intestinalis)		+	Enteric (diarrhea)	Hepatobiliary, renal, nasal, respiratory
Enc. cuniculi	+	+	Ocular	Hepatic, renal, peritoneal
Enc. hellem		+	Ocular	Renal, genitourinary, throat, nasal, respiratory
Trachipleistophora hominis (Pleistophora hominis)	+	+	Muscular	
Nosema connori	+ (athymic)		Corneal	Widely distributed
N. ocularum	+		Corneal	
Vittaforma corneae (Nosema corneum)	+		Corneal	

*Rare.

Enterocytozoon bieneusi has been reported from stool specimens in patients with AIDS in frequencies ranging from 50% to as low as 2%. However, it has been noted that in some 17% of AIDS patients, shedding of spores in the stool is intermittent. In a study from Australia involving 240 consecutive duodenal biopsies from HIV-infected patients with gastrointestinal symptoms, 18% were found to be infected.

As in cryptosporidiosis, the cellular arm of the immune system is most important in controlling microsporidial infection. CD4$^+$ cell counts generally correlate with susceptibility to enteric disease. Chronic diarrhea in HIV-positive patients with counts less than $100/\mu l$ should raise the suspicion of microsporidiosis. A summary of recommendations for the prevention of microsporidiosis was published as a joint report by the Centers for Disease Control and Prevention (CDC) and the Infectious Disease Society of America (IDSA) in mid-1997 (Centers for Disease Control and Prevention, 1997).

Nematoda

The only intestinal nematode that is known to present special pathogenetic (disease) problems in immunocompromised hosts is *Strongyloides stercoralis*. In addition to its free-living cycle, this helminth may undergo endogenous multiplication, so that in the immunocompetent host, a low-level, asymptomatic infection with *S. stercoralis* may persist for many years. Following the advent of HTLV-1 infection, cancer chemotherapy, and the long-term use of corticosteroids for various conditions, it was discovered that the autoinfection cycle could be enhanced and these smoldering and frequently asymptomatic infections could suddenly overwhelm the patient (Adedayo et al., 2002). The tremendous proliferation of the adult worms in the intestine, and the spread of their filariform larvae throughout the body, apparently by lymphohematogenous dissemination after penetration of the thoracic duct (Haque et al., 1994), results in a condition named disseminated strongyloidiasis or "hyperinfection syndrome," in which injury may occur to virtually every organ and tissue. Fatal strongyloidiasis has been reported especially among patients receiving long-term corticosteroid therapy. In one series of autopsied cases with demonstrated overwhelming *S. stercoralis* infection, as many as 24 (57.1%) of 42 patients had been on cancer chemotherapy involving steroids, and 15 (35.7%) had been on high-level corticosteroids alone.

Despite the association of HTLV-1 with strongyloidiasis, there is no evidence of a link to HIV/AIDS. Over 300 cases of opportunistic strongyloidiasis were cited by Liu and Weller (1993). Of these, as few as 15 cases were found in AIDS patients. The remainder were seen in patients with chronic conditions treated with corticosteroids and included those with cardiac and renal transplants, various malignancies, lymphoma, angioimmunoblastic lymphadenopathy, mixed connective tissue disease, inflammatory demyelinating polyradiculoneuropathy, idiopathic polymyositis, hypogammaglobulinemia, periarteritis nodosa, pemphigus erythematosus, relapsing polychondritis, idiopathic pulmonary fibrosis, and chronic obstructive pulmonary disease. Three cases of disseminated strongyloidiasis complicating kala-azar have been reported from India. One study in 287 subjects in rural Tanzania did report a higher prevalence in AIDS and HIV-positive than in HIV-negative patients ($p < 0.01$). Nevertheless, the very few cases of disseminated strongyloidiasis seen in AIDS patients—despite geographic overlap of the two diseases—have led to the exclusion of *S. stercoralis* infection from case definitions of AIDS.

Among infections by the tissue-dwelling nematodes, modification of the host response by concomitant HIV infection has been noted in onchocerciasis. However, this has taken the form of decreased recognition of *Onchocerca volvulus* antigens by IgG antibodies in sera of HIV-positive individuals and of an apparently *lower* dermal microfilaria (mf) density among HIV-positive versus HIV-negative individuals with onchocerciasis (11.9 mf per gram of skin versus 17.7 mf per gram), rather than an increased pathogenetic effect. A possible decrease in reactivity to HTLV-1 antigen(s) in onchocerciasis has also been reported.

Trematoda

The schistosomes appear to have the greatest impact on host immune mechanisms among the trematodes, and it could be suspected that modifications of immune response brought about by HIV infection might have an impact on schistosome pathology and/or epidemiology. Despite the increasing overlap of schistosomiasis and HIV-endemic areas, no significant effects, mutual or unilateral, have been reported. Nevertheless, two intriguing reports have appeared recently to suggest that significant effects may be noted in the future. A cross-sectional study of HIV seroprevalence among 895 adults living in an area of high incidence of urinary schistosomiasis in the Congo found that the incidence of frank schistosome infection was significantly lower in HIV-positive than in HIV-negative patients (3.5 versus 6.7%, respectively), and that the number of eggs shed in the urine was similarly lower in HIV-positive than in HIV-negative persons (3.6 versus 26.6 eggs per ml, respectively). Similar results were reported from western Kenya for *Schistosoma mansoni* coinfections with HIV, in that patients infected with *S. mansoni* and HIV shed far fewer schistosome eggs (34%) in the feces than patients infected with *S. mansoni* but who were seronegative for HIV. These observations support the concept of immune regulation/mediation of excretion of schistosome ova; the correlations with pathologic and epidemiologic study should be most interesting.

Cestoda

Among the cestodes, *Hymenolepis nana* is uniquely capable of completing its life cycle within a single human host, and can produce a hyperinfection syndrome in immunocompetent persons. As with the potentially single-host nematodes, *Strongyloides stercoralis* and *Capillaria philippinensis*, the cestode *H. nana* also might be expected to produce a more intense hyperinfection syndrome in immunocompromised hosts; however, no such instance has yet been reported. In a serologic test for cysticercosis with 70% sensitivity and 90% specificity, false-negative results were reported to be associated with HIV infection among some 630 patients with signs and symptoms compatible with neurocysticercosis in Zimbabwe.

An recent addition to the list of new parasites reported from the immunocompromised host, and yet another capable of lethal infection, is a previously unknown metazoan, presumably a larval cestode and possibly a sparganum that was isolated from an adult male patient with AIDS (Connor et al., 1976; Santamaria-Fries et al., 1996). This as-yet-unnamed organism (Fig. 11-1), tentatively placed taxonomically among the cestodes by construction of phylogenetic trees based on rDNA analysis, produced a rapidly enlarging abdominal mass suggestive of a neoplasm, then invaded the patient's liver and regional lymph nodes, causing his death (Stark, 1998). Subcutaneous infection with the larval form of *Taenia crassiceps* has been seen in three patients with HIV/AIDS (Francois et al., 1998).

Arthropoda

Sarcoptes and *Demodex* are two genera of "human" mites whose manifestations in humans are affected by immunocompromised states. *S. scabiei*, the itch mite, does not produce overwhelming infections in immunocompetent persons under ordinary circumstances. In the immunocompromised, however, whether in patients involved with malignancy, those having undergone organ transplantation and subsequent immunosuppression, or those with AIDS or HTLV-1 infection, so-called Norwegian or crusted scabies may occur as a result of a decreased cutaneous immune response (Brites et al., 2002). The condition is characterized by widespread dissemination of massive numbers of mites, with thick, crusted lesions, and inconsistent pruritus, from intense to absent. It is highly contagious, owing to the extraordinary numbers of mites present, and is usually more difficult to treat.

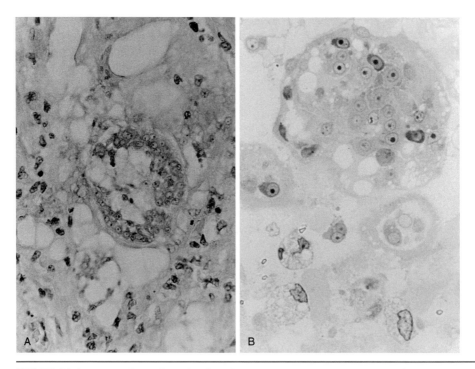

FIGURE 11-1 ■ Sections of previously unknown metazoan parasite isolated from an adult male patient with AIDS and tentatively identified as a cestode. **A,** Paraffin section showing parasite sac (hematoxylin and eosin). **B,** Epon section showing large and smaller sacs (toluidine blue). (Courtesy Prof. L. F. Fajardo, Stanford University School of Medicine, Stanford, CA.)

D. folliculorum and *D. brevis*, normally innocuous commensals that inhabit human skin and hair follicles, can produce pruritic, popular eruptions of head and neck regions in HIV-infected patients (Ray and Gately, 1994).

References

Addo-Yobo EO et al. Malnutrition and malaria gave him anaemia, then blood transfusion gave him HIV. *Trop Doct* 1992; *22*:123.

Adedayo O, Grell G, Bellot P. Hyperinfective strongyloidiasis in the medical ward—review of 27 cases in 5 years. *Southern Med J* 2002; *95*:711–716.

Albrecht H et al. Visceral leishmaniasis emerging as an important opportunistic infection in HIV-infected persons living in areas non-endemic for *Leishmania donovani*. *Arch Pathol Lab Med* 1996; *120*:189–198.

Alvar J, Cañavate C et al. Leishmania and human immunodeficiency virus coinfestation: The first 10 years. *Clin Microbiol Rev* 1997; *10*:298–319.

Atias A. Actualizaciones sobre microsporidios en el hombre. *Rev Med Chil* 1995; *123*:762–772.

Brites C, Weyll M, Pedroso C, Badaro R. Severe and Norwegian scabies are strongly associated with retroviral (HIV-1/HTLV-1) infection in Bahia, Brazil. *AIDS* 2002; *16*:1292–1293.

Centers for Disease Control and Prevention. 1997 USPHS/IDSA guidelines for the prevention of opportunistic infections in persons infected with human immunodeficiency virus. *MMWR* 1997; *46*:suppl RR-12.

Chai-Savaneeyakorn S, Moore JM, Otieno J et al. Impairment of IL-12, not IL-18, and interferon-inducible protein—10 responses in the placental intervillous blood of HIV/malaria coinfected woman. *J Infect Dis* 2002; *185*:127–131.

Chesson HW, Blandford JM, Pinkerton SD. Estimates of the annual number and cost of new HIV infections among women attributable to trichomoniasis in the United States. *Sexually Transmitted Diseases* 2004; *31*:547–551.

Connor DH et al. Disseminated parasitosis in an immunosuppressed patient. Possibly a mutated sparganum. *Arch Pathol Lab Med* 1976; *100*:65–68.

Cotte L et al. Prevalence of intestinal protozoans in French patients infected with HIV. *J Acquir Immune Defic Syndr* 1993; *6*:1024–1029.

DiLorenzo GA et al. Chagasic granulomatous encephalitis in immunosuppressed patients. *J Neuroimaging* 1996; *6*:94–97.

Esfandiari A et al. Prevalence of enteric parasitic infection among HIV-infected attendees of an inner city AIDS clinic. *Cell Mol Biol* (Noisy-le-grand) 1995; *41*(suppl 1):S19–S23.

European Collaborative Study. Low incidence of congenital toxoplasmosis in children born to women infected with human immunodeficiency virus. *Eur J Obstet Gynecol Reprod Biol* 1996; *68*:93–96.

Francois A, Favenneck, Cambon-Michot C et al. *Taenia crassiceps* invasive cysticercosis: A new human pathogen in acquired immunodeficiency syndrome? *Am J Surg Path* 1998; *22*:488–492.

Gatti S et al. Non-pathogenic *Entamoeba histolytica* in Italian HIV-infected homosexuals. *Int J Med Microbiol Virol Parasitol Infect Dis* 1992; *277*:382–388.

Gentry LO et al. Dermatologic manifestations of infectious diseases in cardiac transplant patients. *Infect Dis Clin North Am* 1994; *8*:637–654.

Gunnarsson G et al. Multiorgan microsporidiosis: Report of five cases and review. *Clin Infect Dis* 1995; *21*:37–44.

Haque AK et al. Pathogenesis of human strongyloidiasis: Autopsy and quantitative parasitological analysis. *Mod Pathol* 1994; *7*:276–288.

Haque R et al. Current concepts: Amebiasis. *N Engl J Med* 2003; *348*:1565–1573.

Harms G, Feldmeier H. HIV and tropical parasitic diseases–deleterious interactions in both directions? *Trop Med International Health* 2002; *7*:479–488.

Jackson DJ et al. Lymphadenopathy and hepatosplenomegaly in the first year in children infected with HIV-1 in Zaire. *Ann Trop Paediatr* 1992; *12*:165–168.

Katongole-Mbidde E et al. Blackwater fever caused by *Plasmodium vivax* infection in the acquired immune deficiency syndrome. *Br Med J* (Clin Res Ed) 1988; *296*:827.

Keusch GT. The history of nutrition: malnutrition, infection and immunity. *J Nutrition* 2003; *133*:3365–3405.

Kirchhoff LV. Chagas' disease. American trypanosomiasis. *Infect Dis Clin North Am* 1993; 7:487–502.

Laguna F et al. Gastrointestinal leishmaniasis in human immunodeficiency virus-infected patients: Report of five cases and review. *Clin Infect Dis* 1995; *19*:48–53.

Liu LX, Weller PF. Strongyloidiasis and other intestinal nematode infections. *Infect Dis Clin North Am* 1993; 7:655–682.

Lockwood DNJ, Weber JN. Parasitic infections in AIDS. *Parasitol Today* 1989; *5*:310–316.

Marsh K, Greenwood BM. The immunopathology of malaria. *Clin Trop Med Communic Dis* 1986; *1*:91–125.

Mendez OC et al. Comparacion de indices de infestaciones por enteroparasitos entre poblaciones HIV positivas y negativas. *Medicina* (B Aires) 1994; *54*:307–310.

Murakawa GJ et al. Disseminated acanthamebiasis in patients with AIDS. A report of 5 cases and a review of the literature. *Arch Dermatol* 1995; *131*:1291–1296.

Ortega YR et al. Cyclospora species—a new protozoan pathogen of humans. *N Engl J Med* 1993; *328*:1308–1312.

Ortega YR et al. A new coccidian parasite (Apicomplexa Eimeriidae) from humans. *J Parasitol* 1994; *80*:625–629.

Pape JW et al. *Cyclospora* infection in adults infected with HIV. Clinical manifestations, treatment and prophylaxis. *Ann Int Med* 1994; *121*:654–657.

Poirot JL et al. Broncho-pulmonary cryptosporidiosis in four HIV-infected patients. *J Eukaryot Microbiol* 1996; *43*:78S–79S.

Pratlong F, Dereure J, Denian M et al. Enzymatic polymorphism during leishmame/HIV coinfection. A study of 381 leishmanie strains received between 1986 and 2000 of the international cryobank in Montpelier, France. *Ann Trop Med Parasitol* 2003; *97*(S):1:47–56.

Ray MC, Gately LE III. Dermatologic manifestations of HIV infections and AIDS. *Infect Dis Clin North Am* 1994; *8*:586–606.

Reynolds SJ, Bantle HJG, Quinn TC, Beyrer C, Bolliner RC. Antiretroviral therapy where resources are limited. *N Engl J Med* 2003; *348*:1806–1809.

Samuel R, Betticker RL, Sah B. AIDS related opportunistic infections. Going but not gone. *Arch Pharmacol Res* 2002; *25*:215–228.

Santamaria-Fries M et al. Lethal infection by a previously unrecognized metazoan parasite. *Lancet* 1996; *347*:149–154.

Sargeaunt PG et al. *Entamoeba histolytica* in male homosexuals. *Br J Vener Dis* 1983; *59*:193–195.

Silberman JD et al. Human parasite finds taxonomic home. *Nature* 1996; *380*:398.

Sison JP et al. Disseminated acanthamoeba infection in patients with AIDS: Case reports and review. *Clin Infect Dis* 1995; *20*:1207–1216.

Sorvillo FJ et al. Epidemiology of isosporiasis among persons with acquired immunodeficiency syndrome in Los Angeles County. *Am J Trop Med Hyg* 1995; *53*:656–659.

Stark P. Radiologic features of a fatal platyhelminth (tapeworm) infection in an AIDS patient. *Am J Roentgenol* 1998; *170*:136–138.

Steele RW. Sizing up the risks of pet-transmitted diseases. *Contemp Pediatrics* 1997; *14*:43–68.

Torre-Cisneros J et al. Successful treatment of antimony-resistant visceral leishmaniasis with liposomal amphotericin B in patients infected with human immunodeficiency virus. *Clin Infect Dis* 1993; *17*:635–627.

United Nations Joint Programme of HIV (UNAIDS). *Report on the global HIV epidemic* 2004; Geneva: UNAIDS.

Villanueva MS. Trypanosomiasis of the central nervous system. *Semin Neurol* 1993; *13*:208–218.

Visvesvara GS et al. Polyclonal and monoclonal antibody and PCR-amplified small-subunit rRNA identification of a microsporidian, *Encephalitozoon hellem,* isolated from an AIDS patient with disseminated infection. *J Clin Microbiol* 1994; *32*:2760–2768.

Wittner M et al. Parasitic infections in AIDS patients. Cryptosporidiosis, isosporiasis, microsporidiosis, cyclosporiasis. *Infect Dis North Am* 1993; *7*:5699–5686.

Wong SY et al. AIDS-associated toxoplasmosis. *In* Sande MA, Volberding PA (eds). *The medical management of AIDS*, ed 4, Philadelphia, 1995, WB Saunders.

Signs and Symptoms of Parasitic Disease

Very few of the signs or symptoms evoked by infection with parasitic organisms can be said to deserve that much-abused term *pathognomonic*. There are but a limited number of ways in which the body is able to react to altered conditions, and therefore it is not surprising that few of these reactions are specific. Nevertheless, the presence of certain signs and symptoms should alert the clinician to corresponding diagnostic possibilities, while various constellations of symptoms, or syndromes, are to a greater or lesser degree diagnostic.

It must be emphasized that the following is not intended as a complete differential diagnosis of any of the symptoms discussed. Limitations of space do not permit even mention of the various nonparasitic causes of many of these conditions.

Abdominal Pain

Crampy abdominal pain may characterize amebic colitis, with tenesmus if ulcerations involve the rectal area. Diarrhea or dysentery is usually present when the infection is symptomatic. If hepatic abscess develops, pain is usually felt in the right upper quadrant (left, if the abscess involves the left lobe), and may be referred to the scapular area. Pain in giardiasis is usually mild but may occasionally be severe; it is usually crampy and may be accompanied by steatorrhea and a full-blown malabsorption syndrome. Pain is seldom present in intestinal worm infections. Intestinal or biliary obstruction (the former primarily in smaller children) can be the result of *Ascaris* infection, with signs and symptoms that mimic obstruction of these passages from any other cause. *Strongyloides stercoralis*, invading the mucosal wall, may cause a severe duodenitis or jejunitis, with symptoms suggestive of duodenal ulcer disease. Anisakid larvae, penetrating the wall of the stomach or small bowel, may give rise to symptoms suggestive of gastric or duodenal ulcer or appendicitis, as may *Eustrongylides* in compulsive minnow gobblers. *Angiostrongylus costaricensis* most frequently invades the bowel wall in the region of the appendix, with pain in the right iliac fossa. Moderate to heavy eosinophilia generally accompanies these invasive worm infections.

Abscess, Amebic

Amebic invasion of the liver is characterized by tenderness and enlargement of that organ, progressive malaise, an irregularly spiking fever with night sweats, leukocytosis, elevation and fixation of the right diaphragm (often seen on presenting chest radiograph), and sometimes development of a right lower lobe pneumonitis. With abscess formation, pain becomes more intense and may be referred to the tip of the right (less commonly the left) scapula.

Abscess, Filarial

Abscesses may develop spontaneously or appear shortly after antifilarial treatment is begun. They occur along the course of lymphatics or at lymph nodes and may be distinguished from pyogenic abscesses by the fact that they are generally sterile when first opened and that fragments of the adult worms may be found in the abscess drainage. Filarial abscesses are even more common in *Brugia* infections than in those caused by *Wuchereria*.

Anemia

Most frequently associated with malaria, hookworm, and broad fish tapeworm infections, anemia may be seen in babesiosis, kala-azar, trypanosomiasis, schistosomiasis, fasciolopsiasis, and trichuriasis. In falciparum malaria the red blood cell count may fall to 2.5 to 4.0 million per mm^3 in cases of average severity, and fewer than 1.0 million per mm^3 in severe infections. Anemia is usually not severe in vivax malaria and is still less pronounced in quartan infections. The characteristic microcytic hypochromic anemia of hookworm infection is the result of blood loss and is thus proportional to the severity of infection, although adequate dietary intake of iron may prevent its development in light or moderate infections. The small amount of blood ingested per *Trichuris* worm makes anemia rare except in massive infections. Persons infected with *Diphyllobothrium latum* may develop macrocytic hyperchromic anemia on the basis of vitamin B_{12} deprivation if the worm is attached to the jejunal wall. In kala-azar, and possibly also in Chagas' disease, anemia may be a consequence of proliferation of infected reticuloendothelial cells in the bone marrow. In the other trypanosomiases, schistosomiasis, and certain intestinal helminthic infections such as fasciolopsiasis, anemia may result in part from nutritional causes.

Appendicitis

Amebic ulceration involving the cecal area or appendix may simulate acute appendicitis; when there is extensive cecal ulceration surgical intervention may be disastrous. *Ascaris* may block the lumen of the appendix and give rise to appendicitis; this is reported also for *Trichuris*. *Angiostrongylus costaricensis* infection may also mimic appendicitis, as may the response to a black widow spider bite.

Ascites

Circumoval tissue proliferation leading to extensive fibrosis of the liver in *Schistosoma mansoni* and *S. japonicum* infections may lead eventually to a condition clinically very similar to Laënnec's cirrhosis, with portal hypertension, splenomegaly, and ascites. Although hepatomegaly and splenomegaly occur early in kala-azar, ascites is uncommon. It may occur in chronic cases, probably secondary to a nutritional cirrhosis.

Asthma, Bronchial

Asthmatic attacks may occur in *Ascaris* infection during the stage of migration through the lungs, or later in the course of the infection because of hypersensitization to the absorbed worm antigens. Asthma is not uncommon in visceral larva migrans infections, in which there is usually an accompanying hepatomegaly and marked eosinophilia. House dust mites, belonging to the genus *Dermatophagoides*, are an important cause of nasal allergies and asthma, especially in children. See also tropical eosinophilia, under Eosinophilia.

Blackwater Fever

See Hemoglobinuria.

Calabar Swellings

Circumscribed subcutaneous swellings are seen in loiasis. They are usually intensely pruritic and may be quite painful if they develop in areas where there is little loose subcutaneous tissue, such as the elbows and knees. They appear rapidly, developing within an hour or so to a diameter of several centimeters, and persist for several days; if in an area subject to repeated trauma they may last a week or longer.

Calcifications, Cerebral

Calcification of areas of intracerebral infection in congenital toxoplasmosis may be seen on radiographs, and when intracerebral calcifications are found in a patient who has retinochoroiditis, toxoplasmosis is highly probable. Calcified cysts of *Taenia solium* larvae within the brain may be distinguished by their size and uniform rounded or oval shape, and subretinal lesions may also be observed by funduscopy.

Chagoma

The hard, reddened, raised primary lesion in *Trypanosoma cruzi* infection usually develops on the head or neck, and sometimes on the abdomen or limbs, and may persist for 2 to 3 months. Although it may occur on or about the eye, the chagoma is not to be confused with the unilateral palpebral edema of Romaña's sign (q.v.).

Chyluria

The formation of lymphatic varices, consequent to repeated attacks of filarial lymphangitis and obstruction of lymphatic drainage, may lead to passage of lymphatic fluid in the urine if varices rupture into any part of the urinary tract. Chyluria usually occurs in attacks that last a few days; the urine may be milky white and contain microfilariae.

Coma

The sudden onset of coma in a patient known to be suffering from falciparum malaria, or in an apparently healthy person who is in or has recently returned from a malarious area, should always suggest cerebral malaria and requires emergency treatment. In African trypanosomiasis, coma develops after a protracted period of increasingly severe symptoms of meningoencephalitis. It is also seen in primary amebic meningoencephalitis, in which a history of rapidly developing fever, meningeal signs, confusion, loss of smell, and coma and of recent swimming or diving in fresh water may often be elicited.

Cerebral cysticercosis may be a diagnostic consideration in persons of Mexican or Latin American origin, or in long-time residents of those areas, who present with a variety of neurologic symptoms, including new onset seizures, headache, alteration of consciousness, coma, and internal hydrocephalus. Diagnosis may be difficult, and eosinophilia (either peripheral or of the spinal fluid) is not always present. Serologic tests may be helpful. Computed tomography (CT) often reveals the calcified and uncalcified cysts, and magnetic resonance imaging (MRI) those within the ventricles.

Conjunctivitis

Chronic conjunctivitis is seen in onchocercal infections, with hyperpigmentation of the conjunctiva, photophobia, and gradual development of corneal opacities; acute exacerbations of conjunctivitis and photophobia may be associated with attacks of onchocercal dermatitis. The sheep botfly, *Oestrus ovis*, may lay its eggs in the conjunctivae, and development of the larvae in the conjunctival sac is accompanied by considerable pain, localized swelling, and conjunctivitis. *Thelazia* larvae deposited in the conjunctival sac by flies may mature there and give rise to a severe conjunctivitis.

Convulsions

Focal convulsive seizures of the jacksonian type are seen in a number of parasitic infections that involve the central nervous system. These are discussed under Neurologic Symptoms. Convulsions also may be seen in the malarial paroxysm, in acute toxoplasmosis occurring in newborn children, and in *Ascaris* infection in children.

Dermatitis

Dermal leishmanoid is a secondary cutaneous manifestation of *Leishmania donovani* infection, occurring a year or so after supposedly successful treatment of kala-azar. The lesions may be flattened or depressed depigmented macules, or erythematous nodules that, on the face, often occur in a butterfly distribution reminiscent of lupus erythematosus or Hansen's disease (leprosy). Leishmanial amastigotes are found in the lesions.

Penetration of schistosome cercariae through the skin causes localized edema and pruritus, mild in the case of the human schistosomes, more severe in the swimmer's itch caused by bird schistosome cercariae. A similar localized pruritic reaction occurs with penetration of *Strongyloides* larvae through the skin; the reaction to penetration of hookworm larvae is somewhat more severe, often with the formation of papules or vesicles. It may last a couple of weeks or longer if there is a secondary infection. The cutaneous larva migrans reaction caused by larvae of *Ancylostoma braziliense* or *A. caninum* is characterized by a reddened papule at the site of entry; the larva forms a reddened serpiginous tunnel, at first covered with vesicles, later dry and crusted, often with localized edema at the active end that advances at the rate of a few millimeters to centimeters a day. The area itches intensely; without treatment, infection may persist several weeks or months. *Strongyloides* larvae may produce similar cutaneous lesions, but because of their more rapid subcutaneous movement, they are referred to as larva currens.

Presence of adult *Loa loa* beneath skin may be indicated by a thin, raised reddened line, a few centimeters in length. The adult female *Dracunculus* also may be visible beneath the skin but usually produces no reaction until it is about to larviposit, when a vesicle forms over the point at which the worm will break through the skin. In onchocerciasis, the presence of microfilariae in the skin sometimes elicits an acute pruritic inflammatory reaction resembling erysipelas that is usually confined to the face, neck, and ears. Repeated acute attacks may result in a chronic lichenification, with hyperpigmentation and fissuring. Itching may be intense and scratching almost constant, with skin excoriations present.

The migration of *Sarcoptes scabiei* through the skin produces lesions resembling those of cutaneous larva migrans but frequently seen in parts of the body that have no contact with soil. This organism is highly infectious, and localized hospital epidemics have been reported. The mites invade the upper layers of the epidermis, in which they form sinuous burrows. They seem to have a predilection for the interdigital, popliteal, and inframammary folds and the groin. Intense itching, with formation of small vesicles and crusting of the chronic excoriated lesions, is typical. The larvae of the horse botfly, *Gasterophilus*, produce similar cutaneous lesions in man. Chiggers and other mites attack the skin, evoking a pruritic maculopapular dermatitis. Pediculosis in hypersensitive persons, usually as a result of repeated exposure, may give rise to a severe localized reaction, with reddish papules at the feeding site, and surrounding vesiculation and a weeping dermatitis. Bronzing of the affected area may persist following healing. The chigoe flea, *Tunga penetrans*, produces local pruritus as it lies partly buried in the skin of the toes or elsewhere on the body; secondary infections by clostridia are not uncommon. See also Rash.

Diarrhea

Diarrhea in parasitic diseases may have diverse causes. In kala-azar, infiltration of the submucosa with leishmania-containing macrophages may lead to mucosal ulceration and diarrhea. Plugging of the mucosal capillaries with parasitized red blood cells may lead, in falciparum malaria, to a watery diarrhea so profuse as to suggest cholera. Blood containing parasitized red blood cells may be found in the stools. The diarrhea or dysentery is usually accompanied by nausea and vomiting. Mucosal ulceration in amebiasis or balantidiasis may produce diarrhea or, if the ulceration is more extensive, dysentery (q.v.). *Isospora* develops within the epithelial cells of the lower ileum and cecum. Infection is self-limited, lasting usually a month or less. In some cases there is mild abdominal pain, nausea and vomiting, and diarrhea. *Cryptosporidium* invades the brush border of the epithelial cells of the intestine. In immunocompetent persons it gives rise to a mild and self-limited diarrhea lasting a week or so, whereas in immunodeficient persons, it produces a severe and prolonged infection like that seen in isosporiasis, often with malabsorption.

One of the most recently defined parasitic causes of diarrheal disease is the coccidian *Cyclospora cayetanensis*, which produces a syndrome clinically indistinguishable from those due to *Cryptosporidium* or *Isospora belli*. Uncreated cyclosporiasis encompasses the range of mild to moderate and self-limited (in immunocompetent persons) through profuse, watery diarrhea, frequently prolonged for weeks to months (in patients with AIDS), with an incubation period of 2 to 11 days, and accompanied by a generalized enteropathy manifested by nausea, vomiting, anorexia, abdominal cramping, weight loss, and mild fever (Topazian and Bia, 1994; Wurtz, 1994). In addition, this coccidian has recently demonstrated a significant common source (water-borne) epidemic potential.

The microsporidian *Enterocytozoon bieneusi*, which infects enterocytes, has been shown to cause a persistent watery diarrhea in patients with acquired immunodeficiency syndrome (AIDS). *Giardia* infections may be asymptomatic, accompanied by a mild mucoid diarrhea, or may give rise to a full-blown malabsorption syndrome with steatorrhea.

Development of the cysticercoids of *Hymenolepis nana* within the intestinal villi may elicit a mucous diarrhea. Maturation of *Trichinella* within the wall of the duodenum and jejunum produces nausea, vomiting, colicky abdominal pain, and diarrhea, starting about 24 hours after infection and lasting up to 5 days. In *Strongyloides* infections there may be mild diarrhea alternating with periods of constipation, or the diarrhea may be severe and prostrating. In heavy infections ulceration and sloughing of the intestinal mucosa may take place, with dysentery and often with secondary bacterial infection and fever. *Capillaria philippinensis* infections may result in profuse diarrhea, malabsorption, and protein-wasting enteropathy.

In schistosomiasis mansoni and japonicum, there is diarrhea, presumably of toxic origin, associated with nausea, vomiting, hepatic tenderness, fever, eosinophilia, and urticarial rash during the period when the worms are maturing in the liver sinusoids. Somewhat later, with the beginning of egg deposition in the intestinal wall, there may be profuse diarrhea or dysentery.

In previously uninfected persons, the onset of a heavy hookworm infection may be marked by nausea, vomiting, epigastric or midabdominal tenderness, and diarrhea. The diarrhea is presumably caused by toxicity or hypersensitivity, although mechanical irritation may play some part. The same may be said of the diarrhea in heavy whipworm infections, which may, in children, be accompanied by rectal prolapse. In fasciolopsiasis, diarrhea, which usually has its onset about a month after infection takes place, is characterized by the passage of stools containing much undigested food; severe infections are accompanied by symptoms of severe malnutrition: edema of the face, abdominal wall, and lower extremities; ascites; and prostration. The diarrhea sometimes seen in *Taenia* and broad fish tapeworm infections and in infections with the smaller intestinal flukes may be related to local irritation.

Blastocystis hominis, a frequent, unicellular stool inhabitant of incompletely defined phylogenetic affinity, is mentioned in the context of diarrheal disease for the sake of both completeness and dismissal. Although long the subject of controversy, recent studies have again put to rest any serious consideration of this microorganism as a pathogen (Markell, 1995; Zuckerman et al., 1994).

Dysentery

Acute amebic dysentery is characterized by the passage of six to eight, or sometimes a dozen or more, mucoid, blood-flecked (or more overtly bloody) stools a day. There may be generalized abdominal pain and tenderness if the entire colon is involved, tenderness over McBurney's point, nausea and vomiting with cecal infection, or tenesmus, with relief of the accompanying pain after evacuation if the rectosigmoid is the main diseased area. An untreated attack lasts a few days to several weeks and usually subsides spontaneously to recur after an interval of some days of several years. Between attacks the patient may be constipated. Balantidial dysentery is similar to the amebic type, and as in the latter disease, many infections are asymptomatic. Dysentery accompanying kala-azar, falciparum malaria infections, strongyloidiasis, and schistosomiasis is mentioned in the discussion of Diarrhea.

Edema

Circumorbital edema, possibly resulting from vasculitis provoked by the migrating larvae, is frequently seen in the early stages of trichinellosis; there also may be edema of the hands. Unilateral circumorbital edema, with local pruritus and sometimes intense pain, results from passage of the adult *Loa loa* across the eyeball or lid. Passage of the worm across the eyeball can take less than half a minute to as long as 10 minutes; the resulting inflammatory changes usually persist for several days. Calabar swellings (q.v.) are also seen in loiasis, whereas localized edema of the face, neck, ears, and other parts of the body, accompanied by intense pruritus and erythema, may be recurrent in onchocerciasis. Ocular sparganosis is not uncommon in some areas where eye lesions are poulticed with split raw infected frogs. In the subcutaneous tissues around the eye, the sparganum produces a violent tissue reaction with edema; retrobulbar development of the sparganum may cause protrusion of the eyeball and consequent corneal ulceration. Areas of localized hard edema, of uncertain cause, are frequently seen in Chagas' disease, occurring after appearance of the chagoma (q.v.). The most common type is unilateral edema of the eyelids (Romaña's sign, q.v.). Edematous patches may develop elsewhere on the body, especially involving the abdominal wall, pubic area, scrotum, and legs. Of equally obscure origin is the edema of the hips, legs, hands, and face that may accompany the acute stage of African sleeping sickness. The edema of the face and legs, with a protuberant abdomen seen in severe hookworm infections, fasciolopsiasis, and diphyllobothriasis, may be related to malnutrition.

Elephantiasis

Filarial elephantiasis is a chronic enlargement of a limb, the scrotum, a breast, or the vulva, with hyperplasia of the connective tissue and skin, a woody nonpitting edema, and thickened, coarsened skin, often with verrucous changes. In Malayan and Timoran filariasis, elephantiasis is less severe and generally is confined to the lower limbs below the knees. Elephantiasis of the external genitalia in both sexes, and hypertrophy of the femoral lymph nodes, producing a peculiar condition known as hanging groin, have been reported from some areas in Africa where bancroftian filariasis is unknown and are ascribed to onchocercal infection, in which elephantiasis of the legs may also occur. In schistosomiasis haematobium, extensive egg deposition may lead to fibrosis that blocks the lymphatic drainage, and to subsequent elephantiasis of the penis.

Eosinophilia

A retrospective study of 119 Caucasians returning from the tropics with eosinophilia and referred to the Hospital for Tropical Diseases in London (Harries et al., 1986) found that a parasite was the cause of the eosinophilia in 46 patients (38.7%). Diagnoses and mean eosinophil counts (per mm^3) were as follows:

Loa loa	$6368/mm^3$
Schistosoma mansoni	$3203/mm^3$
Mansonella (Dipetalonema) perstans	$2884/mm^3$
Trichinella spiralis	$2790/mm^3$
Hookworm	$2330/mm^3$
Schistosoma haematobium	$2017/mm^3$
Schistosoma intercalatum	$1500/mm^3$
Cutaneous larva migrans	$1430/mm^3$
Trichuris trichiura	$1408/mm^3$
Onchocerca volvulus	$1353/mm^3$
Strongyloides stercoralis	$978/mm^3$
Ascaris lumbricoides	$760/mm^3$

The proportionate numbers of eosinophils given here may be misleading, as they reflect relatively small numbers of patients. Perhaps more important is the fact that, even in a group of patients referred to a hospital that specialized in tropical diseases, more than 60% were not found to have parasites. These authors suggest that if eosinophilia persists undiagnosed for several months, empirical therapy with a broad-spectrum anthelminthic (they suggest mebendazole or thiabendazole, though recent experience might suggest albendazole; depending on travel history, praziquantel or ivermectin might be added).

Eosinophilia is a consistent finding in helminth infections, though it may be quite variable in degree. In general, tissue parasites provoke more pronounced eosinophilia than those that live only in the lumen of the bowel, nematodes more than cestodes.

As many physicians equate eosinophilia with parasitic disease, it may be well to report the result of a Mayo Clinic study of 418 patients with an eosinophilia of 20% or greater, as quoted by Harris (1979) (Table 12-1), although these data represent a largely U.S.-domiciled population.

A marked eosinophilia (20% to 70% or more) is most frequently seen with trichinosis, strongyloidiasis, hookworm infection, visceral larva migrans, filariasis, schistosomiasis, and fasciolopsiasis, Moderate eosinophilia (6% to 20%) often accompanies trichuriasis, ascariasis, paragonimiasis, taeniasis, and eosinophilic meningitis. It must be realized that eosinophilia is an index of host reaction to the parasite, so it varies considerably from one patient to another.

Eosinophilia is not characteristic of any of protozoan infections with the exception of *Isopora belli* and perhaps *Dientamoeba fragilis*. Tropical eosinophilia or eosinophilic lung disease is characterized by symptoms of chronic bronchitis or asthma, marked eosinophilia, accelerated erythrocyte sedimentation rate, paroxysmal cough or wheezing, malaise, easy fatigability, anorexia, and weight loss. The chest film may show diffuse, patchy mottling and transverse branching striations, most prominent in the midlung and basal lung fields, with enlargement of the hilar shadows. Occasionally there may be unilateral densities in the upper lung field that are suggestive of the picture seen in pulmonary tuberculosis. The disease is reported from such areas as India, Pakistan, Sri Lanka, China, Burma, Thailand, the Philippines, Malaysia, Indonesia, tropical Africa, and the West Indies. Filarial infection is considered to be a common cause of this condition. Other agents may be the pulmonary stages of *Ascaris, Strongyloides, Toxocara,* or other helminths Treatment with conventional doses of diethylcarbamazine (DEC) is often effective; antimonial (stibophen) or arsenical (neoarsphenamine) drugs are sometimes effective when there is no response to DEC.

TABLE 12-1   ■   Diseases with Eosinophilia Greater than 20% (Mayo Clinic, 1944)

Disease	Eosinophils (%)
Atopic diseases (vasomotor rhinitis, asthma, hay fever)	28
Lymphoproliferative diseases (lymphoma)	20
Dermatoses (pemphigus, dermatitis herpetiformis)	10
Nonparasitic infections (principally streptococcal)	11
Periarteritis nodosa (with lung involvement)	10
Parasitic infections	4
Nonlymphatic malignant tumors and leukemia	4
Miscellaneous	13

Data from Harris (1979).

Eosinophilic Cerebrospinal Fluid Pleocytosis

Cerebrospinal fluid eosinophilic pleocytosis is primarily associated with parasitic infection, but a number of other disease entities may evoke this response. The agents (modified from Asperilla, 1989, and Kuberski, 1979) that may result in eosinophils in the CSF are as follows:

A. Parasitic infections

Angiostrongylus cantonensis

Ascaris lumbricoides

Baylisascaris procyonis

Coenurus

Cysticercus

Dirofilaria immitis?

Echinococcus

Fasciola hepatica

       Gnathostoma spinigerum
       Hypoderma bovis
       Onchocerca volvulus?
       Paragonimus spp.
       Schistosoma spp.
       Toxocara spp.
       Toxoplasma gondii
       Trichinella spiralis

B. Fungal infections
   Coccidioides immitis
   Histoplasma capsulatum

C. Bacterial infections
   Treponema pallidum?
   Mycobacterium tuberculosis?

D. Rickettsial infections

E. Viral infections
   Lymphocytic choriomeningitis

F. Miscellaneous
   Malignancies (leukemia, lymphoma, meningeal tumors)
   Allergies?
   Collagen vascular diseases
   Drug hypersensitivity
   Foreign material (dyes, contrast media, etc.) in the central nervous system
   Hypereosinophilic syndrome
   Multiple sclerosis

Eosinophilic Meningitis

While eosinophilic cerebrospinal fluid pleocytosis is seen in a number of parasitic and nonparasitic infections and in some noninfections conditions, when associated with meningitis it is typically associated with certain helminthiases that affect the central nervous system. Important among these are angiostrongyliasis, gnathostomiasis, paragonimiasis, cysticercosis, and schistosomiasis. Table 12–2 lists important features in the diagnosis of the first four conditions.

TABLE 12-2   ■   Differential Diagnosis of Some CNS Parasitic Infections

Feature	Angiostrongyliasis	Gnathostomiasis	Paragonimiasis	Cysticercosis
Patient origin or travel history	Pacific islands, Taiwan, Thailand	Japan, Thailand	Asia, Africa, South America	Latin America, Asia, Africa
Food history	Raw fresh-water snails, shrimps	Raw fresh-water fish, frogs, snakes, etc.	Raw fresh-water crabs, crayfish	Food contaminated with *T. solium* eggs
Symptoms	Headache; rarely sensory impairment	Migratory swellings, severe nerve root pain	Cough, headache	Headache, psychiatric problems
Signs	Onset insidious or sudden, stiff neck, cranial nerve impairment (optic, facial, abducens)	Onset sudden: stiff neck, paraplegia, impaired consciousness, coma	Onset insidious: convulsions, hemiplegia, visual disturbances	Onset insidious: stiff neck, convulsions, movement disorders, cerebellar signs, hydrocephalus
CSF eosinophils	+ + + +	+ + +	+	+
Blood eosinophils	+ + +	+ + + +	Normal	Low
Serologic tests	Blood ELISA	Blood ELISA	Blood and CSF ELISA	CSF ELISA

Adapted from Jaroonvesama N. Differential diagnosis of eosinophilic meningitis. *Parasitol Today* 1988; 4:262–266.

Eosinophiluria

Eosinophils in the urine are not regularly detected by means of Wright's stain, but Hansel's stain (Chapter 15) seems to demonstrate them well. Eosinophiluria, a variable finding in diseases of the urinary tract, is frequently seen in drug-induced acute interstitial nephritis and is absent in acute tubular necrosis. In acute interstitial nephritis, eosinophilia is more often under 5%, but it may range up to 50% of the white cells in the urine. A level of 1% or greater is considered abnormal in these conditions. In urinary schistosomiasis, eosinophiluria is a constant finding; the percentage of eosinophils in the urinary sediment is always higher than that in the blood and can range from 15% to 95% (median of 73%).

Epididymitis

Epididymitis is an early complication of bancroftian filariasis, often associated with orchitis, and with or without accompanying lymphangitis and fever.

Fever

Patterns of fever may be characteristic in malaria and kala-azar, but it is a mistake to suppose that they must conform to the textbook pattern, although a "classical" pattern is more likely to be seen in cases of relapse or even recrudescence. Please see the review article by Ryan et al. (2002) for an in depth analysis of the approach to fever in the returning traveler. A *quotidian fever* is often seen in the initial attack of vivax malaria, two or more broods of parasites completing their pre-erythrocytic phase at different times so that there may be a daily fever peak corresponding to rupture of the infected red cells and liberation of merozoites. Daily fever peaks usually are seen only for a few days; apparently within this time all broods of parasites become synchronized, and thereafter the fever cycle exhibits tertian periodicity. Quartan and falciparum malaria may likewise exhibit quotidian or irregular periodicity during the first few days of the primary attack. *Tertian fever* is characteristic of vivax and ovale malaria. The paroxysm has an abrupt onset, usually initiated with a chill, which varies from a moderate sensation of cold to the intense, bed-shaking chill usually thought typical of malaria. The chill lasts up to an hour and the fever (to 104° or 105°F) for 2 hours or longer, followed by a profuse sweat, during the course of which the temperature falls to normal over a period of an hour or so. The sweating stage is usually followed by sleep, and when the patient awakens he or she generally feels well. The next paroxysm is initiated approximately 48 hours after the onset of the previous one. *Subtertian fever*, seen in falciparum malaria, is so called because the cycle may more nearly approach 36 than 48 hours. There is usually no frank chill, and the febrile stage is prolonged, though the fever is not usually as high as in vivax; it may not fall to normal even in the intervals between paroxysms. There may be double peaks of fever in each 24-hour period, resembling the fever curve in kala-azar. There is often no well-defined sweating stage, though sweating may be continuous, periodic, or completely absent. *Quartan fever* is seen in malaria caused by *Plasmodium malariae*. There is often a regular periodicity from the start; the paroxysms recur at 72-hour intervals; while similar to those of vivax malaria, they are generally more severe. The hot stage often lasts several hours and is frequently accompanied by nausea and vomiting; the sweating stage may be followed by prostration. *Hyperpyrexia* may develop as part of an attack of cerebral malaria or in the course of an apparently uncomplicated attack of falciparum malaria; as the result of injury to the heat-control center in the hypothalamus there is a rapid rise in temperature to 107°F or higher and death quickly ensues.

A *doubly remittent* or "*dromedary*" *fever* is frequently found in kala-azar. Febrile attacks, which last a few days to several weeks, are separated by afebrile periods of equal irregularity.

At some time during the course of a febrile attack there are usually one or more days during which a double or triple rise to a temperature of 103° to 105°F can be demonstrated during a 24-hour period.

An irregularly spiking fever with hepatic tenderness, suggestive of cholangitis, may be seen in amebic hepatitis, fascioliasis, and acute clonorchiasis and opisthorchiasis. The initial period of schistosome infection is likewise marked by irregular fever and hepatic tenderness, with nausea and vomiting, diarrhea, and, often, giant hives. An irregular fever, usually with evening peaks and night sweats, is an early finding in African trypanosomiasis, and a high remittent fever lasting for several weeks occurs early in Chagas' disease. A remittent fever, with temperature to 104° or 105°F, frequently marks the stage of larval migration in trichinosis. *Filarial fever* may occur very early in the course of a filarial infection. There is usually a sudden onset, with fever ranging in the neighborhood of 102° to 104°F and remaining elevated for several hours to a couple of days, and gradually subsiding in the next several days. Attacks of lymphangitis and lymphadenitis (q.v.) usually accompany the febrile episodes.

Funiculitis

Inflammation of the spermatic cord is frequently an early sign of bancroftian filariasis.

Hematuria

In *Schistosoma haematobium* infections, beginning as early as 3 months after infection or sometimes not until several years later, there may be intermittent hematuria. There is no dysuria, but there may be some frequency and also bladder pain following urination. Hematuria is often referred to as terminal hematuria limited to the last few drops of urine, blood being forced out as the bladder wall contracts.

Hemoglobinuria

Blackwater fever usually is seen in conjunction with an attack of falciparum malaria, generally in patients who have had previous attacks of malaria. The passage of reddish or redbrown urine signals a bout of intravascular hemolysis, which may occur once or repeatedly and may lead to severe renal tubular damage and anuria. The cause of blackwater fever is unknown; hypotheses include quinine sensitivity, glucose-6-phosphate dehydrogenase deficiency in persons treated with primaquine and related drugs, and autohemolysis on the basis of antibodies formed against altered infected red blood cells.

Hepatitis

Amebic hepatitis is described under the heading of Abscess, Amebic.

Hepatomegaly

Any parasitic infection involving the liver may result in enlargement of that organ. Thus, amebic hepatitis or liver abscess, visceral larva migrans, liver fluke infections, and early schistosomiasis are all characterized by an enlarged and tender liver, which is also seen in some cases of falciparum malaria and acute neonatal toxoplasmosis as well as in kala-azar and Chagas' disease. Hydatid infections of the liver and *Schistosoma mansoni* and *S. japonicum* infections may result in an enlarged but usually nontender liver. The hepatic fibrosis ("pipestem fibrosis") characteristic of chronic schistosome infections produces a clinical picture similar to that of Laënnec's cirrhosis, often with splenomegaly.

Helminth infections involving the liver are also characterized by eosinophilia. In visceral larva migrans, a leukocytosis of up to 80,000 per mm^3 may be present, with a striking eosinophilia. In amebic abscess of the liver, on the other hand, though the white blood cell count may be in the range of 25,000 per mm^3, there is no eosinophilia.

Hives

Giant hives and other allergic symptoms, such as bronchial asthma, are commonly seen in ascariasis, and hives often appear during the first few weeks of schistosome infections.

Hydatid Thrill

In large unilocular echinococcal cysts of the abdominal viscera that are situated close to the abdominal wall, a characteristic thrill may be elicited by quick palpation or percussion. This phenomenon may be simulated by percussion of a balloon filled with water.

Hydrocele

Hydrocele is a common finding in areas where filariasis is endemic, developing as a sequela to repeated attacks of orchitis. If lymphatic varices develop in the cord and rupture into the scrotal sac, a condition known as lymphocele results.

Hydrocephalus

Although not as intimately associated with congenital toxoplasmosis as are retinochoroiditis and cerebral calcifications, hydrocephalus or microcephaly is commonly seen in this condition. Cysticerci within the ventricular system of the brain may lead to an internal hydrocephalus.

Hyperpigmentation

Kala-azar (Hindi for "black fever") (visceral leishmaniasis) derives its name from intensification of the pigmentation of the skin over the cheeks and temples and around the mouth. It is most obvious in dark-skinned races. In onchocerciasis, repeated attacks of allergic dermatitis may result in hyperpigmentation of the area, usually on the face, neck, or ears. Bronzing and induration of the affected skin areas may occur in chronic pediculosis (vagabonds' disease).

Jaundice

Obstructive jaundice may be seen in severe liver fluke infections but is not characteristic of light infections or those of moderate intensity. The symptoms of the falciparum malaria syndrome known as *bilious remittent fever* include acute epigastric pain, nausea and vomiting, and marked enlargement and tenderness of the liver, with jaundice appearing on about the second day. Diarrhea, a high remittent fever, and oliguria are usually seen, and death may result from renal or hepatic failure.

Kerandel's Sign

Noted in the stage of central nervous system involvement in African sleeping sickness, Kerandel's sign may be elicited by pressure on the palm of the hand or over the ulnar nerve and consists of severe pain that occurs shortly after the pressure has been relieved.

Keratitis

Ocular migration of the microfilariae of *Onchocerca volvulus* frequently produces a character-istic keratitis, or inflammation of the cornea. The keratitis (punctate or sclerosing) may lead to blindness. Uveitis may also occur. Free-living amebae of the genus *Acanthamoeba* are able to penetrate the cornea, which rapidly leads to visual deterioration and blindness. The amebae also cause conjunctivitis, iritis, and uveitis.

Leukocytosis

Leukocytosis seldom continues throughout the course of any of the parasitic infections. In amebic hepatitis or abscess there may be a white blood cell count of 25,000 to 30,000 per mm^3 with 70% to 80% polymorphonuclear neutrophils. In visceral larva migrans a leuko-cytosis of up to 80,000 per mm^3 has been reported, with an eosinophilia of 20% to 80%. Trichinosis may be characterized by a white blood cell count of 30,000 per mm^3 early in the infection, and strongyloidiasis by one nearly as elevated; these usually decline and may be followed by leukopenia. Leukocytosis early in the course of infection, followed by leukopenia with a relative monocytosis, is common to many protozoan and helminth infections.

Leukopenia

A white blood cell count of 4000 per mm^3 or less, with a relative monocytosis, generally is seen throughout the course of kala-azar, sometimes terminating in agranulocytosis.

In malaria, leukopenia of 3000 to 6000 white blood cells per mm^3 with a relative monocytosis may accompany the afebrile periods, only to be replaced by leukocytosis during the paroxysm.

Lymphadenitis

In filariasis, the femoral, inguinal, axillary, and epitrochlear nodes are most commonly involved. The nodes are enlarged, painful, and tender during an acute attack of lymphangi-tis and tend to remain enlarged between attacks. A condition resembling infectious mononucleosis sometimes is seen in the acute stage of toxoplasmosis, with fever, weakness, malaise, generalized adenopathy, and sometimes a rash. There may be generalized lym-phadenitis without fever or other symptoms. In the early stages of African trypanosomiasis, there may be generalized adenopathy; the glands of the posterior cervical triangle are most conspicuously affected (Winterbottom's sign). Generalized adenopathy is seen in the acute stage of Chagas' disease.

Lymphangitis

Acute lymphangitis is an early symptom of lymphatic filarial infection. It usually is accompanied by fever and may affect the limbs, breast, or scrotum. When it occurs in a limb, it is usually centrifugal in development, starting at a lymph node and progressing distally. The course of the lymphatic is readily seen because of local distension and erythema. Centrifugal spread of the lymphangitis is the reverse of that seen in bacterial lymphangitis (blood poisoning), in which the infection extends proximally from the point of origin.

Lymphocytosis

Relative or absolute lymphocytosis, unusual in parasitic infections, is, however, generally seen in Chagas' disease. Initially there may be slight leukocytosis, usually followed by leukopenia. Increased numbers of lymphocytes are seen in the spinal fluid (though not the blood) during central nervous system involvement in African trypanosomiasis.

Lymph Varices

Dilatations of the lymphatic vessels may occur secondarily to lymphatic blockage in filariasis. They are most frequently seen in the inguinal and femoral areas, but other lymphatic tracts may be affected. The soft lobulated swellings may rupture and drain. When this occurs on the scrotum, a chronic condition known as *lymph scrotum* may develop.

Melena

Upper gastrointestinal bleeding of a degree sufficient to produce melena is rare in parasitic disease; it is mentioned here primarily with strongyloidiasis in mind. Infection with *Strongyloides stercoralis* may run the gamut from a complete absence of symptoms to those infections of the duodenum and jejunum that are so extensive as to produce ulceration of the mucosa, with blood loss to the point of clinical anemia, and with melena. Especially in immunosuppressed patients, the coincidental finding of anemia with melena and a significant eosinophilia should stimulate a thorough search for this sometimes elusive parasite.

Meningoencephalitis

Invasion of the central nervous system by trypanosomes is characterized in African sleeping sickness by increasing symptoms of meningoencephalitis. There may be quite variable sensory and motor changes, personality disorders, headache, confusions, drowsiness, and finally coma. Similar but milder symptoms are seen in Chagas' disease. Minor neurologic symptoms are seen during almost any attack of malaria (i.e., headache, disorientation). Cerebral malaria is characteristic of falciparum infection and may develop slowly with increasing headache and drowsiness over several days or present as a coma or mental disturbance of sudden onset. There may be signs of meningeal irritation; symptoms are quite varied, depending on the brain areas affected. If the cord is affected, the symptoms may be suggestive of multiple sclerosis.

Primary amebic meningoencephalitis, caused by invasion of the central nervous system by ordinarily free-living ameboflagellates belonging to the genus *Naegleria*, is an acute, rapidly progressive infection, acquired while swimming or diving in fresh water. It is characterized by fever, headache, mental confusion, and coma; death frequently occurs within a few days of onset. *Acanthamoeba* and *Balamuthia* may produce a more chronic granulomatous meningoencephalitis.

Eosinophilic meningoencephalitis, seen in various Pacific islands as well as Thailand, Taiwan, Central America, and Cuba in recent years, is believed, on strong epidemiologic grounds, to be symptomatic of infection with *Angiostrongylus cantonensis* and thus a form of larva migrans infection. It is characterized by fever, headache, stiff neck, and increased cells (mainly eosinophils) in the spinal fluid. It is generally a mild and self-limited infection. *Micronema deletrix*, ordinarily saprophytic, and *Baylisascaris procyonis*, usually found parasitizing raccoons, are two other nematodes that may produce meningoencephalitis in humans.

Myocarditis

Myocardial infection is characteristic of Chagas' disease and is seen in about 50% of chronic cases. Cardiac failure may come on slowly, although in infants it tends to occur in the early acute stage. There may be pericardial effusion. Congestive heart failure also has been reported in African trypanosomiasis, probably in the Rhodesian form of the disease, but the cause of the heart failure is not as apparent. Myocarditis, occasionally severe enough to cause death, has been reported in trichinosis. It is the result of migration of the larvae through the myocardium, in which they do not encyst. Myocarditis also may be seen in acute toxoplasmosis in both infants and adults, the result of invasion of the myocardium.

Myositis

Although myositis is a nonspecific symptom of many febrile illnesses, severe myositis is characteristic of the stage of larval migration in trichinosis. If accompanied by circumorbital edema, eosinophilia, and a history of consumption of insufficiently cooked pork, the diagnosis may be made with some certainly. Myositis, usually involving a single muscle group, may also occur in *Sarcocystis* infection.

Neurologic Symptoms

Neurologic symptoms in trypanosomiasis, malaria, and amebic and eosinophilic meningoencephalitis are discussed under Meningoencephalitis. Variable neurologic symptoms may occur in schistosomiasis when eggs carried by the bloodstream to the central nervous system lodge there and provoke a granulomatous reaction. Neurologic and other symptoms caused by embolization of eggs are more common in *Schistosoma japonicum* infection than in the other two species, whereas in *S. mansoni* and *S. haematobium*, eggs are found more frequently in the spinal cord than in the brain, perhaps because of ectopic wanderings of the adult worms. In *S. japonicum* infection, there may be severe neurologic symptoms, including coma and paresis, during the incubation period or first few weeks after infection. Transitory neurologic symptoms of a variable nature may be caused by the migration of ascarid and trichina larvae in the central nervous system; hemiplegia and focal epileptic attacks have been reported in trichinosis. Hydatid, coenurus, and cysticercus cysts may develop within the central nervous system, where they may produce symptoms related to a space-occupying lesion or, if within the ventricular system, internal hydrocephalus. Cysticercus larvae may give rise to epileptiform seizures, as may *Sparganum proliferum* and adults of *Paragonimus westermani* that have gone astray.

Nodules, Subcutaneous

Lipoma-like subcutaneous nodules include onchocercomas (q.v.) and cysticercus and coenurus larvae. The cysticercus larva of *Taenia solium* develops most frequently in the subcutaneous tissues, where it forms nodules 0.5 to 3.0 cm in diameter. In almost half the recorded human cases of coenurus infection, the larvae have been found in the subcutaneous tissues; others have been recorded from the brain, spinal cord, and eye. *Echinococcus* cysts also may be found in the subcutaneous tissues. Spargana also form subcutaneous nodules, somewhat elongate and several centimeters in length, which may resemble lipomas, but they may move through the subcutaneous tissues at irregular intervals and often cause pain. *Sparganum proliferum* may develop as branched or multiple nodules and invade the viscera. (See also Edema, for a discussion of ocular sparganosis.) Larvae of the botfly *Hypoderma* migrate through the subcutaneous tissues, finally coming to rest beneath the skin, where they produce elongate nodules several centimeters in length. Considerable pain may accompany migration, but the resting nodule is seldom painful or pruritic. The human botfly, *Dermatobia hominis*, burrows into the skin and subcutaneous tissues, producing an intensely pruritic popular lesion, which has the appearance of a furuncle. There is a small central opening, from which comes a serous exudate and through which the posterior end of the larva may protrude from time to time. Secondary infection is common.

Obstruction, Intestinal

Ascaris, especially in children, may produce complete intestinal obstruction, with accompanying abdominal pain, vomiting, distention, and hyperperistalsis. Partial or complete intestinal obstruction may also characterize infection by *Angiostrongylus costaricensis*.

Onchocercoma

Adult worms of *Onchocerca volvulus* lie in coiled masses beneath the skin, completely enclosed in a fibrous tissue capsule. They are from a few millimeters to several centimeters in diameter, generally freely movable, and resemble lipomas. In Mexico and Guatemala they frequently occur beneath the patient's scalp; in Africa most occur on other parts of the patient's body.

Orchitis

Filarial orchitis may occur early in the disease and at times in the absence of lymphangitis or fever; repeated attacks lead to hydrocele.

Pain

Abdominal pain, generally vague or ill defined, is said to accompany many of the intestinal parasitic infections. The presence or absence of such tenuous pains is of no value from a diagnostic standpoint. Epigastric pain, sometimes with nausea and vomiting, may be seen in giardiasis, cryptosporidiosis (especially in immunodepressed persons), trichinosis, and strongyloidiasis; it is related to the duodenitis and jejunitis provoked by these infections. Moderate to severe abdominal pain is seen in acute amebic colitis; it may be confined to the cecal area or may be generalized. *Angiostrongylus costaricensis* may give rise to similar symptoms, as may *Eustrongylides* larvae. In ascariases, severe pain may signal intestinal obstruction (q.v.), perforation and peritonitis (q.v.), or bile duct blockage.

Muscle pain in trichinosis is discussed under Myositis, and the delayed pain sensation seen in African trypanosomiasis under the heading of Kerandel's Sign.

Peritonitis

Penetration of *Ascaris* through the wall of the intestine usually leads to generalized peritonitis, with pain, marked distension, generalized abdominal tenderness, and free air under the diaphragm, detectable by x-ray. In severe amebic dysentery, ulcers may erode through the wall of the intestine and cause peritonitis. Peritonitis may rarely result from perforation of the bowel wall by, or in the course of infection with, a number of other parasites.

Pica

"A craving for unnatural foods ... as seen in hysteria, preganancy, and in malnourished children": this dictionary definition of pica must be broadened to include among its causes anemia, especially the anemia of hookworm disease, and the realization that the consumption of soil, a frequent form of pica, may increase exposure to such infections as hookworm, ascariasis, toxocariasis, and toxoplasmosis.

Pneumonitis

Pneumonitis is characteristic of severe *Ascaris* infection and is caused when the worm larvae break out of the capillaries into the alveoli, whence they are coughed up to be swallowed, beginning the intestinal phase of the disease. Symptoms and signs, first noted 1 to 5 days after the eggs are ingested, consist of cough, fever, respiratory distress, and the physical and x-ray signs of a bronchopneumonia; in severe cases there may be complete consolidation of one or more lobes. The pneumonitis usually clears within a week or two; it may be accompanied by intense eosinophilia and an urticarial rash. Similar signs and symptoms may accompany the corresponding stage in *Strongyloides* infection, although the pneumonitis is generally not as severe. In hookworm infection there is seldom a clear-cut pneumonitis at this stage, but cough is frequently present. In schistosomiasis there may likewise be a transitory cough, sometimes with hemoptysis and frequently with dyspnea, during the stage of migration through the lungs.

Proteinuria

In falciparum malaria, proteinuria, with hyaline and granular casts in the urine, is common. Rarely there may be oliguria or anuria, usually accompanying an attack of blackwater fever (q.v.). The nephrotic syndrome, with proteinuria, is sometimes seen in quartan malaria.

Pruritus Ani

The nocturnal pruritus that accompanies pinworm infection varies considerably in degree, probably depending upon hypersensitivity of the host. In some persons there is no noticeable itching, whereas in others it may be sufficiently severe to interfere with rest.

Anal pruritus may be associated with active migration of gravid proglottids of *Taenia saginata* out of the anus.

Pulmonary Infiltrates with Eosinophilia (PIE)

A clinical classification of PIE modified from Pierce and Crouch (1989) is as follows:
A. Illnesses in which PIE is a major component:
   Allergic bronchopulmonary aspergillosis
   Chronic eosinophilic pneumonia
   Drug reactions (e.g., nitrofurantoin)
   Hypereosinophilic syndrome
   Parasitic infections (e.g., tropical eosinophilia [q.v.]; strongyloidiasis, ascariasis, and
      hookworm disease [during invasive stage])
   Polyarteritis nodosa
B. Illnesses in which PIE occurs infrequently:
   Bacterial and fungal infections (e.g., tuberculosis, brucellosis, histoplasmosis, coccid-
      ioidomycosis)
   Neoplasms (e.g., Hodgkin's disease)
   Immune disorders (e.g., rheumatoid lung disease, sarcoidosis)

Pulmonary Symptoms, Chronic

In all three types of schistosomiasis, but especially in *Schistosoma haematobium* infections, eggs may be carried to the lungs, where pseudotubercle formation around them may produce a radiologic picture suggestive of miliary tuberculosis, and increasing fibrosis may lead to cor pulmonale. Paragonimiasis is characterized by chronic cough; the production of thick, blood-specked sputum or sometimes frank hemoptysis; and increasing dyspnea. X-ray may show patchy infiltrates, rounded shadows suggestive of coin lesions, calcifications, and pleural thickening or effusion. In pulmonary echinococcosis, cough is usually the first symptom. There may be increasing dyspnea; with erosion of blood vessels there will be hemoptysis, and with obstruction there results secondary bacterial infection and fever. If the cyst ruptures into a bronchus, the contents may be coughed up or the patient may become asphyxiated.

Rash

An allergic urticarial rash or hives (q.v.) is often seen in the early stages of schistosome infection and in ascariasis. A macular or maculopapular eruption may occur early in the course of a trichina infection, and one of the variants of acute toxoplasmosis is a typhuslike fever, with a macular rash, prostration, and sometimes stupor and cardiac decompensation. During attacks of fever in the early stages of African trypanosomiasis there may be an irregular blotchy rash, often annular. The individual patches may be several inches across; they tend to fade in a few hours and reappear at irregular intervals. A petechial rash may occur with high parasitemias in any of the malarias, but especially those due to *P. falciparum* or *P. vivax*.

Retinochoroiditis

Infection of the retina and choroid by *Toxoplasma* or (rarely) *Entamoeba histolytica* may produce visual disturbances, which can be profound if the macula is involved. On ophthalmoscopic examination, a grayish or yellow-white area surrounded by exudate is seen early; with healing this leaves a white, atrophic patch bordered by pigment deposits. Invasion of the eye by microfilariae of *Onchocerca volvulus* or the larvae of *Toxocara* or *Angiostrongylus cantonensis* may also produce a retinochoroiditis.

Romaña's Sign

Unilateral palpebral edema, involving both upper and lower eyelids, appears early in the course of an infection with *Trypanosoma cruzi*. The edema is hard and nonpitting; it may remain confined to the eyelids or may spread to involve the cheek and neck. It may subside promptly or persist for weeks or months.

Shock

When shock complicates falciparum malaria, the patient is pale, with a cold and clammy skin, thin fast pulse, and low blood pressure. There is often acute abdominal pain, vomiting, and diarrhea. The cause may be primary adrenal failure, through parasite-induced ischemia or infarction, or it may be secondary to reduced blood volume and blood pressure caused by widespread vascular injury. Rupture of an echinococcus cyst may lead to anaphylactic shock.

Splenomegaly

As part of generalized lymphoid hyperplasia in both African and American trypanosomiasis, splenomegaly may be observed. In kala-azar the spleen is said to enlarge downward about an inch per month, and it may extend into the pelvis. It is not tender and reverts to normal size after effective therapy. The spleen enlarges during an acute attack of malaria and is usually palpable within 2 weeks after onset, although in some nonimmune individuals, palpable (acute) splenomegaly may appear within a day or two of initially detectable parasitemia (approximately 50 to 100 parasites per µl of blood). Between attacks it may shrink, and in adults it may become fibrotic and smaller than normal. In children, repeated attacks may lead to great enlargement of the organ, which may extend to the pelvis. The "splenic index," a guide to endemicity of malaria obtained by examination of a population for evidence of enlarged spleens, obviously must be derived only through examination of children. The spleen is usually tender during an acute attack of malaria, and tenderness may be apparent before the organ can be palpated. Splenic infarction or rupture is rare and tends not to produce catastrophic bleeding, but rather, an ooze. In *Schistosoma mansoni* and *S. japonicum* infections, splenomegaly is secondary to hepatic fibrosis brought about by egg deposition in the liver, and resulting portal hypertension.

In an area where malaria, schistosomiasis, and kala-azar all are common (Kenya), tropical splenomegaly syndrome (hyperreactive malarial splenomegaly) accounted for 31% of cases of chronic splenomegaly. Hepatosplenic schistosomiasis was the cause in 17.6% of those involved, and visceral leishmaniasis 5.3%. Other common diagnoses were portal hypertension of unknown cause (10.7%) and cirrhosis (6.9%).

Splinter Hemorrhages

Sometimes occurring during the stage of active larval migration in trichinosis, minute linear hemorrhages in the nail beds are a general sign of vascular injury.

Steatorrhea

Malabsorption, characterized by the presence of fat in the stools, is seen in certain parasitic infections. The most common of these is giardiasis, which may make its presence known by flatulence and the production of foul-smelling, fatty stools. Unfortunately, *Giardia*-induced malabsorption does not necessarily disappear with eradication of the infection but may persist some time thereafter. *Strongyloides* infections may also cause steatorrhea, as may infection with *Capillaria philippinensis*, and in immunosuppressed patients, *Cryptosporidium* and *Isospora belli*.

Tachycardia

A fast pulse is noted early in both African and American trypanosomiasis. In Chagas' disease it persists into the subacute and chronic stages, where it may be associated with heart block, Stokes-Adams syndrome, and fibrillation.

Ulcers, Cutaneous

In leishmanial and trypanosomal diseases there is a primary multiplication at the site of infection. In *Leishmania tropica*–complex infections there is first a papule at the site of infection, which gradually transforms into a shallow ulcer with raised edges. The Chiclero ulcer of Southern Mexico and Central America is similar to an oriental sore, except when it occurs on the ear, where it may erode the pinna. *L. braziliensis* first produces cutaneous ulcerations, which may, through extension or metastasis, come to involve the nasal mucosa, the soft and the hard palate, the nasal septum, the pharynx, and the larynx, even after complete healing of the initial cutaneous ulcer. In blacks, granulomatous rather than ulcerative lesions are generally seen. In African sleeping sickness there may be a firm, tender, raised lesion, up to 2 cm or more in diameter, at the site of infection. This "trypanosomal chancre" is painful or pruritic, but like the chagoma (q.v.) it apparently does not ulcerate unless secondarily infected. Ulcerative cutaneous lesions are seen rarely in amebiasis, either in the perianal region or in the skin surrounding fistulas or surgical drainage incisions from hepatic abscesses. A rounded ulcer, 2 mm to several centimeters in diameter, marks the place at which the guinea worm discharges its larvae. In the center of the ulcer, a portion of the worm may be visible. There is often secondary infection, and a painful localized reaction may persist until discharge of the larvae is complete.

Urethritis

Trichomonas vaginalis has been found in up to a third of cases of "nonspecific" urethritis in men.

Vaginitis

A prolific, irritating, thin green or yellowish discharge may be seen in *Trichomonas vaginalis* infection; the vagina may be diffusely congested or covered by punctate hemorrhagic spots. The organisms may be present in asymptomatic persons. Pinworms may migrate from the anus and enter the vagina, where they produce a temporary, intense pruritus in some children.

Visual Difficulties

Vision problems associated with parasitic disease include circumorbital edema (q.v.), conjunctivitis (q.v.), and retinochoroiditis (q.v.). Ascarid larvae (of *Ascaris lumbricoides* and *Toxocara*) may invade the eye, producing iritis or other symptoms. *Angiostrongylus cantonensis* also invades the eye, producing visual impairment, iritis, retinal edema, and other signs and symptoms. Patients infected with *Onchocerca* actually may be aware of the intraocular movement of the microfilariae, and lesions of the anterior chamber, iris, ciliary body, choroid, and retina developing in this condition may lead to diminution of vision or total blindness. *Loa loa* migration may produce ocular pain and conjunctivitis or frank subconjunctival hemorrhage, but not visual difficulty. Cysticercus and coenurus larvae may develop within the eye. Pentastomids may invade the anterior chamber. Ophthalmomyiasis, or invasion of the orbit, is often caused by migratory larvae of *Hypoderma*, the cattle grub. External ophthalmomyiasis is usually caused by larvae of *Oestrus ovis*, the sheep botfly.

Winterbottom's Sign

Posterior cervical lymphadenitis is seen early in African trypanosomiasis. Aspiration of the enlarged nodes may reveal trypomastigotes at a time when none can be found in the peripheral blood.

X-Ray Evidence of Parasitic Disease

Amebiasis: Amebic granulomas of the large bowel simulate carcinoma in barium enema studies. Cecal amebiasis tends to produce a funnel-shaped deformity of that portion of the bowel as seen in barium enema studies. In amebic abscess of the liver there may be elevation of the right diaphragm and sometimes right lower lobe pneumonitis. CT, MRI, and ultrasound are equally sensitive for the detection of liver abscess due to *Entamoeba* or *Echinococcus*. *Giardiasis:* Evidence of intestinal malabsorption. *Toxoplasmosis:* Intracerebral calcifications. *Dracunculiasis, filariasis,* and *loiasis:* Calcified worms may be seen in the tissues. *Ascariasis:* Pneumonitis. Adult worms may be seen as cylindrical empty spaces in the barium-filled bowel or common bile duct in a small bowel series. *Strongyloidiasis* and *hookworm infection:* Pneumonitis. Loss of mucosal markings and a tubular deformity of the duodenum and jejunum may be seen in small bowel studies on patients with strongyloidiasis. *Cysticercosis:* Calcified cysts in the subcutaneous tissues, muscles, brain (MRI is more sensitive than CT for visualizing CNS cysticercosis). *Echinococcosis:* Well-defined, rounded masses may be seen in the lung parenchyma; sometimes a fluid level is visible within them. Hepatic cysts are visible by CT, MRI, or ultrasound. Hydatid cysts of bone produce extensive intramedullary erosion, demonstrable by x-ray. *Paragonimiasis:* Patchy infiltrates or rounded densities in the lung parenchyma, pleural thickening, or fluid. *Schistosomiasis:* Pulmonary fibrosis, or a picture suggestive of miliary tuberculosis. Cor pulmonale with dilation of the pulmonary artery and its main branches, right ventricular hypertrophy. *S. haematobium infections:* Calcification in the wall of the bladder; hydronephrosis, hydroureter. *Pentastomiasis:* C-shaped calcifications, less than 1 cm in diameter, in the viscera or lungs.

References

Asperilla MO. Eosinophilic meningitis associated with ciprofloxacin. *Am J Med* 1989; 87:589–590.
Harries AD et al. Eosinophilia in Caucasians returning from the tropics. *Trans R Soc Trop Med Hyg* 1986; 80:327–328.

Harris ED. Case records of the Massachusetts General Hospital. *N Engl J Med* 1979; *302*:256–263.

Jaroonvesama N. Differential diagnosis of eosinophilic meningitis. *Parasitol Today* 1988; *4*:262–266.

Kuberski T. Eosinophils in the cerebrospinal fluid. *Ann Intern Med* 1979; *91*:70–75.

Markell EK. Is there any reason to continue treating *Blastocystis* infection? *Clin Infect Dis* 1995; *21*:104–105.

Pierce J, Crouch E. Clinicopathologic conference. Asthma and eosinophilia in a 66-year-old woman. *Am J Med* 1989; *87*:439–444.

Ryan ET, Wilson ME, Kain KC. Illness after international travel. *N Engl J Med* 2002; *347*:505–516.

Wurtz R. *Cyclospora:* A newly identified intestinal pathogen of humans. *Clin Infect Dis 1994*; *18*:620–623.

Zuckerman MJ et al. *Blastocystis hominis* and intestinal injury. *Am J Med Sci* 1994; *308*:96–101.

Pseudoparasites
and Pitfalls

It is common experiene that the beginner almost as frequently misidentifies a yeast or other plant cell as an ameba, or a platelet as a malarial parasite, as he or she fails to identify the parasitic organisms actually present in the material examined. A wide variety of objects that resemble parasites may be found in stool specimens or other materials. It would be impractical as well as unprofitable to attempt a complete listing of these diagnostic pitfalls, but a number of the more important types will be briefly considered.

A pseudoparasite is an object that resembles a parasite or the egg of a parasite but is either not a parasite at all or not parasitic in the host under consideration. "Pseudosymbiont" might be a better term in the latter instance, although pseudoparasite has been used by some to designate commensal organisms, such as *Entamoeba coli*. While *E. coli* is not in the strict sense a parasite, it hardly seems necessary to call it a pseudoparasite and thus accuse it of sailing under false colors.

Even inorganic materials may occur in such forms as to suggest parasitic organisms to the unwary. Oil droplets present in the stool because of diet, disease, or drug administration may be small and surprisingly uniform in size. If their lack of internal structure is disregarded, they may suggest amebic cysts. A fat stain reveals their true nature, and fatty materials are eliminated by the ether used in both of the concentration methods described in Chapter 14. Many kinds of yeasts normally present in the stool may be confused with cysts of some of the intestinal protozoa. Figure 13-1 indicates some of the more common types. Yeasts are quite variable in size and shape, although the majority are ovoid, and most fall within the size range of the various protozoan cysts. The nuclei of yeast cells are solid, without obvious internal structure, and stain blue-black or black with hematoxylin stains and dark red with trichrome. It is generally assumed that intestinal yeasts are harmless, but it must be remembered that *Candida* and, rarely, *Blastomyces* may occur in the feces. However, these organisms, like the pathogenic intestinal bacteria, cannot be recognized morphologically and must be isolated and identified by specialized techniques when indicated.

Blastocystis hominis (Figs. 3-35 and 13-1) has a spherical form and ranges from 5 to 30 μm in diameter. It thus resembles amebic cysts in both size and shape, but it differs sharply from them in internal organization. While this organism may assume several different forms, the form most readily identified in stained specimens has a large, central fluid-filled vacuole surrounded by a layer of cytoplasm containing the nuclei. In iodine preparations, the central area does not stain but the peripheral layer is light yellowish, and the peripheral position of the one or more nuclei is clearly indicated. Somewhat ameboid forms may also be seen. With permanent stains, the central material may take an intense stain, stain lightly, or not stain at all; the nuclei stain darkly and may be seen embedded in the peripheral layer of cytoplasm. Generally considered a nonpathogenic yeast in the past, some maintain that this organism has protozoan affinities, although on the basis of rRNA sequencing (Johnson et al., 1989) its phylogenetic affinities are less clear.

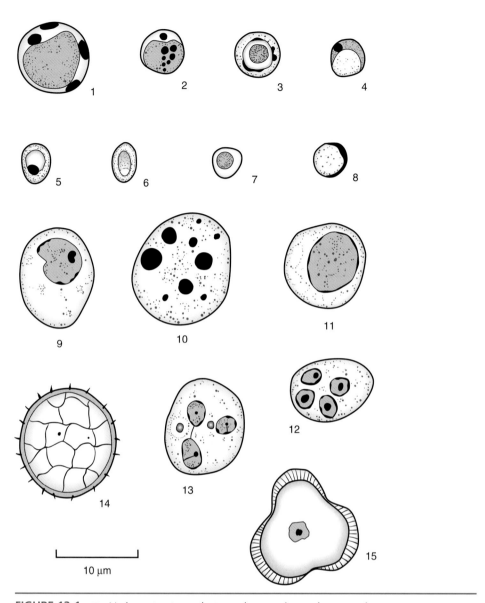

FIGURE 13-1 ■ Various structures that may be seen in stool preparations:
1–4, Blastocystis hominis; 5–8, various yeasts; *9, 11,* squamous cells from rectal mucosa;
10, deteriorated macrophage without nucleus; *12, 13,* polymorphonuclear leukocytes;
14, 15, "pollen grains."

Much attention has been focused on *Blastocystis hominis* in the past two decades, principally because of its classification as a protozoan (perhaps forgetting that a number of intestinal protozoa are definitely nonpathogenic). It is frequently found in patients with gastrointestinal disorders, but as stool examinations are seldom done on asymptomatic patients, any such association must be regarded with caution. Studies by Udkow and Markell (1993) show, in a blinded examination of the stools of approximately 180 asymptomatic persons and a similar number of symptomatic patients, essentially the same prevalence of *Blastocystis* in both groups. Much of the controversy may exist because this is a genetically diverse group of organisms, only some of which might cause illness (Clark 1997). Until there is more convincing evidence of pathogenicity, we do not consider its presence in the stool to be any more significant than that of *Iodamoeba* or *Endolimax.*

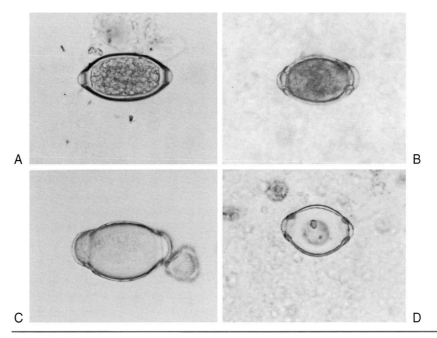

FIGURE 13-2   ■   **A,** *Trichuris* egg. **B–D,** Egglike objects from stools of persons taking "Australian bee pollen" dietary supplement.

Two interesting fungi are occasionally seen as parasites of intestinal amebae: *Sphaerita* invades the cytoplasm, and *Nucleophaga* destroys the nucleus of the ameba. Individual organisms are spherical and about 0.5 to 1 μm in diameter. They usually occur in closely packed masses of varying size. These two organisms seem to be rather invasive, as a large proportion of amebae will be found infected when either organism is found in the stool. The obvious therapeutic potential of this phenomenon has unfortunately failed to materialize!

A variety of the plant materials regularly found in the feces may cause confusion. Pollen grains (Fig. 13-1) and similar structures are very regular in size and often are present in large numbers. Their regularity and abundance may suggest that they are some form of animal parasite; although their structure is generally unlike that of any of the parasitic forms, some may mimic helminth eggs closely enough to confuse the inexperienced observer. A recent pseudo-outbreak of cyclosporiasis was attributed to pollen grain and other artifacts that were similar in size and staining characteristics to *Cyclospora* (Centers for Disease Control and Prevention, 1997). The objects shown in Figure 13-2 have been found in the stools of patients taking "Australian bee pollen" as a dietary supplement, and in samples of the pollen itself. Some more common plant cells, hairs, and fibers are shown in Figure 13-3. Vegetable fibers often have a spiral structure, and frequently a regularly sculpted surface. Plant cells may be recognized by their thick and frequently smooth walls. Some are about the same size and shape as certain helminth eggs, but they seldom possess the regular shape that characterizes the eggs. Vegetable hairs may be confused with larval nematodes but will be seen to have a homogeneous, thick, refractile wall and a minute central canal extending the whole length of the structure. Starch granules may be spherical and, if undigested, can be seen to be composed of concentric layers of white, homogeneous material. Potato starch frequently occurs in irregular saclike aggregates of granules. Undigested starch stains blue when iodine is added to the fecal suspension; partially digested starch stains red. A frequent source of confusion is the presence in the feces of undigested citrus fruit vesicles, the small spindle-shaped individual components of sections of oranges or grapefruit. These resemble in size and general outline the gravid female pinworm. Close observation shows that they do not possess any obvious internal structure.

In areas where fresh-water crayfish (crawfish) are consumed in quantity (e.g., southern Louisiana; northern and central Europe, western Russia), a protistan parasite of these tasty creatures, *Psorospermium haeckelii*, may be simultaneously ingested then passed in the stool. Also known as "beaver bodies" or *corpora parasitica* (Fig. 13-4), they are of a size similar to schistosome ova but have no clinical significance other than of recent diet.

While intestinal myiasis, or the development of fly larvae in the intestinal tract, may occur in humans (Chapter 10), more frequently body parts or whole larval or adult insects in the stool are present as the result of their ingestion with food. Live larvae in a stool specimen may indicate either myiasis or contamination of the specimen. It is important in such cases to ascertain the method of collection of the specimen, particularly if it was obtained outside the laboratory or hospital.

Even if one finds unmistakable helminth eggs in a stool specimen, this does not necessarily indicate infection. Occasionally eggs of the roundworm *Capillaria*, and of certain

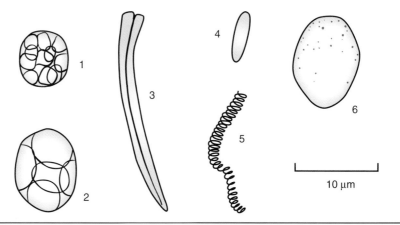

FIGURE 13-3 ■ Plant structures seen in the stool: *1, 2,* aggregates of starch granules; *3,* plant hair; *4, 6,* amorphous vegetable materials, superficially resembling ova or protozoan cysts; *5,* vegetable spiral.

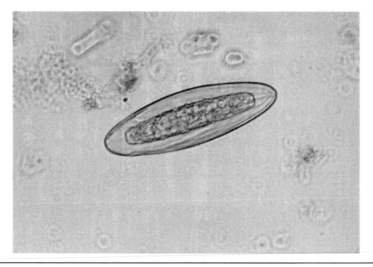

FIGURE 13-4 ■ *Psorospermium haeckelii,* or "beaver body," a protistan parasite of crayfish that may be found in human stools following the consumption of this delicacy. It is of no clinical significance.

trematodes such as *Fasciola*, may be accidentally ingested and pass through the gastrointestinal tract unchanged. The livers of cattle and sheep infected with *Fasciola* are not approved for human consumption if the infection is detected, but if the meat is not inspected or if the infection is light and escapes detection the adult worms may be ingested and their eggs appear in the stools. When there is any question of the possibility of pseudoparasitism of this sort, one should request another specimen, obtained after the diet has been controlled to eliminate any chance of such contamination. Eggs of plant-parasitic roundworms may be ingested with root vegetables and subsequently appear in the feces. One of these, *Heterodera*, is not uncommon and is listed in the key to helminth eggs that appears at the end of Chapter 14.

Mentally disturbed or malingering patients may attempt to feign parasitism by placing various objects in their stools. Earthworms seem to be widely favored for this purpose. The earthworm is an annelid, with a well-developed circulatory system, and the blood vessels can usually be detected under the low power of the microscope. They do bear a superficial resemblance to ascarid nematodes but are generally reddish brown, whereas ascarids are white or pinkish white. The reproductive openings of the earthworm are marked by an annular enlargement of the body, extending for several segments, which is not seen in nematodes.

Various cellular elements in the stool may be mistaken for intestinal amebae. Most important in this regard are polymorphonuclear leukocytes (which have caused false "epidemics" of amebiasis), macrophages, columnar epithelial cells from the intestinal mucosa, or squamous cells from the anal mucosa (Fig. 13-1). Identification of these cells depends on observation of structure and relative size of the nuclei in relation to the cytoplasm. Polymorphonuclear leukocytes, when stained, may show a nucleus divided into four apparently separate spheres, each with peripheral chromatin and an apparent karyosome. However, the nuclear material is larger in proportion to the amount of cytoplasm than in amebic cysts of comparable size, and the shapes of the nuclei are usually more variable. Macrophages may be differentiated from the intestinal amebae by their possession of numerous inclusions within the dark-staining cytoplasm. The nucleus does not appear to have a karyosome but instead has a fine network of chromatin as well as larger particles scattered throughout. Degenerate macropages that have lost their nuclei may also be seen, still containing bits of ingested material.

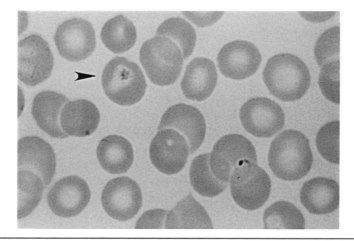

FIGURE 13-5 ■ Platelet, sometimes misidentified as a malaria parasite, overlying a red blood cell *(arrow)* in a Giemsa-stained thin smear. Note true *P. falciparum* ring, to the right and below the platelet-covered red blood cell.

In examining thin blood smears for malaria parasites the novice is often misled by the superimposition of platelets on red blood cells. These may be said to bear a vague resemblance to young trophozoites of *Plasmodium*, but if the slide is correctly stained, their color will be altogether different. While a malaria parasite has blue cytoplasm and red chromatin, the platelet stains in varying shades of purple. So, think "red and blue" when searching for malaria parasites. Platelets are rather fuzzy in outline (Fig. 13-5), whereas the malaria parasite will usually be quite sharp. Careful focusing will help to distinguish the extracellular platelets from intracytoplasmic malaria parasites. Various abnormalities of the red blood cells, such as Howell-Jolly bodies or Cabot's rings, may also be superficially misleading but again do not stain in the same manner as the malaria parasites.

Staining artifacts may fool the unwary. Stages in the life cycle of a presumed helminth ("*Hydatoxi lualba*") were described from the blood of pregnant women with eclampsia or trophoblastic disease, and the "organism" was also purported to cause a toxemia-like syndrome in experimentally inoculated pregnant dogs. Parasitologists were skeptical, and further studies revealed the "helminth" to be an artifact of the toluidine blue O-staining method used to prepare the blood films (Gau et al., 1983; Richards et al., 1983).

References

Centers for Disease Control and Prevention. Outbreaks of pseudoinfection with *Cyclospora* and *Cryptosporidium*. Florida and New York City, 1995. *MMWR* 1997; *46*:354–358.

Clark CG. Extensive genetic diversity in *Blastocystis hominis*. *Molec Bioch Parasitol* 1997; *87*:79–83.

Gau G et al. The worm that wasn't. *Lancet* 1983; *1*:1160–1161.

Johnson AM et al. *Blastocystis hominis:* Phylogenetic affinities determined by rRNA sequence comparison. *Exp Parasitol* 1989; *68*:283–288.

Richards FO et al. The question of a helminthic cause of preeclampsia. *JAMA* 1983; *250*:2970–2972.

Udkow MP, Markell EK. *Blastocystis hominis:* Prevalence in symptomatic versus asymptomatic hosts. *J Infect Dis* 1993; *168*:242–244.

Examination of Stool Specimens

Serologic tests were introduced (see Chapter 16) to identify many intestinal protozoa and helminths but generally have the disadvantage of specificity—that is, they indicate exposure to one particular parasite, but nothing about other organisms that may be present or when the exposure occurred. On the other hand, visual and microscopic examination of the specimen (or of a series of specimens) will in most cases allow the identification of any parasites present, is readily available in most labs, and should precede or accompany serologic examination if the latter seems indicated. On the horizon is the replacement of microscopic examination of stool specimens with antigen- and DNA-detection techniques. These offer increased sensitivity and specificity and are becoming available for many but not all parasites found in the intestine.

Many methods have been described for the examination of stool specimens; some are generally applicable, whereas others serve only limited purposes. Success is directly proportional to the user's familiarity with various methods of examination, thus assuring that those most suitable for a particular specimen or for detection of a particular type of parasite will be employed. For routine examination, it is best to employ certain standard techniques so that one may become familiar with the advantages and limitations of each. Much time may be lost by using a method for purposes for which it was never intended, and identification of a parasite may become difficult or impossible unless the correct method of examination is used.

Physical Characteristics of the Specimen

The consistency of an unpreserved stool specimen is of some importance, giving an indication of the types of organisms that it may contain. Trophozoites of the intestinal protozoa are usually found in liquid or soft stools but almost never in fully formed ones. Protozoan cysts are rarely seen in liquid stools, unless these are the result of administration of a cathartic, in which case both trophic and cystic forms may be present. Cysts are usually found in fully formed specimens. Helminth eggs (see Table 14-1) may be found in either liquid or formed stools, but as the liquid stool is usually very dilute, they are often difficult to detect in such specimens.

If the unpreserved specimen is available, its surface should be examined for macroscopic parasites. Pinworms may be seen on the surface, and tapeworm proglottids can be found there or in the interior. The stool should be broken up with applicator sticks to check for helminths. If bright red blood is seen on the surface of formed stools, it is most frequently a sign of bleeding hemorrhoids; bloody mucus in loose or liquid specimens is highly suggestive of amebic ulcerations in the large intestine, though it may be due to other conditions. Patches of mucus on the surface of a specimen, particularly if blood-tinged, should always be examined with care for trophic amebae. Occult blood in a stool may be a result of intestinal bleeding caused by parasitic organisms, but it is more likely to be indicative of other gastrointestinal disorders.

TABLE 14-1 ■ **Key to the Helminth Eggs**

a. Egg nonoperculate, spherical or subspherical, containing a six-hooked embryo	b
Egg other than above	e
b. Eggs separate	c
Egg in packets of 12 or more	*Dipylidium caninum*
c. Outer surface of egg consists of a thick, radially striated capsule or embryophore	*Taenia* sp.
Outer surface of egg consists of very thin shell, separated from inner embryophore by gelatinous matrix	d
d. Filamentous strands occupy space between embryophore and outer shell	*Hymenolepis nana*
No filamentous strands between embryophore and outer shell	*Hymenolepis diminuta*
	e
e. Egg operculate	f
Egg nonoperculate	j
f. Egg less than 35 μm long	*Clonorchis* or *Opisthorchis sinensis* or *Heterophyes heterophyes* or *Metagonimus yokogawai*
Egg 38 μm or longer	g
g. Egg 38 μm to 45 μm long	*Dicrocoelium dendriticum*
Egg over 60 μm in length	h
h. Egg with shoulders into which operculum fits	*Paragonimus westermani*
Egg without opercular shoulders	i
i. Egg more than 85 μm long	*Faciolopsis buski* or *Fasciola hepatica* or *Echinostoma* sp.
Egg less than 75 μm long	*Diphyllobothrium latum*
j. Egg 75 μm or more in length, spined	k
Egg less than 75 μm long, not spined	m
k. Spine terminal	*Schistosoma haematobium*
Spine lateral	l
l. Lateral spine inconspicuous (perhaps absent)	*Schistosoma japonicum*
Lateral spine prominent	*Schistosoma mansoni*
m. Egg with thick tuberculated capsule	*Ascaris lumbricoides*
Egg without thick tuberculated capsule	n
n. Egg barrel-shaped, with polar plugs	o
Egg not barrel-shaped, without polar plugs	P
o. Shell not striated	*Trichuris trichiura*
Shell often striated	*Capillaria* sp.
p. Egg flattened on one side	*Enterobius vermicularis*
Egg symmetrical	q
q. Egg with large blue-green globules at poles	*Heterodera* sp.
Egg without polar globules	r
r. Egg bluntly rounded at ends, 56 to 75 μm long	Hookworm
Egg pointed at one or both ends, 73 to 95 μm long	*Trichostrongylus* sp.

The age of an unpreserved specimen is an indication of what one may expect to find in it. Freshly passed specimens are essential for the detection of trophic amebae or flagellates. All liquid or soft stools are best examined *within a half hour of the time of passage.* If this is impossible, part of the specimen should be preserved within this period for subsequent examination. Immediate examination of fully formed stools is not as critical, but if they cannot be processed within 3 to 4 hours, they should be preserved.

Examination of a freshly passed stool specimen is impractical or impossible in many instances. For this reason, as well as for the convenience of both the patient and laboratory personnel, most laboratories now rely almost entirely on specimens preserved immediately after passage in various fixative solutions. The specimens may then be submitted to the laboratory for examination at a convenient time. Kits containing these solutions are commercially available or may be prepared by the laboratory for distribution to patients.

Techniques of Stool Examination

Unfortunately, no single technique of stool examination yields entirely satisfactory results, as none of the methods is equally applicable to the detection of trophic protozoa, cysts, and helminth eggs. For this reason, a combination of two or more techniques of examination is desirable. The more useful of these methods are outlined here, with indications of their role in the detection of the various forms of parasites.

DIRECT WET FILM

The *direct* wet film is most useful for the detection of trophic forms of amebae and flagellates, allowing the observer to study the motility of the organisms, which is often characteristic. Wet films are particularly appropriate for immediate examination of bloody mucus and other samples recovered during endoscopic examination of the lower intestinal tract, and for other fresh specimens in which protozoal disease is suspected. It is generally impractical for outpatient use unless special arrangements are made.

In the preparation of a wet film, a small portion of feces is mixed with a drop of normal saline on a clean slide, a coverslip is placed on the preparation, and it is first examined unstained. It is best in making the wet film to take small amounts of material from several parts of the stool specimen. The film should not be too thick. A convenient rule of thumb is to prepare the film just thin enough so that ordinary newsprint can easily be read through it. After the wet film has been thoroughly checked for trophic amebae and flagellates, under low power of the microscope and using a low intensity of illumination, an iodine stain may be prepared.

Iodine stains the cysts of amebae and other protozoa, revealing some details that cannot be seen in the unstained preparation. Trophozoites are rapidly killed and are sometimes unidentifiable after iodine staining; *the stain should not be applied until after the specimen has been thoroughly examined in the unstained condition.* Gram's iodine or Lugol's solution gives satisfactory results, but a modified D'Antoni's iodine solution is preferable.

A separate iodine stain may be prepared by adding a small drop of this reagent to a wet film of fecal material before it is covered, or the iodine may be added to the edge of the coverslip so that it gradually diffuses into the saline mount. The latter technique has the double advantage of not requiring a separate preparation and of staining the fecal material gradually, so that by searching the preparation one may find areas in which the intensity of stain is optimal. A concentrate of the stool may also be stained with iodine and will reveal, in larger numbers, any organisms that may be seen by direct examination of the iodine-stained specimen. Organisms present in such small numbers that they may not be seen at all in direct examination may at times be detected with ease after concentration of the specimen.

CONCENTRATION TECHNIQUES

Many concentration methods have been employed, all of which attempt to separate protozoan cysts and helminth eggs from the bulk of fecal matter through differences in specific gravity. The described methods fall into two general classes: sedimentation and flotation techniques. With the various sedimentation methods, eggs and cysts, which are heavier than the suspending liquid, become concentrated in the bottom of a tube. Flotation involves the use of a heavy liquid, to the surface of which the lighter parasites rise.

The concentrated specimen may be examined directly for protozoan cysts (trophozoites will not be recognizable after concentration) and helminth eggs. Addition of an iodine stain, as discussed under Direct Wet film, may be helpful after the initial examination.

PERMANENT STAINED SLIDES

Frequently it is impossible to make an exact identification of certain protozon on the basis of what is revealed by one or a combination of the preceding techniques. In such cases, the cytologic detail revealed by one of the permanent staining methods is essential for accurate identification. It has been proved that a permanent stain, used alone, reveals a significantly higher percentage of *Entamoeba histolytica* and other protozoan parasites than is detected when only direct examination and concentration methods are used. The use of a permanent stain should be part of any stool examination for protozoa.

When fresh stool specimens are used, a small quantity of feces is transferred to a clean side with an applicator stick. The material is then streaked out in a thin, uniform film, as indicated in Figure 14-1. A little practice will enable one to produce films that are the correct thickness. Generally, formed stools are of the proper consistency for making films, but if the specimen is particularly hard, it may be necessary to add a small amount of saline to a portion of the stool. Liquid stool sometimes fails to adhere to the slide; in such cases a thin layer of serum or of egg albumin, as used in mounting tissue sections, increases adherence. It is essential when using fresh specimens that the film be placed in fixative immediately after it is made; if it dries at any time, it will be useless.

At the present time, the majority of fecal specimens are received in the laboratory in a fixative/preservative solution, which may be of several types. Permanent stained slides (Fig. 14-2) may be made from such material for days or even weeks after they have been placed in the solution, obviating the necessity for immediate processing, which applies to those received fresh. The techniques used in making such slides vary with the type of preservative used and are discussed later.

Number of Specimens to Be Examined

This is a subject over which the laboratory frequently has little or no control, yet a discussion of it may at least have some influence in setting a normal number of stool examinations to be performed on a patient. The number also depends on the purpose for which the examination is made. If one is interested only in determining the presence or absence of helminth parasites, one or two examinations may be sufficient if concentration methods are used, as these methods are very efficient in the detection of small numbers of eggs. On the other hand, Sawitz and Faust (1942) have stated that examination of a single stool will uncover somewhat fewer than 50% of *E. histolytica* infections, and that at least six examinations are necessary if better than 90% accuracy is to be obtained. This is shown graphically in Figure 14-3. These percentages apply to normally passed stools only. Many authorities recommend the routine use of purged stools if one is searching for *E. histolytica*. There is little question that the proper use of purged specimens increases the chances of finding parasites. On the other hand, unless purged specimens are examined immediately they are worthless. If one has the facilities to collect purged specimens *and examine them immediately after they have been passed*, this procedure will probably increase the percentage of positive results. Unless one has such facilities, it is probably best to examine only normally passed stools.

If purgation is to be used, castor and mineral oil should be avoided as they make exmination of the specimen almost impossible. A saline purge of Epsom salts or Fleet Phospho-Soda

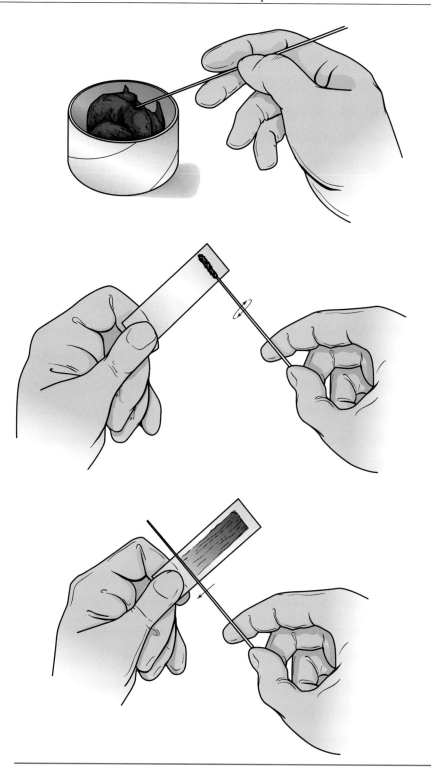

FIGURE 14-1 ■ Preparation of fecal film from fresh specimen, for permanent staining.

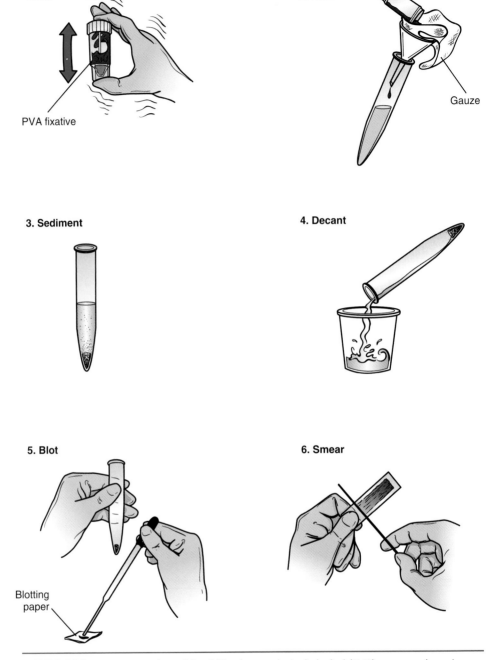

FIGURE 14-2 ■ Preparation of fecal film from polyvinyl alcohol (PVA)–preserved specimen.

is recommended. Parasites in the first bowel movement will probably be distorted; the second and subsequent movements will be most likely to contain recognizable parasites.

Substances that Interfere with Stool Examinations

Castor oil or mineral oil should not be administered prior to the collection of stool specimens. Antibiotics that affect the intestinal flora, administered within the preceding month,

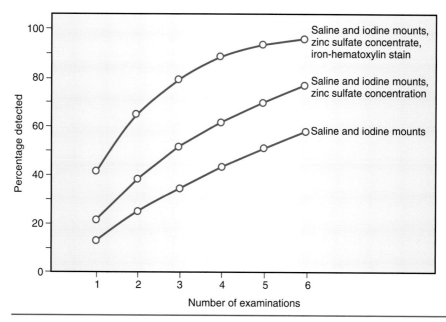

FIGURE 14-3 ■ Probability of detecting *Entamoeba histolytica* by successive stool examinations, using various methods. (Adapted from Sawitz WG, Faust EC. The probability of detecting intestinal protozoa by successive stool examinations. *Am J Trop Med* 1942; *22*:131–136.)

decrease the chances of finding intestinal protozoa, as do antimalarials such as chloroquine. Stools passed for about a week after the administration of barium cannot be examined for parasites, as the barium interferes with microscopy. Enemas of any type should be avoided. Compounds containing kaolin and bismuth, milk of magnesia, and antacids also interfere with the examination for parasites, as does urine in the specimen.

Serologic Testing in Conjunction with Stool Examination

There are specific situations in which serologic testing for intestinal parasites may be necessary on a regular basis. If organisms of the *E. histolytica/dispar* complex are found, serologic testing may be indicated before a precise diagnosis can be given. (Of course, if trophozoites containing ingested red blood cells are found, the diagnosis becomes obvious without further testing.) In some areas where *Giardia* is the most common intestinal protozoan causing diarrheal disease, serologic testing for this organism may be indicated at the time the initial stool specimen is submitted. When *Cryptosporidium* is suspected on epidemiologic grounds, such testing may be performed initially, as microscopic identification is complicated and difficult.

Stains for Direct Smears

MODIFIED D'ANTONI'S IODINE

Distilled water	100 ml
Potassium iodide	1 g
Powdered iodine crystals	1.5 g

The potassium iodide solution should be saturated with iodine, with some excess remaining in the bottle. Store in brown, glass-stoppered bottles in the dark. The solution is ready for use after 4 days, and sufficient quantity for daily use is decanted into a brown glass dropping bottle and discarded after 1 day. The stock solution remains good as long as an excess of iodine remains in the bottle.

LUGOL'S SOLUTION

Distilled water	100 ml
Potassium iodide	10 g
Iodine crystals	5 g

GRAM'S IODINE

Lugol's solution	1 part
Distilled water	14 parts

MIF STAIN (FOR DIRECT SMEARS)

Lugol's solution	0.10 ml
Formaldehyde solution	0.125 ml
Tincture of Merthiolate	0.775 ml

Combine in a small test tube to make sufficient quantity for 25 or 30 preparations. Mixed immunofluorescence (MIF) stain must be made fresh daily, and Lugol's solution should not be over 1 week old. To use the stain, add a small quantity of feces to 1 drop of MIF solution and 1 drop of distilled water, mix thoroughly, and cover with a coverglass.

Preservative Solutions

MIF STAIN-PRESERVATIVE SOLUTION

STOCK MIF SOLUTION:

Distilled water	250 ml
Tincture of Merthiolate	200 ml
Formaldehyde	25 ml
Glycerin	5 ml

This solution is stored in brown glass bottles. For use, it is combined with fresh Lugol's solution (not over 1 week old) in the following manner:

1. Measure 2.35 ml stock MIF solution into a small test tube, and stopper with a cork.
2. Measure 0.15 ml Lugol's solution into a second tube, and close with a rubber stopper.

The two solutions are combined immediately before adding the fecal specimen. The amount of fecal material to be added to this volume of preservative should be about 0.25 g. The specimen is broken up in the MIF solution and mixed thoroughly. The specimen may be examined immediately or stored in a well-stoppered tube; it will retain a good stain for some months. After storage, it will be found that most protozoa and helminth eggs occur in the upper layers of sedimented feces. A drop of mixed supernatant fluid and feces is withdrawn, placed on a slide, and covered with a coverslip.

PVA FIXATIVE SOLUTIONS

The original PVA fixative consists of a mixture of polyvinyl alcohol, glycerin, glacial acetic acid, and Schaudinn's solution. It has the disadvantage of containing mercuric chloride, with consequent disposal problems. Accordingly, it has been modified by the substitution of copper or zinc for the mercury. Although posing less problems of disposal, these modified solutions give less precise preservation of intestinal protozoan morphology than does the mercury-containing solution.

PVA solutions of these three sorts are obtainable in a wide variety of commercial kits, as well as in bulk. If obtained in bulk, it is convenient to dispense the PVA solution in screw-capped vials, in approximate 5-ml quantities. To this volume fixative, about 1 g of formed feces (somewhat more of liquid) may be added. Formed feces must be broken up and mixed thoroughly with the preservative solution. The solution preserves both trophozoites and cysts of protozoa; most eggs are recognizable after PVA preservation, but it is often advisable to include in the packet a second vial containing 10% formalin to allow for concentration for eggs from another aliquot of feces. Protozoa retain their staining quality for at least a month. If a series of stool specimens is desired, the patients may preserve them immediately after passage and bring them all in at one time for processing.

To prepare slides for staining, shake the preserved specimen well, or mix using applicator sticks. Pour some of the PVA mixture onto blotting paper, and allow excess PVA to be absorbed. Apply the preserved stool to the slide in the manner shown in Figure 14-2, and dry for 2 hours at 37°C, or overnight at room temperature. The slides may then be stained with trichrome, but the dry slides may be kept unstained for long periods of time without loss of morphology.

SAF FIXATIVE SOLUTION (YANG AND SCHOLTEN, 1977)

Like PVA, the SAF fixative-preservative may be used for the preservation of material, which can then be concentrated by the formol–ethyl acetate technique or made into permanent stained smears. The fixative is more fluid than PVA, and the preserved specimen must be centrifuged after straining through gauze and the sediment used to prepare smears for staining; adherence to the glass slide may be improved if the slide is coated with albumin. After drying, the slides may be placed in 70% alcohol. The fixative solution is made up as follows:

Sodium acetate	1.5 g
Acetic acid, glacial	2.0 ml
Formaldehyde, 40%	4.0 ml
Distilled water	92.5 ml

SCHAUDINN'S SOLUTION

Schaudinn's solution, a constituent of the original PVA solution, is also used as a fixative and preservative for fresh stool specimens or scrapings from the intestinal mucosa, and as a constituent of the original PVA it carries the same disposal problems because of its mercury content; however, when used on strictly fresh specimens, it provides the optimum in fixation and preservation of structural detail. Liquid or mucoid stool specimens do not adhere well to the slide without the prior application of Meyer's albumin, and specimens preserved in Schaudinn's solution are not suitable for concentration.

Schaudinn's solution may be obtained from a number of commercial sources, or can be prepared as follows:

$HgCl_2$, saturated aqueous solution, 2 parts
95% ethyl alcohol, 1 part

This stock solution keeps indefinitely. Immediately before use, 5 ml of glacial acetic acid is added to each 100 ml of the stock solution.

Meyer's Egg Albumin

This adhesive is prepared from equal parts of fresh egg white and glycerin, mixed thoroughly. A thin layer of albumin is spread on the slide and allowed to dry before Schaudinn-fixed specimens are applied. When used with SAF-preserved specimens, drop-size quantities of albumin and of the concentrated SAF-preserved specimen may be mixed and spread out on the slide. It is unnecessary to use albumin with PVA-preserved specimens.

Concentration Methods

Concentration of stool specimens to demonstrate cysts and eggs present in small numbers shoud be a routine part of the parasitologic examination. The Ritchie sedimentation method is effective for the recovery of most kinds of protozoan cysts and of helminth eggs.

THE RITCHIE CONCENTRATION METHOD (FIG. 14-4)

While this type of concentrate originally employed ether, ethyl acetate is now more commonly substituted. Both work equally well.
1. Emulsify approximately 1 ml feces in 10 to 12 ml normal saline.
2. Filter through two layers of moist gauze into a centrifuge tube.
3. Centrifuge 1 minute at 900 × g; pour off supernatant and resuspend in fresh saline.
4. Centrifuge again 1 minute at 900 × g; if supernatant is still cloudy, repeat.
5. Add 10 ml of 10% formalin to sediment; allow to stand for 5 minutes.
6. Add 3 ml ethyl acetate or ether; shake vigorously.
7. Centrifuge 1½ minutes at 900 × g; loosen "plug" between formalin and ethyl acetate or ether layer, decant supernatant, and examine sediment.

MODIFIED SHEATHER'S SUGAR FLOTATION FOR CRYPTOSPORIDIUM

The sporozoites contained within the rounded oocysts of *Cryptosporidium* (4 to 5 μm in diameter) are well visualized by this method.

SHEATHER'S SUGAR FLOTATION:

Sucrose	500 g
Tap water	320 ml
Phenol	6.5 g

Boil sugar solution until clear. *Carefully* add phenol and stir, using fume hood. Cool to room temperature.
1. Place 1 to 2 ml fecal suspension in 12-ml conical centrifuge tube.
2. Add Sheather's sugar flotation until tube is three-quarters full.
3. Stir vigorously with applicator stick.
4. Fill tube with sugar solution to 1 or 2 cm from top.
5. Centrifuge at 500 × g for 10 minutes.
6. Transfer surface material to microscope slide by means of a wire loop.
7. Cover with coverslip, and observe with phase-contrast microscopy.

MODIFIED RITCHIE'S CONCENTRATION METHOD FOR CRYPTOSPORIDIUM

This modification of the Ritchie formalin–ethyl acetate procedure is said to be capable of detecting oocysts of *Cryptosporidium* at much lower concentrations than the original Ritchie procedure or modified Sheather's sugar flotation (Weber et al., 1992).

1. The sediment produced by the standard Ritchie concentration method, but centrifuged at $500 \times g$ for 5 minutes, is resuspended in 5 ml deionized water and layered *over* 5 ml of saturated NaCl, using a disposable plastic bulb pipette. It is then centrifuged at $500 \times g$ for 10 minutes, at which point the oocysts are concentrated in a layer just above the NaCl, while most fecal debris is at the bottom of the tube.

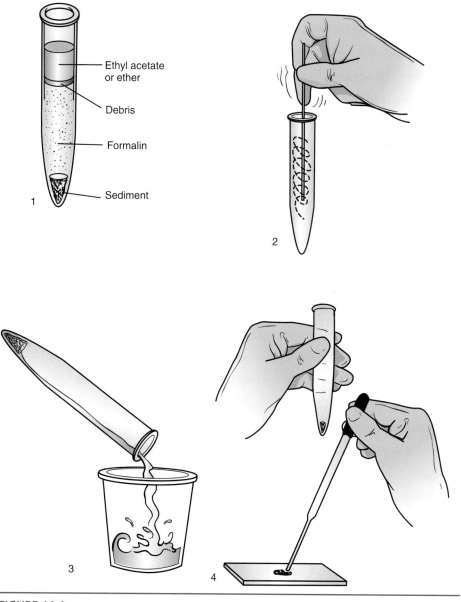

FIGURE 14-4 ■ Preparation of formol-ether or ethyl acetate concentrate. *1*, Appearance of tube after centrifugation; *2*, dislodging debris before decanting; *3*, decanting supernatant; *4*, pipetting sediment for examination.

2. After removal of the uppermost 3.5 or 4 ml of the top layer by pipette, the remainder of that layer plus approximately 0.5 ml of the underlying saline layer is removed using the same pipette, and resuspended in 13 ml of deionized water.

3. Centrifugation at $500 \times g$ for 10 minutes yields a sediment in which the oocysts are concentrated; slides prepared from the sediment are stained with Merifluor *Cryptosporidium* (obtainable from Meridian Diagnostics, Cincinnati, Ohio), and scanned using fluorescence microscopy at a magnification of 400×.

POTASSIUM HYDROXIDE (KOH) CONCENTRATION METHOD FOR CYCLOSPORA (BERLIN ET AL., 1994)

1. Mix specimen well by taking aliquots from several areas.
2. Place 2 ml of specimen in 15-ml centrifuge tube.
3. Add 2 ml of 10% KOH; vortex well.
4. Allow to stand 5 minutes at room temperature.
5. Add 8 to 10 ml saline and mix.
6. Filter through four layers of gauze into a clean centrifuge tube.
7. Centrifuge at 2000 rpm for 2 minutes.
8. Decant and discard the supernatant.
9. Resuspend sediment in approximately 10 ml saline.
10. Centrifuge at 2000 rpm for 2 minutes.
11. Decant and discard supernatant; examine sediment,

Stained Smears

For many years the somewhat laborious iron hematoxylin stain, in various forms, was the only one available for permanent stains of stool specimens. It is a precise when used properly. The one recommended here is the "short method" of the United States Naval Medical School.

IRON HEMATOXYLIN

HEMATOXYLIN STOCK SOLUTION:

Hematoxylin crystals, certified	10 g
Ethyl alcohol, 95%	100 ml

The crystals are dissolved in the alcohol with gentle heating, after which the stock solution must be allowed to ripen for 6 to 8 weeks in a stoppered bottle no more than two-thirds filled. Exposure to sunlight and daily shaking hasten the ripening process. When the solution is fully ripened, a drop added to 100 ml tap water produces a delicate violet color. The unripe solution will turn the water reddish or red-purple.

HEMATOXYLIN WORKING SOLUTION:

Hematoxylin stock solution	1 part
Distilled water	19 parts

Preparations to be stained with iron hematoxylin must be fixed in freshly prepared Schaudinn's fluid while still moist if unpreserved stool specimens are used. If the specimen is preserved in PVA fixative, start with step 2 of the procedure given below; with SAF-preserved material, start with step 4:

1. Fix in Schaudinn's solution with acetic acid 30 minutes.
2. Dehydrate in 70% alcohol 15 minutes.

3. Wash, to remove fixative, in 70% alcohol with iodine added, sufficient to give a port wine color in 3 minutes.
4. Wash in 70% alcohol 3 minutes.
5. Rinse in tap water.
6. Mordant in 4% ferric ammonium sulfate 15 minutes.
7. Rinse in tap water.
8. Stain in hematoxylin working solution 10 minutes.
9. Rinse in tap water.
10. Decolorize in 0.25% ferric ammonium sulfate 12 minutes.
11. Wash in running water at least 5 minutes.
12. Dehydrate in 70%, 95%, and two changes of 100% alcohol, each 5 minutes.
13. Place in xylol, two changes each 5 minutes.
14. Mount in Permount, or other mounting medium, for examination.

The trichrome stain has supplanted iron hematoxylin in most laboratories; the detail obtained is sufficient for diagnostic purposes, and the stain is easier to use.

GOMORI'S TRICHROME STAIN

Chromotrope 2R*	0.6 g
Light green SF*	0.3 g
Phosphotungstic acid	0.7 g
Acetic acid, glacial	1.0 ml
Allow to stand 30 to 60 minutes; add distilled water	100.0 ml

Slides may be prepared from fresh or PVA- or SAF-preserved material. If mercury-containing PVA-preserved material is used, start with step 3 of the procedure; with non-mercury containing PVA or with SAF-preserved stools, start with step 4:

1. Fix in Schaudinn's solution with acetic acid added for 30 minutes.
2. Wash in 70% alcohol 15 minutes.
3. Wash in 70% alcohol, to which sufficient iodine has been added to produce a port wine color 3 minutes.
4. Wash in 70% alcohol, two changes, each 1½ minutes.
5. Stain in Gomori's trichrome 8 to 15 minutes.
6. Rinse in 90% alcohol with 1% acetic acid 1 to 2 seconds.
7. Dip twice in 100% alcohol.
8. Dehydrate in second change of 100% alcohol 30 seconds.
9. Place in xylol 1 minute.
10. Cover with coverslip, using Permount or other mounting medium.

MODIFIED ACID-FAST STAIN FOR CRYPTOSPORIDIUM, CYCLOSPORA, AND ISOSPORA (GARCIA ET AL., 1983)

Coccidia do not stain well with iron hematoxylin or trichrome, but they may be identified using a modified Kinyoun's acid-fast stain, in which they take a pink to red stain, while yeasts and most other material will stain blue.

KINYOUN'S CARBOLFUCHSIN:

Basic fuchsin	4 g
Phenol (liquefied)	8 g
Ethyl alcohol, 95%	20 ml
Distilled water	100 ml

*Manufactured by National Aniline Division, Allied Chemical and Dye Corp., New York, NY.

Dissolve fuchsin in alcohol, add liquefied phenol, and mix well, then add water.

LÖFFLER'S ALKALINE METHYLENE BLUE:

Methylene blue (90% dye content)	0.3 g
Ethyl alcohol, 95%	30 ml
KOH solution, 0.01% by weight	100 ml

Dissolve methylene blue in alcohol, then add KOH.

1. Make fecal smears either from the sediment of a centrifuged formalinized specimen or from the unpreserved stool, and allow to air-dry.
2. Place slide on staining rack and flood with carbolfuchsin.
3. Gently heat slide to steaming with Bunsen burner. Do not boil.
4. Stain for 5 minutes, adding more carbolfuchsin if necessary, without additional heating.
5. Rinse slide with tap water.
6. Decolorize with 1% sulfuric acid for about 2 minutes. Do not overdecolorize.
7. Rinse with tap water. Allow to drain.
8. Flood slide with methylene blue and stain for 1 minute.
9. Rinse with tap water, drain, and air-dry.

RYAN'S TRICHROME BLUE STAIN FOR MICROSPORIDIA (RYAN ET AL., 1993)

Microsporidial spores are difficult to identify because of their small size (*Enterocytozoon bieneusi* about 1 μm by 1.8 μm, *E. intestinalis* about 1.5 μm by 2.5 μm). They may be isolated from the feces as well as from many different bodily fluids. Stained by this technique, the spore wall is a pinkish red, and some will have a diagonal or horizontal line across them (the polar tube); the background will appear blue, though bacteria, some yeasts, and various sorts of debris will also stain red. Control positive slides for comparison are an absolute necessity!

TRICHROME BLUE STAIN:

Chromotrope 2R	6.0 g
Aniline blue	0.5 g
Phosphotungstic acid	0.25 g
Glacial acetic acid	3.0 ml

Mix the preceding ingredients together, and allow to stand for 30 minutes at room temperature. Then add 100 ml distilled water. Adjust pH to 2.5 with 1.0 M HCl. Store in glass or plastic bottle at room temperature, protected from light. Shelf life is at least 2 years.

ACID-ALCOHOL:

Ethyl alcohol	995.5 ml
Glacial acetic acid	4.5 ml

Specimens must be concentrated at $500 \times g$ for 10 minutes, after preservation in formalin of SAF. A 10-μl aliquot of the sediment is spread out over an area 45×25 mm on a glass slide and allowed to air-dry.

1. Immerse in absolute methyl alcohol for 5 to 10 minutes, allow again to air-dry.
2. Stain with trichrome blue for 90 minutes.
3. Rinse in acid-alcohol, not over 10 seconds.
4. Rinse in 95% alcohol by dipping several times (not more than 10 seconds in all).
5. Place in two changes of 95% alcohol, 5 minutes in each, then in 100% alcohol for 10 minutes.

6. Place in xylol for 10 minutes, add coverslip, and mount with Permount or other mounting medium.
7. Examine under oil (1000× magnification).

In cases of suspected disseminated *Encephalitozoon* infection, Weber et al. (1997) suggest examination of urine sediment obtained by centrifugation at 1500 × *g*.

Special Procedures for Recovery of Helminth Larvae and Eggs

BAERMANN APPARATUS FOR RECOVERY OF STRONGYLOIDES LARVAE

Strongyloides larvae do not always concentrate well with either of the concentration techniques, though they may be detected by those methods. The Baermann technique (Fig. 14-5) yields a good concentration of the *living* larvae of *Strongyloides stercoralis*. It should be used when there

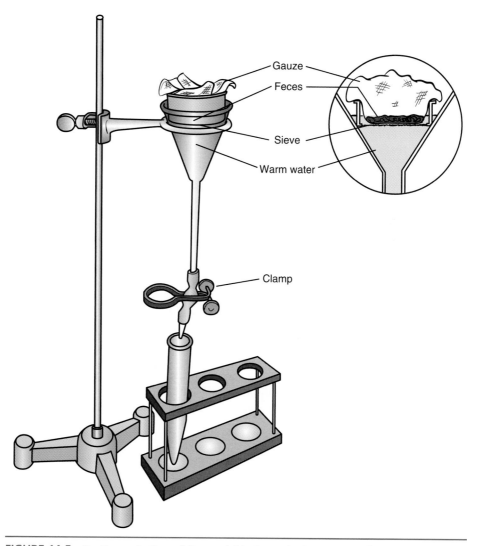

FIGURE 14-5 ■ Concentration of *Strongyloides* larvae by Baermann technique.

is a high index of suspicion and routine stool examinations are negative and for following the results of therapy.

1. A glass funnel with a diameter of 10 cm or greater is set up in a ring stand, with a short piece of rubber tubing attached to its stem and a pinchcock closing the tubing.
2. A wire circle or sieve, of slightly smaller diameter than the top of the funnel, is covered with two layers of gauze.
3. The funnel is filled with lukewarm water to a level just covering the gauze, and a specimen of stool is placed on the gauze, partially in contact with the water.
4. The apparatus is left to stand at room temperature for 8 to 12 hours, then a few drops of fluid are drawn off through the tubing into a small glass dish.
5. Examine for larvae under low power of the microscope.

FILTER PAPER STRIP PROCEDURE FOR RECOVERY OF STRONGYLOIDES OR TRICHOSTRONGYLUS LARVAE

This method takes too long to be clinically useful but is well-adapted for field or survey use, where quick results are not essential. The technique, originally described by Harada and Mori in 1955, requires minimal equipment

A 20- × 13-mm filter paper strip, in the center of which is placed 0.5 to 1.0 g feces, is inserted into a 15-ml centrifuge tube containing 3 to 4 ml distilled water. The tube is placed upright or in a slightly slanted position, so that the filter paper is kept moist by capillary flow. Water may be added as needed to maintain the original fluid level. After 10 days, a small amount of fluid is withdrawn from the bottom of the tube and examined for larvae.

AGAR PLATE METHOD FOR RECOVERY OF STRONGYLOIDES LARVAE

More sensitive than either Baermann or filter paper strip methods, an agar plate method such as that described by Koga et al. (1991) will probably supplant them.

1. Agar medium (1.5% agar, 0.5% meat extract, 1.0% peptone, and 0.5% NaCl) is autoclaved and dispensed in sterilized dishes. (The authors use 8.5 to 9.0 ml of agar in a 9- × 2.5-cm plastic dish.) Plates are dried at room temperature for 4 to 5 days to eliminate excess moisture, and then stored in sealed plastic bags.
2. Approximately 2 g of fresh or refrigerated stool specimen is placed in the center of the plate, which is then sealed with adhesive tape to prevent escape of the infectious larvae, and incubated at room temperature (26° to 33°C) for 48 hours.
3. Plates are then examined macroscopically for the presence of larval tracks or larvae, and if negative they are reexamined under the microscope at low magnification using a green filter. If still negative, plates are washed with 10% formalin, which is collected and its sediment examined under high dry magnification.

The rhabditiform larvae of *Strongyloides* are said to exhibit whiplike movements as they progress, while hookworm larvae glide like a snake. Microscopic examination (see Chapter 8) is necessary for final identification.

CELLOPHANE TAPE SWAB FOR ENTEROBIUS AND TAENIA EGGS

Pinworm eggs, which are generally deposited at night, will be found scattered around the perianal region. The tape should be used in the morning before the patient washes or defecates. A number of commercial pinworm detection kits are now available, but if cellophane is used, the procedure is as follows:

1. Fold together sticky surfaces of a piece of cellophane tape, 1 × 8 cm, for about 1 cm at each end.

2. Stretch tape, sticky side out, over butt end of a test tube or a wooden tongue blade, holding nonsticky ends firmly with thumb and forefinger.
3. Apply tape to anal area, rocking back and forth to cover as much of the mucosa and mucocutaneous area as possible.
4. Remove tape and apply to microscope slide, sticky slide down. Press firmly into position.
5. Examine for eggs under low power of microscope.

Clear cellophane tape is essential. That which has a frosted appearance obscures the eggs. If, however, frosted tape is used, a few drops of xylene introduced under the edge clears the tape so that the eggs can be seen.

SCHISTOSOMAL HATCHING TEST

If feces containing viable schistosome eggs are diluted with approximately 10 volumes of water, the eggs hatch within a few hours, releasing miracidia. The miracidia are positively phototrophic. The following procedure takes advantage of this characteristic.
1. A stool specimen is homogenized by shaking in normal saline and is then strained through two layers of gauze.
2. The material is allowed to sediment, the supernatant is decanted, and the sediment is resuspended in saline. This process is repeated at least twice.
3. The saline is decanted and replaced with distilled water, and the suspension is placed in a side-arm (Fig. 14-6) or Erlenmeyer flask. The side-arm flask is covered with black paper, aluminum foil, or black paint, except for the side arm. If an Erlenmeyer flask is used, it is covered to 1 cm below the level of fluid in the neck of the flask. Additional water is added if necessary.
4. The flask is allowed to stand at room temperature for several hours in subdued light.
5. The side arm, or water in the neck of the flask, is then illuminated strongly from the side.
6. The illuminated area is examined with a magnifying glass to detect the presence of free-swimming miracidia.

Eggs of *Schistosoma haematobium* in the urine may also be hatched in this manner, but they are more easily concentrated by centrifugation or membrane filtration.

Duodenal Sampling and Biopsy

Sampling and examination of duodenal contents are a means of recovery of *Strongyloides* larvae, the eggs of *Clonorchis*, *Opisthorchis*, and *Fasciola*, and other small-intestine parasites such as *Giardia*, *Isospora*, and *Cryptosporidium*. Specimens may be obtained by intubation or by use of the enteric capsule or string test (Enterotest). A number 00 gelatin capsule containing a 90-cm line for children, or a 140-cm line for adults (Fig. 14-7), composed of a 20-cm silicon rubber-covered thread and a 70-cm or 120-cm soft nylon yarn, is swallowed by the patient

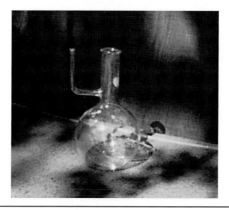

FIGURE 14-6 ■ Side-arm flask used in hatching of miracidia.

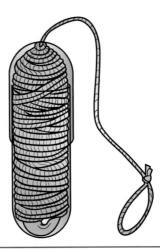

FIGURE 14-7 ■ Enteric capsule used for sampling duodenal parasites.

while the thread, which protrudes from a hole in the capsule, is held firmly. To the end of the nylon yarn is attached a 1-g weight, which eventually helps carry the string into the duodenum. The free end of the line is taped to the patient's neck or cheek, and after 4 hours may be pulled up. The bile-stained mucus adhering to its distal end is examined under the microscope. The weight becomes disengaged in the intestine at the time the thread is withdrawn.

Biopsy of the small intestinal mucosa may reveal *Giardia, Cryptosporidium, Isospora,* and microsporidia, as well as *Strongyloides* larvae.

Culture Methods

Many of the intestinal protozoa have now been successfully cultured. Cultivation of the nonpathogenic amebae, the flagellates, and *Balantidium* falls into the category of research procedures, requiring too much material and time to be of diagnostic usefulness.

Entamoeba histolytica can be cultivated on a variety of media, some of which may be purchased in the dehydrated form and prepared with a minimum of effort. None of the culture media can be used to differentiate between the pathogenic *E. histolytica* and harmless *E. dispar.*

The success with which *E. histolytica* is cultivated depends largely on familiarity with the techniques involved. For this reason, sporadic use of culture techniques is not recommended, and they should be undertaken only in laboratories where the number of specimens examined is sufficiently large to justify a considerable portion of time being spent on their maintenance and examination. Likewise, culture methods should never be used as a substitute for routine and thorough microscopic examination by the various methods outlined previously. Diamond's medium may be obtained freeze-dried for reconstitution as a liquid medium, while Boeck and Drbohlav's Locke-Egg; Serum (LES) medium is solid with a liquid overlay and can be prepared in the laboratory.

DIAMOND'S MEDIUM FOR AXENIC CULTURE OF ENTAMOEBA AND TRICHOMONAS

Now obtainable as TYI-S-33 medium, freeze-dried, from the American Type Culture Collection,* it is prepared as follows:

TYI-S-33 broth base with 10% bovine serum	1 bottle
Distilled water	55 ml

---

*American Type Culture Collection, Manassas, VA 20110; (703) 365-2700.

Dispense 13 ml medium per tube into 16- × 125-mm screw-capped culture tubes. May be stored at ambient temperature (~ 25°C) for up to 90 days, but it is recommended to store at 2° to 8°C for longest shelf life. Some strains of *E. histolytica* require 15% bovine serum, necessitating the addition of an extra 5% by volume of bovine calf serum, inactivated at 56°C for 30 minutes prior to use.

Inoculate with vaginal or prostatic exudate or a portion of stool the size of a small pea, adding to the medium before inoculation 100 units of penicillin and 100 μg of streptomycin per ml of medium. Gentamicin, 50 μg/ml, may substitute for penicillin and streptomycin. Incubate at 37°C and examine after 2, 3, and 4 days' incubation by removing a small amount of sediment with a pipette. The sediment is transferred to a slide, covered, and examined under low power. Primary isolation may yield few organisms, whereas subsequent transfers show a considerable increase in numbers. It should be unnecessary to use antibiotics for successive transfers after primary isolation.

BOECK AND DRBOHLAV'S LOCKE-EGG-SERUM (LES) MEDIUM FOR AMEBAE

BOECK AND DRBOHLAV'S SOLUTION:

NaCl	9.0 g
CaCl$_2$	0.2 g
KCl	0.4 g
NaHCO$_3$	0.2 g
Glucose	2.5 g
Distilled water	1 L

This solution should be autoclaved before storage. LES medium is prepared as follows:
1. Wash four eggs, brush with alcohol to sterilize, and break into a sterile flask containing glass beads.
2. Add 50 ml Locke's solution; shake until homogeneous.
3. Dispense in test tubes sufficient quantity to produce a 2.5- to 3.5-cm slant in bottom of tube.
4. Slant plugged tubes and place in inspissator at 70°C until slants are solidified. If an inspissator is not available, a substitute may be devised by leaving the door of the autoclave partly open.
5. When slants have solidified, autoclave at 15 pounds pressure for 20 minutes. Discard any badly broken slants.
6. Cover slants to a depth of about 1 cm with mixture of 8 parts sterile Locke's solution to 1 part sterile inactivated human blood serum. Sterility or mixture of Locke's solution and serum should be ensured by filtration sterilization followed by incubation at 37°C for 24 hours or longer before use.

A loopful of sterile rice starch or powder is added to each tube before inoculation. Inoculate with a portion of stool the size of a small pea, break up well in medium, and incubate at 37°C. Examine as noted for Diamond's medium. Note that this is not an axenic medium, and antibiotics are not added.

MODIFIED THIOGLYCOLATE MEDIUM FOR CULTURE OF TRICHOMONAS VAGINALIS

A modification of the fluid thioglycolate medium produced by the Difco Laboratories (Detroit, Michigan) is found to be equally effective as Diamond's medium for the cultivation of *Trichomonas*, and can be produced at a lower cost (Poch et al., 1996).

To approximately 1 liter of Difco thioglycolate medium is added:

Yeast extract	7 g

(The medium already contains 5 g yeast extract.) It is then autoclaved, and the following ingredients are added aseptically:

Horse serum	120 ml
Amphotericin B	2 mg
Penicillin G	1,000,000 U
Gentamicin	80 mg

The fluid medium is dispensed in 10-ml quantities in screw-capped tubes, which are stored at 4°C. After inoculation with vaginal (or prostatic) exudate, tubes are incubated at 35°C, and 10 μl aliquots from the bottom of the tube are examined daily for up to 7 days.

Methods for Estimation of Worm Burden

Estimates of daily egg output have been made for a number of hepatic and intestinal worms. If one can estimate the total number of eggs in a 24-hour stool specimen, it is possible to calculate the approximate number of adult worms present. This makes it possible to follow the results of therapy in a somewhat quantitative manner by making periodic egg counts, affording a basis for comparison of the efficacy of various medications.

Estimates of numbers of eggs laid per female worm vary considerably and depend to some extent on the numbers of worms present. The Chinese liver fluke may lay 2400 or so eggs within 24 hours, and an *Ascaris* female about 200,000 during the same time period. Thus, from 1000 to 2000 eggs would be found per gram of feces in a 24-hour specimen from a patient infected with one pair of *Ascaris*. The egg-laying capacity of a single *Necator* female may vary from 12 to 44 eggs per gram of feces in a 24-hour period, and fewer than 2100 eggs per gram usually represents a subclinical infection. *Ancylostoma* females lay about twice as many eggs as *Necator*. *Trichuris* females presumably lay about 14,000 eggs in 24 hours, but egg-laying capacity seems to vary inversely with total numbers of worms present.

STOLL'S EGG-COUNTING TECHNIQUE

1. Save entire 24-hour stool specimen and determine weight in grams.
2. Weigh out accurately 4 g of feces.
3. Place feces in calibrated bottle or large test tube, and add sufficient N/10 NaOH to bring volume to 60 ml.
4. Add a few glass beads and shake vigorously to make a uniform suspension. If specimen is hard, the mixture may be placed in a refrigerator overnight before shaking, to aid in its comminution.
5. With a pipette, remove immediately 0.15 ml suspension and drain onto a slide.
6. Do not use a coverslip; place slide on mechanical stage and count *all* the eggs on the slide.
7. Multiply egg count by 100 to obtain the number of eggs per gram of feces and by weight of specimen to get total number of eggs per 24-hour specimen.

KATO'S THICK-SMEAR TECHNIQUE

This technique has undergone a number of modifications since its introduction. A common method employs the examination of a standard 50-mg sample of fresh feces, pressed between a microscope slide and a strip of wettable cellophane soaked in glycerin. After the fecal film has cleared, eggs in the entire film are counted. The fecal sample may be weighed, but it has been found that with some practice it is possible to estimate sample size with acceptable reliability. Samples taken from various portions of the specimen do not differ greatly in egg content. Materials needed for this method are wettable, medium-thickness cellophane coverslips, 22 × 30 mm. They are soaked for at least 24 hours in a solution of 100 ml pure glycerin, 100 ml water, and 1 ml 3% malachite green (the last is optional).

Feces are transferred to a clean slide and covered with a presoaked cellophane coverslip. The slide is inverted and pressed against an absorbent surface until the fecal mass covers an area 20 to 25 mm in diameter. The preparation is then left for 1 hour at room temperature to allow clearing of the fecal material (but *not* of the eggs) and should then be examined promptly.

For eggs of *Schistosoma mansoni*, a longer period of clearing (24 hours) is needed. To obtain 10-, 20-, or 50-mg samples, metal templates containing holes calibrated to deliver those amounts of feces are utilized.

Special Methods for Intestinal Helminths

CESTODES

If gravid proglottids are found in a stool specimen or brought in for identification, *Diphyllobothrium* can usually be identified by the presence of a uterine rosette in the middle of each segment. If no rosette is seen, the segments are probably those of a *Taenia*. To differentiate between the two species of *Taenia*, segments should be rinsed in tap water and placed between two microscope slides that are separated at the edges by thin pieces of cardboard. The preparation may then be fastened by means of rubber bands at each end of the slides so that the segments become somewhat flattened. The uterine branches should be clearly visible under the low power of a dissecting microscope.

Species identification on the basis of uterine structure of gravid segments may be greatly facilitated by injection of segments with India ink. A little ink is drawn into a 1-ml tuberculin syringe, a No. 26 hypodermic needle is inserted into the distal end of the proglottid or in the central uterine stem, and a small amount of ink is slowly injected. The branches of the uterus become black and can be easily counted. This procedure works best with fresh specimens but may at times be successful with formalin fixed segments if they are first cleared by immersion in glycerin, after transfer to 70% alcohol.

SMALL NEMATODES

Small nematodes, such as anisakids, may be cleared in glycerin for identification. Specimens should be in 70% alcohol before transfer to glycerin. Most nematodes are fixed by immersion in 70% alcohol heated to 75°C. If fixed in formalin, they may be transferred to a mixture of equal parts of formalin and 70% alcohol, and after 3 hours to the first of two changes of 70% alcohol, in each of which they should remain 3 hours or longer. Transfer the specimens from 70% alcohol to a relatively large volume of 10% glycerin in 70% alcohol, in a shallow dish. Leave uncoverd, in a dust-free location, and allow the alcohol to evaporate (several days).

The specimens may be mounted on a slide in glycerin and covered with a coverslip for examination; however, if permanent preparations are desired, it is necessary to use glycerin jelly.

GLYCERIN JELLY:

Gelatin, unflavored (Knox or other)	8 g
Distilled water	52 ml
Glycerin	50 ml
Egg albumin (fresh)	5 ml
Phenol crystals	0.1 g

Soak the gelatin in water for an hour and then dissolve with the application of gentle heat. Add glycerin and white of egg, stir until thoroughly mixed, then heat to 75°C for 30 minutes. Filter through several layers of fine flannel, using a funnel with a hot water jacket if available. Add phenol crystals to the filtrate, and store in tightly stoppered wide-mouthed bottle.

To mount in glycerin jelly, transfer the object to be mounted from glycerin onto a clean glass slide. Cover the specimen with two or three drops of melted glycerin jelly and then with small round coverslip. When the jelly has hardened, a few drops of Permount or similar mounting medium may be placed on top of the round coverslip, and a larger square coverslip used to cover the entire preparation, now sealed on all sides by glass or the mounting medium.

This method is also excellent for preparation of permanent mounts of helminth eggs (Table 14-1).

NEW TECHNIQUES FOR DIAGNOSIS OF INTESTINAL PARASITES.

Robust FDA-approved stool antigen detection tests are available for *Cryptosporidium parvum, Giardia lamblia,* and *Entamoebe histolytica.* Where laboratory technology and finances permit, these tests should be used in place of stool microscopy because of their superior performance (Chen et al., 2002; Haque et al., 2003; Davis et al., 2001; Goodgame, 1996). Even greater sensitivity and specificity are achievable by real-time PCR amplification and detection of parasite DNA in stool, and as this technology evolves and becomes less technically demanding and cheaper it will have a major if not dominant role in reference laboratories and eventually community labs (Verweij et al., 2004; Ward et al., 2002).

References

Berlin OGW et al. Recovery of *Cyclospora* organisms from patients with prolonged diarrhea. *Clin Infect Dis* 1994; *18*:606–609.

Chen XM, Keithly JS, Paya CV, LaRusso NF. Current concepts: Cryptosporidiosis. *N Engl J Med* 2002; *346*:1723–1731.

Davis AN, Haque R, Petri WA Jr. Update on protozoan parasites of the intestine. *Current Opinion in Gastroenterology* 2001; *17*:17–23.

Garcia LS et al. Techniques for the recovery and identification of *Cryptosporidium* oocysts from stool specimens. *J Clin Microbiol* 1983; *18*:185–190.

Goodgame RW. Understanding intestine spore-forming protozoa: Cryptosporidia, microsporidia, isospore and cyclospora. *Ann Intern Med* 1996; *124*:429–441.

Haque R et al. Current concepts: Amebiasis. *N Engl J Med* 2003; *348*:1565–1573.

Harada Y, Mori O. A new method for culturing hookworm. *Yonago Acta Med* 1955; *1*:177–179.

Koga K et al. A modified agar plate method for detection of *Strongyloides stercoralis. Am J Trop Med Hyg* 1991; *45*:518–521.

Poch F et al. Modified thioglycolate medium: A simple and reliable means for detection of *Trichomonas vaginalis. J Clin Microbiol* 1996; *34*:2630–2631.

Ryan NJ et al. A new trichrome-blue stain for detection of microsporidial species in urine, stool and nasopharyngeal specimens. *J Clin Microbiol* 1993; *31*:3264–3269.

Sawitz WG, Faust EC. The probability of detecting intestinal protozoa by successive stool examinations. *Am J Trop Med* 1942; *22*:131–136.

Verweij JJ, Blange RA, Templeton K et al. Simultaneous detection of *Entamoeba histolytica, Giardia lamblia,* and Cryptosporidium parvum in fecal samples by using multiplex real-time PCR. *J Clin Microbiol* 2004; *42*:1220 1223.

Ward PL et al. Detection of eight *Cryptosporidium* genotypes in surface and waste waters in Europe. *Parasitology* 2002; *124*:359–681.

Weber R et al. Improved stool concentration procedure for detection of *Cryptosporidium* oocysts in fecal specimens. *J Clin Microbiol* 1992; *30*:2869–2873.

Weber R et al. Reply to: Cerebral microsporidiosis due to *Encephalitozoon cuniculi*. *N Engl J Med* 1997; *337*:640–641.

Yang J, Scholten T. A fixative for intestinal parasites permitting the use of concentration and permanent staining procedures. *Am J Clin Pathol* 1977; *67*:300–304.

Examination of Blood, Other Body Fluids and Tissues, Sputum, and Urine

Examination of Blood and Spinal Fluid

FRESH BLOOD

Microscopic examination of fresh blood is not undertaken routinely but is useful for the detection of two types of parasites. Trypanosomes and microfilariae may be easily recognized by their characteristic motility in fresh blood. For specific identification of these organisms, however, a permanent stain is essential. When fresh blood is to be examined, it is important to make a sufficiently thin preparation so that the relatively small protozoan parasites are not masked by several layers of blood corpuscles. A small drop of blood is placed on a slide and covered with a coverglass to prevent clotting. If the preparation is too thick, it may be diluted with normal saline. For the detection of trypanosomes, the high-dry objective with reduced illumination is most suitable. During a search for microfilariae, the low power of the microscope should be employed. Whiplike motions of microfilariae and the rapid undulating and twisting movements of trypanosomes are usually seen before the precise shape of the organism is apparent. Organisms may quickly attract attention through their movements even when they are so few that a long search may be required to reveal them in fixed preparations.

PERMANENT PREPARATIONS

The preparation of good blood films depends to a large extent on the cleanliness of microscope slides and coverglasses employed. All glassware must be free of dust and oil. It is essential that both slides and coverglasses be washed in alcohol and dried with a clean towel before a blood film is prepared. New slides should be used for the preparation of permanent stains; it is impossible to make uniform films on old, scratched slides, and they cannot be thoroughly cleaned.

Many methods have been described for the preparation and permanent staining of blood films. Only those most commonly employed in laboratory work are discussed here. It is important to bear in mind that correct initial handling of the blood is essential if good stains are to be obtained, regardless of the specific methods used. The necessity of absolute cleanliness of all equipment has been emphasized. It is preferable to use peripheral blood from the fingertip or earlobe. The skin should be cleansed with alcohol before an incision is made to remove all fatty substances, and the incision should be sufficiently deep so that blood flows freely; appropriate precautions should be taken to prevent infection. Blood that is "milked" from a finger is mixed with tissue fluids, which dilute the parasites and make detection more difficult. Films should be prepared as quickly as possible to prevent clotting. If venous blood must be employed, a small amount of heparin or other anticoagulant must be added, but preparations made from such blood usually show some distortion.

Both thin and thick films may be used for the identification of blood parasites. The advantages and disadvantages of each are discussed next. Newer techniques based on the detection of malaria antigen or DNA in blood are not yet widely available, and examination of blood smears remains the gold standard (Craig and Sharp, 1997).

THIN BLOOD FILMS

Thin blood films are used for the specific identification of malarial parasites, trypanosomes, and microfilariae. It is essential that a thin film be, as the name indicates, really thin. A thin film should consist of *one* layer of evenly distributed blood cells. Since malarial parasites are intracellular, a piling up of red blood cells makes specific identification of these parasites difficult if not impossible. Specific identification of blood parasites rests on their morphologic characteristics. The chief advantage of a thin film is that it preserves the structure of the parasites with a minimum of distortion. If the film is too thick, the structural detail of individual parasites will not be observable.

There are several ways to make a thin blood film, and while the procedure to be adopted will vary with individual preference, the following is recommended: Place a small drop of blood near one end of a microscope slide, as shown in Figure 15-1, *A*. Raise the end of the slide farthest from the drop of blood by placing the end of the slide on your finger, as your hand rests on a table or other steady surface. Take a second slide for a spreader, and rest one end of it against the first slide and one end on the middle finger of the hand that is not supporting the first slide. Hold your hand so that the second slide makes an angle of approximately 30 degrees with the first; do not grasp either slide, but allow gravity to hold the two in contact. Draw back the supporting finger to move the slide back toward the drop of blood until the drop of blood touches the spreader and begins to run out toward the edges. Before the blood has a chance to reach the edges of the spreader, move the finger that supports it forward in an even, quick motion, so that the drop is drawn out into a thin film. Ideally, this should not reach the edges of the slide, and it should taper off into a "comet tail" toward the end of the slide. After the film has been air-dried, it may be stained.

The stains commonly used are of two general types. One of these has the fixative incorporated in the staining solution so that fixation and staining of the dried film are accomplished simultaneously. An example is Wright's stain, in which methyl alcohol acts as a fixative. Wright's stain gives fair results and requires a short staining period but is *not* recommended for parasitologic use. More precise detail is seen in slides prepared with Giemsa's stain. Since this stain does not contain a fixative, thin films must be fixed in absolute methyl alcohol and air-dried before they are placed in the staining solution. It is important to dry slides in a vertical position after removal from either fixative or stain. As soon as the stained films are dry, they may be examined under oil immersion of the microscope. Immersion oil may be placed directly on the uncovered blood film and, when no longer needed, carefully removed with xylene and lens paper. If magnifications lower than oil immersion are to be used, a coverglass should be placed over the film. Slides that one desires to keep for a permanent collection should always have the protection of a coverglass; a mounting medium, such as Permount, should be used. Stains fade in time unless protected by the addition of an antioxidant, such as butylated hydroxytoluene, 1% by volume.★

(*Note*: Microfilariae stained with Giemsa will not show as clear internal detail as those stained with hematoxylin, as can be seen by a comparison of Figures 9-2 and 9-10; however, Giemsa is usually sufficient for identification.)

★May be obtained from Sigma Chemical Company, P.O. Box 14508, St. Louis, MO 63178.

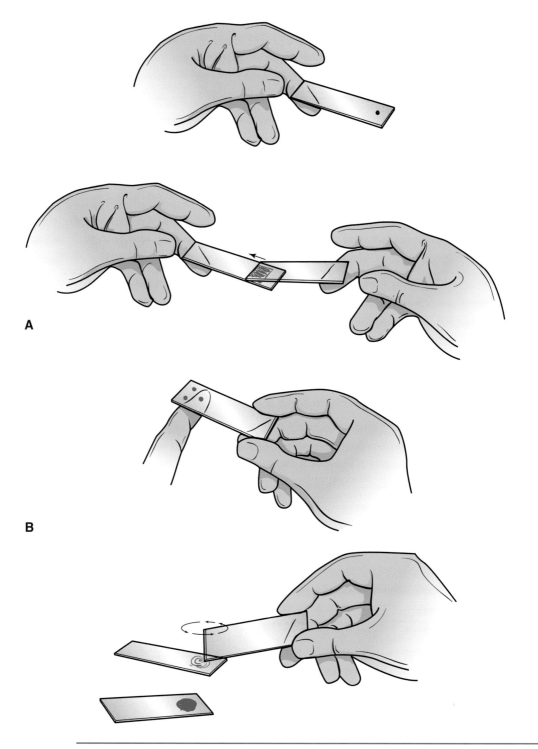

FIGURE 15-1   ■   **A,** Preparation of a thin blood film. **B,** Preparation of a thick blood film.

THICK BLOOD FILMS

The thick film may also be used in identification of malarial parasites, trypanosomes, and microfilariae. As a thick layer of blood is used in this method, many more parasites will be present in each field. Increased distortion of the parasites is a disadvantage of this method, but experience enables one to recognize them as readily as in the thin film.

To make a thick film, place three drops of blood, each about the size that would be used to make a thin film, close together near one end of the slide. With one corner of another absolutely clean slide, stir the blood, mingling the three drops over an area 2 cm in diameter (Fig. 15-1, B). Continue stirring for at least 30 seconds to prevent formation of fibrin strands, which otherwise tend to obscure the parasites. Allow the films to air dry normally or, in very humid conditions, in a 37°C incubator; do not heat, because this will fix the blood. After the films are thoroughly dry, they must be laked to remove the hemoglobin. This can be done by immersion in buffer solution, prior to staining, or in the Giemsa stain itself. Thick films that cannot be stained immediately should be laked in buffer solution before storage, because removal of hemoglobin becomes increasingly difficult with time. When Giemsa's stain is used for thick films, the procedure is exactly the same as that employed with thin films, except that fixation in methyl alcohol is omitted. Staining times for thick and thin films are similar, but if separate preparations are made, different staining times may be required for optimal results. Thick and thin films may, however, be made on the same slide and stained simultaneously with Giemsa. To accomplish this, the thin portion of the slide is fixed for 1 minute in methyl alcohol and then dried before staining.

Field describes another method that may be used in the staining of thick films. It is very rapid and gives satisfactory, though not outstanding, results. Field's stain has been used extensively for survey purposes and when large numbers of slides must be prepared, but it is not recommended for routine use.

BLOOD CONCENTRATION PROCEDURES

The thick film is itself a type of concentration technique, the only one applicable to the identification of parasites within the red blood cell. Buffy coat films serve to concentrate the white blood cells, in which *Leishmania* may be found, and are useful for detection of trypanosomes and microfilariae. A triple centrifugation technique is also used to check for trypanosomes when they are too few in number to be found even in thick blood films. Microfilariae present in the blood in small numbers can be detected by means of a membrane filtration technique.

EXAMINATION OF CEREBROSPINAL FLUID

Trophozoites of *Naegleria* and trypanosomes may be found in the cerebrospinal fluid (CSF). *Trichinella* larvae may be found in the CSF of patients with severe infections; they also may be isolated from the blood. CSF eosinophilia (see Chapter 12) may be caused by parasites such as *Angiostrongylus* and *Gnathostoma*, which will not be found in the blood. Transverse myelitis caused by *Schistosoma mansoni* may result in an eosinophilic pleocytosis. Helminth eggs are very rarely seen in the CSF.

The CSF must be examined promptly, as trypanosomes survive only about 20 minutes, and *Naegleria* may round up and become nonmotile. The CSF may be centrifuged (7000 × *g* for 10 minutes), the supernatant removed, and the sediment examined under reduced illumination. Motility of *Naegleria* may be enhanced by use of a warm stage, and culture of the CSF or its sediment may be effective in isolation of this organism. Examination of the CSF or blood (not a routine diagnostic procedure in suspected trichinosis) may reveal the migrating larvae in severe infections, and filtration of blood or CSF through a membrane filter (discussed later) increases the chances of finding them.

Examination of Tissues and Body Fluids

TISSUE IMPRESSIONS

The detection of intracellular parasites such as *Leishmania* and *Toxoplasma* is greatly facilitated by the examination of tissue impression smears stained with Giemsa's or Wright's stain. Fresh lymph nodes, liver biopsy material, or bone marrow is lightly impressed on a clean microscope slide; the film is allowed to dry at room temperature and is stained in the manner of a thin blood film. Whole cells, with organisms showing little if any distortion, may be clearly distinguished in such preparations (see Figs. 5-19 and 5-27). When dealing with lymph nodes or other fairly solid tissue, it is best to prepare the smear from a freshly cut surface. The remaining tissue can then be fixed for conventional histologic procedures or cultured if sterile techniques have been used and the slides autoclaved.

BIOPSY AND ASPIRATION

Spleen, liver, and bone marrow biopsies are extensively used in the diagnosis of visceral leishmaniasis. Organisms may be demonstrated directly in the biopsy material, which also may be used for culture or animal inoculation. Sternal marrow aspiration is approximately as productive as the more hazardous splenic or hepatic biopsy. *Leishmania tropica* cannot be recovered from the surface of an oriental sore; if a hypodermic syringe is introduced through normal tissue at the side of the ulcer to the area below the ulcer bed, intracellular parasites may be demonstrated in the fluid that is withdrawn after instillation of a few drops of normal saline. Aspiration of enlarged posterior cervical or other involved lymph nodes at times reveals trypanosomes when the blood is apparently free of them. The lymph nodes are less often involved in Rhodesian sleeping sickness than in the Gambian form or in Chagas' disease. Biopsy of enlarged nodes from patients with the latter disease may reveal intracellular (amastigote) forms of the parasite.

Trophozoites or cysts of *Acanthamoeba* may be detected in corneal scrapings or biopsy. Brain biopsy can detect *Toxoplasma, Naegleria, Acanthamoeba, Balamuthia,* and *Entamoeba.* Various developmental stages of *Cryptosporidium* or the microsporidia may be identified in intestinal biopsy material. Aspiration of an amebic liver abscess often demonstrates a thick, reddish brown fluid, but amebae are seldom seen, as they occur chiefly in the tissue surrounding the abscess cavity. *E. histolytica* may be demonstrated by biopsy of colonic ulcers, with periodic acid Schiff stain or immunoperoxidase stains most sensitive for its detection in the biopsy material.

Aspiration of fluid from a hydatid cyst (a dangerous procedure unless done as part of an open surgical operation or perhaps with ultrasonographic guidance) may reveal hydatid sand, but it must be remembered that certain hydatid cysts are sterile, so that the absence of scolices or hooklets from the sediment, centrifuged or put through a membrane filter, is not evidence against the parasitic nature of the cyst.

Eggs of *Schistosoma mansoni* may be found in tissue taken from the rectal mucosa (e.g., with a wooden tongue blade or by biopsy when they cannot be recovered from the stool); mucosa from the bladder wall, taken at cystoscopy, may likewise reveal eggs of *S. haematobium.* Larval *Trichinella spiralis* may be found in any voluntary muscle, but biopsies are usually taken from the gastrocnemius. Larvae may be most abundant in the diaphragm, and they may be sought in this muscle at autopsy. Microfilariae of *Onchocerca volvulus, Mansonella ozzardi,* and *M. streptocerca* may be demonstrated in skin snips or scrapings.

EXAMINATION OF THE SPUTUM

Examination of the sputum is indicated when there is a question of pulmonary paragonimiasis, although the swallowed eggs are often found in the feces. *Entamoeba histolytica* may appear in the sputum of patients with pulmonary abscesses. Migrating larvae of *Ascaris*, hookworm, and *Strongyloides* are rarely seen, as is *Entamoeba gingivalis*, which may multiply in bronchial mucus, but like *Trichomonas tenax* is usually an oral contaminant. *Cryptosporidium* has been found in both sputum and lung biopsy material. Microsporidia have been associated with upper and lower respiratory infections, and spores may appear in the sputum. Ruptured hydatid cysts may be recognized by the presence of hooklets in the sputum.

Sputum specimens should be induced, if possible. Early morning specimens, uncontaminated with saliva, also are acceptable. They should be examined by wet mount while fresh or preserved in PVA fixative for protozoa and formol-saline for other organisms or eggs. If the specimen is very viscid, it may be necessary to dilute with an equal quantity of 3% sodium hydroxide, mix thoroughly, and centrifuge before examination or preservation. Sodium hydroxide, of course, destroys any amebae or flagellates that are present.

EXAMINATION OF URINE AND VAGINAL SECRETIONS

Eggs of *Schistosoma haematobium* and, on occasion, microfilariae of *Wuchereria, Brugia, Loa,* and *Onchocerca* may be found in the urine. *Trichomonas vaginalis* may be found in the urinary sediment of both males and females and in prostatic and vaginal secretions. The spores of microsporidia may also be found in the urine.

Schistosome eggs and microfilariae may best be recovered by examination of centrifuged or membrane-filtered urine specimens. A fresh or midday urine specimen is preferred for *S. haematobium*; microfilariae of *Wuchereria* and *Brugia* may be found in the urine of patients exhibiting chyluria, while those of *Onchocerca* are usually seen immediately following treatment with diethylcarbamazine. The hatching test (Chapter 14) may demonstrate the presence of small numbers of schistosome eggs, if viable.

T. vaginalis may be recognized in a fresh specimen of urine or in vaginal or prostatic exudate by its jerky motility or (under high-dry power) by the movement of its undulating membrane. The flagella and undulating membrane are seen best with phase-contrast microscopy. It may also be seen in Papanicolaou smears.

Blood Films and Tissue Impression Smears

FIELD'S STAIN

Solution A:	
Methylene blue	0.8 g
Azure I	0.5 g
Na$_2$HPO$_4$ anhydrous	5.0 g
KH$_2$PO$_4$ anhydrous	6.25 g
Distilled water	500 ml
Solution B:	
Eosin	1.0 g
Na$_2$HPO$_4$ anhydrous	5.0 g
KH$_2$PO$_4$	6.25 g
Distilled water	500 ml

Dissolve salts first, then add the stains, after grinding the azure I in a mortar. Let the solutions stand for 24 hours, then filter. If a scum forms or if dye precipitates, filter again. The same solutions may be used for many weeks, but the eosin should be renewed when it becomes greenish. The staining procedure is as follows:
1. Dip slides in solution A for 1 second.
2. Rinse by immersion in water, waving gently for a few seconds until stain ceases to flow from film.

3. Dip slides in solution B for 1 second.
4. Rinse as before for 2 to 3 seconds.
5. Place vertically against a rack to drain and dry.

GIEMSA'S STAIN

Giemsa's stain is sold commercially as a concentrated stock solution. The product is quite variable, and each new lot should be thoroughly tested before it is put into use. In general, if the coloration of the red and white blood cells seems satisfactory, it can be assumed that the stain will be adequate for the demonstration of malarial and other parasites. The procedure for use of Giemsa's stain with thin films is as follows:

1. Fix blood films in absolute methyl alcohol for 1 minute.
2. Allow slides to dry.
3. Immerse slides in a solution of 1 part Giemsa stock to 30 to 50 parts buffered water (pH 7.2). Stain 30 minutes to 1 hour.
4. Dip slides briefly in buffered water, drain quickly and thoroughly, and air-dry.

   The procedure to be used with thick films is the same, except that steps 1 and 2 are omitted. If the slide has a thick film at one end and a thin film at the other, fix only the thin portion, then stain both parts of the film simultaneously; dry with the thick end down.

HANSEL'S SECRETION STAIN

Hansel's stain★ has recently been found valuable for demonstrating eosinophils in the urine. Eosinophiluria (Chapter 12) appears to be a constant finding in urinary schistosomiasis. The procedure is as follows:

1. Centrifuge approximately 10 ml of freshly voided urine at $1000 \times g$ for 5 minutes. Decant supernatant.
2. Pipette sediment onto 1 or more slides, spread out thinly with applicator stick, and allow to air-dry.
3. Cover slide with Hansel's stain, and allow to stand for 25 to 30 seconds.
4. Add distilled water, allow to stand for 30 seconds. Pour off stain, and rinse with distilled water to remove excess stain.
5. Rinse with 95% methyl alcohol. Drain and allow slide to air-dry.

   Hansel's stain stains the granules of the eosinophil a very bright red; other cells will stain blue or pink, depending on cell type and degree of destaining with methyl alcohol. Hansel's stain is not suitable for staining blood smears.

Concentration Techniques

MODIFIED KNOTT'S CONCENTRATION FOR MICROFILARIAE

This technique hemolyzes the red blood cells and concentrates leukocytes and microfilariae.

1. Obtain 1 ml blood by venipuncture and deliver it directly into a centrifuge tube containing 10 ml 2% formalin. Mix thoroughly.
2. Centrifuge at $500 \times g$ for 1 minute.
3. Decant supernatant, spread sediment out to approximate thickness of thick films on a slide or slides. Dry thoroughly.
4. Stain with Giemsa's stain.

★Hansel's stain may be obtained from Lide Laboratories, Inc., 15422 Cousteau Drive, Florissant, MO 63034; (314) 831-2933.

MEMBRANE FILTRATION METHOD FOR MICROFILARIAE (Dennis and Kean, 1971)

1. Blood is collected in tubes containing 3.8% sodium citrate (20% by volume of blood specimen).
2. A Nuclepore★ filter of 5 μm pore size is placed in a Swinney adapter; a 20- to 50-ml disposable plastic syringe is attached to the adapter.
3. Several milliliters of normal saline are added to the upright barrel.
4. About 2 to 4 ml of the blood specimen is added to the saline, and the mixture of blood and saline is forced through the filter.
5. Following several washes of small amounts of saline or distilled water, the filter may be removed from the adapter, placed on a microscope slide, and examined for living microfilariae; it can also be dried, fixed, and stained as for a thin blood film.

GRADIENT CENTRIFUGATION TECHNIQUE FOR CONCENTRATION OF MICROFILARIAE (Jones et al., 1975)

1. Thirty ml of 50% Hypaque is mixed with 14 ml distilled water; 1 part of this mixture is added to 2.4 parts of 9% Ficoll.
2. Four ml of the Ficoll-Hypaque mixture is placed in a 17- × 100-mm plastic centrifuge tube and overlaid with 4 ml heparinized venous blood.
3. The tube is centrifuged at 500 × g for 40 minutes.
4. Microfilariae will be found in the middle Ficoll-Hypaque layer, which separates the overlying plasma and white blood cell layers from the underlying red blood cells.

BUFFY COAT FILMS FOR *LEISHMANIA*

This method is useful for the detection of *Leishmania donovani* if present in the circulation, and it will also reveal *Histoplasma capsulatum*, a fungus similar in size and shape to *Leishmania* but differentiated by details of internal structure. Microfilariae and trypanosomes may also be found in the buffy coat.

1. Obtain 5 ml blood and deliver into a tube containing oxalate crystals (prepared as for the Wintrobe hematocrit method).
2. Transfer blood with a capillary pipette into a Wintrobe tube. Cap to prevent evaporation, and centrifuge for 30 minutes at 2000 × g.
3. With a fine capillary pipette, withdraw the layer of cells of the buffy coat, situated between the packed red blood cells and the overlying plasma.
4. Spread out as thin film, dry, and stain with Giemsa's stain.

ACRIDINE ORANGE FOR DETECTION OF BLOOD PARASITES

Microhematocrit tubes were originally modified for quantitative buffy coat (QBC) analysis by the addition of plastic floats that, when inserted into the tubes, leave a layer approximately 40 μm thick, in which the granulocyte, eosinophil, and lymphocyte layers may be distinguished after microhematocrit centrifugation. This detection is possible, using fluorescence microscopy, because the walls of the capillary tubes are precoated with acridine orange. Under ultraviolet illumination, this dye does not stain erythrocytes, but does stain not only white blood cells and platelets but also plasmodia, trypanosomes, and microfilariae. This technique cannot be recommended for laboratories doing small numbers of parasitologic examinations. It requires the following:

1. A fluorescence microscope with a 50-power oil-immersion lens.
2. A microhematocrit centrifuge.

★This method is unsatisfactory for the isolation of *Mansonella perstans* microfilariae because of their small size. Other filters of similar pore size are not as satisfactory as the Nuclepore.

3. Modified QBC tubes and floats.★ (The QBC tubes used for hematologic purposes contain an agglutinating agent that does not allow for the concentration of the less dense parasitized erythrocytes at the top of the erythrocyte column.)
4. Specially constructed lucite blocks to hold the QBC tubes for viewing under the microscope.★

Levine and associates (1989) described the method in some detail, and Wongsrichanalai et al. (1991) consider it sensitive and specific for the detection of plasmodia present in small numbers, some of which could not be found on Giemsa-stained thick smears in their series.

TRIPLE-CENTRIFUGATION METHOD FOR TRYPANOSOMES

1. Deliver 9 ml blood obtained by venipuncture into a centrifuge tube containing 1 ml of 6% citrate solution.
2. Centrifuge at $400 \times g$ for 10 minutes.
3. Remove supernatant fluid to another centrifuge tube; recentrifuge at $500 \times g$ for 10 minutes.
4. Remove supernatant fluid once more to a clean centrifuge tube; centrifuge at $1500 \times g$ for 10 minutes.
5. Examine sediment as a wet film, or make a thin film and stain with Giemsa's stain.

DOUBLE-CENTRIFUGATION TECHNIQUE FOR TRYPANOSOMES IN SPINAL FLUID (WHO, 1986)

1. Centrifuge CSF obtained by spinal puncture for 10 minutes at $900 \times g$. Decant supernatant.
2. Resuspend sediment in the small amount of fluid left in bottom of centrifuge tube.
3. Draw suspension into microhematocrit tube, leaving 1 cm free of CSF.
4. Seal free end of hematocrit tube by inserting in flame of Bunsen burner.
5. Centrifuge sealed tube in microhematocrit centrifuge for 2 minutes.
6. Place microhematocrit tube on microscope slide, with coverslip over sealed end, and flood space between microhematocrit tube and slide (two or more microhematocrit tubes may be needed to stabilize coverslip) with water.
7. Examine sealed end of microhematocrit tube under microscope at 200× magnification for trypanosomes, which will move away from sedimented white blood cells.

Culture Methods

Acanthamoeba and *Naegleria*, the leishmanias, *Trypanosoma cruzi*, and *Toxoplasma* can be cultured with relative case. Cultivation of other blood and tissue parasites either has not been successful or (as in the case of the plasmodia) remains a research procedure.

CULBERTSON'S MEDIUM FOR *ACANTHAMOEBA*

For the isolation of *Acanthamoeba* from tissues, Culbertson and coworkers (1965) recommend the following procedure:

Materials

1. Prepare a neomycin sulfate solution, 0.56% in sterile distilled water. Prepare a sterile nystatin suspension in distilled water to contain 1500 units per milliliter.

★May be obtained from Becton Dickinson and Company, One Becton Drive, Franklin Lakes, NJ 07417.

2. Prepare agar stock, 3 g of Bacto-Agar per 100 ml of 1.7% NaCl.
3. Prepare suspension of *Enterobacter aerogenes* in trypticase soy broth, giving 40% transmission on a Coleman Junior spectrophotometer against uninoculated broth. Since both live and killed bacteria are to be used in medium preparation, place at least 5 ml suspension in a sealed ampule and immerse in a water bath at 65°C for 30 minutes to kill the organisms. Keep refrigerated until use.

Procedure

1. To a mixture consisting of 5 ml of each antibiotic solution, 5 ml killed bacterial suspension, and 85 ml sterile distilled water, add 100 ml melted and cooled 3% agar and combine all ingredients at 56°C in water bath.
2. Pour mixture into Petri plates, 8 ml per plate; allow excess moisture to evaporate by inverting bottom plate and resting it at a slight angle.
3. Place 0.05 ml of live *Enterobacter* suspension in center of plate and spread over an area 25 to 40 mm in diameter. Allow surface to dry at room temperature or at 4°C overnight.

Inoculation

Place drops of fluid or small pieces of tissue suspected of containing amebae near center of plate. Check for presence of amebae at edges of inoculum during the following 4 or 5 days.

MIX AMEBA MEDIUM FOR OPPORTUNISTIC AMEBAE

A variety of free-living amebae, including *Acanthamoeba, Hartmannella,* and *Naegleria,* may be cultivated axenically in a medium consisting of an equal mixture of Balamuth's medium and Nelson's medium supplemented with 4% bovine calf serum and 1 μg hemin/ml (John, 1993).
1. Make up following ingredients in Page's ameba saline (see under Modified Nelson's Culture Medium for *Naegleria*):
   a. 0.55% liver digest
   b. 0.50% proteose peptone
   c. 0.25% yeast extract
   d. 0.30% glucose

Autoclave.
2. Add 4% bovine calf serum to the above before use.
3. Add 1 μg hemin/ml to the above before use.
4. If material to be cultured is a clinical specimen or an environmental sample, add 200 μg streptomycin/ml and 200 U penicillin/ml.

MODIFIED NELSON'S CULTURE MEDIUM FOR *NAEGLERIA FOWLERI*

1. Make up following ingredients in Page's ameba saline:
   a. 0.1% liver infusion (Oxoid, Wilson 1:20)
   b. 0.1% glucose
   Autoclave.
2. Add 0.5 ml inactivated calf serum to 9.5 ml of above before use (5% serum). Inactivate calf serum at 56°C for 30 minutes.

Conditions of Incubation

With pathogenic strains 35° to 37°C works best. Transfer every 2 to 4 weeks, depending on density of the organism.

Page's Ameba Saline Solution (very dilute balanced salt solution [2 mM])

$MgSO_4$ 7 HOH	0.4 mg
$CaCl_2$ 2 HOH	0.4 mg
Na_2HPO_4	14.2 mg
KH_2PO_4	13.6 mg
NaCl	12.0 mg
Distilled water	100.0 ml

Nonnutrient Agar

a. Page's saline	100.0 ml
b. Difco agar	1.5 g

Dissolve agar in Page's saline with gentle heating. Aliquot 20-ml quantities into 20- × 150-mm screw-capped tubes. Autoclave at 15 psi for 15 minutes. Store in refrigerator.

Procedure

1. Prepare nonnutrient agar plates from above as needed, or store in refrigerator (up to 3 months) and warm to 37°C before use.
2. Add 0.5 ml of suspension of *Escherichia coli* or *Enterobacter aerogenes* in Page's saline to the surface of the plate and spread with a glass spreader; allow saline to absorb into the agar.

Inoculation

Inoculate a few drops of CSF sediment onto plate. Incubate at 35° to 37°C, and examine daily under low power. Cysts may appear within 4 to 5 days, and trophozoites earlier. Amebae will grow on the moist agar surface and produce plaques as they consume the bacteria. Once good growth has been achieved on agar, amebae may be transferred to Nelson's medium or Mix ameba medium, with streptomycin added at the rate of 100 μg/ml, for axenic cultivation. *Acanthamoeba*, from a suspected case of keratitis, may be isolated and cultivated in the same manner in Culbertson's medium or Mix ameba medium.

NOVY-MACNEAL-NICOLLE (NNN) MEDIUM FOR *LEISHMANIA* AND *TRYPANOSOMA CRUZI*

Nonnutrient Agar

Agar	14 g
NaCl	6 g
Distilled water	900 ml

The water is brought to the boiling point, and the salt and agar are added and dissolved in it. It is then distributed in test tubes filled to about one-third capacity. The test tubes are plugged and sterilized in the autoclave in the usual manner. Tubes containing the agar base may be stored in the refrigerator and used as needed.

For use, the tubes are placed in hot water to melt the agar, after which they are cooled to 48° to 50°C. To each tube is added approximately one-third as much sterile defibrinated rabbit's blood as the volume of agar. The blood and agar are mixed thoroughly by rapid rotation of the tube, and the tube is then placed in a slanting position, on ice, and cooled. After the tubes are cool, they are placed in an upright position and incubated for 24 hours at 37°C to determine sterility.

Blood is obtained from the rabbit from the ear artery or by cardiac puncture, with sterile precautions being observed. The blood so obtained is placed in a sterile flask containing glass beads and defibrinated by shaking.

Peripheral blood, or material obtained by biopsy or marrow aspiration or from cutaneous ulcers by aspiration from below the ulcer bed, may be cultured on this medium, which gives excellent results. The tubes are kept at room temperature, as close to 22°C as possible. The organisms develop in the water of condensation, which collects at the bottom of the slanted agar. Cultures should be examined every other day for a month before being discarded as negative. If leishmanias are present in the inoculum in some numbers, culture forms will usually be found within 2 to 10 days, but if scarce, leishmanias may require much longer to develop in sufficient numbers to be detected. Leishmanias will not grow in the presence of bacterial contamination.

TISSUE CULTURE OF *TOXOPLASMA GONDII*

A method for culture of *Toxoplasma* described by Shepp and coworkers (1985) is applicable to blood, CSF, and placental and presumably other tissues. The procedure for blood specimens is as follows:
1. Collect 10 ml blood in preservative-free heparin tubes; allow to sediment by gravity.
2. Remove the buffy coat with aseptic precautions; centrifuge at $800 \times g$ for 10 minutes.
3. Wash buffy coat cells three times with Eagle's minimal essential medium.★
4. Inoculate washed buffy coat material onto complete human foreskin (CF-3) fibroblast monolayers and observe weekly for cytopathologic effects.

Other tissues may be inoculated directly onto the tissue culture. If more than 1 ml CSF is available, it may be centrifuged at $500 \times g$ for 10 minutes and the sediment used for the inoculum.

Animal Inoculation

Trypanosoma brucei gambiense and *T. b. rhodesiense* infections can be established in a number of laboratory animals. White rats, white mice, and guinea pigs are most useful for diagnosis and the maintenance of laboratory strains. Young animals are most readily infected, and *T. b. rhodesiense* is more virulent than *T. b. gambiense*. Rats infected with *T. b. gambiense* survive for several months with a low-grade parasitemia; infected with *T. b. rhodesiense*, they die within a short time with an overwhelming parasitemia. *Trypanosoma rangeli* multiplies in common laboratory animals but does not cause apparent disease. Young white rats and white mice can be infected with *T. cruzi*; the white mouse is best for diagnostic inoculation. When first isolated, this trypanosome is quite virulent, but after repeated animal passage it loses its virulence and may become noninfective. Intraperitoneal or subcutaneous inoculation should be used; amounts of blood up to 2 ml are injected, depending on the size of the animal used. It is important to check rats for the presence of their common parasite, *T. lewisi*, before inoculation.

For isolation of leishmanias, the hamster is most satisfactory; other laboratory animals are infected only with difficulty. Following intraperitoneal or intratesticular inoculation, hamsters develop a generalized infection with any form of *Leishmania*, and the organisms may be demonstrated in spleen impression smears or in testicular aspirates. This infection develops slowly, and culture methods are generally regarded as being superior for diagnostic use.

Toxoplasma gondii, a parasite that shows little host specificity, will infect all common laboratory animals. White rats and mice are generally used; rats develop a chronic infection and are good for maintenance of the strain, whereas intraperitoneal infection of mice results in tremendous proliferation of the organisms in the ascitic fluid and death of the mice within a few days. Mouse peritoneal fluid, rich in organisms, is used as a source of toxoplasmas for the dye test and other diagnostic procedures.

★Can be obtained from Grand Island Biological Co., Grand Island, NY.

The pathogenicity of opportunistic amebae may be tested by intranasal inoculation of weanling mice. Amebae are concentrated by centrifugation and a 10-μl drop containing the amebae is introduced into a single naris of an anesthetized mouse using a micropipet. A highly virulent strain of ameba will begin to produce deaths in 5 to 8 days. Amebae may be cultivated from brain tissue in Mix's ameba medium.

Xenodiagnosis may be considered a special case of animal inoculation; the term was originally applied to the diagnosis of Chagas' disease by placing uninfected reduviid bugs on a patient suspected of having the disease and allowing them to feed. Subsequent examination of the bugs reveals developmental stages of the parasites if the test result is positive. Recently the term xenodiagnosis has been used to describe the diagnosis of trichinosis by feeding rats muscle tissue from patients suspected of having the infection.

References

Craig MH, Sharp BL. Comparative analysis of four techniques for the diagnosis of *Plasmodium falciparum* infections. *Trans R Soc Trop Med Hyg* 1997; *91*:279–282.

Culbertson CC et al. The isolation of additional strains of pathogenic *Hartmannella* sp. (*Acanthamoeba*). Proposed culture method for application to biological material. *Am J Clin Pathol* 1965; *43*:383–387.

Dennis DT, Kean BH. Isolation of microfilariae: Report of a new method. *J Parasitol* 1971; *57*: 1146–1149.

John DT. Opportunistically pathogenic free-living amebae. *In* Kreier JP, Baker JR (eds.). *Parasitic Protozoa*, ed 2, vol 3, pp 143–246, San Diego, CA, 1993, Academic Press.

Jones TC et al. A technique for isolating and concentrating microfilariae from peripheral blood by gradient centrifugation. *Trans R Soc Trop Med Hyg* 1975; *69*:243–246.

Levine RA et al. Detection of hematoparasites using quantitative buffy coat analysis tubes. *Parasitol Today* 1989; *5*:132–134.

Shepp DH et al. *Toxoplasma gondii* reactivation identified by detection of parasitemia in tissue culture. *Ann Intern Med* 1985; *103*:218.

Wongsrichanalai C et al. Acridine orange fluorescence microscopy and the detection of malaria in populations with low-density parasitemia. *Am J Trop Med Hyg* 1991; *44*:17–20.

World Health Organization. 1986. *Epidemiology and Control of African Trypanosomiasis*. Technical Report Series 739, p. 127. World Health Organization, Geneva.

CHAPTER

16

Immunodiagnostic Techniques

In the majority of cases, the diagnosis of parasitic disease is made in the clinical laboratory by identification of the parasite itself in body fluids, tissues, or excreta. Clinical signs and symptoms, together with the patient's travel history, may dictate what laboratory tests to employ and may suggest ancillary testing by means such as radiography, ultrasonography, and magnetic resonance imaging. In some cases, parasites may not be found despite careful search, and radiologic findings may be equivocal. In such cases, we may have to rely on immunodiagnostic methods to search for a diagnosis on the basis of clues left either by the parasite itself (antigens) or by the body's response to parasitic invasion (antibodies).

Special Techniques

Most special techniques are at present beyond the scope of even the best clinical laboratories, although for a number of the more common infections, tests are available in kit form. The problem is, of course, that the need for tests for the less common parasitic diseases is so sporadic that it is both economically impractical for them to be made available at a local level and impossible for the laboratory to become proficient in their use. Later in this chapter, we present a list of governmental and some commercial laboratories that perform these tests, but first we discuss the different types of tests and their usefulness. Many tests referred to in the earlier chapters of this book that either are of limited applicability or have not yet come into general use are not discussed here. Readers interested in such tests are referred to the references given in the text.

Tests vary considerably in sensitivity (the percentage of positive results in a group known to have an infection; true positives), in specificity (the percentage of negative reactions in a group known to be uninfected; true negatives), and in reactivity. Reactivity is the amount of antigen or antibody needed to produce a demonstrable serologic reaction. Fortunately, most of the tests in current use have a high degree of reactivity.

A consideration of sensitivity, specificity, and reactivity must be made to determine the diagnostic potential of a specific test, and all of these factors may vary among laboratories. It is essential to take these variations into account in the interpretation of test results. The laboratory to which specimens are sent and the manufacturer of kits sold for antigen detection should be able to supply interpretation criteria for each such test.

The following types of tests are those most frequently used at the present time for diagnosis of parasitic disease. Many of the older ones have been replaced, and some to which reference has been made in the preceding chapters are not yet available for general use.

BENTONITE FLOCCULATION (BF)

This test, of relatively low reactivity, is performed by coating particles of bentonite with the test antigen and observing flocculation on addition of the serum. Titration is achieved by serial dilution of the serum. This test is used primarily for the diagnosis of trichinosis, for which other tests are also available.

DIRECT IMMUNOFLUORESCENCE (DFA)

Fluorescence of parasite antigen is induced by the introduction of monoclonal antibodies (produced in vitro against the parasite in question and fluorescently tagged) into a fluid or applied to a slide containing the parasite. The organism fluoresces when viewed by fluorescence microscopy. This test is used for detection of cryptosporidiosis, giardiasis, and trichomoniasis.

DNA PROBE

Performance of this test involves transfer of DNA-containing material of any sort (insect salivary glands or gut, human serum or feces, etc.) to a nitrocellulose membrane, where it is fixed. A DNA segment of known sequence, characteristic of the parasite DNA (produced by a cloning technique by means of hybridomas and then radioactively labeled), is hybridized to the DNA on the membrane. Radioactivity remaining after the membrane is washed signals the presence of the parasite. This procedure is used primarily for the detection of *Trichomonas vaginalis*.

ENZYME IMMUNOASSAY (EIA)

A general term for several different procedures that determine the presence or absence of a parasite by the reaction between the parasite antigen or antibodies, an enzyme-coupled corresponding antibody or antigen, and the enzyme substrate, with production of a color that may be assayed either qualitatively or quantitatively. Enzyme immunoassay is the most widely used of all the types of tests for detection of parasitic infections.

ENZYME-LINKED IMMUNOSORBENT ASSAY (ELISA)

A specific variation of enzyme immunoassay, the ELISA has become increasingly popular because of sensitivity and ease of interpretation. The appropriate antigen or antibody is bound to a solid support (microtiter wells, beads, test tube walls). The specimen to be tested (serum, cerebrospinal fluid, feces) is added and reacts with the already present antigen or antibody. Washing then removes unbound test material, after which enzyme-linked antibody or antigen is added, which reacts with the antigen or antibody of the test material. An additional washing removes all unbound material, and finally a solution that reacts with the remaining enzyme to produce a color change is added. This change may be measured either visually or colorimetrically ELISA (often listed simply as EIA) is used to diagnose a wide variety of parasitic diseases.

INDIRECT FLUORESCENT ANTIBODY (IFA)

A known parasite antigen (for example, blood smears containing *Plasmodium falciparum* obtained from infected *Aotus* monkeys) is exposed to patient serum suspected of containing antibodies to that parasite. Antibodies in the serum bind to antigen of the parasites, the slide is then washed to remove the serum, and the slide is then covered with a solution containing a fluorescent dye coupled with antihuman globulin. When this is in turn washed, any fluorescent dye remaining indicates the presence of the antibody in the serum specimen.

By use of the appropriate antihuman globulin, one may test for IgG or IgM. This test is used for diagnosis of babesiosis, Chagas' disease, cryptosporidiosis, giardiasis, leishmaniasis, malaria, and toxoplasmosis.

INDIRECT HEMAGGLUTINATION (IHA)

One of the older test modalities, indirect hemagglutination depends on the agglutination (clumping) of antigen-coated sheep erythrocytes by antibodies in the test serum. It may be roughly quantitated by dilution of the test serum, and is used for diagnosis of amebiasis (*E. histolytica/dispar* complex), Chagas' disease, cysticercosis, echinococcosis, filariasis, and toxoplasmosis.

IMMUNOBLOT (IB)

A more sensitive version of the IHA, in which a sample of protein-containing material from serum, cerebrospinal fluid, or other tissue or excreta is electrophoresed onto a poly-acrylamide gel. The electrophoretically separated proteins on the gel are then transferred (by blotting) onto a sheet where they are recognized by radioactively labeled specific anti-bodies, whose presence can be assayed after the sheet is washed. This technique is used primarily for the detection of cysticercosis, echinococcosis, paragonimiasis, and schistosomiasis.

LATEX AGGLUTINATION (LA)

See Bentonite Flocculation. This procedure is the same, with substitution of latex particles for bentonite. Latex agglutination is an older test, but it is still used for diagnosis of *Trichomonas vaginalis* infection.

POLYMERASE CHAIN REACTION (PCR)

A method whereby low levels of specific DNA sequences may be amplified to reach the threshold of detection, through action of the enzyme DNA polymerase. This complicated procedure is used for the diagnosis of babesiosis and toxoplasmosis.

RADIOALLERGOSORBENT TEST (RAST)

Developed as a test for antibodies to certain allergens, RAST tests specifically for IgG and IgE. Known parasite antigen is bound to a complex carbohydrate matrix known as a sorbent. Test serum is then added to the sorbent, which is washed and then allowed to react with a radioactively labeled antibody to human IgG or IgE. After removal of the excess labeled antibody, the presence and amount of radioactivity measure antibody present in the serum. RAST is used for diagnosis of anisakiasis and ascariasis.

WESTERN BLOT (WB)

This type of immunoblot test is used in diagnosis of cysticercosis, echinococcosis, and schistosomiasis.

   The tests listed here include all those performed by the Division of Parasitic Diseases of the Centers for Disease Control and Prevention (Table 16-1) and the three private reference laboratories listed next, as well as those available in kit form at the time of this writing (2005). An excellent overall review of the tests available at the CDC and elsewhere, and their

TABLE 16-1   ■   Antibody and Antigen Detection Tests for Parasitic Diseases

Disease	Antibody Test(s)	Antigen Test(s)
African trypanosomiasis[†]		
Amebiasis	EIA*	EIA
Angiostrongyliasis[†]		
Anisakiasis[†]		
Babesiosis	IFA*	
Baylisascariasis[†]		
Chagas' disease	EIA, IFA*	
Cryptosporidiosis		EIA, DFA, IFA
Cysticercosis	EIA, IB*	
Echinococcosis	EIA*, IB*	
Fascioliasis	EIA	
Filariasis	EIA	
Giardiasis		EIA, DFA, IFA
Leishmaniasis	EIA, IFA*	
Malaria	IFA*	
Paragonimiasis	EIA, IB*	
Schistosomiasis	EIA, ELISA*, IB*	
Strongyloidiasis	EIA*	
Toxocariasis	EIA*	
Toxoplasmosis	EIA*, IFA*	
Trichinellosis	BF, EIA*	
Trichomoniasis		DFA, LA, DNA probe

*Performed at the Division of Parasitic Disease (DPD), Centers for Disease Control and Prevention (CDC). The DPD does not do antigen testing.
[†]Unavailable at CDC but may be available elsewhere in the United States. If suspected, call Division of Parasitic Diseases, Centers for Disease Control and Prevention, at (770) 488-4431 for information.
Adapted from Wilson M et al. Clinical immunoparasitology. *In* Rose NR et al. (eds). *Manual of Clinical Laboratory Immunology*, ed. 6, Herndon, VA, 2002, ASM Press.

interpretation, is given by Wilson et al. (2002). They consider parasite-specific tests for IgA and IgE as generally not useful for diagnosis and suggest that specific IgM only be considered when attempting to determine the approximate time of initial infection with *Toxoplasma gondii*.

Reference Laboratories

In the United States, if a physician wishes to obtain a serologic test through the CDC, a serum specimen must be drawn and sent, along with details of patient history, to the state public health laboratory (in some states it first must go to the county public health department). If the county or the state does not perform the required test, the specimen is sent to the CDC, where the test is performed, and the report comes back to the physician through the same channels. This may at times be a lengthy process.

In Canada, much the same procedure is followed. With the exception of British Columbia and Ontario, where the provincial laboratories do most of their own parasite serology, specimens for serologic testing are sent to the National Center for Parasitology (Serology) at the McGill Centre for Tropical Diseases, 1650 Cedar Avenue, D71523, Montreal, Quebec, H3G 1A4.

Several commercial laboratories in the United States perform a wide variety of immunodiagnostic tests in parasitology. Important among these are as follows:
Focus Technologies, Inc. (formerly MRL)
5785 Corporate Avenue
Cypress, California 90630
(800) 445-4032

Quest Diagnostics, Nichols Institute
33608 Ortega Highway
San Juan Capistrano, California 92690
(800) 553-5445

Specialty Laboratories
2211 Michigan Avenue
Santa Monica, California 90404-3900
(800) 421-4449

Tests performed by these laboratories are summarized in Table 16-2. Results are usually obtainable within a few days. There are no private reference laboratories in Canada.

Kit Tests

Kit tests for the diagnosis of a number of parasitic diseases have come on the market within the past few years. By far the largest number are for the serodiagnosis of toxoplasmosis. An algorithm for diagnosis of time of infection with *Toxoplasma*, employing tests for both IgG and IgM antibodies, is given in Chapter 5. Kits testing for both types of antibody by EIA* and by IFA are available. Kit tests for other parasitic diseases are listed in Table 16-3. These latter kits employ several different modalities to identify parasitic antigen or antibodies.

TABLE 16-2   ▒   **Serologic Tests Offered by Listed Laboratories†**

Disease	Focus	Quest	SL
Amebiasis	EIA (antigen), ELISA		EIA (antigen and antibody), ELISA
Anisakiasis			RAST
Ascariasis			RAST
Babesiosis	IFA, PCR	IFA	IFA, PCR
Chagas' disease	IFA		IFA
Cryptosporidiosis	EIA (antigen)	DFA and EIA (antigen)	DFA and EIA (antigen)
Cysticercosis	ELISA	ELISA	ELISA, WB
Echinococcosis	ELISA	ELISA, WB	EIA, RAST
Filariasis	ELISA		ELISA
Giardiasis	EIA (antigen), IFA	EIA (antigen)	DFA and EIA (antigen), IFA
Leishmaniasis	IFA		IFA
Malaria speciation			IFA
Paragonimiasis	ELISA		EIA
Schistosomiasis	ELISA		ELISA
Strongyloidiasis	ELISA		ELISA
Toxocariasis			CF
Toxoplasmosis	DFA, ELISA, PCR	ELISA	EIA, DFA, PCR
Trichinellosis	ELISA		ELISA

*Companies producing EIA tests for toxoplasmosis:
Abbott Laboratories, Diagnostics Division, 100 Abbott Park Rd., Abbott Park, IL 60064; Bio-Medical Products Corp. 10 Halstead RD., Mendham, NJ 07945; Bio-Rad Laboratories, 4000 Alfred Nobel Dr., Hercules, CA 94547; Biotecx Laboratories Inc., 6023 South Loop East, Houston, TX 77033; Biotest Diagnostics Corp., 66 Ford Rd., Suite 220, Denville, NJ 07834; Diamedix Corp., 2140 N. Miami Ave., Miami, FL 33127; DiaSorin Inc., 1951 Northwestern Ave, P.O. Box 285, Stillwater, MN 55082; Gen Bio, 15222 Avenue of Science, Suite A, San Diego, CA 92131; Hemagen Diagnostics Inc., 34-40 Bear Hill Rd., Waltham, MA 02154; INOVA Diagnostics Inc., 10180 Scripps Ranch Blvd., San Diego, CA 92131; KMI Diagnostic Inc., 8201 Central Ave. NE, Suite P, Minneapolis, MN 55423; Labsystems, 8 E. Forge Pkwy., Franklin, MA 02038; Meridian Bioscience (formerly Meridian Diagnostics Inc.), 3471 River Hills Dr., Cincinnati, OH 45244; Sigma Diagnostics, P.O. Box 14508, St. Louis, MO 63178; Wampole Laboratories, Half Acre Rd., P.O. Box 1001, Cranbury, NJ 08512. (Adapted from Wilson M et al. Clinical immunoparasitology. *In* Rose NR et al. (eds). *Manual of Clinical Laboratory Immunology*, ed. 6, Herndon, VA, 2002, ASM Press.
†Focus, Focus Technologies, Inc.; Quest, Quest Diagnostics, Nichols Institute; SL, Speciality Laboratories.

TABLE 16-3 ■ **Commercially Available Kits for Immunodetection of Parasite Antibodies and Antigens**

Organism and Kit Name	Manufacturer-Distributor*	Test[†]
Babesia microti		
Babesiosis	Immunetics	IB[†]
Cryptosporidium parvum		
ProSpecT	Alexon-Trend	EIA
Crypto-CELISA	Cellabs	EIA
Premier	Meridian	EIA
Cryptosporidium	Novocastra	DFA
Cryptosporidium	TechLab	EIA
RIM Cryptosporidium	Remel	EIA
C. parvum/G. lamblia		
ProSpecT	Alexon-Trend	EIA
ColorPAC	Becton Dickinson	Rapid[‡]
Crypto/Giardia-Cel	Cellabs	IFA
Merifluor	Meridian	DFA
C. parvum/G. lamblia/E. histolytica		
Triage	BioSite	Rapid
Cysticercus cellulosae		
Cysticercosis	Alexon-Trend	EIA[†]
Cysticercosis	Chemicon	EIA[†]
Cysticercosis	Immunetics	IB[†]
Cysticercosis	IVD Research	EIA[†]
Echinococcus granulosus		
Echinococcosis	Alexon-Trend	EIA[†]
Echinococcosis	Bordier Affinity	EIA[†]
Echinococcosis	Immunetics	IB[†]
Echinococcosis	IVD Research	EIA[†]
Echinococcus multilocularis		
Echinococcosis	Bordier Affinity	EIA[†]
Entamoeba histolytica		
Amebiasis	Alexon-Trend	EIA[†]
Amebiasis	Chemicon	EIA[†]
Amebiasis	IVD Research	EIA[†]
Amebiasis	Sigma Diagnostics	EIA[†]
ProSpecT	Alexon-Trend	EIA
Entamoeba-CELISA	Cellabs	EIA
E. histolytica	TechLab	EIA
E. histolytica	Wampole	EIA
Giardia lamblia		
ProSpecT	Alexon-Trend	EIA
ProSpecT	Alexon-Trend	Rapid
Giardia-CELISA	Cellabs	EIA
Giardia-Cel	Cellabs	IFA
Premier	Meridian	EIA
Giardia	Novocastra	DFA
RIM Giardia	Remel	EIA
Giardia	TechLab	EIA
Giardia	Wampole	EIA
Leishmania spp.		
Leishmaniasis	Acon Laboratories	Rapid[†]
Leishmaniasis	Amrad ICT	Rapid[†]
Leishmaniasis	Immunetics	IB[†]
Leishmaniasis	InBios	Rapid[†]
Plasmodium falciparum		
Malaria	Cellabs	EIA[†]
ICT Malaria P.f.	Amrad ICT	Rapid

TABLE 16-3 ■ Commercially Available Kits for Immunodetection of Parasite Antibodies and Antigens—cont'd

Organism and Kit Name	Manufacturer-Distributor*	Test[†]
Plasmodium spp.		
ICT Malaria P.f./P.v.	Amrad ICT	Rapid
ParaSightF	Becton Dickinson	Rapid
Malaria-Ag	Cellabs	EIA
OptiMAL	Flow	Rapid
Toxocara canis		
Toxocariasis	Alexon-Trend	EIA[†]
Toxocariasis	Bordier Affinity	EIA[†]
Toxocariasis	IVD Research	EIA[†]
Trichinella spiralis		
Trichinellosis	Alexon-Trend	EIA[†]
Trichinellosis	IVD Research	EIA[†]
Trichomonas vaginalis		
T. Vag.	Chemicon	DFA
Quick-Trich	PanBio InDx	LA
Trypanosoma cruzi		
Chagas' disease	Abbott Laboratories	EIA[†]
Chagas' disease	Hemagen Diagnostics	EIA[†]
Chagas' disease	Meridian Diagnostics	EIA[†]
Wuchereria bancrofti		
ICT Filariasis	Amrad ICT	Rapid
TropBio	TropBio, JCU	EIA

*Addresses: Abbott Labs, Diagnostics Division, North Chicago, IL 60064; Acon Laboratories, 115 Research Dr., Bethlehem, PA 18015; Alexon-Trend, 14000 Unity St. NW, Ramsey, MN 55303; Amrad ICT, 13 Rodborough Rd., French Forest, NSW 2086, Australia; Becton Dickinson, 1 Becton Dr., Franklin Lakes, NJ 07417; BioSite, 11030 Roselle St., San Diego, CA 92121; Bordier Affinity Products, Chatanerie 2, CH-1023, Crissier Switzerland; Cellabs, PO Box 421, Brookvale, NSW 2100, Australia; Chemicon, 28835 Single Oak Dr., Temecula, CA 92590; Flow, Inc., 6127 SW Corbett, Portland, OR 97201; Hemagen, 34-40 Bear Hill Rd., Waltham, MA 02154; Immunetics, 380 Green St., Cambridge, MA 02139; InBios, 562 1st Ave. South, Suite 600, Seattle, WA 98104; IVD Research, 5909 Sea Lion Pl., Suite D, Carlsbad, CA 92008; Meridian Diagnostics, 3471 River Hills Dr., Cincinnati, OH 45244; Novocastra, 30 Ingold Rd., Bulingame, CA 94010; PanBio InDx, 1756 Sulfur Rd., Baltimore, MD 21227; Remel, PO Box 14428, Lenexa, KS 66215; Sigma Diagnostics, PO Box 14508, St. Louis, MO 63178; TechLab, VPI Research Park, 1861 Pratt Dr., Blacksburg, VA 24060; TropBio Pty Ltd, James Cook University, Townsville, Queensland 4811, Australia; Wampole Laboratories, PO Box 1001, Cranbury, NJ 08512.
[†]Antibody detection kits; all others listed are antigen detection.
[‡]Rapid, rapid immunoassay.
Table adapted from Wilson M et al. Clinical immunoparasitology. *In* Rose NR et al. (eds.). *Manual of clinical laboratory immunology*, ed 6, Herndon, VA, 2002, AMS Press.

In general, antibody tests are performed on serum and antigen tests on *unpreserved* fecal specimens; specific instructions for collection of specimens will accompany each type of kit.

Another development is the production of a monoclonal EIA test for the rapid detection of the adhesin specific for *Entamoeba histolytica* in fecal specimens. This "*E. histolytica* test" (produced by TechLab), with its accompanying "*Entamoeba* test," which recognizes the *E. histolytica/dispar* complex, has the reliability of zymodeme analysis for the differentiation of the pathogenic and nonpathogenic species and is much more rapidly performed (Haque et al., 1995). A second-generation test, "*E. histolytica* II test" (TechLab), has higher sensitivity (Haque et al., 2000).

IMMUNODIAGNOSIS (PLASMODIUM FALCIPARUM)

At least three malaria antigen detection systems are available. ParaSight-F (Becton Dickinson) and ICT Malaria (Amrad ICT) detect histidine-rich protein-2 (HRP-2), and OptiMAL (Flow, Inc.) detects plasmodial lactate dehydrogenase (pLDH). The tests based on the detection of HRP currently have the highest sensitivity and specificity (Grobusch et al., 2003; Moody, 2002).

Skin Tests

At one time skin tests were a very important adjunct to the diagnosis of parasitic disease, and a number are still in use in European countries and other parts of the world. At the present time, none of the skin test antigens is available in the United States.

References

Grobusch MP et al. Comparison of three antigen detection tests for diagnosis and follow-up of falciparum malaria in travellers returning to Berlin, Germany. *Parasitol Res* 2003; *89*:354–357.

Haque R et al. Rapid diagnosis of *Entamoeba* infection by using *Entamoeba* and *Entamoeba histolytica* stool antigen detection kits. *J Clin Microbiol* 1995; *33*:2558–2561.

Haque R et al. Diagnosis of amebic liver abscess and intestinal infection with the Techlab *Entamoeba histolytica* II antigen detection and antibody tests. *J Clin Microbiol* 2000; *38*:3235–3239.

Moody A. Rapid diagnostic tests for malaria parasites. *Clin Microbiol Rev* 2002; *15*:66–78.

Wilson M et al. Clinical immunoparasitology. *In* Rose NR et al. (eds.). *Manual of Clinical Laboratory Immunology*, ed 6, Herndon, VA, 2002, ASM Press.

Index

Page numbers followed by *f* indicate illustrations; *t* indicates tables.